Cardiac Biomarkers
in Clinical Practice

EDITED BY

James L. Januzzi, Jr., MD
Director
Cardiac Intensive Care Unit
Massachusetts General Hospital
Associate Professor of Medicine
Harvard Medical School
Boston, MA

JONES AND BARTLETT PUBLISHERS
Sudbury, Massachusetts
BOSTON TORONTO LONDON SINGAPORE

World Headquarters
Jones and Bartlett Publishers
40 Tall Pine Drive
Sudbury, MA 01776
978-443-5000
info@jbpub.com
www.jbpub.com

Jones and Bartlett Publishers
Canada
6339 Ormindale Way
Mississauga, Ontario L5V 1J2
Canada

Jones and Bartlett Publishers
International
Barb House, Barb Mews
London W6 7PA
United Kingdom

Jones and Bartlett's books and products are available through most bookstores and online booksellers. To contact Jones and Bartlett Publishers directly, call 800-832-0034, fax 978-443-8000, or visit our website, www.jbpub.com.

Substantial discounts on bulk quantities of Jones and Bartlett's publications are available to corporations, professional associations, and other qualified organizations. For details and specific discount information, contact the special sales department at Jones and Bartlett via the above contact information or send an email to specialsales@jbpub.com.

Production Credits
Senior Acquisitions Editor: Alison Hankey
Senior Editorial Assistant: Jessica Acox
Production Editor: Daniel Stone
Production Director: Amy Rose
V.P., Manufacturing and Inventory Control: Therese Connell
Manufacturing and Inventory Control Supervisor: Amy Bacus
Assistant Print Buyer: Jessica DeMarco
Cover Design: Kristin E. Parker
Printing and Binding: Malloy, Inc.
Cover Printing: Malloy, Inc.
Cover/Title Page Image: @ Vikashu/Dreamstime.com

Library of Congress Cataloging-in-Publication Data
Januzzi, James L.
Cardiac biomarkers in clinical practice / James L. Januzzi, Jr.
p. ; cm.
Includes bibliographical references.
ISBN-13: 978-0-7637-6161-5
ISBN-10: 0-7637-6161-3
1. Heart—Diseases—Diagnosis. 2. Biochemical markers—Diagnostic use. 3. Clinical chemistry. I. Title.
[DNLM: 1. Biological Markers. 2. Cardiovascular Diseases—diagnosis. 3. Cardiovascular Diseases—prevention & control. 4. Risk Assessment. WG 141 J35c 2010]
RC683.5.C5J36 2010
616.1'2075—dc22

2009022814

6048

Printed in the United States of America
13 12 11 10 09 10 9 8 7 6 5 4 3 2 1

Contents

Contributors

Tariq Ahmad, MD
Center for Cardiovascular Disease Prevention
Brigham and Women's Hospital
Boston, MA

Fred S. Apple, PhD
Hennepin County Medical Center
Laboratory Medicine and Pathology
University of Minnesota School of Medicine
Minneapolis, MN

Aarti Asnani, BS
Department of Medicine
Massachusetts General Hospital
Boston, MA

Michael R. Banihashemi, MD
Department of Medicine
University of Maryland
Baltimore, MD

Richard C. Becker, MD
Division of Cardiology
Department of Internal Medicine
Duke University Medical Center
Durham, NC

Luigi M. Biasucci, MD
Department of Cardiology
Catholic University
Rome, Italy

Michael J. Blaha, MD
Johns Hopkins Ciccarone Center for the Prevention of Heart Disease
Baltimore, MD

Roger S. Blumenthal, MD
Johns Hopkins Ciccarone Center for the Prevention of Heart Disease
Baltimore, MD

Biykem Bozkurt, MD
Section of Cardiology
Michael E. DeBakey V.A. Medical Center
Winters Center for Heart Failure Research and Section of Cardiology
Department of Medicine
Baylor College of Medicine
Houston, TX

John C. Burnett, Jr., MD
Cardiorenal Research Laboratory
Division of Cardiovascular Diseases
Departments of Medicine and Physiology
Mayo Clinic
Rochester, MN

Naima Carter-Monroe, MD
CVPath Institute, Inc.
Gaithersburg, MD

Robert H. Christenson, PhD, DABCC, FACB
Department of Laboratory Medicine
University of Maryland
Baltimore MD

Paul O. Collinson, MD, FRCP
Departments of Chemical Pathology and Cardiology
St George's Hospital and Medical School
London, UK

Sabe De, MD
Department of Cardiovascular Medicine
Heart and Vascular Institute
Cleveland Clinic
Cleveland, OH

James A. De Lemos, MD
Department of Medicine
University of Texas Southwestern Medical Center
Dallas, TX

Christopher R. DeFilippi, MD, FACC
Division of Cardiology
University of Maryland School of Medicine
Baltimore, MD

Anita Deswal, MD, MPH
Section of Cardiology
Houston Center for Quality of Care and Utilization Studies
Michael E. DeBakey V.A. Medical Center
Winters Center for Heart Failure Research and Section of Cardiology
Department of Medicine
Baylor College of Medicine
Houston, TX

Estelle Docteur, MD
Department of Medicine
Massachusetts General Hospital
Boston, MA

Kai M. Eggers, MD
Department of Cardiology
University Hospital
Uppsala, Sweden

Robert E. Gerszten, MD
Cardiology Division
Massachusetts General Hospital
Boston, MA

Evangelos Giannitsis, MD
Medizinische Universitätsklinik Heidelberg
Department of Cardiology
Im Neuenheimer Feld
Heidelberg, Germany

Nitin K. Gupta, MD
Department of Medicine
University of Texas Southwestern Medical Center
Dallas, TX

Rajat Gupta, MD
Department of Medicine
Massachusetts General Hospital
Boston, MA

Per Hildebrandt, MD
Section of Cardiology
Glostrup University Hospital
Copenhagen, Denmark

Tomoko Ichiki, MD, PhD
Cardiorenal Research Laboratory
Division of Cardiovascular Diseases
Departments of Medicine and Physiology
Mayo Clinic
Rochester, MN

Erik Ingelsson, MD, PhD
Department of Medical Epidemiology and Biostatistics
Karolinska Institutet
Stockholm, Sweden

Anand V. Iyer, MD
Keck School of Medicine
University of Southern California
Los Angeles, CA

Allan S. Jaffe, MD
Mayo Clinic and Medical School
Rochester, MN

James L. Januzzi Jr., MD
Cardiac Intensive Care Unit Massachusetts General Hospital
Department of Medicine Harvard Medical School
Boston, MA

Sekar Kathiresan, MD
Department of Medicine and Division of Cardiology
Massachusetts General Hospital
Boston, MA

Hugo A. Katus, MD
Medizinische Universitätsklinik Heidelberg
Department of Cardiology
Heidelberg, Germany

Walter E. Kelley, DO
Department of Laboratory Medicine
University of Maryland
Baltimore, MD

Natalie Khuseyinova, MD
Department of Internal Medicine II—Cardiology
University of Ulm Medical Center
Ulm, Germany

Wolfgang Koenig, MD, PhD
Department of Internal Medicine II—Cardiology
University of Ulm Medical Center
Ulm, Germany

Frank Kolodgie, PhD
CVPath Institute, Inc.
Gaithersburg, MD

Elena Ladich, MD
CVPath Institute, Inc.
Gaithersburg, MD

Roberto Latini, MD
Department of Cardiovascular Research
Istituto di Ricerche Farmacologiche "Mario Negri"
Milan, Italy

Candace Y.W. Lee, MD, PhD
Cardiorenal Research Laboratory
Division of Cardiovascular Diseases
Departments of Medicine and Physiology
Mayo Clinic
Rochester, MN

Milena Leo, MD
Department of Cardiology
Catholic University
Rome, Italy

Gregory D. Lewis, MD
Department of Medicine and Division of Cardiology
Massachusetts General Hospital
Boston, MA

Bertil Lindahl, MD
Department of Cardiology
University Hospital
Uppsala, Sweden

Alan S. Maisel, MD, FACC
University of California
San Diego, CA

Douglas L. Mann, MD
Section of Cardiology
Michael E. DeBakey V.A. Medical Center
Winters Center for Heart Failure Research and Section of Cardiology
Department of Medicine
Baylor College of Medicine
Houston, TX

Serge Masson, PhD
Department of Cardiovascular Research
Istituto di Ricerche Farmacologiche "Mario Negri"
Milan, Italy

T. McDonagh, MD, FRCP
Department of Cardiology
Royal Brompton Hospital
London, UK

Javier Mercé-Muntañola, MD
Biochemistry Department
Hospital de Sant Pau
Barcelona, Spain

Asim A. Mohammed, MD
Department of Medicine and Division of Cardiology
Harvard Medical School
Massachusetts General Hospital
Boston, MA

Christopher P. Moriates, MD
University of California, San Diego
School of Medicine
San Diego, CA

M. Gary Nicholls, MD
Cardioendocrine Group
Christchurch University
Christchurch, New Zealand

Torbjørn Omland, MD, PhD, MPH, FESC
Division of Medicine
Akershus University Hospital
University of Oslo
Oslo, Norway

Jordi Ordóñez-Llanos, MD, PhD
Biochemistry Department
Hospital de Sant Pau
Biochemistry and Molecular Biology Department
Universitat Autònoma
Barcelona, Spain

Mahesh J. Patel, MD
Division of Cardiology
Department of Internal Medicine
Duke University Medical Center
Durham, NC

W. Frank Peacock, MD, FACEP
Vice Chair, Emergency Medicine Institute
Cleveland Clinic Foundation
Cleveland, OH

Yigal M. Pinto, MD, PhD
Heart Failure Research Center
Academic Medical Centre
Amsterdam, the Netherlands

A. Mark Richards, MD, PhD
Cardioendocrine Group
Christchurch University
Christchurch, New Zealand

Paul Ridker, MD
Center for Cardiovascular Disease Prevention
Brigham and Women's Hospital
Boston, MA

Sonal Sakariya, MD
University of California
School of Medicine
San Diego, CA

Victor L. Serebruany, MD, PhD
Department of Medicine
Johns Hopkins University
Baltimore, MD

W. H. Wilson Tang, MD
Department of Cardiovascular Medicine
Heart and Vascular Institute
Cleveland Clinic
Cleveland, OH

Richard W. Troughton, MB, ChB, PhD
Cardioendocrine Group
Christchurch University
Christchurch, New Zealand

Roland R.J. van Kimmenade, MD, PhD
Department of Cardiology
University Hospital Maastricht
Maastricht (Limburg), the Netherlands

Ramachandran S. Vasan, MD, PhD
The Framingham Study
Boston University School of Medicine
Framingham, MA
Evans Memorial Department of Medicine and Whitaker Cardiovascular Institute of the Boston University School of Medicine
Boston, MA

Renu Virmani, MD
CVPath Institute, Inc.
Gaithersburg, MD

Thomas J. Wang, MD
Massachusetts General Hospital
Boston, MA

Alan H.B. Wu, PhD
Department of Laboratory Medicine
University of California, San Francisco
San Francisco General Hospital
San Francisco, CA

Preface

Measurement of biomarkers for the evaluation of patients at risk for heart disease, or those who actively have the disease, has evolved dramatically since the first measurements of white blood cell count as an indirect marker for size and severity of myocardial infarction. Indeed, since the 1980s, the field of "cardiac biomarkers" has evolved dramatically and the clinician now has a broad range of blood-based tests for a number of cardiac-related applications—from assessment of the "apparently well" patient, to those with end-stage heart disease. With this rapid advancement has come a degree of uncertainty and confusion among clinicians with respect to *which* markers should be used, *why* they should be used, *when* they should be used, and *how* they might be used.

As a practicing clinician myself, I truly understand this dilemma and it is in this spirit that the concept for *Cardiac Biomarkers in Clinical Practice* was developed. This text, written by some of the most established clinician/researchers in the area of cardiac biomarkers, represents a clearly stated summary of up-to-date knowledge regarding biomarkers in medicine. Spanning the range of blood tests for cardiac ischemia and necrosis, heart failure, inflammation, lipids, thrombosis, and even impending tests for genomics and metabolomics, the hope is for this text to be presently useful to the clinician, laboratorian, trainee, and medical student, but also to maintain its forward-looking nature for years to come. Indeed, in writing the text, the authors focused not only on "where we've been" and "where we are now," but also offered a healthy dose of "where we are going" with cardiac biomarker testing.

I am eternally grateful to all of the authors—experts whom I have grown to know and respect quite greatly as my career in cardiac biomarker research has progressed. These authors not only represent the best and brightest in cardiac biomarker research, but are also outstanding physicians and valued colleagues. It is an honor and an inspiration for me to work side by side with them.

Along these lines, I would like to dedicate this book to my father, James L. Januzzi, Sr., MD, a man who first inspired me to take up the calling of medicine and someone whose brilliance with respect to the factual basis of medicine paled in comparison to his humanism and practical application of his knowledge. Dad, growing up it may not have seemed like I was listening, but I can assure you that I learned more from you than you may realize!

James L. Januzzi, Jr., MD

Section I

Necrosis Markers

1 ▪ Biology of Standard Necrosis Markers: Troponins, Creatine Kinase, and Myoglobin

Fred S. Apple, PhD

Introduction

Cardiac troponin (cTn) has evolved to be the standard biomarker for detection of myocardial injury and myocardial infarction (MI).[1,2] Over the past several years, international guidelines in the fields of laboratory medicine, cardiology, emergency medicine, and epidemiology have all endorsed cTn (either I or T), therefore replacing both creatine kinase MB (CK-MB) and myoglobin, necrosis biomarkers that were the standards prior to 2000.[3] This chapter will address the biology of cTn, CK-MB, and myoglobin pertaining to cellular distribution (Figure 1–1) and tissue specificity of these three biomarkers and their release into the circulation following irreversible, myocardial cell necrosis.

Cardiac Troponin I and T

The contractile proteins of the myofibril include the regulatory protein troponin. Troponin is a complex of three protein subunits: troponin C (the calcium-binding component; molecular mass 18 kDa), troponin I (TnI, the inhibitory component; molecular mass 22.5 kDa), and troponin T (TnT, the tropomyosin-binding component; molecular mass 37 kDa). The subunits exist in a number of isoforms. The distribution of these isoforms varies between cardiac muscle and slow- and fast-twitch skeletal muscle. Only two major isoforms of troponin C are found in human heart and skeletal muscle. These are characteristic of slow- and fast-twitch skeletal muscle. The heart isoform is identical with the

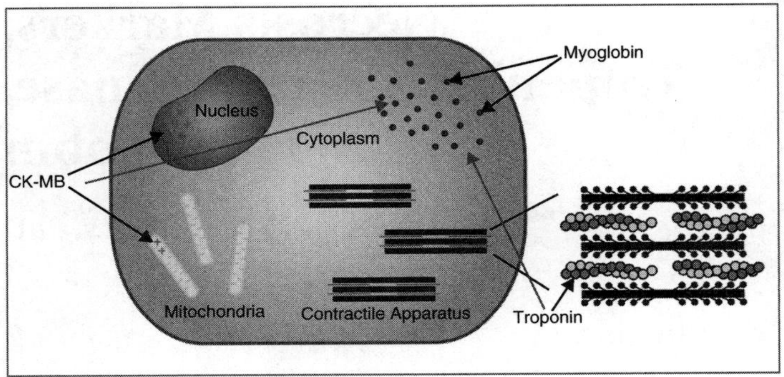

■ **Figure 1–1** Cellular distribution of cardiac troponin, creatine kinase MB and myoglobin in structural and cytoplasm components. **See Plate 1 for color image.**

slow-twitch skeletal muscle isoform. Isoforms of cardiac-specific TnT (cTnT) and cardiac-specific TnI (cTnI) have been identified. Troponin is localized primarily in the myofibrils (94–97%), with a smaller cytoplasmic fraction (3–6%).[4]

Cardiac troponin subunits I and T have different amino acid sequences encoded by different genes. Human cTnI has an additional posttranslational 31-amino acid residue on the amino terminal end compared to skeletal muscle TnI, giving it unique cardiac specificity. Only one isoform has been identified. Neither cTnI nor the mRNA for cTnI has been shown to be expressed in human or animal fetal, regenerating, or diseased skeletal muscle. This includes studies of human skeletal muscle obtained from Duchenne muscular dystrophy, polymyositis and chronic renal failure patients, long-distance runners, as well as in diseased and injured animal skeletal muscle.[4]

Expression of cTnT isoforms in diseased heart and skeletal muscle has been described, however the isoforms detected are not measurable using clinically available methods for cTnT.[4,5] Several studies have demonstrated that one to four cTnT isoforms can be detected in human skeletal muscle obtained from patients with

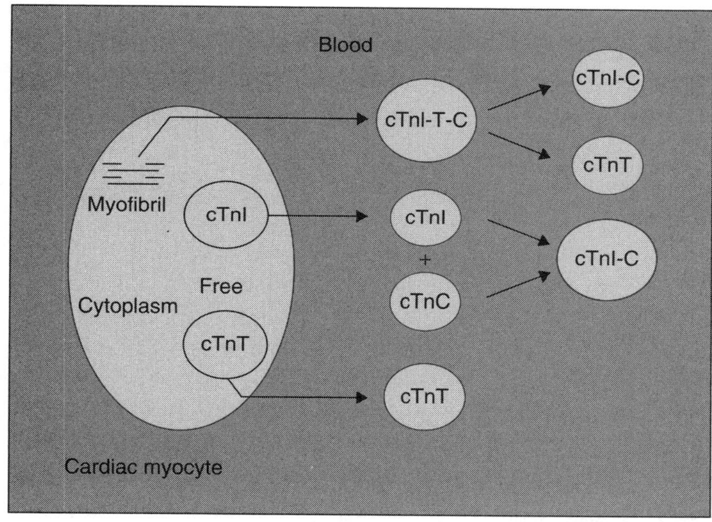

■ **Figure 1–2** Western immunoblots of nondiseased human heart muscle (NHHM; lanes 1–3), nondiseased human skeletal muscle (NHSM; lanes 4–6), and skeletal muscle from chronic renal disease (CRD) patients (lanes 7–13) probed with cardiac-specific TnT MAbs M11.7 (A) and M7 (B). Positions of the molecular mass standards (MW) are shown on the left.

Duchenne muscular dystrophy, polymyositis, and chronic renal disease. Re-expression of multiple cTnT isoforms in diseased human skeletal muscle parallels the expression of cTnT isoforms in differentiating myotubules. This is consistent with the expression of developmentally-expressed fetal isoforms as described for both cTnT and CK isoenzymes. The cTnT isoforms detected on different gels (whether true isoforms or degradation products) have been dependent on the antibodies utilized in the Western blot experiments. As schematically demonstrated in Figure 1–2, the 39 kDa isoforms found in the human heart and recognized equally by monoclonal antibodies M7 and M11.7, were not the same 39 kDa isoforms only recognized in the chronic renal disease skeletal muscles by M7. These findings demonstrate that release of any cTnT isoforms (detected in diseased or injured skeletal muscle) into the circulation would not be detected by the current generation Roche cTnT immunoassay because they are not recognized equally by the M11.7 and M7 antibodies. Thus, detection of circulating cTnT following concomitant injury of heart and skeletal muscle will be 100% specific for the heart.

Acute coronary occlusions in a dog model or in ischemic and necrotic myocardial tissue from humans result in a decrease of cTnT and cTnI compared to normal myocardium.[4] In this study, cTnT was noted to decrease 38–50% in infarcted human right- and left-ventricle tissue, respectively. By analogy, both cTnI and cTnT were decreased 87% and 60%, respectively, following three weeks of acute occlusion of the left anterior descending coronary artery in left ventricular tissue in dogs. Furthermore, in pig hearts with severe left ventricular remodeling two months postinfarction, both cTnI and cTnT were decreased 80% and 40%, respectively, compared with nondiseased normal myocardium. These data demonstrate that loss of cardiac troponins from necrotic myocardium is not replenished through re-expression of genes that might increase protein synthesis. Thus, leakage of cardiac troponins from myocardium to the circulation appears to represent irreversibly damaged myocardium. Finally, immunohistochemical staining techniques have demonstrated cTnT and cTnI loss from myocardium from experimental animal models of myocardial ischemia.[6] Loss of cTn occurs very early (within 30 minutes) following ischemic injury and may precede histological evidence of necrosis, but does not occur in myocardium that is not necrotic. This supports the irreversible injury mechanism of cardiac troponin release into the circulation.

Cardiac troponin I exists as a part of the troponin T-I-C ternary complex as a structural and regulatory component of the myofibril. A substantial body of evidence now exists that shows following myocardial injury or due to genetic disposition, multiple troponin forms are elaborated both in tissue and in blood. Figure

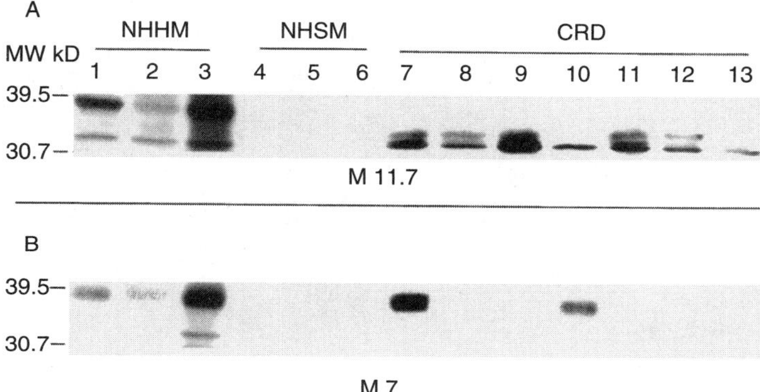

■ **Figure 1–3** Biology of multiple cardiac troponin I and T isoforms released from the myocardium after cell necrosis into the circulation.

1–3 describes the multiple forms of cTnI and T that can be found in both the myocardium and circulating in blood after release from irreversible myocardial cell necrosis.[7] These include the following: T-I-C ternary complex, IC binary complex, free I and T. Multiple modifications of these three forms can also exist, involving oxidation, reduction, phosphorylation and dephosphorylation, as well as both C and N terminal degradation. Seven different cTnI forms in an injured human heart have been described.[8] Figure 1–4 shows a schematic of the cTnI molecule and what epitope locations are more prone to alterations and what regions are most stable. The conclusions from these observations are that immunoassays need to be developed in which the antibodies recognize epitopes in the stable region of cTnI and ideally demonstrate an equimolar response to the different cTnI forms that do circulate in the blood.

Creatine Kinase (CK) Isoenzymes and Isoforms

CK isoenzymes consist of CKMM, CK-MB, CKBB, and mitochondrial CK. Each subunit of the dimeric CK is regulated by a distinct

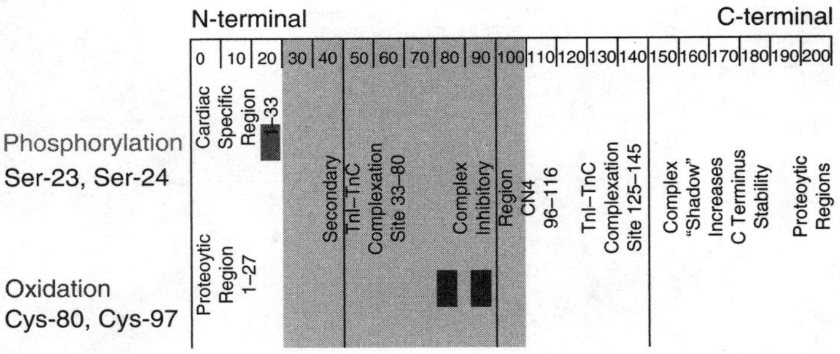

■ **Figure 1–4** Molecular epitope structure of cardiac troponin I demonstrating sites and regions of variability and potential interferences for immunoassay antibody sandwich design.

gene, and expressed in a tissue-specific manner.[9] In humans and animals, CK-MB is found predominantly in the myocardium, with concentration ranges from 10–30% of the total CK activity of the heart. The largest portion of CK in the heart is composed of CKMM (>70%). In contrast, skeletal muscle is typically comprised of 98 to 99% CKMM, with <2% CK-MB. CK-MB may be found in the gastrointestinal tract (typically in the capsules of hollow viscera) from mouth to rectum, in the tongue, as well as in the genitourinary system, including the bladder, uterus, and prostate.

The content of CK-MB in the myocardium has always been thought to be 10 to 30% of the total CK activity, based on the studies performed at autopsy from hearts obtained from patients who expired from MI.[10] Ingwall et al. demonstrated in histologically normal hearts that the CK-MB composition was <2%. In comparison, hearts examined from patients with known chronic coronary disease were found to contain >20% CK-MB. Studies in normal and diseased human heart tissues show a fourfold increase in CK-MB in diseased left ventricles compared to normal myocardium[4]; confirming Ingwall's earlier report. Thus, the concept of dynamic changes in CK-MB in human heart disease has stood the test of time and has been substantiated in several ischemic myocardial animal models.[10]

Canine models involving both acute (5 hour) and chronic (3 week) coronary artery occlusion involving the left anterior descending (LAD) and right coronary artery (RCA) have been studied to monitor CK-MB alterations over time.[4] In the acute LAD occlusion study, myocardial CK-MB globally increased threefold at five hours after occlusion. However, in the chronic three-week occlusion model, increases in CK-MB content were only observed in ischemic myocardium, demonstrating a fourfold increase in the ischemic LAD myocardium and a sevenfold increase in ischemic RCA myocardium, respectively. Comparable alterations have been described using a postinfarction left ventricular remodeling pig model. At two months after infarction, the CKB subunit increased 80% compared with the control tissues. Since CK gene expression is developmentally regulated, where proliferating myoblasts express the B subunit and differentiated muscle cells express the M subunit, it appears that myocardial ischemia induces an increase in the myocardial CKB subunit mRNA. This would translate to an increase in CKB subunit (therefore increase in CK-MB). This hypothesis is supported by a study that demonstrated an acute increase in mRNA for CKB in ischemic dog myocardium.[11]

The dynamics of CK-MB alterations have also been examined in skeletal muscle, in diseases, such as muscular dystrophy and chronic renal disease, and following exercise in marathon runners.[4,12] It has long been recognized that the CK-MB content of the skeletal muscle in patients' with Duchenne's muscular dystrophy and end-stage renal disease was increased at >10% of the total CK activity (Figure 1–5).

Studies from our laboratory have attempted to explain possible mechanisms responsible for these CK isoenzyme alterations. Studying highly-trained athletes (marathon runners) as subjects, we investigated the effects of ten weeks of chronic, long distance running (greater than 50 miles per week) on the CK-MB content of skeletal muscle. Biopsies obtained from the gastrocnemius

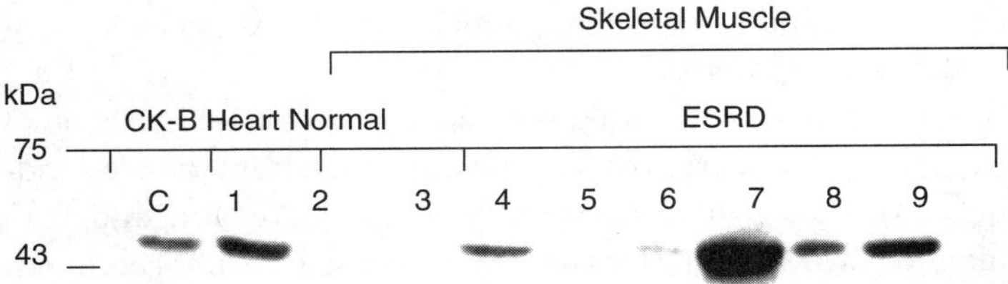

■ **Figure 1–5** Western immunoblot of CKB control (lane C), human heart (lane 1), nondiseased human skeletal muscle (normal lanes 2–3), and skeletal muscle from end-stage renal disease (ESRD) patients (lanes 4–9) probed with CKB monoclonal antibody. Positions of the molecular mass standards (MW) are shown on the left.

muscle (the most metabolically active muscle during running) were obtained at the start and end of the ten-week training period. The CK-MB content of skeletal muscle from the runners increased twofold, from 5.3% to 10.5%, compared to <1% in sedentary control muscle.[12] Findings were similar for both men and women runners over the ten-week period. The dynamic alterations for CK-MB observed are likely explained as follows. Stress-induced skeletal muscle injury, followed by degeneration and regeneration of muscle, allowed the CK isoenzyme composition to differentiate through a pattern similar to embryonic skeletal muscle formation: CKBB and CK-MB to CKMM. Thus, the repetitive stress of intense exercise caused a chronic state of fiber necrosis, with regeneration, leading to increased CK-MB content. Supporting the human findings, a chronic exercise model in rats demonstrated that increased CKB subunits in skeletal muscle were shown to be at least partially controlled by an increase in the mRNA for CKB.[13] Energetically, increased CK-MB in both heart and skeletal muscle following the stress of ischemia and injury would be beneficial in the muscle, playing an important role in the intracellular transport of energy (ATP and creatine phosphate) through the creatine kinase-phosphocreatine shuttle.[14] Finally, the mechanism responsible for increased CK-MB in skeletal muscle following chronic muscle disease or injury is thought to also be due to the regeneration process of muscle, with re-expression of CKB genes similar to those found in the heart; thus giving rise to increased CK-MB levels in skeletal muscle. Thus, skeletal muscle can become like heart muscle in its CK isoenzyme composition, with up to 50% CK-MB in some patients with severe polymyositis.

Numerous investigators have shown that electrophoresis of CK isoenzymes, using extended electrophoresis times or electrophoresis at higher voltages, further separates the bands of CKMM and CK-MB. At least three CKMM isoforms and at least four CK-MB isoforms (subtypes of the individual isoenzymes) exist.[15] The tissue isoform (gene product) of CKMM is designated $CKMM_3$. When this protein/enzyme is released into the circulation, a time-mediated carboxypeptidase hydrolysis of C-terminal lysine residues occurs, giving rise to at least two posttranslational products, $CKMM_2$ and $CKMM_1$. Similarly, following release of the CK-MB tissue isoform into the circulation, carboxypeptidase cleavage of the CKB carboxy-terminal lysine residue gives rise to a B-chain negative product and then a product devoid of lysines on both chains. There are only tiny amounts of the M-chain positive, B-chain negative form produced. Because only two forms are separated by electrophoresis, (the B-chain negative/M-chain positive form comigrates with the tissue form and the small amount of the M-chain negative/B-chain positive form migrates with the ultimate conversion product), only two forms have been used diagnostically and have been labeled CK-MB_2 and CK-MB_1. Studies in an experimental animal model and in humans have shown that posttranslational modifications of isoforms occur in blood, are unidirectional, and do not occur in the lymphatic system or necrotic tissue.

Clinically, CK-MB is detectable within peripheral blood specimens within 4–6 hours of necrosis onset; it peaks within 12–18 hours, and tends to fall within 24–36 hours. Although traditionally used for detection of acute myocardial infarction, CK-MB is both less sensitive and less specific than the troponins for detection of myocardial necrosis, hence its role in clinical use should be on the wane. There may be specific "niche" applications for CK and CK-MB measurement relative to cTnT or cTnI, which include detection of very small reinfarctions, reassessment of patients who represent with symptoms after a period of discharge from the hospital (when the daily trend of troponin is not available), as well as in those with end-stage renal disease.

Myoglobin

Myoglobin is an oxygen-binding protein of cardiac and skeletal muscle with a molecular mass of 17.8 kDa. The protein's low molecular weight and cytoplasmic location probably account for its early appearance in the circulation following muscle (heart or skeletal) injury.[16] There is no difference in the myoglobin protein localization in the heart versus skeletal muscle. Increases in serum myoglobin occur after trauma to either skeletal or cardiac muscle, as in crush injuries or MIs. Serum myoglobin methods are unable to distinguish the tissue of origin, as the proteins are identical. Even minor injury to skeletal muscle may result in elevated concentrations of serum myoglobin, which may lead to the misinterpretation for myocardial injury. Because myoglobin is cleared renally, changes in glomerular filtration rate (GFR) will cause increases.

Clinically, myoglobin has been shown to appear within an hour of myocardial necrosis, and falls rather rapidly following release. There has been great enthusiasm to utilize myoglobin to correctly identify acute myocardial infarction in those patients presenting with an uninterpretable electrocardiogram (e.g., a left bundle branch block of indeterminate duration) and negative troponin; in light of the extreme sensitivity of the high-sensitivity troponin assays (wherein a rise in cTn will be evident very early after necrosis onset), this advantage of myoglobin may be less evident. Indeed, the use of myoglobin has dropped considerably, given clinician frustration with its lack of specificity. In addition to its diagnostic value, myoglobin has been shown to be profoundly prognostic, even in the context of cTn results; again, whether these results will remain significant relative to the high sensitivity troponins is not clear.

Conclusion

Increased cTnI or cTnT in the circulation reflects heart injury. Normal cTnI and cTnT in the presence of increased CK-MB, myoglobin, and total CK reflects noncardiac injury, likely skeletal muscle injury. Both cTnT and cTnI immunoassays can also be used as reliable biomarkers for cardiac tissue-specific injury in the majority of laboratory animals.[17] The tissue evidence of alterations in CK-MB, cTnI, and cTnT presented supports the implementation of cardiac troponins testing in clinical laboratories for the specific tissue detection of myocardial injury, replacing CK-MB and myoglobin, proteins that are not 100% myocardial specific.

References

1. Thygesen K, Alpert JS, White HD, et al., on behalf of the Joint ESC/ACCF/AHA/WHF Task Force for the redefinition of myocardial infarction. Universal definition of myocardial infarction. *J Am Coll Cardiol.* 2007;50:2173–2195.
2. Morrow DA, Cannon CP, Jesse RL, et al. National Academy of Clinical Biochemistry practice guidelines: clinical characteristics and utilization of biomarkers in acute coronary syndromes. *Clin Chem.* 2007;53:552–574.
3. Wu AHB, Apple FS, Gibler WB, Jesse RL, Warshaw MM, Valdes Jr R. National academy of clinical biochemistry standards of laboratory practice: recommendations for use of cardiac markers in coronary artery diseases. *Clin Chem.* 1999;45:1104–1121.
4. Apple FS. Tissue specificity of cardiac troponin I, cardiac troponin T, and creatine kinase MB. *Clin Chim Acta.* 1999;284:151–159.
5. Gaze DC, Collinson PO. Multiple molecular forms of circulating cardiac troponin: analytical and clinical significance. *Ann Clin Biochem.* 2008;45:349–355.
6. Fishbein MC, Wang T, Matijaevic M, Hong L, Apple FS. An immunohistochemical study in experimental models of myocardial ischemia. *Cardiovas Path.* 2003;12:65–71.

7. Wu AHB, Feng YJ, Moore R, et al. Characterization of cardiac troponin subunit release into serum after acute myocardial infarction and comparison of assays for troponin T and I. *Clin Chem.* 1998; 44:1198–1208.
8. Katrukha AG, Bereznikova AV, Filatov VL, et al. Degradation of cardiac troponin I: implications for reliable immunodetection. *Clin Chem.* 1998;44:2433–2440.
9. Lang H. *Creatine Kinase Isoenzymes: Pathophysiology and Clinical Application.* Berlin: Springer-Verlag; 1981.
10. Ingwall JS, Kramer MF, Fifer MA, et al. The creatine kinase system in normal and diseased human myocardium. *N Engl J Med.* 1985;313:1050–1054.
11. Mehta HB, Popovich BK, Dilman WH. Comparison of creatine kinase M and B subunit mRNAs and isoenzyme activity in ischemic dog myocardium. *J Moll Cell Cardiol.* 1987;19 Suppl: 522.
12. Apple FS, Rogers MA, Casal, DC. Skeletal muscle creatine kinase MB alterations in women marathon runners. *Eur J Appl Physiol.* 1987;56:49–52.
13. Ricchiuti V, Apple FS. RNA expression of cardiac troponin T isoforms in diseased human skeletal muscle. *Clin Chem.* 1999;45:2129–2135.
14. Bessman SP, Geiger PJ. Transport of energy in muscle, the phospocreatine shuttle. *Science.* 1981;221:448–452.
15. Holt DW. Creatine kinase isoforms. In: Kaski JC, Holt DW, eds. Myocardial Damage: Early Detection By Novel Biochemical Markers. London: Kluwer Academic Publishers; 1998:17–25.
16. Mair J. Myoglobin. In: Kaski JC, Holt DW, eds. Myocardial Damage: Early Detection By Novel Biochemical Markers London: Kluwer Academic Publishers; 1998:53–60.
17. Apple FS, Murakami MM, Ler R, Walker D, York M, for the HESI Technical Committee on Biomarkers Working Group on Cardiac Troponin. Analytical characteristics of commercial cardiac troponin I and T immunoassays in serum from rats, dog and monkeys with induced acute myocardial injury. *Clin Chem.* 2008;54:1982–1989.

2 ■ The Evolution and Revolution of Necrosis Markers in Modern Cardiology for the Diagnosis of Acute Myocardial Infarction: The Search for Specificity

Allan S. Jaffe, MD

History of the Diagnosis of Acute Myocardial Infarction with Biomarkers

For many years, the diagnosis of acute myocardial infarction (AMI) was made almost exclusively based on clinical findings, such as chest pain and electrocardiographic changes as suggested by the original World Health Organization (WHO) criteria.[1] In 1954, Karmen and colleagues reported the release of aspartate aminotransferase, known at that time as glutamate oxaloacetate transaminase (SGOT), into the blood of patients with AMI.[2] A year later, it was appreciated that additional analytes, such as lactate dehydrogenase (LDH), were also elevated in these patients.[3] Both markers lacked cardiac specificity, although later, LD1 and LD2 isoenzymes were identified as being somewhat more specific for the heart.[4] Given this lack of specificity, it should not be surprising that the WHO criteria for the diagnosis of myocardial infarction did not include biomarkers or even mention them in the first iteration of their guidelines in 1959.[1] At that time and subsequently, it has been clear that the emphasis of the WHO criteria was in diagnosing clinical events with a high degree of specificity so that the epidemiology of the disease could be tracked. Thus, only overt cases were included. There were also criteria indicated as "indeterminate" or "indefinite" for myocardial infarction at that time.[1] Thus, it should not be surprising that in his textbook, *Clinical Heart Disease*, published in 1958, Dr. Levine did not even mention the use of biomarkers for the diagnosis of myocardial infarction.[5]

It was not until the development of assays for creatine kinase (CK) published by Rosalki[6] in 1967 after several years of work[7] that the use of biochemical tests was seriously considered for the diagnosis of myocardial infarction. The work of Rosalki has been reviewed elsewhere,[7] but the basic structure of the test and the reagents he used are very similar to those still used today for the measurement of CK activity. This breakthrough allowed one to begin to utilize biochemical measures for detection of myocardial infarction, as well as quantitation of its extent.[7] CK was first described as being released from skeletal muscle[8] and only subsequently (by one year) from cardiac tissue.[9] Thus, it also lacked absolute cardiac specificity for cardiac tissue, but it was a marked improvement compared to SGOT and LDH. A discussion of these biomarkers was incorporated into the 1968 textbook by Noble Fowler.[10] It starts with discussion of SGOT and LDH. It is noted that SGOT begins to rise within 6 to 12 hours, reaching a maximum of 1 to 3 days and that marked increases are found in 97% of patients with myocardial infarction. Thus, it has excellent specificity. It is noted as well that LDH was elevated for longer periods of time than SGOT and that fact could be helpful in making a diagnosis of AMI even days after its occurrence. It was also indicated that quantitative measures of these analytes could be used to anticipate complications, such as cardiogenic shock, no doubt because there was a relationship between peak values and infarct size. However, it is noted that liver disease, infection, hepatitis, pulmonary embolism, pericarditis, malignant myocarditis, mesenteric infarction, and renal and pancreatic disease would also cause marked increases. It is suggested even then that CK might eventually be a better marker because of its improved specificity. These comments are similar to those made by Charles Friedberg in 1966.[11] In his book, *Diseases of the Heart*, he describes the kinetics of SGOT, LDH, and CK release, but also opines "I have found them of little clinical help and not infrequently misleading . . . ." and "I have been called frequently to see patients in whom serum enzyme levels were determined and found to be increased, although the clinical history gave little or no reason for the diagnosis of acute infarction, and the electrocardiogram showed no changes or minor ones. Careful study of these cases revealed that the elevated serum enzymes led to a false diagnosis of acute myocardial infarction." Dr. Friedberg then goes on to describe the other etiologies for elevations, the fact that laboratory errors can occur, and opines that there is substantial difficulty in distinguishing between myocardial ischemia and necrosis. Thus, he suggests that, "my diagnoses of acute myocardial infarction depend almost entirely on the clinical history and electrocardiograms." In regards to CK, he indicates: "in the absence of damage to skeletal muscle or brain, it [CK] is diagnostically more specific than other serum enzymes; and its level is elevated very early, e.g., six hours after infarct." However, he seems to imply without saying it directly that he feels the same way in terms of the specificity of the diagnosis about CK as he thinks about SGOT and LDH.

The specificity of CK, and for that matter LDH and SGOT, was inhibited initially by the common practice of giving intramuscular morphine for pain relief to patients with acute myocardial infarction. Once this practice was halted and if patients were selected carefully, there was improved specificity, especially for CK. The marker was helpful diagnostically, but was also shown to be useful to measure infarct size,[12] which was the most important determinant of prognosis.[13] However, it was also clear that increases in CK activity were common and elevations were even more sensitive for skeletal muscle damage than for cardiac abnormalities.[8] This fact led to the development of more specific probes such as CK-MB.[14]

CK is a dimer, composed of B and M chains. There are three isoenzymes of CK: CKBB, CKMM, and CK-MB.[7] The tissue distributions of these are broad, but there are high quantities of CKBB in the brain and some in the GI tract and prostate. CKMM is abundant in skeletal muscle, but also the most prevalent form in heart muscle and many other solid organs. CK-MB is found in abundance in the heart where up to 15% of the CK is thought to be attributable to CK-MB,[15] but it is also found in skeletal muscle and the GI tract. Some of the investigations in the early 1970s underestimated the extent of CK-MB elevations that could occur due to skeletal muscle abnormalities because of the use of Rosalki-type activity assays. These assays, in order to obtain adequate signals, have to ensure that substrate availability is appropriate for the reagents of the assay. This often means that one has to dilute CK activity to make sure this is the case. If, as was the case with original assays, sensitivity is in the range of 5 to 10 IU and such levels are not detected by electrophoresis, for example, one would have to say that there was no CK-MB in the sample. However, if one had diluted the activity from 3000 IU to 300 IU to optimize substrate concentrations for the assay and failed to detect CK-MB, it may have been because it was below the level of detection of the assay system. If only four units were detectable and one had diluted the sample tenfold, then one could have missed a total CK-MB of as much as 40 IU, clearly an elevated value. With less sensitive assay detection systems, one could even miss 80 units. Thus, initial activity assays exaggerated the apparent specificity of CK-MB for the myocardium. This was rapidly unmasked when mass assays were developed by Ladenson et al.,[16] which substantially improved the ability to quantify the true amount of CK-MB. Whether antibodies were used to capture the CK-MB and then measure its activity or used to measure it directly, it then became clear that skeletal muscle damage caused substantial elevations of CK-MB, as well as increases in total CK.[17] This was thought to be the etiology of the elevations observed in 20% of patients with renal failure.[18] Because in the situation of skeletal muscle injury alone without myocardial injury, the percentage of CK-MB with respect to total CK was low reflecting the modest percentages of CK-MB compared to total CK in skeletal muscle compared to that in the heart, the suggestion was made to use a "relative index" to distinguish between CK-MB release from skeletal muscle and that which came from myocardial injury. The hypothesis was that low values would come from skeletal muscle and high values from the heart. This approach was utilized for many years until it was shown convincingly with the use of troponin as a gold standard that the improvement seen in specificity was counterbalanced by a marked loss of sensitivity.[19,20] Because of the huge amount of CK in skeletal muscle, modest amounts of skeletal injury could mask the release of CK-MB from cardiac injury. Thus, it became clear that the use of such criteria would not and should not be used for the detection of myocardial infarction.

Nonetheless, in the appropriate clinical setting, CK-MB provided improvement in specificity because of its relatively beneficial tissue distribution in the absence of concomitant skeletal muscle abnormalities. However, over time, it became clear that CK-MB increases were observed in patients who had both chronic and acute skeletal muscle injury.[19] These phenomena represent the re-expression of gene products that were present during neonatal development as part of the reparative processes. Thus, patients with either chronic or acute skeletal muscle disease will have substantial elevations of CK-MB related to re-expression of the B chain protein in that tissue in response to tissue injury because most skeletal muscle CK is of the B chain variety until late in the process of embryogenesis. Thus, when injury occurs, the B chain is re-expressed, increasing the amount of CK-MB in the tissue. In some situations, CK-MB can be as much as 50% of the CK found in the damaged muscle.[21] This confound obviously impairs the diagnostic specificity of CK-MB for the detection of cardiac injury.

Because of these substantial issues related to the specificity of CK-MB, additional efforts were necessary to attempt to develop markers that were more specific for the heart and that would alleviate the problems of tissue specificity. This has led to the development of cardiac troponin cTn as the biomarker of choice for the diagnosis of acute myocardial infarction.

It should be of no surprise that given this evolution and particularly given the problems with the specificity that biomarkers were included in a relatively modest way in the subsequent WHO criteria. In 1973, the criteria mention that one could take into account increases in enzymes that had been measured locally.[22] It was not at all clear at that time that there was any suggestion that these should or could be used consistently or what values should be relied on. It was not until the 1979 MONICA criteria[23] from the WHO that suggestions for the use of biomarkers became codified. At that time, it was suggested in keeping with the concept of trying to achieve high degrees of specificity that only marked elevations be included and thus, a criterion of a twofold increase in CK-MB in the appropriate setting was advocated. However, elevations were not essential for the diagnosis which could be made based on history and ECG alone. However, with time, the idea that CK-MB was essential for the clinical diagnosis of acute infarction has become clear.[17] With that concept, absolute increases above the upper bound of the reference limits for a given assay were considered indicative of cardiac injury in the appropriate situation. Because it was clear that chronic elevations occurred, a rising pattern of CK-MB activity or mass was considered essential for the diagnosis. The WHO has not updated its criteria to incorporate troponin since 1979.

The situation at present is even more complex because multiple parts of the world do not have access to blood testing of any kind. Thus, it may well be that one will need criteria that are optimized for use in countries where there are sufficient resources to provide accurate diagnoses and alternative criteria will need to be used for those areas where the diagnosis is infrequent or where resources preclude the use of the sophisticated measures used in other countries.[24] The only caveat about the latter approach is that it will impair the ability to compare incidence rates with any degree of sensitivity and specificity. These would obviously be severely compromised if one were comparing data from areas with higher specificity approaches to those utilizing progressively less specific criteria. However, such an approach might become the most practice clinical compromise.

With this background, it was then in the late 1980s and early 1990s that assays for troponin were developed. At that time, it was clear that there was a need for more cardiac specificity because of the large number of circumstances in which CK-MB could be elevated in the absence of cardiac injury.[19–21] In many instances, it was not clear if there was or was not cardiac injury in any given patient leading to diagnostic confusion. Accordingly, several groups began to embark on the development of more specific assays. The cardiac troponin T (cTnT) assay was originally developed by Katus and colleagues.[25] Their initial attempts focused on myosin light chains in experimental myocardial infarction.[26] However, these astute investigators rapidly recognized that cTnT was highly specific for the heart, and this led to the development of the cTnT assays by Katus.[27] Subsequently, antibodies that permitted the development of cardiac troponin I assays were developed by Ladenson et al.[28] The potential utility of cardiac troponin I assays had been reported previously utilizing polyclonal sera by Cummins et al. in the 1970s,[29] an observation that at the time was not actively pursued, but in retrospect was highly prescient for what subsequently developed with these markers. Both cTnI and cTnT were much more specific and much more sensitive than CK-MB.

With the development of this newer iteration of more specific assays, attention turned to the development of criteria for acute myocardial infarction. The first such criteria were proposed by the National Academy of Clinical Biochemistry in 1998–99.[30] The group suggested that rather than increase the sensitivity of new markers, one might have a two-stage process. One phase would include the diagnosis of myocardial infarction by utilizing a value for cTn that would provide similar sensitivity to CK-MB. This approach would take advantage of the improved specificity for cTn, but would not change sensitivity. There would then be a second category of patients who were deemed to have unstable angina with "minimal myocardial necrosis" predicated on elevations in cardiac troponin values. This approach was due to concern that clinicians would have difficulty distinguishing minor elevations that previously had not been called myocardial infarction from those that had. It was an attempt to maintain the sensitivity at a set value not realizing that with time the changes depicted above—first in total CK and then to CK-MB—had over time already markedly improved the sensitivity for detection of AMI. The proposal by the National Academy of Clinical Biochemistry[30] was debated and subsequently approved until it was superseded by the ESC/ACC Conference for the Redefinition of AMI in Nice in 1999.[31]

At that time, the European Society of Cardiology (ESC) and the American College of Cardiology (ACC), recognizing the importance of cTn measurements and their facile use, impaneled a group to decide how best to use this new analyte. A decision then was made to utilize only one cutoff for troponin in the interest of simplicity and to remove the concept that there would be an increasing number of patients with unstable angina with "minimal myocardial necrosis" because it was clear even at that point in time that new iterations and more sensitive troponin assays were being developed.[32] Thus, those guidelines advocated that the 99th percentile of a reference range be utilized to make the diagnosis of cardiac injury with the concept that when one had such injury in the appropriate clinical setting, e.g., acute ischemic heart disease, that the diagnosis of myocardial infarction would be made.[31,32] The biochemistry group advocated for the use of the 99th percentile as a way of reducing the number of increases that one would diagnose compared to the conventionally used 97.5th percentile. This led to substantial unhappiness on the part of the laboratory medicine community, but the 99th percentile has persisted as the appropriate criteria for the diagnosis of myocardial infarction, again in the interest of improving the specificity of the measure for cardiac injury. Intrinsic to this consideration was the understanding that troponin could be elevated in a large number of additional circumstances in which myocardial infarction was not present.[32] In essence, troponin unmasked the fact that there are substantial numbers of other circumstances over and above acute ischemic heart disease where cardiac injury occurs. This has led to continual difficulty with clinicians unhappy over the lack of clinical specificity for the diagnosis of an ischemic mechanism for troponin elevations.

Present-Day Diagnosis of Acute Myocardial Infarction

Given the improved clinical sensitivity and specificity of cTn, these measurements are the markers of choice for the diagnosis of AMI.[24] The cardiac isoforms of both cTnI and cTnT come from unique cardiac genes and therefore should have the potential for increased specificity for cardiac injury per se.[33,34] The situation for cTnI[35,36] is simpler than for cTnT.[35,37,38] None of the cTnI isoforms have been reported to exist outside of the heart.[33,34] Furthermore, elevations of cTnI concentrations from tissue outside of the heart have not been reported suggesting nearly perfect specificity for its release from myocardium. The situation for cTnT is somewhat more complex, but ends at the same place. Some of the fetal cardiac isoforms of cTnT are expressed in skeletal muscle during neonatal development,[38] and the first iteration of the troponin T assay detected some of these isoforms, as well as some cross-reacting skeletal muscle isoforms.[27] This led to the idea that there was a lack of specificity of cTnT due to skeletal muscle. This concern was particularly focused on inpatients with renal failure because of the frequent elevations of cTnT in that circumstance.[39] It is now clear that these findings represented the lack of antibody specificity of the so-called tag antibody.[27,40] When this antibody was replaced with a more specific one, it was shown that the previously-captured cardiac isoforms and the cross-reacting skeletal muscle proteins, though captured, were no longer both captured and tagged.[40–42] Thus, the functional specificity of cTnT remains similar to that of cardiac troponin I, i.e., highly specific. It should be noted

Table 2–1: Criteria for acute myocardial infarction.
Detection of rise and/or fall of cardiac biomarkers (preferably troponin) with at least one value above the 99th percentile of the upper reference limit together with evidence of ischemia with at least one of the following:
Symptoms of ischemia
ECG changes of new ischemia (new ST-T changes or new LBBB)
Development of pathological Q waves in the ECG
Imaging evidence of new loss of viable myocardium or new regional wall motion abnormality

that with new, more sensitive assays all of these evaluations for cTnI and cTnT will require reevaluation since the evaluations done previously were done at a different level of sensitivity.[43] Nonetheless, given the specificity of cTn, it is clear that elevations in the appropriate clinical setting can be relied on to diagnose AMI.

The 99th percentile is the cutoff value of choice and was predicated on the initial ESC/ACC guidelines document[31] and that cutoff has been retained in the 2007 revision.[24] There has always been a strong advocacy that this level of marker should be measurable with a high degree of precision.[24,31] In general, this has been considered coefficient variability (CV) of no more than 10% at the 99th percentile value. This high degree of precision was initially advocated for because of concern that analytic variability in the biochemical determinations could lead to false positives. This concept is not correct.[44] Lack of precision does not lead to false positive signals; it simply induces a loss of sensitivity of the assay involved, assuming the assay has been properly validated. There is not now—nor has there ever been—an advocacy that if for some reason a given assay does not have a 10% CV at the 99th percentile value that the value should be changed to a higher value. The one circumstance where this may be different is with cTnT where the 99th percentile is undetectable. Thus, in order to observe a rising pattern, a higher value may need to be used. However, even with the cTnT assay, it should be clear that the prognostically important value is still the 99th percentile value, while for assays where the "normal" cTn value is undetectable.[45]

The appropriate evaluation of patients with possible myocardial infarction always should include an initial troponin. If the patient is having a classic AMI and that cTn value is above the 99th percentile, no further values are necessary for diagnosis. If, on the other hand, the patient is not totally typical, then subsequent values may be necessary. With the original iterations of the troponin assays, most elevations represented acute disease because relatively substantial elevations were required to reach the threshold where these assays were being measured. With modern-day assays, which are far more sensitive, this is no longer the case. Indeed, it is now clear that substantial numbers of patients with heart disease will harbor chronic elevations of troponin.[46–49] In a study from Dallas,[48] 0.7% of individuals in the general population had elevations of cTnT. All had underlying cardiovascular disease or comorbidities (e.g., renal failure) associated with cardiac disease. Thus, it is clear that a substantial number of individuals who are not acutely ill harbor chronic elevations in cTn that are detectable with the present day iterations of troponin assays. If this number is 0.7% in the general population, this is very likely a higher percentage in the emergency room where many patients with cardiovascular disease are seen and higher still in hospitalized patients. This has led to the concept that changes in cTn indicative of acute events should have a rising pattern.[50–52] This may cause some delays in emergency departments (EDs) because the idea of a rising pattern precludes taking any elevation of troponin as indicative of disease and therefore as a reason for acute admission. This is a critical issue as assays become still more sensitive and larger. A larger number of elevations in troponin are likely to be unmasked that are chronic[46–49] and not indicative of acute heart disease and thus, not an indication for hospital admission. It is important to not lose sight of the fact that these cTn elevations are an adverse

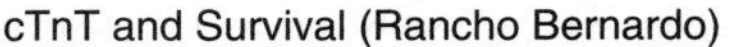

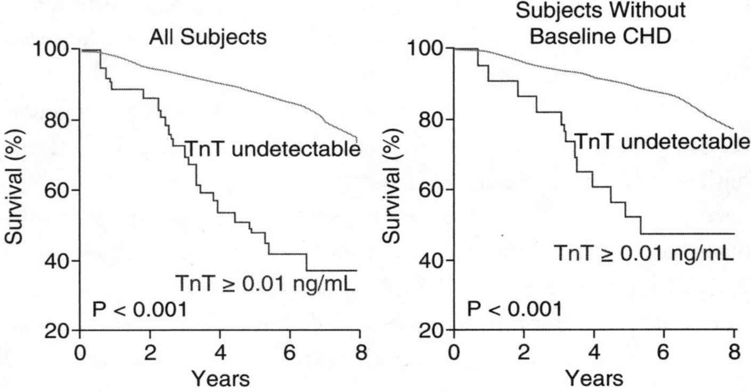

■ **Figure 2–1** Adverse effects of minor troponin increases on the prognosis of individuals who were stable and doing well in the Rancho Bernardo study.

Reproduced with permission of Wallace TW, Abdullah SM, Drazner MH, Das SR, Khera A, McGuire DK, Wians F, Sabantine MS, Morrow DA, de Lemos JA. Prevalence and determinants of troponin T elevation in the general population. *Circulation.* 2006;113:1958–1965.

prognostic signal (Figure 2–1) and that these patients require evaluation and thoughtful treatment.

Determining whether a rising pattern is present is not simple. Significant differences between biochemical values require that there be at least three standard deviations of the variance of the analytic measurement between such values.[53] This is the most important reason why high levels of precision for cTn assays are critical. At present, the newest guidelines[24] suggest that at least a 20% change be utilized to distinguish patients with a changing pattern if the value is already elevated. Others have suggested a value of 30%.[52] At the low end of assay sensitivity, however, it may well be greater depending upon the assay that is used. In addition, when we are aware of biologic variability, this too should be taken into account. Recent data from Wu and colleagues[54] defining biologic variability suggest that the values for biologic variability may be as high as 47% in the short term and still higher long term. There is a need to refine these criteria. At present, it appears that patients whose cTn values are chronically elevated can be identified when they have acute problems if they have a rising pattern of cTn values.[55] This suggestion is best supported by the data in the renal failure patients[55] who are known to have chronic cTnT elevations.

The diagnosis of AMI requires more than just cTn elevations. It requires that the clinical setting in which the elevations occur is one of ischemic heart disease.[24] Obviously, that is easy in some cases and more difficult in others. However, given the data that individuals with spontaneous non-ST segment elevation myocardial infarction (STEMI, a so-called type 1 MI) benefit from aggressive anticoagulation, IIB/IIIA antiplatelet agents, and an early invasive strategy[56] because cTn seems to mark those who have more severe coronary artery disease (Figure 2–2),[57,58] many patients

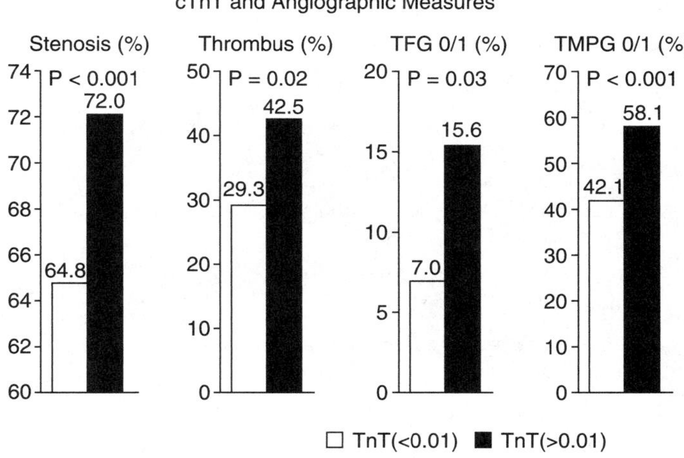

■ **Figure 2–2** Relationship of troponin elevations to coronary anatomy in patients presenting with acute coronary syndromes.

Reproduced with permission from *Prog Cardiovasc Dis* 47 2004.

now will have angiographic data, as well as clinical and ECG information. Often imaging data will be available as well. Patients who have rising troponin values all probably have an acute process that is ongoing. This, however, is not synonymous with a diagnosis of coronary artery disease. cTn elevations can be present for a large number of reasons (Table 2–2),[59] many of which can be readily

Table 2–2: Elevations of troponin in the absence of overt ischemic heart disease.

- Cardiac contusion, or other trauma including surgery, ablation, pacing, etc.
- Congestive heart failure—acute and chronic
- Aortic dissection
- Aortic valve disease
- Hypertrophic cardiomyopathy
- Tachy- or brady arrhythmias, or heart block
- Apical ballooning syndrome
- Rhabdomyolysis with cardiac injury
- Pulmonary embolism, severe pulmonary hypertension
- Renal failure
- Acute neurological disease, including stroke, or subarachnoid haemorrhage
- Infiltrative diseases, e.g., amyloidosis, haemochromotosis, sarcoidosis, and scleroderma
- Inflammatory diseases, e.g., myocarditis or myocardial extenstion of endo-/pericarditis
- Drug toxicity or toxins
- Critically ill patients, especially with respiratory failure, or sepsis
- Burns, especially if affecting > 30% of body surface area
- Extreme exertion

diagnosed clinically. There will, however, be some patients in whom the etiology of a given cTn elevation is unclear. Those patients may require additional evaluation. Recent data would suggest that some such patients have myocardial infarction that can be documented by MRI despite normal coronary arteries.[60–62] It has long been known[63] that 10 to 15% of patients with a diagnosis of non-STEMI have normal or near normal coronary angiograms and an adverse prognosis. This could occur because the timing of the angiogram is such that a significant thrombotic occlusion is missed or perhaps because the etiology of the AMI is due to endothelial dysfunction. Interestingly, most of the patients so far described are women. In addition, it is now clear that myocarditis can be a common mimicker now that we can diagnose it with MRI. In the Assomoll series,[62] 50% of the patients who presented with probable acute coronary syndromes clinically and had elevated cTn but normal coronary arteries had myocarditis by MRI. It is likely that other disease entities will be described which will add to this number as well. However, the diagnosis of myocardial infarction is and should continue to be a clinical one. In the appropriate setting, patients who have elevated cTn with a rising pattern should be diagnosed as having AMI. Recent data support the idea that the prognosis in these patients is similar to those with previously diagnosed non-STEMI and that the time course of subsequent events is also similar.[64,65]

It is of some importance to understand, however, that some of the patients with stable ischemic heart disease can also have detectable or minor elevations in cTns[47,66] so one should not assume that the fact that a cTn elevation is not rising eliminates the possibility of coronary artery disease. In this situation, it is likely that coronary artery disease is not acute, and therefore it may not be necessary, assuming these patients appear stable, for all such patients to be admitted. However, it is clear that some of these individuals can be induced to release cTn. Some of the events can be due to plaque rupture, but the guidelines[24] also recognize what is called a type 2 AMI, which is one that is not associated with acute plaque rupture, but is due to coronary artery disease. If one thinks that endothelial dysfunction is a cause, then it alone or supply-demand abnormalities in the presence of coronary artery disease could fit the classification of a type 2 AMI.

Some mention should be made of attempts to make the diagnosis of AMI earlier with either nonspecific markers of cardiac injury or panels of biomarkers. The approach has been advocated for with myoglobin[67] and then CK isoforms[68] even before the introduction of cTn measurements. Initial data with using relatively insensitive cTn assays as comparators suggested that these approaches may be beneficial in providing an earlier diagnosis and this approach provided some prognostic data as well. However, as cTn assays became more sensitive, it became clear that these markers no longer added very much.[69,70] In addition, the prognostic information turned out to be related to noncardiac, rather than cardiac, morbidity.[71] Recently, similar data have been published with heart fatty acid binding protein. If one uses the lowest and least specific cutoff value, it appears that heart type fatty acid binding protein (HFABP) provides earlier diagnosis than the use of a modestly sensitive, but not highly sensitive, cTnT assay when used with a cutoff value higher than suggested.[72] The differences are not large, thus even if one believes the data totally, it is likely that the number of patients one would need to monitor and the false positive rate due to the lack of specificity of HFABP would make this approach cost effective. Similar information has been published about prognosis using peak values of HFABP, but not peak values of cTn.[73] Finally, it does appear that panels of markers can anticipate the eventual development of cTn elevations.[74,75] Whether the number of patients identified earlier justifies the expense is unclear.

Diagnosis of AMI in Special Circumstances

The diagnosis of myocardial infarction in a multitude of other clinical circumstances can be far more complex. Several are considered here:

Renal Failure

Patients with renal failure often have elevations in troponin. These elevations are highly prognostic[39,76,77] and should lead to scrutiny of the underlying disease process. Recent data suggest that it is not always coronary artery disease that is involved,[78] although there is a relationship between elevations in troponin and the presence of coronary disease.[76] Despite that, left ventricular hypertrophy is another potent determinant,[79] and it is unclear that coronary disease alone can be used to explain the adverse prognosis.

Because the elevations associated with renal failure are chronic[39] and are very common with cTnT, one can and should have baseline values in all patients who are on dialysis.[80] This approach has been approved for cTnT because it is elevated so much more frequently than cTnI despite comparable prognostic significance when elevations occur. When patients on dialysis present with chest discomfort, recent data support the concept that a rising pattern can be used to identify those with acute disease and to distinguish them from patients who have elevations that are simply chronic.[55] These patients are at very high risk.[81] All patients with elevated cTn require evaluation, but those with a rising pattern almost all require inpatient evaluation, whereas the vast majority of those with chronic elevations can probably be evaluated as outpatients.

Post PCI

The literature regarding biomarkers following percutaneous coronary intervention (PCI) initially relied on CK-MB.[82,83] Multiple studies were done to validate that increases in CK-MB post-PCI were of prognostic importance.[84,85] However, when cTn became the marker of choice, the field became confounded by the fact that investigators did not utilize sensitive cutoffs pre-PCI circumstance to define inclusion in the groups until a paper in 2006.[86] These and more recent data suggest that the prognostic significance demonstrated for elevations of CK-MB was likely a reflection of the fact that often cTn is elevated acutely at baseline in these patients, but that these elevations were missed because of the

Table 2–3: Criteria for acute myocardial infarction after PCI.

For PCI in patients with normal baseline troponin values, elevations of biomarkers above the 99th percentile the upper reference limit (URL) are indicative of periprocedural necrosis.

By convention, increases of biomarkers > 3 × 99th percentile URL have been defined as PCI-related myocardial infarction. A subtype related to a documented stent thrombosis is recognized.

relative insensitivity of CK-MB or if high cutoff values are used for cTn.[66,86,87] Recent data would indicate that there is very little, if any, prognostic significance to biomarker elevations post-PCI over and above those which can be gleaned from the baseline troponin values[66,86,87] when the 99th percentile values are used as the cutoff values as suggested by all the guideline groups.[24] In a recent analysis of several thousand patients, elevations of cardiac troponin at baseline were highly prognostic.[86,87] When elevations were present at baseline, there was no additional prognostic significance of subsequent elevations post-PCI.[86] When values were normal, there was some short-term significance to post-PCI elevations,[87] but the significance was marginal and occurred predominantly in patients who had overt complications associated with the procedures. More importantly, this effect seems also to be the case in patients with putatively stable angina.[66] Accordingly, the present standards suggest that one should not make the diagnosis of periprocedural myocardial infarction if the baseline troponin is elevated.[24] In the absence of a baseline troponin elevation, one can make the diagnosis if a post-PCI elevation is present. In fact, any elevation is a marker of cardiac injury. The appropriate criteria for this diagnosis have not been defined scientifically, so a threefold increase based on previous literature was embraced by the recent Universal Definition Task Force.[24] Even in these circumstances, it is unclear that these elevations have prognostic significance and may therefore only be useful for quality assurance of procedure skills.

Table 2–4: Criteria for acute myocardial infarction after cardiac surgery.

For CABG in patients with normal baseline troponin values, elevations of biomarkers above the 99th percentile URL are indicative of periprocedural necrosis.
By convention, increases of biomarkers > 5 × 99th percentile URL plus either new Q waves or new LBBB, or angiographically documented new graft or native coronary artery occlusion, or imaging evidence of new loss of viable myocardium have been defined as CABG-related myocardial infarction.

Post CABG

The diagnosis of myocardial infarction is difficult post–cardiac bypass surgery (CABG). Elevations of biomarkers, whether CK-MB or cTn, occur as part of the procedure due to cross-clamp time, direct invasion of the heart due to trauma, as well as abnormalities related to preservation of the heart and cardioplegia.[24] In general, the more marked the elevations, the worse the prognosis.[85,88,89] However, less complex procedures, such as those done off-pump, compared to, for example, CABG and valve replacement, elaborate less of the biomarkers. Thus, a solitary cutoff value cannot be defined.[24] If one were to choose a low threshold only, one would diagnose a large number of patients undergoing CABG and/or valve replacement as having a periprocedural AMI. If one chose a very high threshold, one would allow patients undergoing off-pump procedures to rarely be diagnosed with AMI. Accordingly, a low threshold was advocated,[24] along with imaging evidence of myocardial injury, which could be present by ECG, by magnetic resonance imaging (MRI), or other imaging technologies. It appears that much of the injury is not transmural[90] and therefore is unlikely related to graft or native-vessel occlusion, but rather to abnormalities related to anesthesia or cross clamp-time. Using MRI, lesions are often found at the cardiac apex.[90] The larger the cTn signal, the more likely the lesion is to be due to a primary vascular event, but there is marked overlap in the present studies so that a discrete cutoff value for vascular complications cannot be defined.[91] These data suggest that improvements in anesthetic and preservation techniques may be more efficacious because there is a relationship between the magnitude of elevations and long-term prognosis.

Critically-Ill Patients

Although the cTn criteria are identical, the most recent criteria distinguishes among patients who have spontaneous myocardial infarction due to plaque rupture from patients who may have coronary artery disease and who may—in response to a stressful circumstance, whether related to tachycardia, hypertension, hypotension, or a variety of other insults—develop some degree of troponin elevation due to supply-demand imbalance.[24] Also included are patients who might have endothelial dysfunction vasospasm, but in whom the primary abnormality is not an atherosclerotic plaque rupture. This then allows all patients who are critically ill and have elevations of troponin to potentially be included as having AMI. One could argue that the patient who is hypotensive has supply-demand imbalance and subendocardium hypoperfusion or that the patient with sepsis has supply-demand imbalance due to tachycardia. Alternatively, patients with sepsis may have cardiac toxicity due to circulating toxins elaborated by the septic process as well. Markers with greater specificity for specific disease entities would clearly help in this area. However, an extensive use of the designation of type 2 AMI would distort its meaning and such an approach is not advocated. But it is clear that regardless of the etiology, elevations of cTn in critically ill patients independently predict both an adverse short- and long-term prognosis even after correction for the severity of illness.[92] The tension in this situation is between the diagnosis of AMI (see Figure 2–3) and treatment of the patient. Certainly, one needs to scrutinize patients who may have cTn elevations to make sure they are not having a spontaneous AMI, e.g., a plaque rupture event. If acute plaque rupture is not present, many of these abnormalities

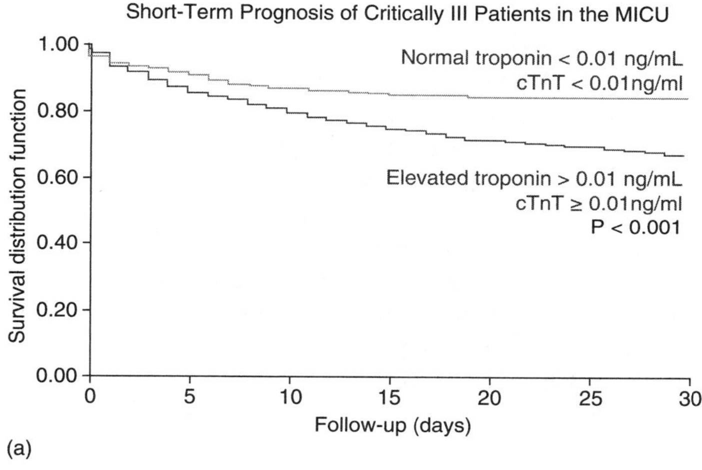

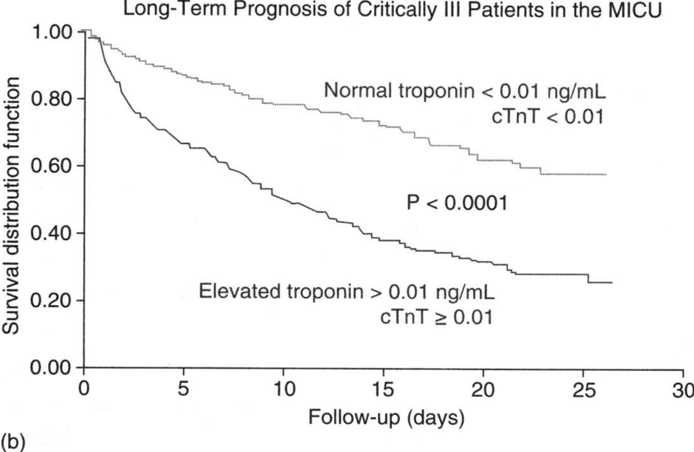

■ **Figure 2–3** Short- (a) and long- (b) term prognosis of patients with and without troponin elevations who were critically ill.

Reproduced with permission from Babuin L, Vasile VC, Rio Perez JA, Alegria JR, Chai HS, Afessa B, Jaffe AS. Elevated cardiac troponin is an independent risk factor for short- and long-term mortality in medical intensive care unit patients. *Critical Care Medicine.* 2008;36:759–765.

will likely be due to supply-demand abnormalities with or without underlying coronary artery disease. The issues related to this area are more clearly observed at present in the post-op surgical circumstance where there are data to suggest that a substantial percentage of these individuals have supply-demand imbalance and elevations in troponin.[93,94] Despite these data, recent trial information suggests that some of the therapies that are used to reduce myocardial oxygen consumption in the surgical situation may be problematic[95,96] and may even increase the frequency of stroke, presumably due to hypotension, and/or mortality related to inhibition of compensatory responses to the supply-demand abnormalities, making such circumstances even more complex. Research is necessary to define individual subsets of patients and to define the best therapeutic options.

Conclusion

The history and present circumstances related to the use of biomarkers are those of a need for increasing specificity. The initial markers were not specific for the heart. Now we have specific markers for the heart, but clinicians would like markers that are more directed at specific pathophysiologies. These may be developed with time, but at present, biomarkers, and particularly cTn, serve as the basis for the diagnosis of myocardial infarction, and a clear understanding of how to use them is critical.

References

1. WHO Expert Committee on Cardiovascular Disease and Hypertension. Hypertension and coronary heart disease: classification and criteria for epidemiological studies. *World Health Organ Tech Rep Ser.* 1959;168:3–28.
2. Karmen A, Wroblewski F, Ladue J. Transaminase activity in human blood. *J Clin Invest.* 1955;34:126–133.
3. Wroblewski F, LaDue J. Lactic dehydrogenase activity in blood. *Pro Soc Exp Biol Med.* 1955;90:210–213.
4. Rosalki SB, Wilkinson JH. Reduction of -ketobutyrate by human serum. *Nature.* 1960;188:1110–1111.

5. Levine SA. *Clinical Heart Disease.* 5th ed. Philadelphia and London: WB Saunders Company; 1963.
6. Rosalki SB. An improved procedure for serum creatinine phosphokinase determination. *J Lab Clin Med.* 1967;69:696–705.
7. Rosalki SB, Roberts R, Katus HA, Giannitsis E, Ladenson JH. Cardiac biomarkers for detection of myocardial infarction: perspective from past to present. *Clin Chem.* 2004;50:2205–2213.
8. Ebashi S, Toyokura Y, Momoi H, Sugita H. High creatine phosphokinase activity of sera of progressive muscular dystrophy. *J Biochem.* 1959;46:103–106.
9. Dreyfus JC, Schapira G, Rasnais J, Scebat L. La creatine-kinase serique dans le diagnostic de l'infarctus myocardique *Rev Fran Etud Clin Biol.* 1960;5:386–390.
10. Fowler NO. Myocardial infarction and coronary aneurysm. In: Noble O. Fowler, ed. *Cardiac Diagnosis.* Hagerstown, MD: Harper & Row; 1968.
11. Friedberg CK. *Diseases of the Heart.* 3rd ed. Philadelphia: WB Saunders Company; 1966.
12. Shell WE, Kjekshus JK, Sobel BE. Quantitative assessment of the extent of myocardial infarction in the conscious dog by means of analysis of serial changes in serum creatine phosphokinase activity. *J Clin Invest.* 1971;50:2614–2617.
13. Geltman EM, Ehsani AA, Campbell MK, Schechtman K, Roberts R, Sobel BE. The influence of location and extent of myocardial infarction on long-term ventricular dysrhythmia and mortality. *Circulation.* 1979;60:805–814.
14. van der Veen KJ, Willebrands AF. Isoenzymes of creatine phosphokinase in tissue extracts and in normal and pathological sera. *Clin Chim Acta.* 1966;13:312–317.
15. Roberts R, Gowda KS, Ludbrook PA, Sobel BE. Specificity of elevated serum MB creatine phosphokinase activity in the diagnosis of acute myocardial infarction. *Am J Cardiol.* 1975;36:433–438.
16. Vaidya HC, Maynard Y, Dietzler DN, Ladenson JH. Direct measurement of creatine kinase-MB activity in serum after extraction with a monoclonal antibody specific to the MB isoenzyme. *Clin Chem.* 1986;32:657–662.
17. Jaffe AS. Biochemical detection of acute myocardial infarction. In: Gersh B, Rahimtoola S, eds. *Acute Myocardial Infarction.* New York: Elsevier; 1997:136–162.

18. Jaffe AS, Ritter C, Meltzer V, Harter H, Roberts R. Unmasking artifactual increases in creatine kinase isoenzymes in patients with renal failure. *J Lab Clin Med.* 1984;104:193–202.
19. Adams 3rd JE, Bodor GS, Davila-Roman VG, et al. Cardiac troponin I: a marker with high specificity for cardiac injury. *Circulation.* 1993;88:101–106.
20. Adams 3rd JE, Schechtman KB, Landt Y, Ladenson JH, Jaffe AS. Comparable detection of acute myocardial infarction by creatine kinase MB isoenzyme and cardiac troponin I. *Clin Chem.* 1994;40: 1291–1295.
21. Tzvetanova E. Creatine kinase isoenzymes in muscle tissue of patients with neuromuscular diseases and human fetuses. *Enzyme.* 1971;12: 279–288.
22. Anonymous. The pathological diagnosis of acute myocardial infarction: preliminary results of a WHO cooperative study. *Bull World Health Organ.* 1973;48:23–25.
23. Tunstall-Pedoe H, Kuulasmaa K, Amouyel P, Arveiler D, Rajakangas AM, Pajak A. Myocardial infarction and coronary deaths in the World Health Organization MONICA project: Registration procedures, event rates, and case-fatality rates in 38 populations from 21 countries in four continents. *Circulation.* 1994;90:583–612.
24. Thygesen K, Alpert JS, White HD, for the Joint ESC/ACCF/AHA/WHF Task Force for the Redefinition of Myocardial Infarction, et al. Universal definition of myocardial infarction. *Circulation.* 2007;116: 2634–2653.
25. Katus HA, Remppis A, Scheffold T, Diederich KW, Kuebler W. Intracellular compartmentation of cardiac troponin T and its release kinetics in patients with reperfused and nonperfused myocardial infarction. *Am J Cardiol.* 1991;67:1360–1367.
26. Katus HA, Diederich KW, Hoberg E, Kubler W. Circulating cardiac myosin light chains in patients with angina at rest: identification of a high risk subgroup. *J Am Coll Cardiol.* 1988;11:487–493.
27. Katus HA, Looser S, Hallermayer K, et al. Development and in vitro characterization of a new immunoassay of cardiac troponin T. *Clin Chem.* 1992;38:386–393.
28. Bodor GS, Porter S, Landt Y, Ladenson JH. Development of monoclonal antibodies for an assay of cardiac troponin-I and preliminary

results in suspected cases of myocardial infarction *Clin Chem.* 1992;38:2203–2214.

29. Cummins B, Auckland ML, Cummins P. Cardiac-specific troponin-I radioimmunoassay in the diagnosis of acute myocardial infarction. *Am Heart J.* 1987;113:1333–1344.
30. Wu AHB, Apple FS, Gibler WB, Jesse RL, Warshaw MM, Valdes RJ. National Academy of Clinical Biochemistry standards of laboratory practice: recommendations for the use of cardiac markers in coronary artery diseases. *Clin Chem.* 1999;45:1104–1121.
31. Alpert JS, Thygesen K, Antman EM, Bassand JP. Myocardial infarction redefined—a consensus document of The Joint European Society of Cardiology/American College of Cardiology Committee for the redefinition of myocardial infarction. *J Am Coll Cardiol.* 2000; 36:959–969.
32. Jaffe AS, Ravkilde J, Roberts R, et al. It's time for a change to a troponin standard. *Circulation.* 2000;102:1216–1220.
33. Cummins B, Perry SV. Troponin I from human skeletal and cardiac muscles. *Biochem J.* 1978;171:251–259.
34. Perry SV. Troponin T: genetics, properties, and function. *J Muscle Res Cell Motil.* 1998;19:575–602.
35. Toyota N, Shimada Y. Differentiation of troponin in cardiac and skeletal muscles in chicken embryos as studied by immunofluorescence microscopy. *J Cell Biol.* 1981;91:497–504.
36. Bodor GS, Porterfield D, Voss EM, Smith S, Apple FS. Cardiac troponin-I is not expressed in fetal and healthy or diseased adult human skeletal muscle tissue. *Clin Chem.* 1995;41:1710–1715.
37. Anderson PA, Greig A, Mark TM, et al. Molecular basis of human cardiac troponin T isoforms expressed in the developing, adult, and failing heart. *Circ Res.* 1995;76:681–686.
38. Bodor GS, Survant L, Voss EM, Smith S, Porterfield D, Apple FS. Cardiac troponin T composition in normal and regenerating human skeletal muscle. *Clin Chem.* 1997;43:476–484.
39. Apple FS, Murakami MM, Pearce LA, Herzog CA. Predictive value of cardiac troponin I and T for subsequent death in end-stage renal disease. *Circulation.* 2002;106:2941–2945.
40. Muller-Bardorff M, Hallermayer K, Schroder A, et al. Improved troponin T ELISA specific for cardiac troponin T isoform: assay

development and analytical and clinical validation. *Clin Chem.* 1997;43:458–466.

41. Ricchiuti V, Voss EM, Ney A, Odland M, Anderson PA, Apple FS. Cardiac troponin T isoforms expressed in renal diseased skeletal muscle will not cause false-positive results by the second generation cardiac troponin T assay by Boehringer Mannheim. *Clin Chem.* 1998;44:1919–1924.
42. Ricchiuti V, Apple FS. RNA expression of cardiac troponin T isoforms in diseased human skeletal muscle. *Clin Chem.* 1999;45:2129–2135.
43. Wu AH, Jaffe AS. The clinical need for high-sensitivity cardiac troponin assays for acute coronary syndromes and the role for serial testing. *Am Heart J.* 2008;155:208–214.
44. Apple FS, Parvin CA, Buechler KF, Christenson RH, Wu AHB, Jaffe AS. Validation of the 99th percentile cutoff independent of assay imprecision (CV) for cardiac troponin monitoring for ruling out myocardial infarction *Clin Chem.* 2005;51:2198–2200.
45. James S, Armstrong P, Califf R, et al. Troponin T levels and risk of 30-day outcomes in patients with the acute coronary syndrome: prospective verification in the GUSTO-IV trial. *Am J Med.* 2003;115: 178–184.
46. Zethelius B, Johnston N, Venge P. Troponin I as a predictor of coronary heart disease and mortality in 70-year-old men. *Circulation.* 2006;113:1071–1078.
47. Schulz O, Paul-Walter C, Lehmann M, et al. Usefulness of detectable levels of troponin, below the 99th percentile of the normal range, as a clue to the presence of underlying coronary artery disease. *Am J Cardiol.* 2007;100:766–771.
48. Wallace TW, Abdullah SM, Drazner MH, et al. Prevalence and determinants of troponin T elevation in the general population. *Circulation.* 2006;113:1958–1965.
49. Daniels LB, Laughlin GA, Clopton P, Maisel AS, Barrett-Connor E. Minimally elevated cardiac troponin T and elevated N-terminal pro-B-type natriuretic peptide predict mortality in older adults: results from the Rancho Bernardo Study. *J Am Coll Cardiol.* 2008;52: 450–459.
50. Jaffe AS. Chasing troponin. how long can you go if you see the rise? *J Am Coll Cardiol.* 2006;48:1763–1764.

51. Macrae AR, Kavsak PA, Lustig V, et al. Assessing the requirement for the 6-hour interval between specimens in the American Heart Association classification of myocardial infarction in epidemiology and clinical research studies. *Clin Chem.* 2006;52:812–818.

52. Apple FS, Pearce LA, Smith SW, Kaczmarek JM, Murakami MM. Use of VITROS troponin I ES assay for early diagnosis of myocardial infarction and predicting risk of adverse events: role of following deltas. *Clin Chem.* 2009:In press.

53. Westgard JO, Klee GG. Quality management. In: Burtis CA, Ashwood ER, Bruns DE, eds. *Tietz Textbook of Clinical Chemistry and Molecular Diagnostics.* 4th ed. St. Louis, MO: Elsevier Saunders; 2006:498–499.

54. Wu AHB, Lu QA, Todd J, Moecks J, Wians F. Short- and long-term biological variation in cardiac troponin I measured with a high-sensitivity assay: implications for clinical practice. *Clin Chem.* 2009;55: 52–58.

55. Ie EH, Klootwijk PJ, Weimar W, Zietse R. Significance of acute versus chronic troponin T elevation in dialysis patients. *Nephron Clin Pract.* 2004;98:c87–c92.

56. Anderson JL, Adams CD, Antman EM, et al. ACC/AHA 2007 guidelines for the management of patients with unstable angina/non ST-elevation myocardial infarction: a report of the American College of Cardiology/American Heart Association Task Force on Practice Guidelines (Writing Committee to revise the 2002 Guidelines for the Management of Patients with Unstable Angina/Non-ST elevation Myocardial Infarction). *Circulation.* 2007;116:e148–304.

57. Lindahl B, Diderholm E, Lagerqvist B, Venge P, Wallentin L. Mechanisms behind the prognostic value of troponin T in unstable coronary artery disease: a FRISC II substudy. *J Am Coll Cardiol.* 2001;38: 979–986.

58. Heeschen C, van Den Brand MJ, Hamm CW, Simoons ML. Angiographic findings in patients with refractory unstable angina according to troponin T status. *Circulation.* 1999;100:1509–1514.

59. Jaffe AS, Babuin L, Apple FS. Biomarkers in acute cardiac disease—The present and the future. *J Am Coll Cardiol.* 2006;48:1–11.

60. Martinez MW, Babuin L, Syed IS, et al. Myocardial infarction with normal coronary arteries: a role for MRI? *Clin Chem.* 2007;53: 995–996.

61. Christiansen JP, Edwards C, Sinclair T, et al. Detection of myocardial scar by contrast-enhanced cardiac magnetic resonance imaging in patients with troponin-positive chest pain and minimal angiographic coronary artery disease. *Am J Cardiol.* 2006;97:768–771.

62. Assomull RG, Lyne JC, Keenan N, et al. The role of cardiovascular magnetic resonance in patients presenting with chest pain, raised troponin, and unobstructed coronary arteries. *Eur Heart J.* 2007;28: 1242–1249.

63. Dokainish H, Pillai M, Murphy SA, et al. Prognostic implications of elevated troponin in patients with suspected acute coronary syndrome but no critical epicardial coronary disease: a TACTICS-TIMI-18 substudy. *J Am Coll Cardiol.* 2005;45:19–24.

64. Roger VL, Killian JM, Weston SA, et al. Redefinition of myocardial infarction: prospective evaluation in the community. *Circulation.* 2006;114:790–797.

65. Salomaa V, Koukkunen H, Ketonen M, et al. A new definition for myocardial infarction: what difference does it make? *Eur Heart J.* 2005;26:1719–1725.

66. Jeremias A, Kleiman NS, Nassif D, et al. Prevalence and prognostic significance of preprocedural cardiac troponin elevation among patients with stable coronary artery disease undergoing percutaneous coronary intervention: results from the evaluation of drug eluting stents and ischemic events registry. *Circulation.* 2008;118:632–638.

67. McCord J, Nowak RM, Hudson MP, et al. The prognostic significance of serial myoglobin, troponin I, and creatine kinase-MB measurements in patients evaluated in the emergency department for acute coronary syndrome. *Ann Emerg Med.* 2003;42:343–350.

68. Zimmerman J, Fromm R, Meyer D, et al. Diagnostic marker cooperative study for the diagnosis of myocardial infarction. *Circulation.* 1999;99:1671–1677.

69. Eggers K, Oldgren J, Nordenskjjold A, Lindahl B. Diagnostic value of serial measurement of cardiac markers in patients with chest pain: limited value of adding myoglobin to troponin I for exclusion of myocardial infarction. *Am Heart J.* 2004;148:574–581.

70. Ilva T, Eriksson S, Lund J, et al. Improved early risk stratification and diagnosis of myocardial infarction, using a novel troponin I assay concept. *Eur J Clin Invest.* 2005;35:112–116.

71. Jaffery Z, Nowak R, Khoury N, et al. Myoglobin and troponin I elevation predict 5-year mortality in patients with undifferentiated chest pain in the emergency department. *Am Heart J.* 2008;156:939–945.

72. McCann CJ, Glover BM, Menown IBA, et al. Novel biomarkers in early diagnosis of acute myocardial infarction compared with cardiac troponin T. *Eur Heart J.* 2008;29:2843–2850.

73. Kilcullen N, Viswanathan K, Das R, et al. Heart-type fatty acid-binding protein predicts long-term mortality after acute coronary syndrome and identifies high-risk patients across the range of troponin values. *J Am Coll Cardiol.* 2007;50:2061–2067.

74. Mockel M, Danne O, Muller R, et al. Development of an optimized multimarker strategy for early risk assessment of patients with acute coronary syndromes. *Clin Chim Acta.* 2008;393:103–109.

75. Kavsak PA, Ko DT, Newman AM, et al. "Upstream markers" provide for early identification of patients at high risk for myocardial necrosis and adverse outcomes. *Clin Chim Acta.* 2008;387:133–138.

76. deFilipi C, Wasserman S, Rosanio S, et al. Cardiac troponin T and C-reactive protein for predicting prognosis, coronary atherosclerosis, and cardiomyopathy in patients undergoing long-term hemodialysis. *JAMA.* 2003;290:353–359.

77. Apple FS, Murakami MM, Pearce LA, Herzog CA. Multi-biomarker risk stratification of N-terminal pro-B-type natriuretic peptide, high-sensitivity C-reactive protein, and cardiac troponin T and I in end-stage renal disease for all-cause death. *Clin Chem.* 2004;50:2279–2285.

78. Hickson LJ, Cosio FG, El-Zoghby ZM, et al. Survival of patients on the kidney transplant wait list: relationship to cardiac troponin T. *Am J Transplant.* 2008;8:1–8.

79. Mallamaci F, Zoccali C, Parlongo S, et al. Troponin is related to left ventricular mass and predicts all-cause and cardiovascular mortality in hemodialysis patients. *Am J Kidney Dis.* 2002;40:68–75.

80. NACB Writing Group, Wu AHB, Jaffe AS, et al. National Academy of Clinical Biochemistry laboratory medicine practice guidelines: use of cardiac troponin and B-type natriuretic peptide or N-terminal pro B-type natriuretic peptide for etiologies other than acute coronary syndromes and heart failure. *Clin Chem.* 2007;53:2086–2096.

81. Aviles RJ, Askari AT, Lindahl B, et al. Troponin T levels in patients with acute coronary syndromes, with or without renal dysfunction. *N Engl J Med.* 2002;34:2047–2052.

82. Oh JK, Shub C, Ilstrup DM, Reeder GS. Creatine kinase release after successful percutaneous transluminal coronary angioplasty. *Am Heart J.* 1985;109:1225–1231.

83. Spadaro JJ, Ludbrook PA, Tiefenbrunn AJ, Kurnik PB, Jaffe AS. Paucity of subtle myocardial injury after angioplasty delineated with MB CK. *Cathet Cardiovasc Diagn.* 1986;12:230–234.

84. Califf RM, Abdelmeguid AE, Kuntz RE, et al. Myonecrosis after revascularization procedures. *J Am Coll Cardiol.* 1998;31:241–251.

85. Brener SJ, Lytle BW, Schneider JP, Ellis SG, Topol EJ. Association between CK-MB elevation after percutaneous or surgical revascularization and three-year mortality. *J Am Coll Cardiol.* 2002;40: 1961–1967.

86. Miller WL, Garratt KN, Burritt MF, Lennon RJ, Reeder GS, Jaffe AS. Baseline troponin level: key to understanding the importance of post-PCI troponin elevations. *Eur Heart J.* 2006;27:1061–1069.

87. Prasad A, Rihal CS, Lennon RJ, Singh M, Jaffe AS, Holmes DRJ. Significance of periprocedural myonecrosis on outcomes after percutaneous coronary intervention. *Circulation: Cardiovascular Interventions.* 2008;1:10–19.

88. Januzzi JL, Lewandrowski K, MacGillivray TE, et al. A comparison of cardiac troponin T and creatine kinase-MB for patient evaluation after cardiac surgery. *J Am Coll Cardiol.* 2002;39:1518–1523.

89. Croal BL, Hillis GS, Gibson PH, et al. Relationship between postoperative cardiac troponin I levels and outcome of cardiac surgery. *Circulation.* 2006;114:1468–1475.

90. Selvanayagam JB, Pigott D, Balacumaraswami L, Petersen SE, Neubauer S, Taggart DP. Relationship of irreversible myocardial injury to troponin I and creatine kinase-MB elevation after coronary artery bypass surgery: insights from cardiovascular magnetic resonance imaging. *J Am Coll Cardiol.* 2005;45:629–631.

91. Thielmann M, Massoudy P, Marggraf G, et al. Role of troponin I, myoglobin, and creatine kinase for the detection of early graft failure following coronary artery bypass grafting. *Eur J Cardiothorac Surg.* 2004;26:102–109.

92. Babuin L, Vasile VC, Rio Perez JA, et al. Elevated cardiac troponin is an independent risk factor for short- and long-term mortality in medical intensive care unit patients. *Crit Care Med.* 2008;36: 759–765.

93. Landesberg G, Mosseri M, Zahger D, et al. Myocardial infarction after vascular surgery: the role of prolonged stress-induced, ST depression-type ischemia. *J Am Coll Cardiol.* 2001;37:1839–1845.

94. Landesberg G, Shatz V, Akopnik I, et al. Association of cardiac troponin, CK-MB, and postoperative myocardial ischemia with long-term survival after major vascular surgery. *J Am Coll Cardiol.* 2003;42:1547–1554.

95. POISE Study Group, Devereaux PJ, Yang H, et al. Effects of extended-release metoprolol succinate in patients undergoing non-cardiac surgery (POISE) trial; a randomised controlled trial. *Lancet.* 2008;371:1839–1847.

96. Kaafarani HM, Atluri PV, Thornby J, Itani KM. Beta-blockade in noncardiac surgery: outcome at all levels of cardiac risk. *Arch Surg.* 2008;143:940–944.

3 ■ Biochemical and Analytical Laboratory Issues for Cardiac Troponin

Alan H.B. Wu, PhD

Introduction

Cardiac troponin has become the main serologic biomarker for detection of myocardial injury. Its use has largely replaced the need for other serologic markers, such as lactate dehydrogenase, myoglobin, and creatine kinase (CK)-MB isoenzyme. While there is debate as to the continued value of CK-MB, and many laboratories continue to offer this test, this practice is becoming more difficult to justify in the current medical economic climate. The transition from a nonspecific relative insensitive marker (CK-MB) to a specific highly-sensitive marker (cardiac troponin) continues to evolve. The clinical laboratory has requested and manufacturers of commercial troponin assays have delivered more robust assays with better sensitivity and precision at the low end, resulting in lower decision limits for acute coronary syndromes (ACS). However, not all physicians have embraced these next-generation assays and use of contemporary cutoff concentrations, i.e., the 99th percentile limit. It is important to understand that troponin is a marker of myocardial injury, not necessarily of ACS alone. Therefore, an assessment of results must be within the context of the patient's clinical presentation. Serial testing will become increasingly important to evaluate values that are just above the cutoff. A management decision to perform acute revascularization based on a single marginally-increased troponin value is potentially problematic. In contrast, the proper use of low cutoff concentrations using state-of-the-art assays will enable clinicians to make earlier diagnoses and improve risk stratification predictions for short-term adverse cardiac events (i.e., 30 days).

Biochemistry of Cardiac Troponin

Troponin is a regulatory protein that is part of the contractile apparatus of striated muscle. Within the myocyte, it exists as a ternary complex of three subunits: troponins T, I, and C. This complex, with a combined molecular weight of about 77 kDa, is bound to tropomyosin, which in turn coils around actin, the thin filament of muscle. Individual troponin subunits also exist within the cytoplasm as free forms (Figure 3–1).[1] Troponin T functions to bind the ternary complex to tropomyosin, has a molecular weight of 37 kDa, and 6–8% of the total is present in the cytosol as a free subunit. Troponin I inhibits ATPase, has a molecular weight of about 24 kDa, and has a 2–4% cytosolic component. The cardiac and skeletal isoforms of troponins T and I are structurally different, and antibodies raised to the cardiac forms do not cross-react with the corresponding skeletal forms. Troponin C is a calcium-binding subunit with a molecular weight of 18 kDa. Cardiac

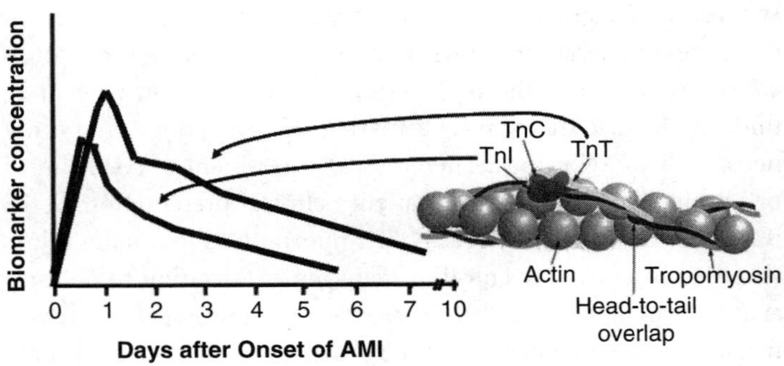

■ **Figure 3–1** Troponin T and I subunits and release kinetics into blood following myocardial injury. Troponin T has a higher relative concentration at peak, a more exaggerated second release phase, and remains increased in blood after AMI longer than troponin I.

subunits are identical to skeletal muscle troponin C. Thus, there is no clinical interest in an assay for troponin C, as positive results will occur in both cardiac and skeletal muscle diseases.

Injury to the cardiac myosite releases troponin in two distinct phases. The initial release is due to the free cytosolic component. Both cardiac troponin T (cTnT) and I (cTnI) appear in blood 3–6 hours after the onset of chest pain (Figure 3–1). Earlier detection of troponin is possible with use of high-sensitivity troponin assays and use of the 99th percentile cutoff concentration. When contemporary troponin cutoff concentrations are used, some investigators have shown that the release of troponin occurs as early as myoglobin, a marker characterized by its earlier release pattern after acute myocardial infarction (AMI).[2] Given that the molecular weight of myoglobin at 17 kDa is near that of the troponins, particularly cTnI, a release pattern similar to myoglobin is not an unreasonable finding. It does question the clinical need for myoglobin use as an early AMI marker, given its noncardiac specificity.

There is also prolonged release of troponin due to the gradual breakdown of the myofibrils. The serum half-life of cTnT is longer at 5–7 days than for cTnI at 3–5 days (Figure 3–1). cTnT also has a higher tissue content at 10.8 mg/g wet weight than cTnI at 4–6 mg/g wet weight. By comparison, CK-MB is entirely found within the cytoplasm and has a tissue content of only 1.4 mg/g wet weight. Therefore, after myocardial injury, more troponin T and I are released, which explains why these biomarkers have higher sensitivity towards myocyte injury. Once released into blood, troponin undergoes degradation and modification. The T-I-C ternary complex breaks down into a binary complex of I-C and free troponin T.[3] Free troponin cannot be recovered in serum or plasma, as it is highly lipophilic and binds to other proteins including troponin C. The individual troponin subunits break down into small fragments at the amino- and carboxy-terminal sequences. The central amino acids of both cTnT and cTnI are described as the stable portion, i.e., the epitopes are conserved and may be present in blood for longer than the N- and C-terminal fragments.

Troponin also undergoes posttranslational phosphorylations and exists as oxidized and reduced forms. The clinical significance of these forms is unknown. It is important that clinical assays have equal molar reactivities to as many of the complexed, free, fragments, and posttranslational forms as possible.[4]

Cardiac Troponin Assays

The International Federation of Clinical Chemistry (IFCC) Committee on Standardization of Markers of Cardiac Damage (C-SMCD) has established quality specification for cTnT and cTnI assays.[5] For cTnI, they recommend standardization to the newly-created troponin I reference material, available through the National Institute on Standards and Technology.[6] They also recommend that antibodies are directed towards the central (stable) portion of the troponin molecule.

Current Central Laboratory Assays

The majority of the testing for cardiac troponin occurs within a hospital's central laboratory using serum or heparinized plasma. Samples must be delivered to the laboratory (within 1–30 mins), centrifuged (5–10 mins), loaded onto and tested with an automated immunochemistry analyzer (15–20 mins), and results verified and reported (5–10 mins). The overall turnaround time from blood collection to testing ranges from 45–90 minutes.

Cardiac troponin T is available through a single manufacturer who owns intellectual property rights (Roche Diagnostics). Cardiac troponin I is not licensed and is freely available to any manufacturer who chooses to produce an assay. While there are some very minor differences in the use of these markers, the clinical utility is largely interchangeable. The selection of one marker versus the other by a clinical laboratory is usually dictated by the availability of the automated immunoassay instrumentation that exists in the laboratory and not a specific preference between the markers themselves.

All commercial cardiac troponins are measured using a sandwich immunoassay with a minimum of two sites. Figure 3–2a

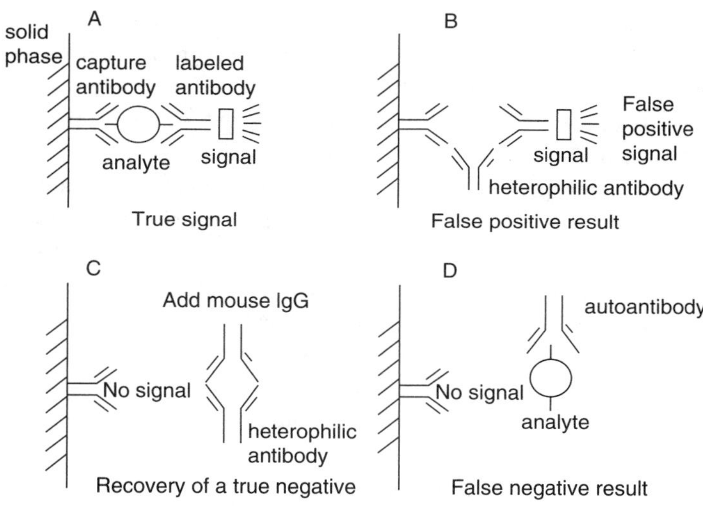

■ **Figure 3–2** A. Sandwich-type immunoassay for cardiac troponin. Two antibodies are used. The target analyte is represented as a circle (the lines coming from the circle represents the two epitopes). The "capture antibody" is bound to a solid surface (test tube, bead, microparticle), which binds to one epitope of the antigen. A second "labeled antibody" is linked to a signaling molecule (fluorophore, chemiluminescent tag, etc) and binds to another epitope of the antigen. Unbound proteins and antibodies are removed and the resulting signal is due to the presence of the analyte alone. B. A heterophile or human anti-mouse antibody (HAMA) interferes with the sandwich assay by binding to both the capture and labeled antibodies. In the absence of the analyte, a false positive signal is produced. C. The addition of a blocking reagent can eliminate antibody interferences, e.g., adding mouse IgG will bind to HAMA (left side of figure) thereby preventing its binding to the anti-troponin antibodies. D. The presence of an autoantibody can produce a false negative result. This interfering antibody binds to troponin near one of the epitopes thereby preventing the recognition of the analyte by the assay's antibodies, and a falsely negative signal occurs.

shows a schematic for this assay. The capture antibody is directed towards one epitope and immobilizes the target protein. For most automated immunoassay analyzers, the capture antibody is linked to a paramagnetic particle. A second labeled antibody directed towards a different epitope is added to create a "sandwich" surrounding the analyte. The use of an electromagnet enables adherence of the particles and the bound analyte to the side of a reaction tube, enabling unbound proteins and labeled antibodies to be rinsed away. The magnet is removed and the labeled antibody is measured. Some manufacturers have added a third antibody to the reagent mixture. This adds to the sensitivity of the assay by detecting additional troponin moieties whose epitope for one of the other antibodies may be blocked by binding to other proteins or antibodies.

Of the variety of tags that have been used for immunoassays, the most sensitive and therefore the most widely used for cardiac troponin is a chemiluminescent label. All troponin assays have an upper limit of the reportable range, and many have on-board dilution capabilities to measure samples with high analyte concentrations.

Point-of-Care Troponin Assays

Results of cardiac troponin are critical to the diagnosis and management of patients who present to the emergency department with chest pain. National and international societies within the disciplines of emergency medicine, cardiology, and laboratory medicine have made recommendations as to the ideal turnaround time for reporting results of cardiac markers. Defined as the time from blood collection to reporting of results, there is a consensus that results should be available within 60 minutes. In emergency departments that have accelerated protocols for rule-out of patients (e.g., "chest pain ER"), a turnaround time of 30 minutes is desirable. If a laboratory can receive samples quickly from the emergency department, such as with pneumatic tubes, it is realistic for a central laboratory to consistently meet the 60-minute objective.

If there are delays in sample delivery, or if a 30-minute reporting time is needed, point-of-care testing (POCT) or testing at an on-site satellite laboratory will be necessary. In a Q-probe conducted by the College of American Pathologists, 159 participating hospitals were questioned as to their turnaround time for cardiac marker testing.[7] Results from the central laboratory required roughly 90 minutes for 90% compliance. For many hospitals, these results do not meet goals established by the ED and cardiology communities and POCT may be necessary. Turnaround times from the central laboratory may have improved since the publication of this survey in 2004.

Qualitative and quantitative POCT devices for cardiac markers based on passive lateral flow technology have been available for over ten years and are used to deliver results of cardiac markers in a more facile manner. A summary of commercially-available devices is presented in Table 3–1.[8–11] All of these devices use whole blood and are either read manually or through an inexpensive portable reader. An instrument-based system that uses whole blood is also available for satellite laboratory applications. There have been several reports that have shown that by using POCT devices, assay turnaround times can be lowered on average from 87 minutes from the central laboratory to 25 minutes (Table 3–2)—sufficient to meet international guidelines.

As with any alternate technology, there are limitations associated with the use of POCT. Devices are approximately ten times more expensive than liquid reagents used on chemistry analyzers, and the analytical sensitivity and precision is not as high as the central laboratory. The use of insensitive assays reduces the clinical sensitivity of troponin for early diagnosis of AMI relative to sensitive central laboratory assays. In addition, POCT assays will reduce the effectiveness of troponin measurements for 30-day risk stratification for major adverse cardiac events.[12] Currently, there have been no prospective randomized trials that have demonstrated that implementation of POCT leads to quicker management decisions and improved outcomes. There may be some economic

Table 3–1: Point-of-care, satellite testing, and other whole blood devices for cTnI and cTnT and other cardiac markers.[1]

VENDOR	NAME	TYPE	FEATURES
cTnI			
Abbott	iSTAT	Reader	Separate assays for CK-MB and BNP.
Biosite	Triage	Reader	Integrated with CK-MB and myoglobin. BNP also available.
Response	RAMP	Reader	CK-MB, myoglobin and NT-proBNP also available.
Nanogen	Status	Reader	Qualitative and quantitative devices. NT-proBNP also available.
Siemens	Stratus CS	Bench	CK-MB, myoglobin and NT-proBNP also available.
cTnT			
Roche	Cardiac T	Reader	CK-MB, myoglobin and NT-proBNP also available.

[1]BNP, B-type natriuretic peptide. NT-proBNP, N-terminal proBNP.

Table 3–2: Published studies documenting improvement in assay turnaround times for cardiac markers.

STUDY	POCT*	CENTRAL LAB	Δ, ↓
Caragher et al., 2002	38	87	56%
Lewandrowski et al., 2003	17	110	85%
Collinson et al., 2004	20	79	75%
McCord et al., 2001	24	71	66%
Average	25	87	70%

*POCT, Point-of-care testing.

advantages, however, in faster triage of patients from overcrowded emergency departments.

Next-Generation "High Sensitivity" Troponin Assays

The current generation of troponin assays has a limit of detection of about 10–50 pg/mL and a 99th percentile cutoff of 50–100 pg/mL. These assays therefore do not have the sensitivity to reliably detect troponin of blood of healthy individuals. Prototype troponin assays have been developed with detection limits of under 1 pg/mL. Testing a cardiac healthy population using this assay resulted in a parametric distribution of data with a 99th percentile cutoff of 10 pg/mL.[13] Use of these ultra high-sensitivity troponin assays will detect even more cases of myocardial injury. Figure 3–3 shows the result of patients presenting to an emergency department with chest pain. Two different groups of patients are

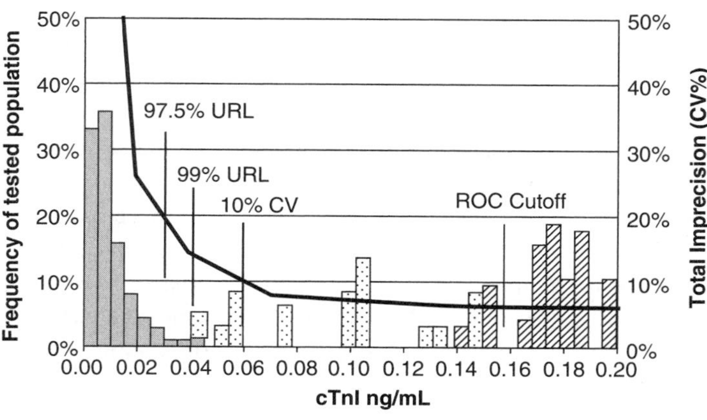

■ **Figure 3–3** Use of a high sensitivity troponin assay were used to test 51 patients who presented to an emergency department with chest pain. Patients with results below 10 pg/mL had a non-cardiac cause of troponin and the remaining had mild myocardial injury. These patients would have been classified as normal using other troponin assays with less analytic sensitivity.

evident. Those with values below 10 ng/mL have a noncardiac source of their symptoms. Those between 10 and 30 ng/mL have minor myocardial injury. These low troponin concentration cases would have been missed with use of a troponin assay of a lower analytic sensitivity. On the other hand, ultra-high sensitivity troponin methods will also increase the number of troponin positive cases due to nonischemic cardiac injury. Serial testing will be important for the proper interpretation of these low level results.[14] This requires knowledge of the analyte's biological variation, which has recently been determined.[15] Values that are acutely rising increase the likelihood of AMI, while those that are falling might suggest an old AMI. Patients with chronic myocardial damage, such as with renal failure, heart failure, and cardiac valve disease, will more likely have troponin results that are stable and unchanging.

Troponin Assay Interferences

A major issue of troponin assays is the potential to produce false positive results due to the presence of atypical antibodies. Heterophile antibodies are antibodies that have multispecificities and weak avidity towards antigens and may exhibit rheumatoid factor activity.[16] In contrast, human antianimal antibodies are produced in response to direct exposure of that species' immunoglobulin. Human antimouse antibodies (HAMA) are the most important subgroup because most the antibodies used in commercial immunoassays are monoclonal, i.e., they are raised against murine cell lines. Both heterophile and HAMA interfere with sandwich-type immunoassays, as they can bind to the two antibodies used in the assay. Thus, in the absence of the analyte, these interferents simulate the analyte, and produce a false positive result (Figure 3–2b). False positive results can also occur with incomplete centrifugation of plasma samples due to the presence of fibrin strands.

As summarized in Table 3–3, there are several ways that a clinical laboratory scientist or clinician can detect the presence of heterophile and HAMA antibodies. Because the antibody titer within

Table 3–3: Methods to detect interferents.

Heterophile or HAMA

1. Serial testing from the sample patient demonstrates a consistent result
2. Testing the sample on an alternate cardiac troponin platform for the same analyte
3. Testing the sample for the alternate troponin analyte (T or I)
4. Demonstrating the lack of recovery when the sample is diluted
5. Adding a blocking reagent such as IgG to bind the interfering antibody

Fibrin strands

1. Centrifugation of the plasma

a subject is consistent in time, the resulting troponin concentration is also roughly the same from sample to sample. This is in contrast to a patient with ACS where the troponin result is acutely rising and falling. The degree of heterophile interference among different troponin assays differs: a sample that interferes in one assay might not necessarily interfere in another, and vice versa. Therefore, retesting the suspicious sample on another testing platform, or testing for troponin T when the original result was for troponin I (and vice versa), is useful to provide evidence of an interferent. When samples containing these antibodies are diluted, the recoveries are usually less than 100%. Finally, in the case of HAMA interference, the laboratory can preincubate the sample with mouse immunoglobulin G. This will bind to the interfering antibody instead of the antibodies used in the assay (Figure 3–2c), preventing the binding of the labeled antibody (i.e., no analytical signal). With regards to fibrin interferences, repeat testing after recentrifugation is effective in correcting these problems.

False negative interferences also occur with some commercial troponin assays. Erikkson et al. identified the presence of circulation troponin autoantibodies that bind to troponin, obscuring the epitope and preventing the binding of the analyte to the antibodies used in some assays (Fig. 3–2d).[17] The prevalence of autoantibodies has been estimated to be about 3–6%. Because the autoantibody titers are usually low, large releases of troponin can overcome the interference, and, while the true results may be slightly lower than that recovered, it does not produce a false negative result. When the troponin concentration is low and only marginally increased, the autoantibody can produce a completely negative result. Troponin assays have been developed with use of antibodies directed away from the binding due to autoantibodies. With the recognition of this phenomenon, it is anticipated that next-generation troponin assays will be immune from this problem.

While the responsibility for generating accurate results for troponin lies with directors and supervisors of the clinical laboratory, cardiologists and other physicians who order this test and interpret results should be aware of the potential analytical limitations of measurements. Results that do not correlate with clinical findings should be questioned. Close communications between the laboratory and medical staff is necessary to ensure optimum use of this test, which has become vital in the management strategies used for patients with ACS.

Cutoff Concentrations for Cardiac Troponin

The cutoff concentration for cardiac troponin is a critical determinant as to the test's clinical usefulness. As with any laboratory test, there is a tradeoff between high clinical sensitivity with low cutoffs and clinical specificity with high cutoffs. There are several strategies in selecting cutoffs for laboratory tests. For physiologic markers, such as glucose or sodium, the central 95% of values from a healthy population (mean ± 2 standard deviation if the distribution is parametric) is used for tests where both abnormally high and low results are clinically important (2-tailed test). For tests where only low or high values are important (1-tailed test), the upper 97.5% or lower 97.5% are used, respectively (or mean +2SD or mean -2SD if parametric). When a biomarker is used to detect the presence of a specific disease, receiver operating characteristic (ROC) curve analysis is used. In this method, data from a diseased population is compared against a population that must be ruled out from that disease. The clinical sensitivity and specificity is computed at varying cutoff concentrations to determine the value that optimizes both of the test's attributes.

Since the first implementation of troponin, there have been changes in the approach towards assigning cutoff concentrations and a reduction in absolute cutoff concentrations. This is due to improvements in analytical sensitivity and precision and the clinical knowledge of the significance of minor myocardial damage that has become evident through clinical trials. Figure 3–4 illustrates the strategies for determining cutoff levels. Initially, troponin cutoff concentrations were set to separate patients with unstable angina from acute myocardial infarction using ROC analysis. At the time, the clinical significance of unstable angina was not fully appreciated, therefore the cutoff was established to differentiate this from acute myocardial infarction. Because unstable angina can produce minor myocardial injury, a relatively high cutoff concentration was produced, and the performance of cardiac troponin mimicked that of CK-MB. With the finding that minor myocardial injury, as reflected by release of troponin, was associated with adverse cardiac outcomes, it became necessary to alter the approach taken for setting cutoff concentrations. Unlike CK-MB, which is a test configured to diagnosis AMI, troponin is a test of myocardial injury, irrespective of the underlying mechanism. Therefore, cutoff concentrations are now set to differentiate health from heart damage. Unfortunately, when this concept was proposed, analytical assays did not have the sensitivity and precision to reliably detect troponin in healthy subjects. Analytical noise from imprecise assays can produce false positive results when low cutoff concentrations are used. Therefore, the clinical laboratory community proposed a troponin cutoff with a maximum imprecision of 10%. This cutoff separated many cases of unstable angina from healthy subjects (Figure 3–4).

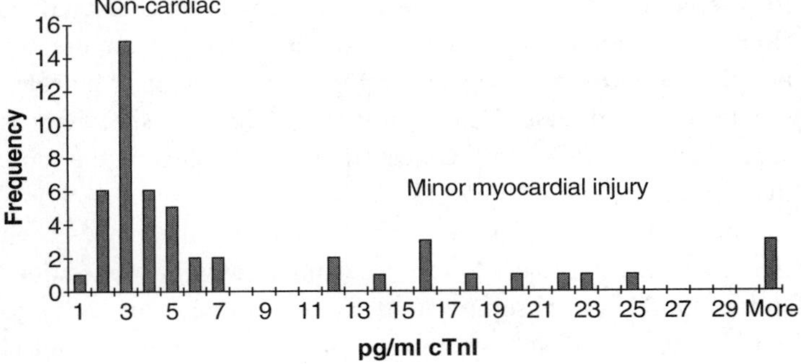

■ **Figure 3–4** Strategies for cutoff concentrations for cardiac troponin for a representative assay. The dark solid line represents the assay precision at various troponin concentrations (x-axis, in ng/mL). The ROC cutoff separated patients with unstable angina (dotted bars) from acute myocardial infarction (cross-hatch bars). The 10% CV cutoff separated healthy patients (gray bars) from unstable angina while maintaining a minimum assay precision (10%). The 99th and 97.5th percentile cutoff characterizes all but the top 1% and 2.5% of troponin values from a healthy population, respectively. The ESC/ACC has recommended the 99th percentile as the cutoff concentration for AMI diagnosis while the 1-tailed 97.5th percentile is the limit typically used for most other clinical laboratory tests. The imprecision for this particular troponin assay is higher than 10% at the 99th or 97.5th percentile cutoff limits. Some overlap in the various groups with the cutoffs selected is noted.

There have been continued improvements in assay quality for troponin. Today, the 99th percentile cutoff of a healthy population is the recommendation made by the European Society of Cardiology (ESC)/American College of Cardiology (ACC) redefinition of AMI.[18] This low cutoff concentration of troponin identifies most patients who present with cardiac symptoms who are at risk for future cardiovascular events. As the sensitivity of troponin becomes even lower with next generation assays, a consideration can be placed to lowering the cutoff concentration to the 97.5th percentile.

References

1. Dean KJ. Biochemistry and molecular biology of troponins I and T. In: Wu AHB, ed. *Cardiac Markers.* Totowa, NJ: Humana Press; 1998;193–204.
2. Eggers KM, Oldgren J, Nordenskjold A, et al. Diagnostic value of serial measurement of cardiac markers in patients with chest pain: limited value of adding myoglobin to troponin I for exclusion of myocardial infarction. *Am Heart J.* 2004;148:574–581.
3. Wu AHB, Feng YJ. Biochemical differences between cTnT and cTnI and its significance for the diagnosis of acute coronary syndromes. *Eur Heart J.* 1998;19 Suppl N:25–29.
4. Wu AHB, Feng YJ, Moore R, et al. Characterization of cardiac troponin subunit release into serum following acute myocardial infarction, and comparison of assays for troponin T and I. *Clin Chem.* 1998;44:1198–1208.
5. Panteghini M, Gerhardt W, Apple FS, et al. Quality specifications for cardiac troponin assays. *Clin Chem Lab Med.* 2001;39:174–178.
6. Christenson RH, Duh SH, Apple FS, et al. for the American Association for Clinical Chemistry Cardiac Troponin I Standardization Committee. Toward standardization of cardiac troponin I measurements part II: assessing commutability of candidate reference materials and harmonization of cardiac troponin I assays. *Clin Chem.* 2006; 52:1685–1692.
7. Novis DA, Jones BA, Dale JC, et al. Biochemical markers of myocardial injury test turnaround time. A College of American Pathologists Q-Probe Study of 7070 troponin and 4368 creatine kinase-MB determinations in 159 institutions. *Arch Pathol Lab Med.* 2004;128: 158–164.
8. Caragher TE, Fernandez BB, Jacobs FL, et al. Evaluation of quantitative cardiac biomarker point-of-care testing in the emergency department. *J Emerg Med.* 2002;22:1–7.
9. Lee-Lewandrowski E, Corboy D, Lewandrowski K, et al. Implementation of a point-of-care satellite laboratory in the emergency department of an academic medical center. Impact on test turnaround time and patient emergency department length of stay. *Arch Pathol Lab Med.* 2003;127:456–460.
10. McCord J, Nowak RM, McCullough PA, et al. Ninety-minute exclusion of acute myocardial infarction by use of quantitative

point-of-care testing of myoglobin and troponin I. *Circulation.* 2001;104:1483–1488.

11. Collinson PO, John C, Lynch S, et al. A prospective randomized controlled trial of point-of-care testing on the coronary care unit. *Ann Clin Biochem.* 2004;41:397–404.
12. James SK, Lindahl B, Armstrong P, et al. GUSTO-IV ACS Investigators. A rapid troponin I assay is not optimal for determination of troponin status and prediction of subsequent cardiac events at suspicion of unstable coronary syndromes. *Int J Cardiol.* 2004;93:113–120.
13. Wu AHB, Fukushima F, Puskas R, et al. Development and preliminary clinical validation of a high sensitivity assay for cardiac troponin using a capillary flow (single molecule) fluorescence detector. *Clin Chem.* 2006;52:2157–2159.
14. Wu AHB, Apple FS, Jaffe AS, et al. National Academy of Clinical Biochemistry Laboratory Medicine Practice Guidelines: use of cardiac troponin and the natriuretic peptides for etiologies other than acute coronary syndromes and heart failure. *Clin Chem.* 2007;53:2086–2096.
15. Wu AHB, Lu A, Todd J, et al. Short- and long-term biological variation for cardiac troponin I using a high sensitivity assay: implications for clinical practice. *Clin Chem.* 2009;55:52–58.
16. Kaplan IV, Levinson SS. When is a heterophile antibody not a heterophile antibody? When it is an antibody against a specific immunogen. *Clin Chem.* 1999;45:616–618.
17. Eriksson S, Halenius H, Pulkki K, et al. Negative interference in cardiac troponin I immunoassays by circulating troponin autoantibodies. *Clin Chem.* 2005;51:839–847.
18. Thygesen K, Alpert JS, White HD, et al. Universal definition of myocardial infarction. *Circulation.* 2007;116:2634–2653.

4 ■ Utility of Troponin Testing for Risk Stratification and Treatment Decision Making in Acute Coronary Syndromes

Kai M. Eggers, MD
Bertil Lindahl, MD

Introduction

An acute coronary syndrome (ACS) is the manifestation of a sudden rupture of a plaque in the coronary arteries with occlusive or subocclusive thrombus formation leading to distal cardiomyocyte ischemia and/or necrosis. A total obstruction of the infarct-related artery results in most cases in a transmural myocardial infarction, accompanied by ST-segment elevation on the ECG (STEMI). However, partial or temporary occlusion of the infarct-related artery is more common. In this situation, distal myocardial ischemia and/or necrosis is caused by microembolization of thrombotic particles formed at the site of rupture. The clinical manifestation in this situation is a non-ST-segment elevation acute coronary syndrome (NSTE-ACS), either as non-ST-segment elevation myocardial infarction (NSTE-MI) or as unstable angina, depending on whether biochemical markers of myonecrosis are elevated or not (Figure 4–1).

The Importance of Risk Prediction

The purpose of early assessment of patients with chest pain suggestive of an ACS is not only to establish the diagnosis of myocardial infarction, but also to predict the risk for cardiac events in the near future. Traditionally, risk assessment has been based on the patient's medical history, the physical examination, and ECG findings without taking biochemical markers into consideration. In the early 1990s, first reports were published

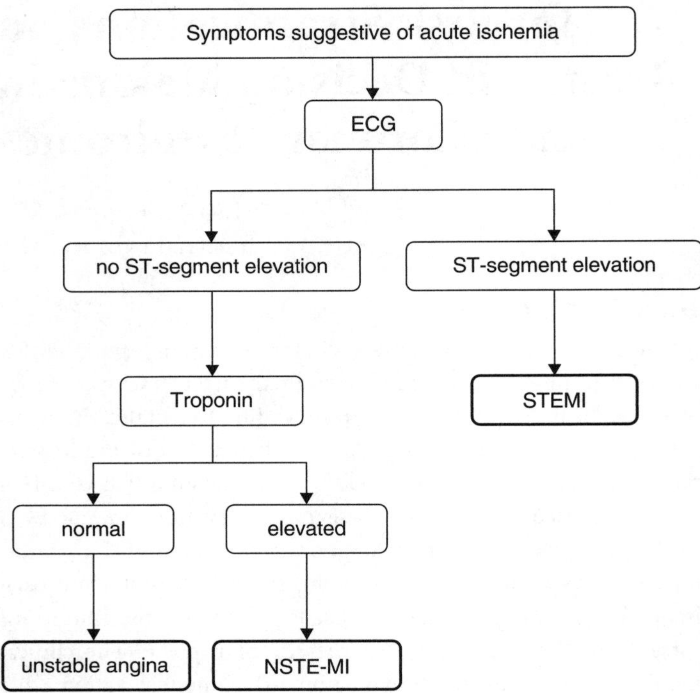

■ **Figure 4–1** Definition of acute coronary syndrome. STEMI: ST-segment elevation myocardial infarction. NSTE-MI: Non-ST-segment elevation myocardial infarction.

demonstrating a prognostic value of creatine kinase (CK)-MB (mass) levels in patients who, at that time, were regarded having unstable angina.[1,2]

Following the introduction of assays for measurement of cardiac troponin T (cTnT) and I (cTnI), it soon became clear that up to 25% of patients being considered as having CK-MB negative unstable angina had elevated cardiac troponin, and that these patients had an increased event rate.[2,3] This issue, together with the high cardiospecificity of the troponins, was anticipated by the ESC/

ACC Joint Committee in 2000, recommending troponin results as the marker of choice for risk prediction with the 99th percentile derived from a healthy reference population as prognostic cutoff.[4] It is noteworthy that this is different compared to the application of troponin results for the diagnosis of myocardial infarction. For that purpose, the lowest concentration measurable with a <10% coefficient of variation (10% CV) should be used as the alternative decision level, given the relative analytical imprecision of most available troponin assays at the 99th percentile.[5]

Relation of Troponin to the Risk for Adverse Events

To be prognostically useful, a risk marker should not only be precise and reliable, but also offer insights regarding its relation to risk. This is particularly important in the broad spectrum of patients with ACS, as their clinical presentation, prognosis, and response to treatment can vary considerably among certain subgroups. Furthermore, the number of treatment options available for ACS patients continues to evolve at a rapid pace. Physicians must choose from a wide array of antiplatelet and antithrombotic therapies, and also determine which patients would benefit from an early coronary revascularization. However, some of these treatments are rather costly or have potential serious side effects. The chosen management strategy must therefore be particularly applied to the patient group in which the most pronounced prognostic benefit is expected. Considering this issue, it is worthwhile to have a closer look at the relationships between troponin and the risk for cardiovascular events. This chapter will focus on the implications of troponin levels in patients with NSTE-ACS. The role of troponin in STEMI is dealt with in depth in Chapter 5.

The prognostic implications of elevated troponin in patients with NSTE-ACS can be attributed to pathological features and underlying mechanisms specifically associated with abnormal troponin results. Several studies have consistently demonstrated that troponin levels in NSTE-ACS reflect the instability of coronary

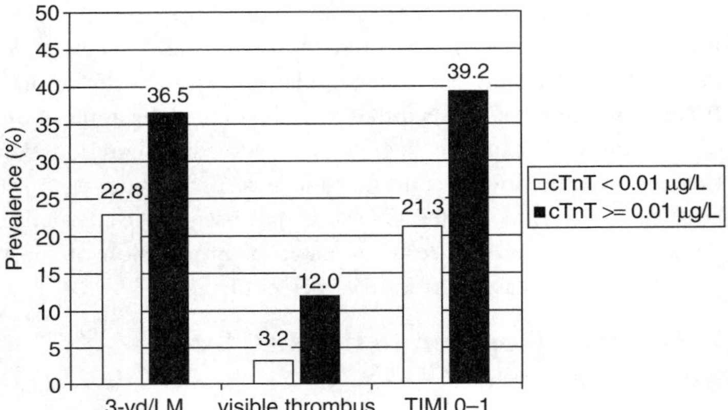

■ **Figure 4–2** Increased thrombus burden and impaired TIMI flow in patients with elevated cTnT. 3vd-LM: 3-vessel disease or left main stenosis.

Source: Lindahl B, Diderholm E, Lagerqvist B, et al. Mechanisms behind the prognostic value of troponin T in unstable coronary artery disease: a FRISC II substudy. *J Am Coll Cardiol.* 2001;38:979–986.

lesions in terms of more severe stenoses and a greater burden of intracoronary thrombus (Figure 4–2).[6,7] Troponin levels do also correlate with impaired tissue-level myocardial perfusion[8] and infarct size.[9] Accordingly, a meta-analysis demonstrated that patients with elevation of cTnT or cTnI had a significantly higher risk of mortality and death or recurrent myocardial infarction with relative odds ratios (OR) of 3.1 (95% CI 2.3–4.1) and 2.5 (95% CI 2.0–3.1), respectively.[10] The event rates in relation to troponin status in studies including more than 300 patients are demonstrated in Figures 4–3a and 4–3b. There is also a gradient of risk for mortality following increasing troponin levels as shown by results from the FRISC II and GUSTO IV substudies (Figure 4–4a).[7,20]

In addition to risk for mortality, it has been unmistakably shown that the risk for recurrent myocardial infarction is also higher in cases of troponin elevation. However, the relation of risk appears to be inversely U-shaped, with a higher number of events in case of minor troponin elevation compared to major elevation

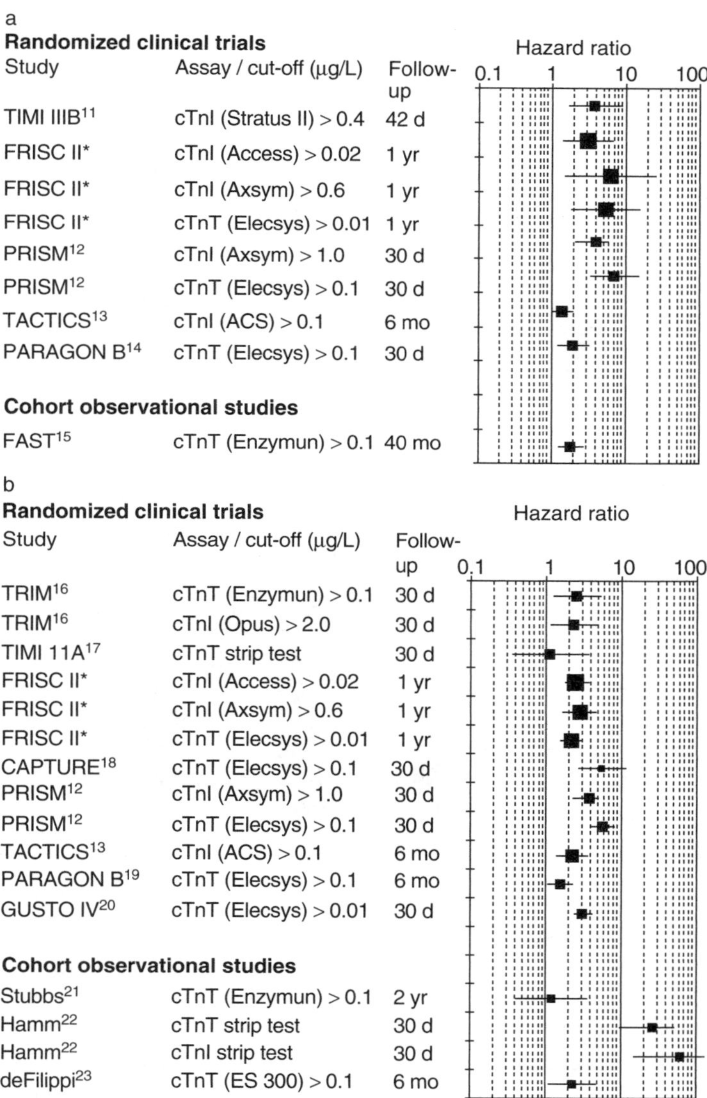

■ **Figure 4–3** Event rates by troponin status for A) mortality and B) death or recurrent AMI.

*unpublished data. The size of the rectangles represents the number of patients included in the studies.

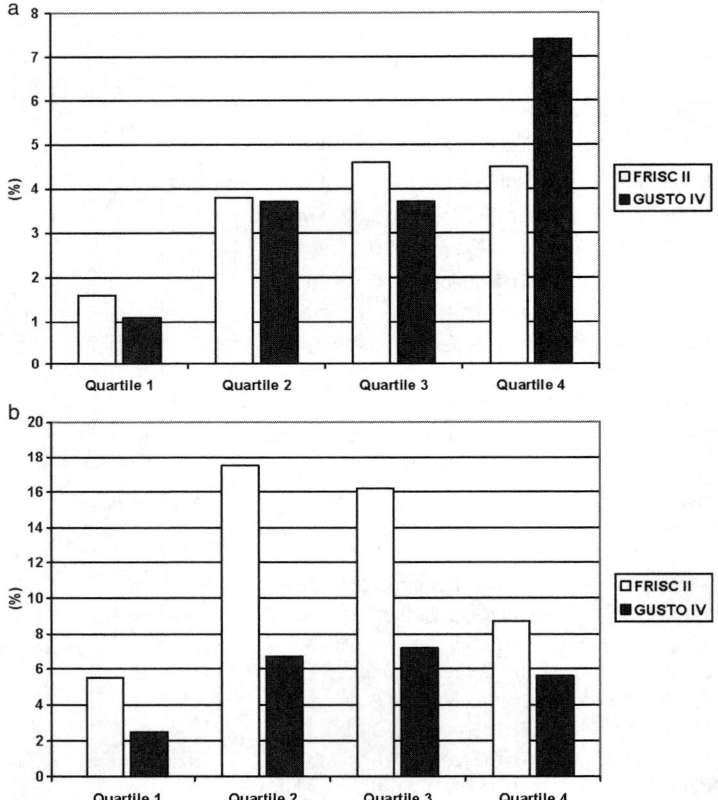

■ **Figure 4–4** A) One-year and 30-day mortality in relation to quartiles of cTnT in the FRISC II and the GUSTO IV studies. B) Rates of AMI at one year and 30 days in relation to quartiles of cTnT in the FRISC II and the GUSTO IV studies.

which contrasts to the linear risk gradient for mortality (Figure 4–4b). The explanation for this is probably that low-level troponin increases are usually not associated with a completed infarction, but reflect an unstable plaque in the culprit vessel with a high risk of new myocardial damage in the jeopardized territory. In patients with higher troponin elevation, a greater proportion will have a persistent occlusion of the infarct-related artery and may have completed the infarction, resulting in a lower risk of new myocardial injury in the same area.

Even though troponin levels correlate well with the final infarct size,[9] there are only limited data regarding the risk of developing heart failure in relation to troponin levels during the index event. At present, only one study has suggested an increased rate of admissions for heart failure in troponin-positive patients.[24]

Troponin Results for Treatment Decisions

Given the association between troponin levels and risk, it seems logical that troponin-positive patients with NSTE-ACS would benefit particularly from more aggressive therapies, such as intensive anticoagulation and/or early coronary revascularization. This was first proven in the FRISC study, which demonstrated a significantly lower incidence of adverse events in cTnT-positive patients treated with the low-molecular weight heparin (LMWH), dalteparin, during both the first 5–7 days of high-dose treatment and the following low-dose treatment.[25] Similar findings were made in patients participating in the TIMI 11-B substudy, who were treated with another LMWH, enoxaparin.[26]

Even for glycoprotein IIb/IIIa inhibitors, a considerable treatment effect exists in case of troponin-positivity. Newby and colleagues performed a meta-analysis of the PRISM, CAPTURE, and PARAGON B troponin substudies to define the interaction of troponin status with treatment on the endpoint of death or infarction.[14] None of these studies revealed a treatment effect with any of the tested glycoprotein IIb/IIIa antagonists in troponin-negative patients (pooled OR 1.1; 95% CI 0.8–1.4), while troponin-positive patients had a significant treatment effect with regard to improved outcome (pooled OR 0.3; 95% CI 0.2–0.6).

During the last years, the spectrum of antithrombotic therapies in NSTE-ACS has been broadened with the introduction of thienopyridines, factor Xa, and thrombin inhibitors. However, at

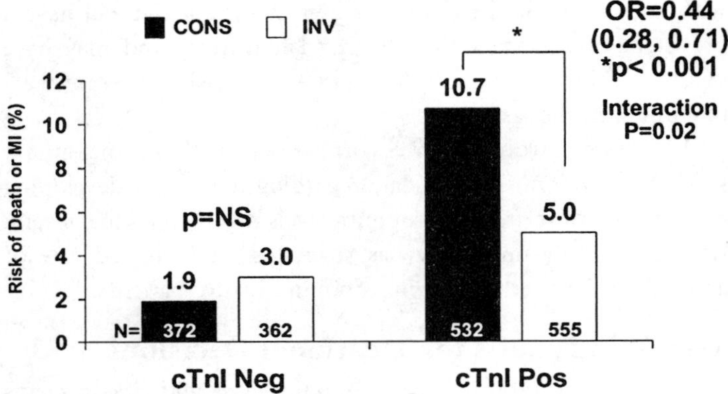

■ **Figure 4–5** Benefit of an early invasive (inv) vs conservative (cons) management strategy on the risk of death and new/recurrent myocardial infarction at 6 months in NSTE-ACS patients from TACTICS-TIMI 18 trial.

Reprinted with Courtesty of Clinical Chemistry.

present, it is not clear whether troponin status may be useful for the decision of whether or not to treat patients with these agents as this issue has not been specifically evaluated.

According to current recommendations, NSTE-ACS patients should be targeted for early coronary revascularization,[27] and there is strong and consistent evidence that the greatest beneficial effects of an invasive strategy are confined to troponin-positive patients (Figure 4–5), in particular in cases of ST-segment depression.[13,29] As demonstrated by results from the FRISC II study, an early invasive approach nearly halved the 1-year risk for death or myocardial infarction in patients with both elevated cTnT and ST-segment depression from 22% to 13%.[29] Similar findings were made in a GUSTO IV substudy regarding the combination of cTnT and NT-pro BNP. In this study, the greatest reduction of mortality by early revascularization was noted in the cohort with abnormal results for both markers (OR 0.6; 95% CI 0.4–0.7), whereas patients with normal cTnT and NT-pro BNP had an increased mortality (OR 10.8; 95% CI 2.1–56.0) due to a higher rate of periprocedural complications, outweighing the potential benefit of treatment.[30]

Determination of troponin might also be useful for the identification of patients needing angiotensin-converting enzyme (ACE) inhibitor treatment after the initial stabilization, given the correlation of troponin levels measured 12–72 hours after the index event to infarct size.[9] However, this issue has at present not been further evaluated as it is not clear whether troponin levels are more appropriate for this purpose than other markers of left-ventricular dysfunction postinfarction, such as echocardiographic findings or the natriuretic peptides.

Taken together, current evidence clearly demonstrates that troponin is useful for guiding treatment decisions in NSTE-ACS in order to maximize the benefit of antithrombotic therapies or early coronary revascularization. Hence, in recent guidelines, troponin testing has been recommended together with the evaluation of ST-T-segment changes as a useful measure for the identification of patients who should be targeted for aggressive therapies.[27]

Practical Issues

Troponin T or Troponin I?

In the past, there has been controversy over which biomarker is preferable for clinical purposes, cTnT or cTnI. Despite some differences in biochemical and analytical characteristics, there is currently no convincing evidence that one troponin is superior to the other. Assay-related issues, such as the analytical sensitivity and imprecision, appear to determine the information obtained from troponin results to a greater extent than the chosen troponin. In this context, it is noteworthy that in contrast to cTnT, cTnI results from one assay cannot be extrapolated to another depending on different normal ranges, detection limits, and medical decision cutoffs. Clinicians, therefore, need to understand which cTnI assay is being used at their facility in order to interpret obtained results correctly.

Timing of Troponin Measurement for Risk Assessment

Current guidelines recommend repetitive troponin testing in patients with suspected NSTE-ACS in order to optimize the diagnostic sensitivity. At present, testing upon admission and after 6–12 hours is recommended.[27,28] This recommendation will probably change with the advent of "high-sensitivity" troponin methods, whose ability to detect minute changes in troponin concentrations from hour to hour is far superior to older versions of their corresponding method.[31]

While the diagnosis of myocardial infarction by troponin results clearly is cutoff-dependent, the situation regarding prognostication is different as there is a gradient of risk with increasing troponin levels starting at concentrations slightly above the lower level of detection.[32,33] This issue is discussed in detail below. With the implementation of assays with improved analytical sensitivity, it has become clear that, besides ACS, subtle troponin elevation may occur in a variety of nonischemic or chronic etiologies that may mimic unstable coronary disease (Table 4–1). This poses a dilemma for clinicians as a single sample with small troponin elevation does not reveal the underlying cause, acute (e.g., ACS) or chronic (e.g., congestive heart failure), and the different mechanisms of troponin leakage might reflect different prognostic patterns. To detect a significant rise or fall of troponin levels indicative of acute myocardial damage, repetitive testing is therefore required, i.e., upon presentation and after six hours. Later troponin samples do not provide a better risk stratification.[34] The sampling interval could be shortened by the combination of troponin with other risk indicators (e.g., ECG findings, natriuretic peptides).[34] However, the use of multimarker strategies for rapid risk prediction is not widely adopted due to the heterogeneity of clinical studies addressing this issue.

Are the Troponins the Ultimate Solution for Risk Prediction?

To be useful for risk assessment in ACS, a marker should be cardiospecific, reliably measurable, and useful for identifying

Table 4–1: Causes and mechanisms of troponin elevation.

Diagnosis	Mechanism
Myocardial infarction	Thrombotic/embolic coronary occlusion
Coronary intervention (PCI, CABG)	
Coronary vasospasm	Coronary vasoconstriction
Increased sympathetic activity (cocaine, catecholamine storm)	
Left ventricular hypertrophy	Increased oxygen demand
Hypertensive crisis	
Prolonged tachyarrhythmia	
Sepsis	
Hypotension	Decreased oxygen supply
Aortic dissection	
Congestive heart failure	Myocardial strain
Pulmonary embolism	
Pulmonary hypertension	
Strenuous exercise	
Cardiac trauma	Direct myocardial damage
Direct current cardioversion	
Infiltrative diseases (amyloidosis, sarcoidosis)	
Myocarditis	
Sepsis	
Drugs (chemotherapy, alcohol)	

appropriate therapies for patients. The troponins meet almost all of these requirements when determined on contemporary assays. However, their predictive value is not absolute. First, troponin levels may be normal in high-risk patients presenting very early, i.e., before troponin levels have risen above commonly-accepted decision thresholds, but at a stage where the initiation of treatments aimed at restoring coronary flow and reducing infarct size are deemed valuable. Second, even though troponin elevation indicates cardiac damage, it does not define its nature as it also may occur in conditions other than ACS. Finally, the emphasis on the use of the troponin 99th percentile as cutoff for decision making is presently problematic, as most commercially-available assays perform with insufficient analytical precision at this low threshold with the risk for false-positive results in patients without ongoing myocardial damage.

Troponin results should thus be used in conjunction with other validated risk indicators. In particular, the clinical history, the physical examination, and the standard 12-lead ECG are all cornerstones for assessment of risk. A thoughtful interpretation of the patient's history and symptoms is essential as previous manifestations of ischemic heart disease and comorbidities, such as heart failure, diabetes mellitus, or renal dysfunction, are associated with a higher event rate independent of troponin. The physical examination may reveal abnormal vital signs, indicating an increased risk, e.g., rales or hypotension. The standard 12-lead ECG is an indispensable prognostic tool: it is inexpensive, rapid, and widely available and provides incremental prognostic information to that obtained from troponin results.[15,29] However, the information obtained from the ECG may be obscured due to pre-existing ST-T-segment abnormalities (e.g., in case of left-ventricular hypertrophy), confounding patterns (e.g., pacing, bundle branch block) and the fact that a single ECG only is a momentary sample and therefore, unable to mirror dynamic coronary blood flow changes in ACS.

Complementary testing for other biochemical markers might, therefore, be an option to improve risk assessment early after patient admission. Different biomarkers clearly reflect different components of the pathophysiology of ACS and may provide additive prognostic information when used as a panel. Some authors have advocated the use of other biomarkers of cardiomyocyte necrosis, e.g., myoglobin or CK-MB, in conjunction with troponin results.[35] However, others were not able to reproduce these findings, probably because CK-MB and myoglobin are less sensitive and specific for myocardial damage compared to troponin.[36]

Markers of inflammation (e.g., C-reactive protein) and hemodynamic stress (e.g., the natriuretic peptides) are elevated in ACS and there is strong evidence that they add prognostic information to that obtained from troponin results.[37,38] These markers are dealt with in depth in Chapter 14. However, the efficiency of any multimarker strategy will depend on the sensitivity and specificity regarding events determined by the selected biomarkers, applied decision levels, and the timing of testing. Simply adding up the number of elevated biomarkers does not take full advantage of the wealth of information provided by them. With regard to this, multimarker strategies are not uncontroversial and, at present, not commonly recommended for prognostication.

Taken together, none of the aforementioned risk indicators should be considered in isolation. Instead, all available information needs to be integrated in order to achieve a proper risk assessment. A proposal for a simple management algorithm for patients with suspected ACS and without diagnostic ECG changes is given in Figure 4–6. An alternative is to use one of the scoring systems, which have been developed and validated on the basis of the clinical history, ECG findings, the markers of myocardial damage, and different populations with ACS.[39,40]

Future Directions

Chasing the Optimal Troponin Cutoff—How Low Can One Go?

The ESC/ACC Joint Committee has recommended the use of the 99th percentile value of troponin as the cutoff for clinical decision

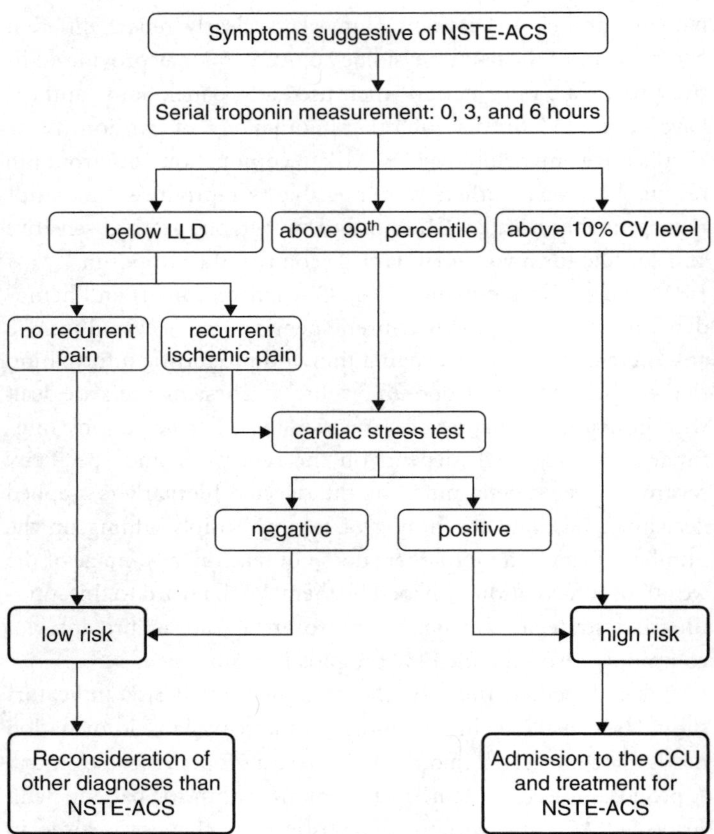

■ **Figure 4–6** Simple algorithm for assessment of patients with suspected NSTE-ACS and without diagnostic ST-segment elevation. LLD: Lower level of detection. CV: Coefficient of variation. CCU: Coronary care unit.

making in patients with NSTE-ACS,[4] or, alternatively, the lowest concentration measurable at the 10% CV level.[5] However, consistent data from studies that include both clinical trials and unselected patients with suspected NSTE-ACS demonstrate that

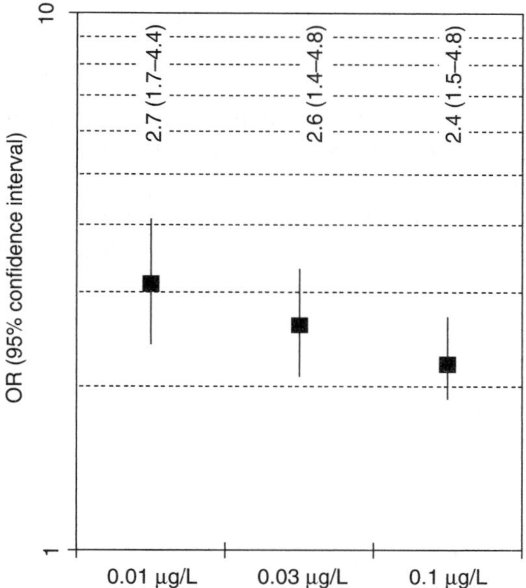

■ **Figure 4–7** 30-day risk for death and recurrent myocardial infarction by baseline troponin T levels in NSTE-ACS patients from the GUSTO IV trial.[41]

troponin levels between the 99th percentile and the 10% CV level are independently associated with a higher risk of recurrent cardiovascular events.[13,32,33] An example comes from the GUSTO IV study. In this study, three cTnT thresholds were compared regarding their ability to predict the risk of death and recurrent myocardial infarction at 30 days. The odds ratios were highest for the 99th percentile, suggesting that this cutoff detected most patients with true cardiovascular risk (Figure 4–7).[41] This underlines that minor troponin elevation, even if it does not meet the criteria for myocardial infarction, still reflects an adverse prognosis which emphasizes the need for assays with improved analytical precision at low troponin levels.

Recent studies, furthermore, suggest that any troponin concentration above the lower level of detection implies an increased risk for complications.[32,33] This poses a dilemma for clinicians as they should consider such subtle troponin elevation as an indicator of risk in subjects with a high probability of ACS, but at the same time be aware of the possibility of false troponin elevation due to imperfect assay performance. It is likely that the prognostic information obtained from very low troponin elevations will become more valid in the near future following the implementation of high-sensitivity troponin assays, allowing for a more reliable determination of very low troponin concentrations.[31,42,43]

Beyond Acute Coronary Syndrome

In patients with confirmed NSTE-ACS, the rationale of risk stratification by troponin measurement is to identify subjects who are most likely to benefit from specific therapeutic interventions aimed at reducing morbidity and mortality, e.g., medical treatment with LMWH, use of glycoprotein IIb/IIIa inhibitors, or early coronary revascularization.

In contrast to the acute situation, there are only a few studies which evaluated whether troponin testing might be relevant for risk prediction in the stable phase after NSTE-ACS.[43,44] Recent results from the FRISC II trial demonstrated that elevated cTnI levels are rather common after a NSTE-ACS when determined with a highly sensitive assay, and that subjects with persistent cTnI elevation had a considerably increased 5-year mortality (HR 1.8; 95% CI 1.3–2.4).[43] As in other populations with stable coronary artery disease and heart failure, persistent cTnI elevation late after NSTE-ACS appears to reflect the presence of coronary atherosclerosis and the degree of left-ventricular dysfunction.[45–47] There were no indications supporting an association between cTnI positivity and ongoing coronary plaque instability.[47] This explains the lack of an independent association between persistent cTnI elevation after NSTE-ACS and recurrent myocardial infarction (HR 1.3; 95% CI 1.0–1.7),[43] which contrasts with the prognostic information provided by troponin results in the acute situation.

Troponin testing might thus be regarded as an option for improving risk stratification in subjects with stable coronary artery disease or during follow-up after an episode of NSTE-ACS. Current routine management at this stage of disease focuses on symptomatic assessment and the modification of cardiovascular risk factors in order to halt the progression of atherosclerosis. However, these measures partly depend on the skills of the attending physician and traditional risk factors do not completely account for the individual risk profile. Thus, complementary measurement of biomarkers appears to be an attractive option, as this may allow for the identification of prognostic features thereby resulting in an ability to tailor treatments. However, to what extent risk prediction incorporating troponin results might perform better than conventional standards, and if so, when and who to test for the risk, remain to be further validated.

Conclusion

Applied in conjunction with the clinical history, physical examination, and interpretation of the ECG, cardiac troponin is a cornerstone for risk assessment of patients presenting with ACS. Troponin provides insights into mechanisms mediating morbidity and mortality and is therefore valuable for targeting of high-risk patients for more aggressive therapies. The forthcoming implementation of high-sensitivity assays will most likely broaden the applicability of troponin results for risk assessment to populations with stable coronary artery disease.

References

1. Pettersson T, Ohlsson O, Tryding N. Increased CK-MB (mass concentration) in patients without traditional evidence of acute myocardial infarction: a risk of coronary death. *Eur Heart J.* 1992;13:1387–1392.
2. Hamm CW, Ravkilde J, Gerhardt W, et al. The prognostic value of troponin T in unstable angina. *N Engl J Med.* 1992;327:146–150.

3. Ravkilde J, Horder M, Gerhardt W, et al. Diagnostic performance and prognostic value of serum troponin T in suspected acute myocardial infarction. *Scand J Clin Lab Invest.* 1993;53:677–685.
4. Alpert JS, Thygesen A, Antman EM, et al. Myocardial infarction redefined—a consensus document of the joint European Society of Cardiology/American College of Cardiology Committee for the Redefinition of Myocardial Infarction. *J Am Coll Cardiol.* 2000;36:959–969.
5. Apple FS, Wu AH, Jaffe AS. European Society of Cardiology and American College of Cardiology guidelines for redefinition of myocardial infarction: How to use existing assays clinically and for clinical trials. *Am Heart J.* 2002;144:981–986.
6. Heeschen C, van den Brand MJ, Hamm CW, et al. Angiographic findings in patients with refractory unstable angina according to troponin status. *Circulation.* 1999;104:1509–1514.
7. Lindahl B, Diderholm E, Lagerqvist B, et al. Mechanisms behind the prognostic value of troponin T in unstable coronary artery disease: a FRISC II substudy. *J Am Coll Cardiol.* 2001;38:979–986.
8. Wong GC, Morrow DA, Murphy S, et al. Elevations in troponin T and I are associated with abnormal tissue level perfusion: a TACTICS-TIMI 18 substudy. Treat Angina with Aggrastat and Determine Cost of Therapy with an Invasive or Conservative Strategy-Thrombolysis in Myocardial Infarction. *Circulation.* 2002;106:202–207.
9. Gibbons RJ, Valeti US, Araoz PA, et al. The quantification of infarct size. *J Am Coll Cardiol.* 2004;44:1533–1542.
10. Heidenreich PA, Alloggiamento T, Melsop K, et al. The prognostic value of troponin in patients with non-ST elevation acute coronary syndromes: a meta analysis. *J Am Coll Cardiol.* 2001;38:478–485.
11. Antman EM, Tanasijevic MJ, Thompson B, et al. Cardiac-specific troponin I levels to predict the risk of mortality in patients with acute coronary syndromes. *N Engl J Med.* 1996;335:1342–1349.
12. Heeschen C, Hamm CW, Goldmann B, et al. Troponin concentrations for stratification of patients with acute coronary syndromes in relation to therapeutic efficacy of tirofiban. PRISM Study Investigators. Platelet Receptor Inhibition in Ischemic Syndrome Management. *Lancet.* 1999;354:1757–1762.
13. Morrow DA, Cannon CP, Rifai N, et al. Ability of minor elevations of troponin I and T to predict benefit from an early invasive strategy

in patients with unstable angina and non-ST elevation myocardial infarction: results from a randomized trial. *JAMA*. 2001;286: 2405–2412.

14. Newby LK, Ohman EM, Christenson RH, et al. Benefit of glycoprotein IIb/IIIa inhibition in patients with acute coronary syndromes and troponin T-positive status: the PARAGON B troponin T substudy. *Circulation*. 2001;103:2891–2896.
15. Jernberg T, Lindahl B. A combination of troponin T and 12-lead electrocardiography: a valuable tool for early prediction of long-term mortality in patients with chest pain without ST-segment elevation. *Am Heart J*. 2002;144:804–810.
16. Lüscher MS, Thygesen K, Ravkilde J, et al. Applicability of cardiac troponin T and I for early risk stratification in unstable coronary artery disease. *Circulation*. 1997;96:2578–2585.
17. Antman EM, Sacks D, Rifai N, et al. Time to positivity of a bedside assay for cardiac-specific troponin T predicts prognosis in acute coronary syndromes: a TIMI 11A substudy. *J Am Coll Cardiol*. 1998;31: 326–330.
18. Hamm CW, Heeschen C, Goldmann B, et al. Benefit of abciximab in patients with refractory unstable angina in relation to serum troponin T levels. c7E3 Fab Antiplatelet Therapy in Unstable Refractory Angina (CAPTURE) Study Investigators. *N Engl J Med*. 1999;340: 1623–1629.
19. Kaul P, Newby LK, Fu Y, et al. Troponin T and quantitative ST-segment depression offer complementary prognostic information in the risk stratification of acute coronary syndrome patients. *J Am Coll Cardiol*. 2003;41:371–380.
20. James SK, Armstrong P, Barnathan E, et al. Troponin and C-reactive protein have different relations to subsequent mortality and myocardial infarction after acute coronary syndrome. *J Am Coll Cardiol*. 2003;41:916–924.
21. Stubbs, Collinson P, Moseley D, et al. Prospective study of the role of cardiac troponin T in patients admitted with unstable angina. *B Med J*. 1996;313:262–264.
22. Hamm CW, Goldmann BU, Heeschen C, et al. Emergency room triage of patients with acute chest pain by means of rapid testing for cardiac troponin I or T. *N Engl J Med*. 1997;337:1648–1653.

23. deFilippi CR, Tocchi M, Parmar RJ, et al. Cardiac troponin T in chest pain unit patients without ischemic electrocardiographic changes: angiographic correlates and long-term clinical outcomes. *J Am Coll Cardiol.* 2000;35:1827–1834.

24. Ottani F, Galvani M, Nicolini FA, et al. Elevated cardiac troponin levels predict the risk of adverse outcome in patients with acute coronary syndromes. *Am Heart J.* 2000;140:917–927.

25. Lindahl B, Venge P, Wallentin L. Troponin T identifies patients with unstable coronary artery disease who benefit from long term anti-thrombotic protection. *J Am Coll Cardiol.* 1997;29:43–48.

26. Morrow DA, Antman EM, Tanasijevic M, et al. Cardiac troponin I for stratification of early outcomes and the efficacy of enoxaparin in unstable angina—a TIMI-11B substudy. *J Am Coll Cardiol.* 2000;36:1812–1817.

27. The Task Force for the Diagnosis and Treatment of Non-ST-Segment Elevation Acute Coronary Syndromes of the European Society of Cardiology, Bassand JP, Hamm CW, et al. Guidelines for the diagnosis and treatment of non-ST-segment elevation acute coronary syndromes. *Eur Heart J.* 2007;28:1598–1660.

28. Morrow DA, Cannon CP, Jesse RL, et al. National Academy of Clinical Biochemistry Laboratory Medicine Practice Guidelines: Clinical characteristics and utilization of biochemical markers in acute coronary syndrome. *Clin Chem.* 2007;53:552–574.

29. Diderholm E, Andren B, Frostfeldt G, et al. The prognostic and therapeutic implications of increased troponin T levels and ST depression in unstable coronary artery disease: the FRISC-II invasive troponin T electrocardiogram substudy. *Am Heart J.* 2002;143:760–767.

30. James SK, Lindbäck J, Tilly J, et al. Troponin-T and N-terminal pro-B-type natriuretic peptide predict mortality benefit from coronary revascularization in acute coronary syndrome. A GUSTO-IV substudy. *J Am Coll Cardiol.* 2006;48:1146–1154.

31. Melanson SE, Morrow DA, Jarolim P. Earlier detection of myocardial injury in a preliminary evaluation using a new troponin I assay with improved sensitivity. *Am J Clin Pathol.* 2007;128:282–286.

32. Kontos MC, Shah R, Fritz LM, et al. Implication of different cardiac troponin I levels for clinical outcomes and prognosis of acute chest pain patients. *J Am Coll Cardiol.* 2004;43:958–965.

33. Kavsak PA, Newman AM, Lustig V, et al. Long-term health outcomes associated with detectable troponin I concentrations. *Clin Chem.* 2007;53:220–227.

34. Eggers KM, Oldgren J, Nordenskjöld A, et al. Risk prediction in patients with chest pain: early assessment by the combination of troponin I results and electrocardiographic criteria. *Coron Artery Dis.* 2005;16:181–189.

35. Newby LK, Storrow AB, Gibler WB, et al. Bedside multimarker testing for risk stratification in chest pain units: The chest pain evaluation by creatine kinase-MB, myoglobin, and troponin I (CHECKMATE) study. *Circulation.* 2001;103:1832–1837.

36. Eggers KM, Oldgren J, Nordenskjöld A, et al. Combining different biochemical markers of myocardial ischemia does not improve risk stratification compared to troponin I alone. *Coron Artery Dis.* 2005;16:315–319.

37. James SK, Lindahl B, Siegbahn A, et al. N-terminal pro-brain natriuretic peptide and other risk markers for the separate prediction of mortality and subsequent myocardial infarction in patients with unstable coronary artery disease: a Global Utilization of Strategies To Open occluded arteries (GUSTO)-IV substudy. *Circulation.* 2003;108: 275–281.

38. Heeschen C, Hamm CW, Bruemmer J, et al. Predictive value of C-reactive protein and troponin T in patients with unstable angina: a comparative analysis. *J Am Coll Cardiol.* 2000;35:1535–1542.

39. Antman EM, Cohen M, Bernink PJ, et al. The TIMI risk score for unstable angina/non-ST elevation MI: a method for prognostication and therapeutic decision making. *JAMA.* 2000;284:835–842.

40. Eagle KA, Lim MJ, Dabbous OH, et al. A validated prediction model for all forms of acute coronary syndrome: estimating the risk of 6-month postdischarge death in an international registry. *JAMA.* 2004;291:2727–2733.

41. James S, Armstrong P, Califf R, et al. Troponin T levels and risk of 30-day outcomes in patients with acute coronary syndrome: Prospective verification in the GUSTO-IV trial. *Am J Med.* 2003;115: 178–184.

42. Wu AH, Jaffe AS. The clinical need for high-sensitivity cardiac troponin assays for acute coronary syndromes and the role for serial testing. *Am Heart J.* 2008;155:208–214.

43. Eggers KM, Lagerqvist B, Venge P, et al. Persistent cardiac troponin I elevation in stabilized patients after an episode of acute coronary syndrome predicts adverse long-term outcome. *Circulation.* 2007; 116:1907–1914.

44. Shimizu M, Sato H, Sakata Y, et al. Effect on outcome of an increase of serum cardiac troponin T in patients with healing or healed ST-elevation myocardial infarction. *Am J Cardiol.* 2007;100:1723–1726.

45. Horwich TB, Patel J, MacLellan WR, et al. Cardiac troponin I is associated with impaired hemodynamics, progressive left ventricular dysfunction, and increased mortality rates in advanced heart failure. *Circulation.* 2003;108:833–838.

46. Schulz O, Paul-Walter C, Lehmann M, et al. Usefulness of detectable levels of troponin, below the 99th percentile of the normal range, as a clue to the presence of underlying coronary artery disease. *Am J Cardiol.* 2007;100:764–769.

47. Eggers KM, Lagerqvist B, Oldgren J, et al. Pathophysiologic mechanisms of persistent cardiac troponin I elevation in stabilized patients after an episode of acute coronary syndrome. *Am Heart J.* 2008;156: 588–594.

5 ■ Use of Cardiac Troponins in ST-Segment Elevation Myocardial Infarction

Hugo A. Katus, MD
Evangelos Giannitsis, MD

Introduction

In symptomatic patients, the diagnosis of myocardial infarction (STEMI) is straightforward in the presence of ST-segment elevations in at least two contiguous leads or a newly-developed left bundle branch block. Due to the fact that cardiac markers appear in blood several hours after onset of symptoms, cardiac markers are neither helpful for early diagnosis nor should their results be awaited before initiation of reperfusion therapy. This applies also to earlier markers of myocardial ischemia, such as ischemia-modified albumin, fatty-acid binding protein, or myoglobin, as a positive test is present in no more than 50% of patients at presentation. Therefore, the most established indications to measure cardiac troponins in the context of STEMI will be outlined in the following:

- Retrospective confirmation of diagnosis
- Estimation of short- and long-term outcomes
- Diagnosis of infarct-related artery reperfusion after thrombolysis
- Cardiac troponins for management of STEMI
- Cardiac troponins for assessment of microvascular reperfusion after successful direct PCI
- Cardiac troponins for identification of reinfarction
- Estimation of infarct size
- Prediction of microvascular obstruction

Retrospective Confirmation of Diagnosis

According to the most recent "universal definition of MI," acute myocardial infarction is defined as an elevated cardiac troponin with at least one value above the 99th percentile of a reference control group, showing a rise and/or fall pattern together with evidence of myocardial ischemia.[1] Evidence of myocardial ischemia should be indicated by at least one of the following: symptoms of ischemia, ECG changes indicative of new ischemia, new Q-waves or imaging evidence of new loss of viable myocardium, or new regional wall motion abnormality.

Cardiac troponin appears in blood with a time delay that partly depends on the elapsed time to presentation, the magnitude of injury, quality of reperfusion, and the selected cutoff for cTn. Older studies using higher cutoffs were not able to demonstrate an appearance of cardiac troponin until two to three hours after the index event. The advent of more sensitive assays is believed to enable earlier detection of cardiac troponin in blood, which may be detectable within an hour of onset of necrosis. After the initial release of unbound troponin, there is a continuous proteolytic degradation of troponin that is structurally bound to the myofilament.[2] Cardiac troponin may be measurable in blood for three weeks, and even longer with more sensitive troponin assays. Typically, a rise and subsequent fall of cardiac troponin is diagnostic for an acute myocardial infarction. Due to the cardiospecificity and their long diagnostic window, cardiac troponins are ideally suited for retrospective confirmation of myocardial infarction.

Estimation of Short-Term and Long-Term Outcomes

Several randomized trials and observational studies have conferred evidence that cardiac troponin levels on admission allow for short-term and long-term risk stratification in patients with STEMI (Table 5–1). In the GUSTO IIa study, 30-day mortality was 13% among patients with ST-segment elevation and positive admission cTnT, as compared to only 4.7% among patients with a negative test result.[3] In the GUSTO III cTnT substudy, which enrolled 12,666 patients, 30-day mortality rates were 15.7 % in patients

Table 5–1: Overview of clinical trials on outcomes among admission cTn positive versus admission cTn negative patients with STEMI.

Trial	Ref	Endpoint	cTn Positive	cTn Negative
GUSTO–IIA	3	Death at 30 days	13%	4.7%
GUSTO–III	4	Death at 30 days	15.7%	6.2%
Trop-T-Substudy		Death/MI at 30 days	18.8%	9.3%
Stubbs	5	Death at 30 days	14%	7%
		Death at 1 year	20%	10%
		Death at 3 years	32%	13%
		Death/MI at 3 years	35.5%	21.2%
Matetzky	7	Death at 426 days	11%	0%
		Death/MI at 426 days	19%	5.4%
		Death/MI/TVR at 426 days	32%	14%
Giannitsis	6	Death at 30 days	17.2%	4.5%
		Death/MI/TVR at 30 days	30.1%	24.2%
Bjorklund	8	Death at 30 days	9.5%	2.0%
		Death at 1 year	14%	4%
Frostfeldt	9	Death at 3 weeks	14%	4%
		Death at 2.5–4.5 yrs	25%	9%
		MI at 2.5–4.5 yrs	24%	14%

tested positive on admission compared to only 6.2% among patients tested negative.[4] The predictive value of cTnT was independent of age, infarct location, Killip class, and systolic blood pressure, and independent of whether patients were reperfused with alteplase or reteplase as fibrinolytic agents. Consistently, Stubbs et al. reported an increased short- and long-term mortality in cTnT-positive patients treated with streptokinase.[5] Mortality rates at 30 days were threefold higher in patients with a positive cTnT on admission as compared to patients tested negative (11% versus 4%). A positive cTn result at admission was also found to be associated with a trend to higher mortality rates after four years (28% versus 7.5%).

Two very recent studies confirmed the adverse prognostic impact of a positive cTnT or cTnI test even for patients with STEMI undergoing primary PCI.[6,7] Giannitsis et al. reported on a series of 159 patients with acute inferior myocardial infarction in whom cardiac mortality rates were significantly higher (10.8% versus 1.5%) when patients had already detectable cTnT levels at admission.[6] Consistently, Matetzky et al. tested the predictive value of cTnI in a cohort of 110 patients with AMI undergoing primary PCI.[7] A positive cTnI test was associated with a higher cardiac mortality rate and a significantly higher incidence of the combined endpoint consisting of death, heart failure, and shock. Thus, unequivocally, detectable amounts of troponins in blood of patients admitted for STEMI are associated with adverse outcomes and higher cardiac event rates.

The exact mechanism for the adverse prognosis associated with a positive cTn at admission is unsettled and may involve several mechanisms. First, time delays between onset of symptoms and admission are longer for troponin-positive than for troponin-negative patients. However, even after adjustment for time delay and other potential confounders, cardiac troponin kept its independent predictive power suggesting a different potential pathomechanism.[6] Therefore, it was tempting to speculate that cardiac troponin elevation might reflect a combination of time and actual myocardial damage and may overcome some shortcomings associated with perception of pain, ischemic preconditioning, or collateral flow to the infarcted area.[4] Moreover, complete epicardial reperfusion is obtained less frequently in patients with already elevated cardiac troponin on admission, both after fibrinolytic therapy[4,5,8,9] and after primary PCI.[6,7] Stubbs et al. reported on lower rates of successful reperfusion following thrombolytic therapy with streptokinase.[5] Successful reperfusion was reported in 50% of patients who tested positive and 72% of patients who tested negative for cTnT on admission. Consistently, others reported on lower rates of TIMI 3 flow following thrombolysis in patients with a positive troponin T result on admission.[4,8,9] Very recent findings suggest that even primary PCI results in significantly lower rates of successful restoration of normal antegrade epicardial flow (TIMI 3) in troponin-positive patients.[6,7] Giannitsis et al. found that TIMI 3 flow grade was achieved in only 77.9% of patients with a positive admission cTnT versus 96.9% with a still negative cTnT on admission.[6] Coronary stenting reduced cardiac mortality and rates of reinfarction and target vessel reintervention in the entire cohort.

Likewise, Matetzky et al. reported on a cohort of 110 patients who were stratified by troponin I at presentation.[7] Consistently, cTnI-positive patients had lower rates of TIMI 3 flow following primary PCI than cTnI-negative patients (76% versus 96%). Whether a positive cTn result at presentation indicates the presence of a thrombus that is more resistant to lysis or mechanical fragmentation, or indicates the presence of microvascular obstruction, is unclear. Even after successful restoration of TIMI 3 flow with primary PCI, the prognosis remains less favorable in patients with elevated cTnT levels before the procedure.[10] It appears tempting to speculate that this finding might be linked to microvascular obstruction.

Patients with detectable cTnT levels at admission were found to retain a more severely impaired microvascular flow despite successful restoration of normal epicardial flow (TIMI 3 flow) as indicated by less washout of cardiac markers 60 minutes after successful PCI.[11]

Cardiac Troponins for Management of STEMI

Diagnosis of Infarct-Related Artery Reperfusion After Thrombolysis

Early and complete patency of infarct-related coronary arteries is an important therapeutic goal. Unlike direct PCI, fibrinolytic therapy is associated with significantly lower rates of complete reperfusion and does not provide visualization of the reperfusion success. Among many methods used to assess infarct artery patency after thrombolytic therapy, resolution of ST segment elevation is the most widely used.[12,13] Cardiac markers can be used complementarily to assess the success or failure of such therapy, as patients with acute myocardial infarctions who develop patent coronary circulation will release a bolus amount of enzymes and proteins into the circulation ("washout phenomenon") when compared with patients with permanent occlusions.[2] Rapid washouts of myoglobin, cTnT or cTnI, or CK-MB have positive predictive values >90% for infarct artery patency.[14,15]

Different cardiac marker proteins and enzymes and numerous algorithms have been proposed for prediction of reperfusion following fibrinolytic therapy.[16] Almost all algorithms require at least two blood samples, one obtained on initiation of fibrinolytic therapy and a second 60 or 90 minutes thereafter. In brief, shorter times to peak values, steeper upslopes, or greater relative increases of cardiac markers have been found to be associated with a successful infarct reperfusion.[16] Cardiac troponins have at least some theoretical advantages over the other soluble markers like myoglobin or CK-MB, including an exclusive cardiospecificity, the largest tissue-to-circulation gradient generating an excellent signal, and a rapid random-access laboratory platform allowing point-of-care and 24-hour laboratory testing with short turnaround times.[16] However, monitoring with biochemical marker strategies has not been successful in distinguishing between TIMI grade 3 and TIMI grade 2 flow patients, rendering the utility of these measurements clinically problematic for determining complete reperfusion.

Cardiac Troponins for Assessment of Microvascular Reperfusion after Successful Direct PCI

As noted, successful reperfusion of the infarct-related coronary artery is associated with a rise in blood concentrations ("washout"); this washout is more brisk after mechanical reperfusion than after fibrinolytic therapy.[17] Because this washout phenomenon reflects reperfusion at the myocardial tissue level rather than only epicardial coronary artery reperfusion, it was tempting to speculate that marker kinetics might be helpful for assessment of microvascular reperfusion.

Frostfeldt et al. found a significantly higher relative increase in myoglobin concentrations and a trend toward higher rates of complete resolution (>70 %) of ST segments in patients who tested negative for cTnT at presentation, suggesting normal microvascular reperfusion.[9] Consistently, Lehrke et al. could demonstrate that abciximab administered during direct PCI improved the early wash-out of cTnT in patients who tested positive for troponin at admission, in diabetics, and in older patients, suggesting a higher propensity for impaired microvascular perfusion in some subsets of patients.[11] A close association between elevations of troponin and abnormal tissue level reperfusion was also found in patients with an acute coronary syndrome without ST segment elevation.[18] Thus, there is increasing evidence that elevations of troponin T resulting from embolization of platelet microaggregates may not only be a surrogate for active plaque, but also imply microvascular obstruction. Along these lines, Kurowski et al. reported higher mortality rates for patients with elevated cTnT levels at admission, despite successful restoration of TIMI 3 grade flow.[10] Cardiac troponin T remained independently predictive even after adjustment for longer time delays from onset of symptoms to admission and for infarct location. These findings underscore the adverse prognostic impact that has been attributed to microvascular dysfunction.[19,20] In randomized trials, however, GP IIb/IIIa inhibitors did not improve mortality rates, suggesting a need for individualized therapy.[21] Selected clinical variables, including measurement of cardiac troponins on admission or infarct scores, may prove more useful for identification of patients who will benefit from adjunctive administration of GP IIb/IIIa inhibitors during direct PCI. Further studies, however, are necessary to prove whether troponin testing could also be helpful to monitor effects of glycoprotein IIb/IIIa inhibitors or other drugs on microvascular reperfusion.

Cardiac Troponins for Identification of Reinfarction

Traditionally, CK-MB has been used to detect reinfarction as elevated values return to normal within 24 to 48 hours after the index event. According to the recommendations of the National Academy for Clinical Biochemistry (NACB), CK-MB is the preferred marker for detection of reinfarction early after the index event when the concentration of cardiac troponin is still increased.[22] However, recent data suggest that serial measurements of troponin provide similar information.[23] In patients in whom recurrent myocardial infarction is suspected from clinical signs or symptoms following the initial infarction, an immediate measurement of the employed cardiac marker is recommended. A second sample should be obtained 3–6 hours later. Recurrent infarction is diagnosed if there is a ≥20% increase of the value in the second sample, and when the value itself exceeds the 99th percentile URL.[1]

Estimation of Infarct Size

Several methods are currently used for estimation of infarct size including: technetium (Tc)-99m, sestamibi single-photon emission computed tomography (SPECT), magnetic resonance tomography, and serum markers.[24] In clinical practice, the measurement of biochemical markers is most readily available. Measurement of maximum enzyme values of CK or CK-MB proves convenient, but has a propensity to overestimate infarct size, particularly when spontaneous reperfusion, PCI, or thrombolysis-induced reperfusion leads to an earlier and higher maximum CK level at identical amounts of left ventricular impairment.

The introduction of cardiac troponins may overcome some of the limitations because troponin T and I are exclusively cardiac-specific and are almost completely bound to the contractile apparatus.[25] With cardiac troponins, particularly cTnT, only the initial rapid peak (which is due to release of the cytoplasmatic pool) depends on the reperfusion status, whereas the later release (due to degradation from the contractile apparatus) is independent of the reperfusion status.[2,26] Due to the short half-life of cTnT in blood of only about 90 minutes, the cTnT blood levels on day 3 or 4 reflect degradation of the contractile apparatus, which is a hallmark of irreversible cell injury. Thus, a cTnT elevation on day 3 or 4 after symptom onset may be taken as definite proof of irreversible myocardial injury.

With this in mind, associations between troponin values following STEMI and infarct size have been made. Animal studies first established a significant correlation between cTnT and infarct size. In an experimental study on 16 beagles[27] undergoing left anterior descending artery (LAD) ligation, the pathoanatomically-measured infarct size correlated significantly with a single troponin measurement after 96 hours ($p = 0{,}0010$). Using SPECT to show perfusion defect size in patients 72 hours after myocardial infarction, Panteghini et al.[28] found a significant correlation between cTnT at 72 hours and both the peak CK-MB concentrations ($r = 0.76$; $P < 0.001$) and the perfusion defect size ($r = 0.62$; $P < 0.001$). For this same time point, Licka et al.[29] also found a significant correlation with scintigraphic infarct size.

Studies using cardiac MRI have illuminated the relationship between troponin and infarct size in STEMI (Figure 5–1). A recent study on 44 patients with STEMI[30] with measurement of cTnT and quantification of infarct size using MRI 72–96 hours after the index event showed a highly significant correlation between cTnT and infarct size ($r_{Spearman} = 0.883$; $P < 0.0001$). More recently, in another MRI study on 61 patients, the performance of single

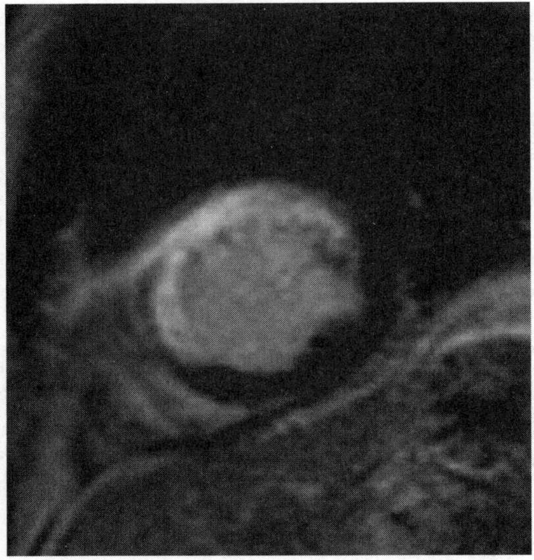

■ **Figure 5–1** Short-axis view of contrast-enhanced cardiac MRI showing infarcted myocardium (bright area).

points versus serial measurements of cTnT for estimation of infarct size was assessed using contrast-enhanced MRI.[31] The results showed that a single troponin value on any of the first four days or using the peak-value correlates well with infarct mass determined by contrast-enhanced cardiac magnetic resonance imaging (CE-MRI) (Figure 5–2). In large STEMI, single values of cTnT performed better than in small MI or non-ST segment elevation MI (NSTEMI), reflecting heterogeneity of cTnT release in NSTEMI due to the variety of pathophysiologies that exist in patients with this affliction. Microinfarcts associated with minor elevations of cTnT may escape visualization with CE-MRI or be difficult to quantify owing to poor image contrast or artifacts.

In aggregate, the data would suggest that a single measurement for cTnT at 96 hours for estimation of infarct size in STEMI would be convenient to use clinically and would also be helpful in a

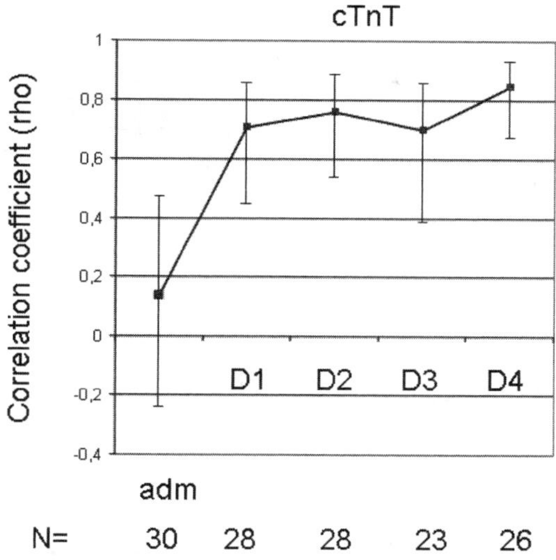

■ **Figure 5–2** Relationship between cTnT concentrations and infarcted myocardial mass (gram infracted tissue) on single point measurements after admission.

standardized protocol for clinical trials. For cTnI (AccuTnI Assay, Beckman-Coulter), a comparable performance was found in the same subset of patients with STEMI who had been tested earlier with cTnT.[32] Spearman analysis demonstrated a strong correlation between cTnI values and infarct mass at 24 (n = 24), 48 (n = 26), 72 (n = 23), and 96 (n = 28) hours after onset of symptoms (Figure 5–2). Thus, as with cTnT (30, 31), cTnI correlated with infarct size in reperfused STEMI patients at 24–96 hours, indicating that clinicians can rely on values on days 1–4 to provide an approximation to MRI-determined reperfused infarct size.[32]

Microvascular Obstruction

After successful revascularization of the infarct-related artery, many patients with acute myocardial infarction (AMI) manifest abnormal tissue level nutritive perfusion despite normal

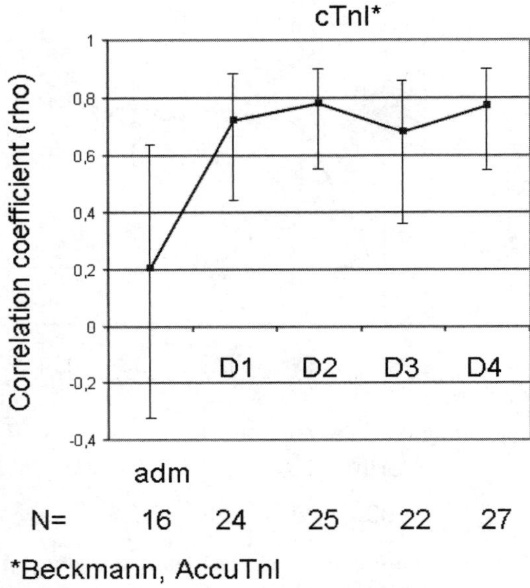

■ **Figure 5–3** Relationship between cTnI concentrations and infarcted myocardial mass (gram infracted tissue) on single point measurements after admission.

thrombolysis in myocardial infarction (TIMI) flow grades.[20] Microvascular obstruction (MVO) after AMI identifies a group of patients with persistently higher mortality rates despite successful reperfusion of the epicardial coronary artery.[19,20] Identification of MVO is difficult and requires the use of sophisticated techniques, including myocardial contrast echocardiography, myocardial blush grade from coronary angiography, and MRI (Figure 5–3). Recent data confirm that the presence and maximal extent of MVO can be best evaluated on early postcontrast MRI.[33,34] Unfortunately, the use of MRI is expensive, requires expert skills, and therefore lacks broad availability. More recently, we and others studied whether the use of cardiac biomarkers, particularly cardiac troponins, might be helpful as there is a close relationship between infarct size and the extent of MVO.

Several studies have reported higher maximum concentrations of creatine kinase, cTnT, or cTnI in the presence of MVO.[35,36] Tarantini et al. reported a progressive increase of peak cTnI with lowest values in those patients without transmural necrosis or severe MVO, intermediate values in those with transmural necrosis without MVO, and highest values in patients with transmural necrosis and MVO (35). Regarding the optimal point for prediction of MVO by a single measurement, there is some controversy. Younger et al.[36] found a close relationship between a single measurement of cTnI at 72 hours, infarct size, and extent of MVO. In this study of ninety-three patients, cTnI at 72 hours correlated better with the presence and the extent of MVO than cTnI at 12 hours. Our unpublished data demonstrate that cTnT values between 24 and 96 hours after AMI are significantly higher in the presence of MVO. We studied 61 consecutive patients with reperfused ST-elevation myocardial infarction (STEMI). cTnT was measured serially at admission and after 24, 48, 72, and 96 hours. Contrast-enhanced cardiac MRI was performed on a 1.5T MR-scanner 4 ± 1 days after STEMI. The best single value for the prediction of MVO was a cTnT concentration > 2.52 μg/L at 24 hours after admission (Figure 5–4). The discrepancy between our findings and the results from Younger et al. may be explained by differences with respect to the cardiac troponin used (cTnT versus cTnI) and by the type of reperfusion therapy (primary PCI versus fibrinolytic therapy) provided.

References

1. Thygesen K, Alpert JS, White HD on behalf of the Joint ESC/ACCF/AHA/WHF Task Force for the Redefinition of Myocardial Infarction. Universal definition of myocardial infarction. *Circulation*. 2007;116: 2634–2653.
2. Katus HA, Remppis A, Scheffold T, et al. Intracellular compartmentation of cardiac troponin T and its release kinetics in patients with

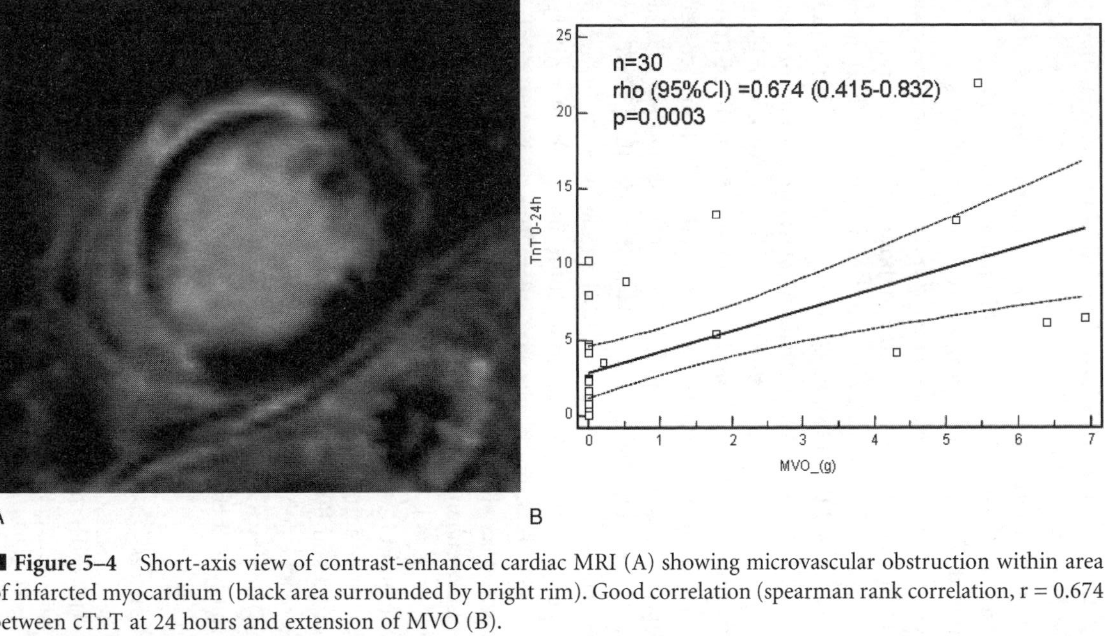

■ **Figure 5–4** Short-axis view of contrast-enhanced cardiac MRI (A) showing microvascular obstruction within area of infarcted myocardium (black area surrounded by bright rim). Good correlation (spearman rank correlation, r = 0.674 between cTnT at 24 hours and extension of MVO (B).

reperfused and nonreperfused myocardial infarction. *Am J Cardiol.* 1991;67:360–367.

3. Ohman EM, Topol EJ, Califf RM, et al. for the GUSTO-IIa investigators. Cardiac troponin T levels for risk stratification in acute myocardial ischemia. *N Engl J Med.* 1996;335:1333–1341.
4. Ohman EM, Armstrong PW, White HD, for the GUSTO-III Investigators. Risk stratification with a point-of-care cardiac troponin T test in acute myocardial infarction. *Am J Cardiol.* 1999;84:1281–1286.
5. Stubbs P, Collinson P, Moseley D, et al. Prognostic significance of admission troponin T concentrations in patients with myocardial infarction. *Circulation.* 1996;94:1291–1297.
6. Giannitsis E, Lehrke S, Wiegand U, et al. Risk stratification in patients with inferior acute myocardial infarction treated by percutaneous coronary interventions—the role of admission troponin T. *Circulation.* 2000;102:2038–2044.
7. Matetzky S, Sharir T, Domingo M, et al. Elevated troponin I level on admission is associated with adverse outcome of primary angioplasty in acute myocardial infarction. *Circulation.* 2000;102:1611–1616.
8. Bjorklund E, Lindahl B, Johanson P, et al. Admission Troponin T and measurement of ST-segment resolution at 60 min improve early risk stratification in ST-elevation myocardial infarction. *Eur Heart J.* 2004;25:113–120.
9. Frostfeldt G, Gustafsson G, Lindahl B, Nygren A, Venge P, Wallentin L. Possible reasons for the prognostic value of troponin-T on admission in patients with ST-elevation myocardial infarction. *Coron Artery Dis.* 2001;12:227–237.
10. Kurowski V, Hartmann F, Killermann DP, et al. Prognostic significance of admission cardiac troponin T in patients treated successfully with direct percutaneous interventions for acute ST-segment elevation myocardial infarction. *Crit Care Med.* 2002;30:2229–2235.
11. Lehrke S, Katus HA, Ciannitsis E. Admission troponin T, advanced age, and male gender identify patients with improved myocardial tissue perfusion after abciximab administration for ST-segment elevation myocardial infarction. *Thromb Haemost.* 2004;92:1214–1220.
12. Krucoff MW, Croll MA, Pope JE, et al. For the TAMI 7 study: performance of a noninvasive method for real-time detection of failed myocardial reperfusion. *Circulation.* 1993;88:437–446.

13. Langer A, Krucoff MW, Klootwijk P, et al. Noninvasive assessment of speed and stability of infarct-related artery reperfusion. Results of the GUSTO ST segment monitoring study: global utilization of streptokinase and tissue plasminogen activator for occluded coronary arteries. *J Am Coll Cardiol.* 1995;25:1552–1557.
14. Stewart JT, French JK, Theroux P, et al. Early non-invasive identification of failed reperfusion after intravenous thrombolytic therapy in acute myocardial infarction. *J Am Coll Cardiol.* 1998;31:1499–1505.
15. Tanasijevic MJ, Cannon CP, Antman EM, et al. for the TIMI 10B Investigators. Myoglobin, creatine kinase MB and cardiac troponin I 60-minute ratios predict infarct-related artery patency after thrombolysis for acute myocardial infarction. *J Am Coll Cardiol.* 1999;34:739–747.
16. Apple FS. Value of soluble markers in the diagnosis of reperfusion. In: Kaski JC, and Holt DW, eds. *Developments in Cardiovascular Medicine: Myocardial Damage: Early Detection by Novel Biochemical Markers.* New York: Springer; 1998:149–157.
17. Laperche T, Steg PG, Dehoux M, et al. A study of biochemical markers of reperfusion early after thrombolysis for acute myocardial infarction. The PERM Study Group. Prospective Evaluation of Reperfusion Markers. *Circulation.* 1995;92:2079–2086.
18. Wong GC, Morrow DA, Murphy S, et al. Elevations in troponin T and I are associated with abnormal tissue level perfusion: a TACTICS-TIMI 18 substudy. Treat Angina with Aggrastat and Determine Cost of Therapy with an Invasive or Conservative Strategy-Thrombolysis in Myocardial Infarction. *Circulation.* 2002;106:202–207.
19. Ito H, Tomooka T, Sakai N, et al. Lack of myocardial perfusion immediately after successful thrombolysis: a predictor of poor recovery of left ventricular function in anterior myocardial infarction. *Circulation.* 1992;85:1699–1705.
20. Wu KC, Zerhouni EA, Judd RM, et al. Prognostic significance of microvascular obstruction by magnetic resonance imaging in patients with acute myocardial infarction. *Circulation.* 1998;97:765–772.
21. Kandzari DE, Hasselblad V, Tcheng JE, et al. Improved clinical outcomes with abciximab therapy in acute myocardial infarction: a systematic overview of randomized clinical trials. *Am Heart J.* 2004;147:457–462.

22. Morrow DA, Cannon CP, Jesse RL, et al. National Academy of Clinical Biochemistry Laboratory Medicine Practice Guidelines: Clinical characteristics and utilization of biochemical markers in acute coronary syndromes. *Circulation*. 2007, Apr 3;115(13):e356–375.

23. Apple FS, Murakami MM. Cardiac troponin and creatine kinase MB monitoring during in-hospital myocardial reinfarction. *Clin Chem*. 2005;51:460–463.

24. Gibbons RJ, Valeti US, Araoz PA, Jaffe AS. The quantification of infarct size. *J Am Coll Cardiol*. 2004;44:1533–1542.

25. Katus HA, Remppis A, Scheffold T, et al. Intracellular compartmentation of cardiac troponin T and its release kinetics in patients with reperfused and nonreperfused myocardial infarction. *Am J Cardiol*. 1991;67:1360–1367.

26. Katus HA, Diederich KW, Scheffold T, Uellner M, Schwarz F, Kübler W. Non-invasive assessment of infarct reperfusion: the predictive power of the time to peak value of myoglobin, CK-MB, and CK in serum. *Eur Heart J*. 1988;9:619–624.

27. Remppis A, Ehlermann P, Giannitsis E, et al. Cardiac troponin T levels at 96 hours reflect myocardial infarct size: a pathoanatomical study. *Cardiology*. 2000;93:249–253.

28. Panteghini M, Cuccia C, Bonetti G, Giubbini R, Pagani F, Bonini E. Single-point cardiac troponin T at coronary care unit discharge after myocardial infarction correlates with infarct size and ejection fraction. *Clin Chem*. 2002;48:1432–1436.

29. Licka M, Zimmermann R, Zehelein J, Dengler TJ, Katus HA, Kubler W. Troponin T concentrations 72 hours after myocardial infarction as a serological estimate of infarct size. *Heart*. 2002;87:520–524.

30. Steen H, Giannitsis E, Futterer S, Merten C, Juenger C, Katus HA. Cardiac troponin T at 96 hours after acute myocardial infarction correlates with infarct size and cardiac function. *J Am Coll Cardiol*. 2006;48:2192–2194.

31. Giannitsis E, Steen H, Kurz K, et al. Cardiac Magnetic Resonance Imaging Study for Quantification of Infarct Size Comparing Directly Serial Versus Single Time-Point Measurements of Cardiac Troponin T. J *Am Coll Cardiol*. 2008;51:307–314.

32. Vasile VC, Babuin L, Giannitsis E, Katus HA, Jaffe AS. Relationship of MRI-determined infarct size and cTnI measurements in patients

with ST-elevation myocardial infarction. *Clin Chem.* 2008;54: 617–619.

33. Bogaert J, Kalantzi M, Rademakers FE, Dymarkowski S, Janssens S. Determinants and impact of microvascular obstruction in successfully reperfused ST-segment elevation myocardial infarction. Assessment by magnetic resonance imaging. *Eur Radiol.* 2007;17: 2572–2580.
34. Jesel L, Morel O, Ohlmann P, et al. Role of pre-infarction angina and inflammatory status in the extent of microvascular obstruction detected by MRI in myocardial infarction patients treated by PCI. *Int J Cardiol.* 2007;121:139–147.
35. Tarantini G, Razzolini R, Cacciavillani L, et al. Influence of transmurality, infarct size, and severe microvascular obstruction on left ventricular remodeling and function after primary coronary angioplasty. *Am J Cardiol.* 2006;98:1033–1040.
36. Younger JF, Plein S, Barth J, Ridgway JP, Ball SG, Greenwood JP. Troponin-I concentration 72 hours after myocardial infarction correlates with infarct size and presence of microvascular obstruction. *Heart.* 2007;93:1547–1551.

6 ▪ Interpretation of Cardiac Troponin Elevation in Patients with End-Stage Renal Disease

Michael R. Banihashemi, MD
Christopher R. DeFilippi, MD, FACC

Nearly 500,000 people in the United States suffer from end-stage renal disease (ESRD), defined as glomerular filtration rate <15 ml/min/1.73 m^2.[1] Cardiovascular disease is the major cause of death in ESRD, accounting for close to 50% of all mortality.[1] Given the renal-dependent nature of many cardiac biomarkers for clearance, interpretation of such markers may be challenging in those with impaired renal function. However, use of markers such as troponin is still possible, not just for evaluation of acute presentation, but also for screening and prognosticating cardiovascular disease in the ESRD population.[2–10]

Cardiac troponins are regulatory proteins that control the interaction between actin and myosin. Troponin T binds to tropomyosin, facilitating muscle contraction. Troponin I binds to actin, inhibiting the interaction between actin and myosin. Troponin C binds to calcium ions, resulting in a conformational change from the "closed" to "open" state.[11] The conformational change initiates a series of events culminating in the inhibition of actin-myosin interaction and subsequent muscle contraction.

Conditions, such as coronary artery occlusion, inflammation, toxin exposure, and trauma, lead to myocyte damage, which results in the release of cardiac troponin into the bloodstream.[12] Detection of cardiac-specific troponin T (cTnT) and troponin I (cTnI) by monoclonal antibody-based assays is made possible by the different amino acid sequences of their respective cardiac and skeletal muscle isoforms.[13,14] Identical amino acid sequences of troponin C in cardiac and skeletal muscle precludes its use as a cardiac specific marker.[15]

Diagnosis and Prognosis of Acute Coronary Syndromes (ACS) in Patients with ESRD

It is well understood that troponin values are frequently elevated in those with ESRD in the absence of clear myocardial necrosis. Despite this, such elevations may have prognostic import, and will be discussed shortly. Nonetheless, it does render the use of cTnT and cTnI challenging in the context of ESRD for the acute evaluation of those with symptoms suggestive of an acute coronary syndrome.

The magnitude of the issue is not small: Apple et al. studied 733 patients using three cutoffs for cTnT and cTnI.[2] This included the 99th percentile of a normal reference population, the lowest concentration associated with a 10% coefficient of variation, and the receiver operator characteristic curve determined value optimized for diagnostic sensitivity and specificity in the detection of myocardial infarction. cTnT was predictive of increased mortality using all cut points, but cTnI was only predictive above the 99th percentile (0.1 ng/mL) cut point. Importantly, using the cTnT 99th percentile cutoff of 0.01 ng/mL, 82% of patients had evidence of myocardial injury versus only 6% for cTnI using this assay's 99th percentile cutoff of 0.1 ng/mL for cTnI. This result, similar to findings from other studies, suggested there could be a different pathophysiology between cTnT and cTnI allowing for either decreased clearance of cTnT or increased degradation of cTnI.

Thus, it can be reasonably expected—particularly with the change over to higher sensitivity troponin methods—that near-universal elevation in cTnT (and possibly cTnI) will be seen. This leads to some important considerations for the clinician.

For ESRD patients with signs and symptoms suggestive of an acute coronary syndrome, it is important to emphasize that cardiac troponin elevation has an important role in the diagnosis of myocardial infarction. In patients with previously undetectable levels of cardiac troponins on presentation, a change in such markers allows for a presumptive diagnosis of myocardial infarction to be made.

In those with ESRD, with an elevated cTnT or cTnI and acute symptoms from an acute coronary syndrome, it was shown that such elevations are even more prognostically meaningful than in those without ESRD. The prognostic significance of troponin elevation in patients with renal disease and acute coronary syndromes has been examined in a large cohort by Aviles et al. using data from the 7033 patients enrolled in the Global Use of Strategies to Open Occluded Arteries IV (GUSTO IV) trial. An elevated cTnT (above the 10% coefficient of variation for the assay) was an independent predictor of myocardial infarction or death risk across the entire spectrum of renal function, even when controlling for potential confounders (Figure 6–1).[16] However, a caveat is that the study included few patients on dialysis. Recent registry data

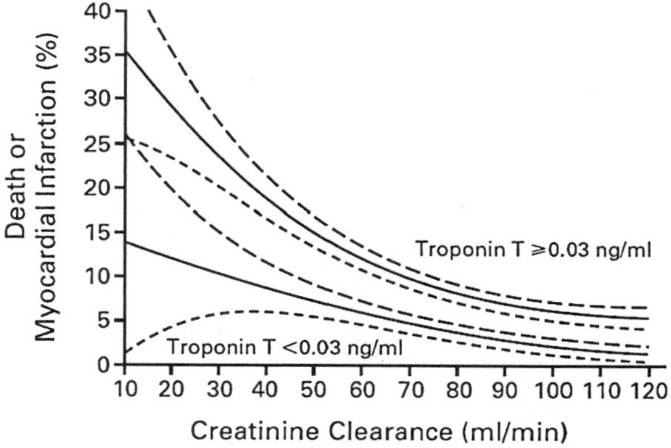

■ **Figure 6–1** The rate of death or myocardial infarction is significantly higher among patients with an acute coronary syndrome and a baseline troponin T level of 0.03 ng per milliliter or higher across the entire spectrum of creatinine clearance rates. However, higher rates of events were seen among those with impaired renal function. The dashed lines indicate the 95 percent confidence intervals.

Reproduced from: Aviles RJ, Askari AT, Lindahl B, et al. Troponin T levels in patients with acute coronary syndromes, with or without renal dysfunction. *N Engl J Med.* 2002;346:2047–2052.

did examine patients with acute coronary syndromes and severe chronic kidney disease (estimated glomerular filtration rate [eGFR] <30 mL/min/1.73 m^2) and found only major elevations (>3x upper limit of normal) of either troponin T or I predicted a higher mortality.[17]

Nonetheless, many patients with ESRD and an elevated troponin level may not have an acute coronary syndrome. As stressed in the 2007 revised definition of myocardial infarction, a change in troponin level between blood draws separated by six or more hours would have the highest accuracy for the diagnosis of myocardial infarction.[18] Though there is no definitive data to recommend a specific percent change threshold, an elevated value with a subsequent change of at least 20% has been recommended.[18,19] Thus, serial measurements—perhaps even sooner than six or more hours—may be the appropriate approach for those with ESRD and diagnostic uncertainty for acute myocardial infarction.

Prognostic Value of cTnT and cTnI

Elevated levels of cTnT and cTnI are associated with increased all-cause mortality in asymptomatic patients with ESRD.[2–10] Apple and colleagues[2] showed that both tests were predictive of mortality, independent of the presence of known heart disease: the relative risk of death associated with elevated (>99th percentile) cTnT at 2-year follow-up was 5.0 (95% Confidence Interval (CI), 2.5–10), while that of cTnI was 2.0 (95% CI, 1.3–3.3). Both relationships remained statistically significant after adjustment for potential confounders including age, history of coronary artery disease or diabetes, and time since initial hemodialysis.

The association between cardiac troponin and mortality has been best summarized in a meta-analysis of 28 studies from 1999–2004 by Khan et al.[9] The analysis included 3931 ESRD patients on hemo- or peritoneal dialysis not suspected of having an acute coronary syndrome. All studies used cardiac-specific troponin assays and evaluated long-term risk of death or cardiac events. According to the 17 studies assessing cTnT, elevated levels

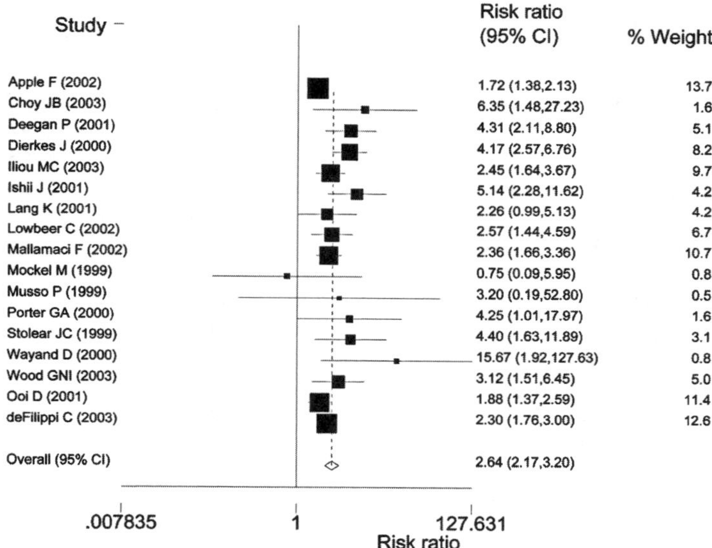

■ **Figure 6–2** Forest plot of primary studies demonstrating the relationship between abnormally elevated cTnT and all-cause mortality. Heterogeneity $x^2 = 30.55$ ($df = 16$); p = 0.015.

Reproduced from: Khan NA, Hemmelgarn BR, Tonelli M, Thompson CR, Levin A. Prognostic value of troponin T and I among asymptomatic patients with end-stage renal disease: a meta-analysis. *Circulation.* 2005;112:3088–3096.

(>0.1 ng/ml) were significantly associated with increased all-cause mortality (Relative Risk (RR), 2.64; 95% CI, 2.17–3.20; [Figure 6–2]). The majority of the studies controlled for advanced age and presence of cardiovascular disease or diabetes, all factors strongly associated with mortality in these patients. According to the 12 studies assessing cTnI, elevated levels were also associated with increased mortality (RR, 1.74; 95% CI, 1.27–2.38; [Figure 6–3]). However, Khan et al. caution that studies involving cTnI included a wide array of assays and different cut points. Also, when controlling for potential confounders, cTnI only remained independently associated with mortality in two of the eight studies. Thus, there

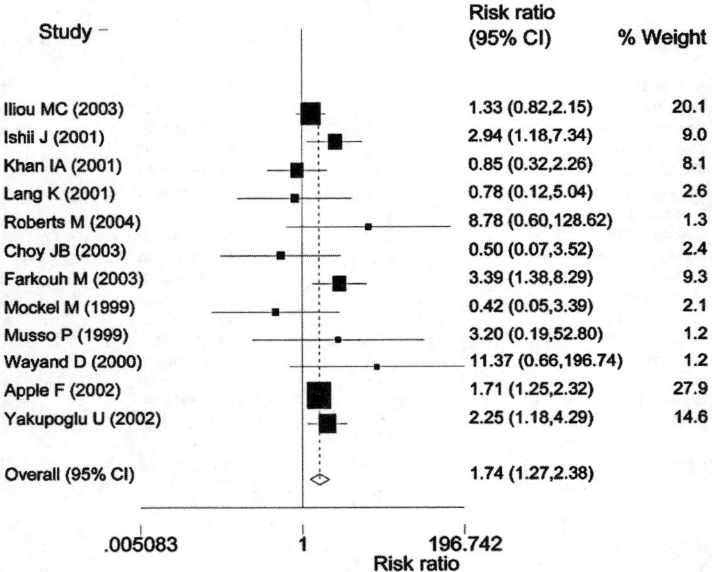

■ **Figure 6–3** Forest plot of primary studies demonstrating the relationship between abnormally elevated cTnI and all-cause mortality. The x^2 test for heterogeneity was nonsignificant.

Reproduced from: Khan NA, Hemmelgarn BR, Tonelli M, Thompson CR, Levin A. Prognostic value of troponin T and I among asymptomatic patients with end-stage renal disease: a meta-analysis. *Circulation*. 2005;112:3088–3096.

is strong evidence that elevated cTnT is associated with increased mortality, however there is less support for cTnI.

The increased mortality associated with elevated cTnT may in part be attributed to an increased risk of cardiac death. In the meta-analysis by Khan et al., all eight studies assessing the association between elevated cTnT (>0.1 ng/ml) and cardiac death demonstrated a significant relationship.[9] When collectively pooled, cTnT was strongly associated with increased long-term cardiac death (RR, 2.55; 95% CI, 1.93–3.37; [Figure 6–4]). On the other hand, no statistically significant association was found

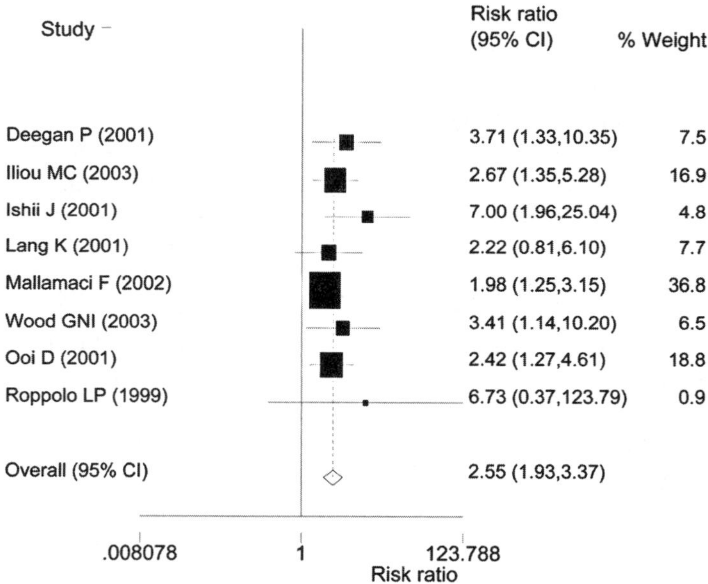

Study
Risk ratio (95% CI)
% Weight
Deegan P (2001)
3.71 (1.33,10.35)
7.5
Iliou MC (2003)
2.67 (1.35,5.28)
16.9
Ishii J (2001)
7.00 (1.96,25.04)
4.8
Lang K (2001)
2.22 (0.81,6.10)
7.7
Mallamaci F (2002)
1.98 (1.25,3.15)
36.8
Wood GNI (2003)
3.41 (1.14,10.20)
6.5
Ooi D (2001)
2.42 (1.27,4.61)
18.8
Roppolo LP (1999)
6.73 (0.37,123.79)
0.9
Overall (95% CI)
2.55 (1.93,3.37)
.008078
1
123.788
Risk ratio

■ **Figure 6–4** Forest plot of primary studies demonstrating the relationship between elevated cTnT and cardiac death.

Reproduced from: Khan NA, Hemmelgarn BR, Tonelli M, Thompson CR, Levin A. Prognostic value of troponin T and I among asymptomatic patients with end-stage renal disease: a meta-analysis. *Circulation.* 2005;112:3088–3096.

between cTnI and cardiac death in the six studies assessing the relationship.

Since Khan's meta-analysis, assay- and population-specific questions have remained. Introduction of newer generation cTnI assays with improved lower-end sensitivity have identified that cTnI elevation is also common in patients with renal disease.[20] In one study of chronic kidney disease patients not on dialysis, the cTnI Ultra assay (Siemens) was elevated (≥0.040 ng/mL) in 33% of patients versus 26% for cTnT (≥0.03 ng/mL), with both being predictors of mortality. In contrast, only 18% of patients had elevated cTnI values (≥0.07 ng/mL) as measured by a standard assay. Additional studies will be needed to determine if these high-sensitivity cTnI assays will have the same prognostic potential in ESRD as do those of cTnT. For now, the Food and Drug Administration has approved only cTnT for mortality risk stratification in ESRD. Furthermore, cTnT has been incorporated into the Kidney Disease Outcomes Quality Initiative (KDOQI) and both cTnI and cTnT into the National Academy of Clinical Biochemistry (NACB) guidelines.[19,21] With respect to additional ESRD populations, one study has also reported that elevated cTnT levels (≥0.03 ng/mL) are predictive of all-cause and cardiac mortality in renal transplant recipients.[22] Though, interestingly, only 21 of 372 transplant patients (5.7%) had cTnT values ≥0.03 ng/mL.

Potential Pathophysiological Mechanisms for Elevated Cardiac Troponin Levels in ESRD

In asymptomatic ESRD patients, elevated cTnT levels and the associated increased risk of cardiac death may in part be explained by an increased incidence of multivessel coronary artery disease, subclinical microinfarctions, and left ventricular hypertrophy.

Multivessel Coronary Artery Disease

Elevated cTnT levels in asymptomatic ESRD patients may indicate the presence of multivessel coronary artery disease. In a prospective study by deFilippi et al., a serum cTnT measurement and coronary angiogram were performed in 67 ESRD patient volunteers without clinical indications for the procedure and an absence ischemic symptoms.[5] Coronary artery disease (CAD) was defined as 50% or greater luminal narrowing in a major epicardial artery or its branches. An elevated cTnT level across was strongly associated with a progressively higher prevalence of multivessel CAD (0%, 25%, 50%, and 62% respectively; $p < 0.001$, [Figure 6–5]). Other studies have also evaluated the association of CAD with elevated cTnT in this setting. Sharma et al. found less compelling results.[23] They studied 126 renal transplant candidates over a 2-year period in which clinical, biochemical, echocardiography, coronary

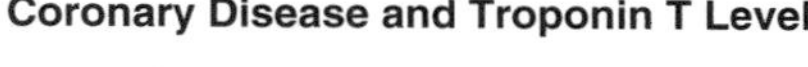

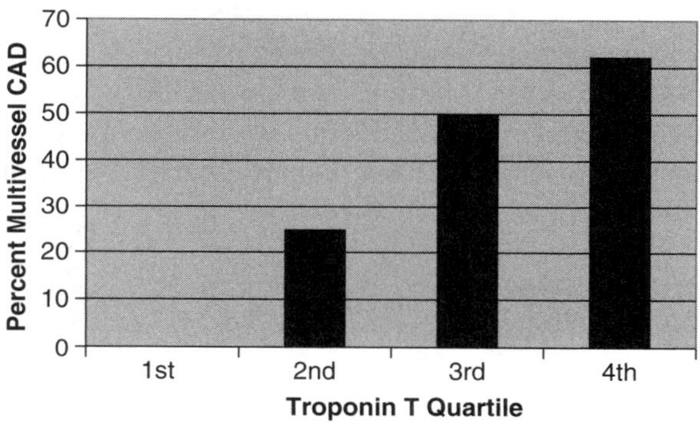

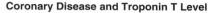

■ **Figure 6–5** Graph depicting the relationship between increasing cTnT quartiles and progressively higher prevalence of multivessel CAD.

Data from: deFilippi C, Wasserman S, Rosanio S, et al. Cardiac troponin T and C-reactive protein for predicting prognosis, coronary atherosclerosis, and cardiomyopathy in patients undergoing long-term hemodialysis. *JAMA*. 2003;290: 353–359.

angiography, and dobutamine stress echocardiography data were compared using cTnT cut points of 0.04 ng/mL and 0.10 ng/mL. Patients with cTnT ≥0.04 ng/mL were more likely to have multivessel CAD (number of diseased arteries, 1.24 ± 1.02) than those with cTnT <0.04 ng/mL (number of diseased arteries, 0.83 ± 0.63). However, no statistically significant relationship was found using the higher (0.10 ng/mL) cut point. More recently, Hayashi et al. found that an elevated cTnT level had a sensitivity of 93% with a specificity of 64% to predict multivessel coronary disease in patients referred for coronary angiography or CT coronary angiography just prior to initiating dialysis.[24] The disparate results of deFilippi et al. and Sharma et al. may be explained by differences in patient selection with older "all-comers" in the deFilippi cohort and younger patients referred for renal transplant evaluation in the Sharma study. Advanced age is associated with an increased risk of progression to multivessel CAD. The Hayashi study, while compelling to suggest ischemic heart disease is a major etiology for cTnT elevation in their patients, needs to be interpreted in light of the fact that these were high-risk ESRD patients being referred for coronary angiography based on clinical high-risk characteristics. More studies are needed at this time to determine whether the increased incidence of cardiac death seen in asymptomatic ESRD patients with elevated cTnT may in part be attributed to an association between cTnT and multivessel CAD.

Microinfarctions

Consistent with the association between elevated cTnT levels and multivessel coronary disease, elevated cTnT levels may indicate subclinical microinfarctions, which are presumably the result of coronary plaque rupture with embolization into the distal microcirculature.[25] Until recently, the relationship could not be demonstrated because microinfarctions were often undetectable due to the limited spatial resolution using nuclear imaging techniques, such as Single Photon Emission Computed Tomography (SPECT), which is routinely used to diagnose myocardial infarction. However, microinfarctions can now be visualized using contrast-enhanced cardiovascular magnetic resonance (CMR) imaging. With the higher spatial resolution of CMR imaging, microinfarction may be identified as a pattern of small subendocardial myonecrotic foci in coronary vascular territories.[26]

Cardiovascular magnetic resonance imaging has been used to study the relationship between cTnT elevation and microinfarction in asymptomatic patients with ESRD in 26 asymptomatic hemodialysis patients with a left ventricular ejection fraction >40% and no known history of CAD.[27] Patients were divided into presumed low-risk (cTnT, <0.03 ng/mL; mean, 0.01 ± 0.01 ng/mL; n = 13) and high-risk (cTnT, ≥0.07 ng/mL; mean, 0.18 ± 0.16 ng/mL; n = 13). CMR patterns consistent with microinfarctions were detected in three (23%) high-risk patients and zero low-risk patients ($p = 0.22$). Although not statistically significant in this small patient population, the data suggest that microinfarction is present in just a minority of asymptomatic hemodialysis patients with elevated cTnT, and therefore additional etiologies must explain the majority of patients with cTnT elevation. This study was underpowered to determine if there is a significant association with microinfarction by CMR and elevated cTnT. Unfortunately, such studies are not forthcoming due to the recent identification of nephrogenic systemic fibrosis or nephrogenic fibrosing dermopathy in patients with renal disease exposed to intravenous gadolinium contrast used in magnetic resonance imaging.[28]

Left Ventricular Hypertrophy

Elevated cTnT levels may also indicate the presence of left ventricular hypertrophy (LVH).[7,29–33] According to a cross-sectional study of 258 asymptomatic hemodialysis patients, LVH was more prevalent in patients with elevated (>0.10 ng/ml) cTnT ($p < 0.05$).[29] In addition, left ventricular mass index (LVMI) was independently associated with cTnT concentration (Odds Ratio (OR), 1.01; 95% CI, 1.0–1.02; $p = 0.05$). Mallamaci et al. had similar findings in a cohort of 199 hemodialysis patients without acute coronary syndrome or heart failure.[32] They found that cTnT level was directly related to LVMI (Pearson's correlation coefficient ($r = 0.45$; $p < 0.001$). By multivariate analysis, LVMI was one of the strongest independent predictors of cTnT level, second to age ($\beta = 0.28$; $p < 0.001$). Further recent support was found in another study of 150 patients with LVMI being higher among those with cTnT levels above the median compared to those below.[33]

However, the association with LVH does not account for the increased incidence of all-cause and cardiac death in asymptomatic ESRD patients with cTnT elevation. In the Mallamaci et al. study, cTnT levels remained a significant and independent predictor of all-cause and cardiovascular mortality in multivariate Cox regression models—including LVMI—suggesting the cTnT level is also related to these outcomes independently of its link to cardiac mass.[32] Moreover, in the aforementioned meta-analysis by Khan et al., elevated cTnT was independently associated with mortality after adjustment for the presence of LVH.[9] Lastly, not all studies have found significant association between LVMI and cTnT.[5] This may be based in part on the limitations of the accuracy of echocardiography estimated LV mass compared to a high resolution technique, such as CMR.[34] However, even when assessing LVMI by CMR, there was not an association between greater LVMI and higher cTnT values, suggesting limits to this association.[27]

Other Potential Etiologies for Troponin Elevations

Reversible myocardial ischemia may play a role in causing cardiac troponin increases in ESRD patients. Patients with ESRD have an increased risk of cardiac ischemia due to increased left ventricular filling pressures, LVH, microvascular disease, decreased capillary density, anemia, excessive sympathetic tone, and impaired insulin-dependent glucose uptake.[35] Although typically believed to represent irreversible injury, increased cardiac troponin has been observed in animal models after transient coronary occlusion in the absence of histologic evidence of infarction.[36] Frequent episodes of silent ischemia in ESRD patients may result in release of cytosolic troponin T. Another possibility is that uremia-induced myocardial fibrosis is the link between increased troponin T and poor prognosis in this population. In ESRD patients with depressed left ventricular systolic function without coronary disease, the presence of ≥30% fibrosis on myocardial biopsies was associated with a poor prognosis.[37]

Future Perspective

The recent development of high-sensitivity troponin I assays may eliminate the perceived differences in mortality and cardiac death between cTnT and cTnI. Interestingly, a high sensitivity cTnT assay has also been developed, but not yet studied in patients with renal disease. In a study by Latini et al., plasma troponin T levels were compared using the conventional cTnT assay and new highly-sensitive (hsTnT) assay in 4053 patients with chronic heart failure in the Valsartan Heart Failure Trial (Val-HeFT).[38] Troponin T was detectable in 10.4% of the population using the current cTnT assay (detection limit 0.01 ng/mL), compared to 92.0% with the high-sensitivity cTnT assay (detection limit 0.001 ng/mL). High-sensitivity TnT was associated with risk of death in unadjusted analysis for the highest seven deciles of concentrations and in multivariable models in this stable heart failure population. Thus, using the new highly-sensitive assay, troponin T retains prognostic value at concentrations tenfold lower than the detection limit of the traditional assay. It might be expected that nearly all ESRD patients would have elevated levels using such an assay. The prognostic importance of such low-range troponin detection in the ESRD population will need to be determined. Lastly, the primary etiology for troponin release in ESRD patients has yet to be determined. Promising new techniques to noninvasively detect cardiac fibrosis are being developed using CMR, but may have limited application until a less toxic substitute for gadolinium is developed.[39]

Conclusion

Cardiovascular disease is the leading cause of death in patients with end-stage renal disease.[1] Universal screening is an impractical strategy considering the cost of diagnostic tests and size of the ESRD population. Cardiac troponin has emerged as a serum biomarker with the potential to identify patients at highest risk for cardiovascular disease.

Elevated levels of cardiac troponin T have been associated with increased all-cause and cardiac mortality. Several potential mechanisms have been proposed to explain these associations. There is evidence that cTnT is associated with multivessel coronary artery disease and left ventricular hypertrophy. However, data showing associations with cardiac troponins and both of the pathologies is not consistent between studies. Additional forms of cardiac pathology, such as uremic cardiomyopathy, may also play a role. It is also likely that as more sensitive cTnI assays are adapted, frequent elevations will be found with these tests. Though it is not yet determined, similar prognostic information may be provided.

A better understanding of the diagnostic implications of cTnT may enable the development of therapeutic strategies targeted to cTnT levels. For instance, ESRD patients with elevated cTnT may experience improved mortality from medications like aspirin and beta blockers initiated even before documented cardiac pathology. More research is needed at this time to define the role of cardiac troponin in this high cardiovascular risk population. New developments in cTnI and cTnT assays will facilitate this endeavor.

References

1. System USRD. USRDS 2008 Annual Data Report: Atlas of Chronic Kidney Disease and End-Stage Renal Disease in the United States. National Institutes of Health–National Institute of Diabetes and Digestive and Kidney Diseases. Available at: www.usrds.org/2008/view/default.asp. Accessed December 1, 2008.
2. Apple FS, Murakami MM, Pearce LA, Herzog CA. Predictive value of cardiac troponin I and T for subsequent death in end-stage renal disease. *Circulation.* 2002;106:2941–2945.
3. Conway B, McLaughlin M, Sharpe P, Harty J. Use of cardiac troponin T in diagnosis and prognosis of cardiac events in patients on chronic haemodialysis. *Nephrol Dial Transplant.* 2005;20:2759–2764.
4. Deegan PB, Lafferty ME, Blumsohn A, Henderson IS, McGregor E. Prognostic value of troponin T in hemodialysis patients is independent of comorbidity. *Kidney Int.* 2001;60:2399–2405.
5. deFilippi C, Wasserman S, Rosanio S, et al. Cardiac troponin T and C-reactive protein for predicting prognosis, coronary atherosclerosis, and cardiomyopathy in patients undergoing long-term hemodialysis. *JAMA.* 2003;290:353–359.
6. Dierkes J, Domrose U, Westphal S, et al. Cardiac troponin T predicts mortality in patients with end-stage renal disease. *Circulation.* 2000;102:1964–1969.
7. Duman D, Tokay S, Toprak A, et al. Elevated cardiac troponin T is associated with increased left ventricular mass index and predicts mortality in continuous ambulatory peritoneal dialysis patients. *Nephrol Dial Transplant.* 2005;20:962–967.
8. Ishii J, Nomura M, Okuma T, et al. Risk stratification using serum concentrations of cardiac troponin T in patients with end-stage renal

disease on chronic maintenance dialysis. *Clin Chim Acta.* 2001; 312:69–79.

9. Khan NA, Hemmelgarn BR, Tonelli M, Thompson CR, Levin A. Prognostic value of troponin T and I among asymptomatic patients with end-stage renal disease: a meta-analysis. *Circulation.* 2005;112:3088–3096.
10. McLaurin MD, Apple FS, Voss EM, Herzog CA, Sharkey SW. Cardiac troponin I, cardiac troponin T, and creatine kinase MB in dialysis patients without ischemic heart disease: evidence of cardiac troponin T expression in skeletal muscle. *Clin Chem.* 1997;43:976–982.
11. Higgins JP, Higgins JA. Elevation of cardiac troponin I indicates more than myocardial ischemia. *Clin Invest Med.* 2003;26:133–147.
12. Jeremias A, Gibson CM. Narrative review: alternative causes for elevated cardiac troponin levels when acute coronary syndromes are excluded. *Ann Intern Med.* 2005;142:786–791.
13. Katus HA, Looser S, Hallermayer K, et al. Development and in vitro characterization of a new immunoassay of cardiac troponin T. *Clin Chem.* 1992;38:386–393.
14. Adams JE III, Bodor GS, Davila-Roman VG, et al. Cardiac troponin I. A marker with high specificity for cardiac injury. *Circulation.* 1993;88:101–106.
15. Van de Werf F. Cardiac troponins in acute coronary syndromes. *N Engl J Med.* 1996;335:1388–1389.
16. Aviles RJ, Askari AT, Lindahl B, et al. Troponin T levels in patients with acute coronary syndromes, with or without renal dysfunction. *N Engl J Med.* 2002;346:2047–2052.
17. Melloni C, Alexander KP, Milford-Beland S, et al. Prognostic value of troponins in patients with non-ST-segment elevation acute coronary syndromes and chronic kidney disease. *Clin Cardiol.* 2008;31:125–129.
18. Thygesen K, Alpert JS, White HD, et al. Universal definition of myocardial infarction. *Circulation.* 2007;116:2634–2653.
19. Wu AH, Jaffe AS, Apple FS, et al. National Academy of Clinical Biochemistry laboratory medicine practice guidelines: use of cardiac troponin and B-type natriuretic peptide or N-terminal proB-type natriuretic peptide for etiologies other than acute coronary syndromes and heart failure. *Clin Chem.* 2007;53:2086–2096.

20. Lamb EJ, Kenny C, Abbas NA, et al. Cardiac troponin I concentration is commonly increased in nondialysis patients with CKD: experience with a sensitive assay. *Am J Kidney Dis.* 2007;49:507–516.

21. K/DOQI clinical practice guidelines for cardiovascular disease in dialysis patients. *Am J Kidney Dis.* 2005;45(4 Suppl 3):S1–153.

22. Connolly GM, Cunningham R, McNamee PT, Young IS, Maxwell AP. Troponin T is an independent predictor of mortality in renal transplant recipients. *Nephrol Dial Transplant.* 2008;23:1019–1025.

23. Sharma R, Gaze DC, Pellerin D, et al. Cardiac structural and functional abnormalities in end stage renal disease patients with elevated cardiac troponin T. *Heart.* 2006;92:804–809.

24. Hayashi T, Obi Y, Kimura T, et al. Cardiac troponin T predicts occult coronary artery stenosis in patients with chronic kidney disease at the start of renal replacement therapy. *Nephrol Dial Transplant.* 2008; 23:2936–2942.

25. Ooi DS, Isotalo PA, Veinot JP. Correlation of antemortem serum creatine kinase, creatine kinase-MB, troponin I, and troponin T with cardiac pathology. *Clin Chem.* 2000;46:338–344.

26. Wagner A, Mahrholdt H, Holly TA, et al. Contrast-enhanced MRI and routine single photon emission computed tomography (SPECT) perfusion imaging for detection of subendocardial myocardial infarcts: an imaging study. *Lancet.* 2003;361:374–379.

27. deFilippi CR, Thorn EM, Aggarwal M, et al. Frequency and cause of cardiac troponin T elevation in chronic hemodialysis patients from study of cardiovascular magnetic resonance. *Am J Cardiol.* 2007;100:885–889.

28. Nephrogenic fibrosing dermopathy associated with exposure to gadolinium-containing contrast agents—St. Louis, Missouri, 2002–2006. *MMWR Morb Mortal Wkly Rep.* 2007;56:137–141.

29. Iliou MC, Fumeron C, Benoit MO, et al. Factors associated with increased serum levels of cardiac troponins T and I in chronic haemodialysis patients: Chronic Haemodialysis And New Cardiac Markers Evaluation (CHANCE) study. *Nephrol Dial Transplant.* Jul 2001;16:1452–1458.

30. Jeon DS, Lee MY, Kim CJ, et al. Clinical findings in patients with cardiac troponin T elevation and end-stage renal disease without acute coronary syndrome. *Am J Cardiol.* Sep 15 2004;94:831–834.

31. Lowbeer C, Ottosson-Seeberger A, Gustafsson SA, Norrman R, Hulting J, Gutierrez A. Increased cardiac troponin T and endothelin-1 concentrations in dialysis patients may indicate heart disease. *Nephrol Dial Transplant.* 1999;14:1948–1955.
32. Mallamaci F, Zoccali C, Parlongo S, et al. Troponin is related to left ventricular mass and predicts all-cause and cardiovascular mortality in hemodialysis patients. *Am J Kidney Dis.* 2002;40:68–75.
33. Satyan S, Light RP, Agarwal R. Relationships of N-terminal pro-B-natriuretic peptide and cardiac troponin T to left ventricular mass and function and mortality in asymptomatic hemodialysis patients. *Am J Kidney Dis.* 2007;50:1009–1019.
34. Stewart GA, Foster J, Cowan M, et al. Echocardiography overestimates left ventricular mass in hemodialysis patients relative to magnetic resonance imaging. *Kidney Int.* Dec 1999;56:2248–2253.
35. Dikow R, Zeier M, Ritz E. Pathophysiology of cardiovascular disease and renal failure. *Cardiol Clin.* 2005;23:311–317.
36. Feng YJ, Chen C, Fallon JT, et al. Comparison of cardiac troponin I, creatine kinase-MB, and myoglobin for detection of acute ischemic myocardial injury in a swine model. *Am J Clin Pathol.* 1998; 110:70–77.
37. Aoki J, Ikari Y, Nakajima H, et al. Clinical and pathologic characteristics of dilated cardiomyopathy in hemodialysis patients. *Kidney Int.* 2005;67:333–340.
38. Latini R, Masson S, Anand IS, et al. Prognostic value of very low plasma concentrations of troponin T in patients with stable chronic heart failure. *Circulation.* 2007;116:1242–1249.
39. Iles L, Pfluger H, Phrommintikul A, et al. Evaluation of diffuse myocardial fibrosis in heart failure with cardiac magnetic resonance contrast-enhanced T1 mapping. *J Am Coll Cardiol.* 2008;52: 1574–1580.

7 ■ Necrosis Marker Testing in Heart Failure

Roberto Latini, MD
Serge Masson, PhD

Introduction

Myocyte cell death occurs either acutely, such as in acute myocardial infarction, or chronically, such as in chronic cardiomyopathy. Loss of cardiac myocytes decreases cardiac function and structure, leading—with different time courses—to dysfunctional, dilated hearts.[1,2]

The fact that intracellular proteins are released from damaged (either reversibly or irreversibly) cardiac myocytes constitutes the basis for estimating extent of cardiac damage through the assay of circulating molecules. Though it is still unclear whether apoptotic myocytes can release troponins, it has been repeatedly shown that they can be released from necrotic myocytes.[3,4] The evidence for this comes mostly from animal models of acute cardiac injury commonly induced by isoproterenol,[3–5] and, although there is no quantitative correlation between the number of cardiac myocytes undergoing necrotic death and circulating concentrations of cardiac troponins, still the relationship between the histologically-assessed extent of cardiac injury and circulating cardiac troponins (cTn) is convincing. With the development of new pharmaceutical agents, cTn measurement in serum has become an important support to histological studies of the myocardium for detection of myocardial injury.[6] At present, cTn is the preferred translational cardiac safety biomarker widely used in the preclinical evaluation of several classes of drugs, such as anthracyclines and other anticancer agents, phosphodiesterase inhibitors, and antiretroviral agents.[5]

However, while our understanding of the relationship between acute myocardial injury and troponin release is well understood in situations such as myocardial infarction or toxicity, there are no experimental studies focused on slowly-progressing nonischemic cardiac damage, such as the underlying worsening of chronic heart failure (HF).

The Prognostic Role of Circulating Cardiac Troponins in Heart Failure

Though extremely rare, the release of cardiac troponins may be detected in the plasma of apparently healthy subjects with traditional analytical methods. In a population-based study, cTnT was elevated (≥0.01 ng/mL) in 0.7% of 3557 residents of Dallas County and this was statistically associated with a high-risk cardiovascular profile (diabetes mellitus, left ventricular hypertrophy, chronic kidney disease, heart failure).[7] However, this observation might represent only the tip of the iceberg. In fact, new automated assays for circulating cardiac troponins are currently being developed by different manufacturers with much higher sensitivity and limits of detection in the range of a few picograms per milliliter.[8] With these new assays, the proportion of subjects with detectable cTn is likely to increase drastically, even in the general population. For instance, circulating cTnI is detectable with a high-sensitivity immunoassay in three out of four healthy Caucasian subjects for whom the presence of cardiac or systemic acute or chronic disease was excluded.[9]

Circulating cardiac troponins are occasionally detectable in patients with heart disease, but without typical symptoms of acute coronary syndromes. The interpretation for their elevation in this context is challenging to the physician and to the scientist. The first evidence that myofibrillar cTns are released into the bloodstream of patients with HF was published almost simultaneously in 1997 by two independent groups.[10,11] La Vecchia and collaborators were able to detect circulating cTnI (limit of detection 0.3 ng/mL) in a small group of patients with acute HF or severe decompensation in chronic HF. They showed that follow-up measurement of cTnI in these patients was associated with improvement or deterioration of their clinical status, including death. Missov and collaborators studied a larger group of patients with severe congestive HF (n = 35) and provided evidence for ongoing myofibrillar degradation and increased serum levels of cTnI with a highly sensitive assay (limit of detection 3 pg/mL). Two other markers of myocyte injury were assayed, CK-MB isoenzyme mass and myoglobin concentration. However, both remained within the normal range. Since these pioneering studies, our knowledge on the clinical utility of measuring circulating cTn is growing steadily. Due to the very low levels of circulating cTn compared to the limit of detection of the analytical methods available at that time, most of the following clinical investigations were confined to patients with acute decompensation or severe HF because a sizeable fraction of these patients had high (measurable) levels of plasma cTn that were positively correlated to the severity of the disease and unfavorable prognosis.[12–15] Repeated measurement over time of cTn is useful for identifying and monitoring high-risk patients[16] and can be effectively combined with another well-established cardiac marker (natriuretic peptides) to improve risk stratification in patients with HF.[17,18] The largest source of data on the prognostic role of cardiac troponins in acute heart failure comes from a recent report from the Acute Decompensated Heart Failure National Registry (ADHERE).[19] The authors analyzed more than 67,000 patients who were hospitalized for acute decompensated HF and had cTn (either cTnI or cTnT) measured within 24 hours after admission and serum creatinine level of less than 2.0 mg/dL. Overall, 6.2% of the patients were positive for troponin (≥1 ng/mL for cTnI or ≥0.1 ng/mL for cTnT). On admission, patients with elevated troponins had lower systolic blood pressure and lower left ventricular ejection fraction and were less likely to suffer from atrial fibrillation compared to patients negative for troponins. Troponin-positive patients had a higher rate of in-hospital mortality (8.0%) than troponin-negative patients (2.7%, $p < 0.001$), with an adjusted odd ratio of 2.55 (95% CI 2.24–2.89, $p < 0.001$). Ischemic etiology of HF was not a useful determinant of troponin status and did not predict mortality. A negative troponin test may therefore aid in the identification of patients with acute HF for whom less intense monitoring and therapy could be appropriate.

In patients with milder chronic and stable HF, lower levels of cTn should be expected, so that the proportion of patients with elevated cTn should be lower than in acute or severe HF. For instance, only 24% had abnormal cTnT (≥0.02 ng/mL) in a recent study[20] that enrolled 136 ambulatory and stable patients with chronic HF (NYHA II–IV), a prevalence lower than observed in more instable patients (30–83%).[12–15] As already noted in acute HF, cTn concentration was similar in chronic HF patients with or without ischemic etiology, suggesting that troponin release was not related to ischemic events, but rather to ongoing myocardial damage or leakage of myofibrillar proteins reflecting loss of viable cardiac myocytes characteristic of progressive HF.[20] Elevated cTn was an independent predictor of death or readmission for HF at one year after enrollment.

The prognostic value of circulating troponin in patients with stable chronic HF has recently been defined in the Valsartan Heart Failure trial (Val-HeFT).[21] The plasma concentrations of cTnT and various other biomarkers were measured at study entry in more than 4000 patients with chronic and symptomatic HF with depressed systolic function.[22] Using a classical assay with a limit of detection of 0.01 ng/mL, cTnT was measurable in 10.4% of the patients. The median concentration (0.027 ng/mL) was lower than the diagnostic cutoff for acute myocardial infarction. Patients with elevated cTnT were more severely ill than those with undetectable cTnT. They were older and more symptomatic: they had more depressed left ventricular function, suffered more frequently from comorbidities (e.g., diabetes and atrial fibrillation), and had a more compromised renal function and more pronounced neurohormonal activation (higher levels of natriuretic peptides, norepinephrine, renin, and aldosterone). Over a mean follow-up of two years, mortality was almost three times higher in patients with elevated cTnT (43%) than in those with undetectable levels (16%). Elevated cTnT was the strongest predictor of death in multivariable models adjusted for all traditional risk factors.[21]

The threshold for detecting myocyte necrosis has been continuously lowered and a new generation of highly-sensitive troponin assays with improved analytical sensitivity and precision are ready for clinical use (Apple et al., 2008).[6] In the Val-HeFT trial, a precommercial version of a high sensitivity cTnT assay (hsTnT) was evaluated and compared to the traditional assay.[21] The new reagents improved the sensitivity by five- to tenfold, lowering the limit of detection to 1–2 pg/mL, and with this, the fraction of patients with detectable plasma troponin T increased dramatically—from 10% with the traditional assay to 90% with hsTnT reagents. As already observed with the traditional assay, patients with elevated hsTnT (above the median concentration of 12 pg/mL) were more compromised. The circulating concentrations of hsTnT were directly related to left ventricular internal diameter and inversely proportional to the ejection fraction (Figure 7–1). A similar association between the release of cTnI (measured with a highly-sensitive assay) and echocardiographic parameters of increased wall stress (relative left ventricular wall thickness and mitral E/A ratio) has been observed in 71 patients with severe nonischemic HF.[23]

In Val-HeFT, the risk of adverse clinical events increased steadily with hsTnT concentration, even in a range of very low concentrations that were not previously measurable with the traditional assay.[21] In other words, the prognostic accuracy of cardiac troponins was greatly increased with higher sensitivity in those patients with chronic and stable HF. A striking parallel can be made with natriuretic peptides (BNP or NT-proBNP), markers that show good prognostic performance in patients with cardiovascular diseases at concentrations well below their respective diagnostic threshold for the exclusion of HF.

Natriuretic peptides are currently the most powerful biomarkers for risk stratification in HF.[24] Sophisticated statistical analyses were carried out in the Val-HeFT trial to compare the prognostic value of B-type natriuretic peptide and hsTnT.[21] It was concluded

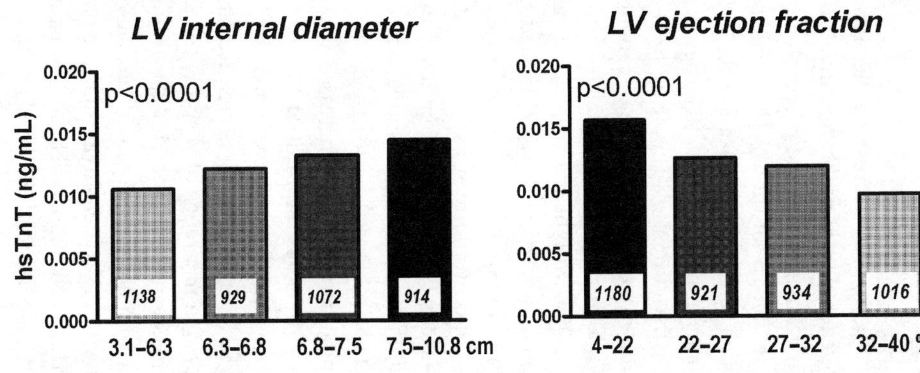

■ **Figure 7–1** Relationship between high sensitive cardiac troponin T concentration and left ventricular diameter and ejection fraction in the Val-HeFT trial. Left ventricular ejection internal diameter in diastole and ejection fraction were measured by echocardiography at randomization in patients with chronic HF enrolled in the Valsartan Heart Failure trial (Val-HeFT). The graphs show the association between quartiles of these two variables and baseline plasma high sensitive troponin T (Roche Elecsys, pre-commercial assay), expressed as median value. The number of patients in each quartile is reported.

that the two cardiac markers had substantially similar prognostic discrimination in these patients with chronic HF. However, patients with both cardiac markers elevated (a natriuretic peptide—either BNP or NT-proBNP—and hsTnT) had a worse prognosis than those with a single elevated marker (Figure 7–2). In addition, we tested whether serial measurement of hsTnT over time could improve its prognostic value and found that the last determination in a sequence of repeated measurements was the best predictor of future adverse events. Similarly, persistently increased cTnT levels were predictive of clinical events (death or hospital readmission for decompensated HF) in a study that enrolled a cohort of 62 patients with decompensated HF in whom cTnT was measured within four days of hospital admission and again seven days later (Del Carlo et al., 2004).[25]

Causes for Elevated Circulating Cardiac Troponins in HF

What is the physiological significance of circulating cardiac troponins in chronic HF? The main issues regard the origin of circulating cardiac troponins and the mechanisms responsible for their release into the bloodstream in chronic HF. A continuous release of troponins from the myocardium might reflect ongoing cardiomyocyte death, as seen in animal models of postmyocardial infarction LV dysfunction[26] and in patients with chronic HF.[27,28] If ongoing cardiac damage is assumed to be a determinant of circulating troponins, this phenomenon seems to be independent of an ischemic etiology of the disease. Stretch of cardiac myocytes might lead to leakage of the cytosolic pool of troponins by transient loss of cell-membrane integrity. This reversible damage may contribute to the increase in circulating cTn caused by irreversible injury of cardiac myocytes. It is unknown to what extent, if any, apoptosis contributes to troponin T elevation in chronic HF.[29] There are, however, alternative causes for elevated cardiac troponin levels including cardiopulmonary disease and chronic renal insufficiency.[30] In addition, several neuroendocrine systems

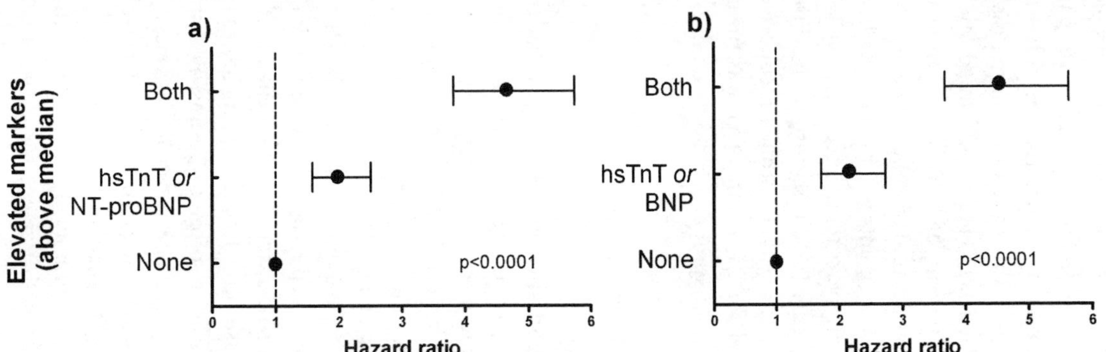

■ **Figure 7–2** The additive prognostic value of cardiac markers in patients with chronic heart failure. Two circulating B-type natriuretic peptides (BNP, IRMA Shionogi and NT-proBNP, Roche Elecsys) and high sensitive cardiac troponin T (hsTnT, pre-commercial assay, Roche Diagnostics) were measured in more than 4,000 patients at randomization in the Val-HeFT trial. The plots show the risk for all-cause mortality (median follow-up time 24 months) according to the number of elevated biomarkers (above median concentration) with the combinations of hsTnT and NT-proBNP (a) or hsTnT and BNP (b). Median concentrations of BNP, NT-proBNP and hsTnT were 97 pg/mL, 895 pg/mL, and 0.012 ng/mL, respectively. 0 = patients with both cardiac markers (a natriuretic peptide and hsTnT) below median concentration, reference category; 1 = patients with one elevated biomarker (either a natriuretic peptide or hsTnT); 2 = patients with two markers elevated (a natriuretic peptide and hsTnT). The univariate hazard ratio [95% confidence interval] for the single markers divided by median concentrations were 2.47 [2.13–2.87], 2.76 [2.37–3.22], and 2.98 [2.55–3.50] for BNP, NT-proBNP, and hsTnT, respectively.

(renin-angiotensin-aldosterone, sympathetic, endothelin) and inflammatory mechanisms are also chronically activated in patients with HF and might contribute to myocyte injury and cell death. Clearly, we need to gain more basic knowledge on the respective role of these mechanisms. Experimental investigations using well-characterized animal models of cardiac damage (myocardial infarction, cardiac overload, diabetes, renal dysfunction, neuroendocrine activation) and/or cultured isolated myocytes (hypoxia, hyperglycemia, hormonal stimulation) will probably help in deciphering the biological complexity behind the apparently naïve measurement of a cardiac contractile protein in the blood of patients with HF.

Alternative Biochemical Markers of Myocyte Injury in Heart Failure

Myocardial cell death can be recognized by the appearance of proteins in the blood released into the circulation from the damaged myocytes. The preferred biomarker for myocardial necrosis is cardiac troponin (I or T) because of its nearly absolute myocardial tissue specificity and high clinical sensitivity.[31] However, other proteins are released by injured myocytes and their clinical utility has been evaluated in patients with chronic HF. The circulating concentrations of cardiac proteins correlate with the severity of HF.[32] However, some of them present a low cardiac specificity in the presence of skeletal muscle injury or renal insufficiency. Fatty-acid binding proteins are small cytosolic proteins that bind long-chain fatty acids and function as the principle transporter of long-chain fatty acids in the cardiomyocyte. Heart-type fatty acid binding protein (H-FABP) is present abundantly in the myocardium and is released into the circulation when the myocardium is injured. Serum levels of H-FABP are elevated in patients with HF compared to control subjects and increase with the severity of the disease and may be an independent risk factor in these patients.[13,33] Serial measurements and changes in the levels of H-FABP may be associated with corresponding changes in the outcome of HF patients.[34] The prognostic value of cardiac troponins and H-FABP have been compared[35] or combined with troponin[36] in single-center studies that enrolled a limited number of patients (~100) with chronic HF. Larger collaborative studies are required to reach more robust conclusions about the role of H-FABP as a prognostic marker in HF.

In acute coronary syndromes, when cardiac troponin assay is not available, the next best alternative as a marker of myocardial necrosis is creatine kinase isoenzyme (CK-MB) measured by mass assay.[37] The circulating levels of CK-MB, together with several other myocardial proteins, such as myosin light chain-I (MLC-I), can predict acute worsening of HF.[38] In an ancillary study of the Prospective Randomized Flosequinan Longevity Evaluation (PROFILE) trial, a multicenter randomized trial comparing the direct vasodilator flosequinan with placebo in patients with severe chronic HF (NYHA III–IV, left ventricular ejection fraction ≤0.35), MLC-1 was measured at baseline and after one month in a subgroup of 218 patients.[39] MLC-1 was increased in more than half of the patients and this was associated with increased age, NYHA class IV, and higher serum creatinine levels. Over a mean follow-up of 302 days, elevated levels of MLC-1 predicted mortality in the patients randomized to placebo, but not in the flosequinan arm. There is unfortunately no clear interpretation for such interaction between a marker of cardiac integrity and a vasodilator. Overall, elevation of MLC-1 was a weak independent predictor of mortality, significant only if NYHA class was excluded from the multivariable logistic model.

References

1. Anversa P, Kajstura J, Olivetti G. Myocyte death in heart failure. *Curr Opin Cardiol.* 1996;11:245–251.
2. Mudd JO, Kass DA. Tackling heart failure in the twenty-first century. *Nature.* 2008;451:919–928.
3. Fishbein MC, Wang T, Matijasevic M, Hong L, Apple FS. Myocardial tissue troponins T and I. An immunohistochemical study in

experimental models of myocardial ischemia. *Cardiovasc Pathol.* 2003;12:65–71.

4. Zhang J, Knapton A, Lipshultz SE, Weaver JL, Herman EH. Isoproterenol-induced cardiotoxicity in Sprague-Dawley rats: correlation of reversible and irreversible myocardial injury with release of cardiac troponin T and roles of iNOS in myocardial injury. *Toxicol Pathol.* 2008;36:277–278.
5. O'Brien PJ. Cardiac troponin is the most effective translational safety biomarker for myocardial injury in cardiotoxicity. *Toxicology.* 2008;245:206–218.
6. Apple FS, Smith SW, Pearce LA, Ler R, Murakami MM. Use of the Centaur TnI-Ultra assay for detection of myocardial infarction and adverse events in patients presenting with symptoms suggestive of acute coronary syndrome. *Clin Chem.* 2008;54:723–728.
7. Wallace TW, Abdullah SM, Drazner MH, et al. Prevalence and determinants of troponin T elevation in the general population. *Circulation.* 2006;113:1958–1965.
8. Wu AH, Fukushima N, Puskas R, Todd J, Goix P. Development and preliminary clinical validation of a high sensitivity assay for cardiac troponin using a capillary flow (single molecule) fluorescence detector. *Clin Chem.* 2006;52:2157–2159.
9. Clerico A, Fortunato A, Ripoli A, Prontera C, Zucchelli GC, Emdin M. Distribution of plasma cardiac troponin I values in healthy subjects: pathophysiological considerations. *Clin Chem Lab Med.* 2008;46: 804–808.
10. La Vecchia L, Mezzena G, Ometto R, et al. Detectable serum troponin I in patients with heart failure of nonmyocardial ischemic origin. *Am J Cardiol.* 1997;80:88–90.
11. Missov E, Calzolari C, Pau B. Circulating cardiac troponin I in severe congestive heart failure. *Circulation.* 1997;96:2953–2958.
12. Sato Y, Yamada T, Taniguchi R, et al. Persistently increased serum concentrations of cardiac troponin T in patients with idiopathic dilated cardiomyopathy are predictive of adverse outcomes. *Circulation.* 2001;103:369–374.
13. Setsuta K, Seino Y, Ogawa T, Arao M, Miyatake Y, Takano T. Use of cytosolic and myofibril markers in the detection of ongoing myocardial damage in patients with chronic heart failure. *Am J Med.* 2002;113:717–722.

14. Ishii J, Nomura M, Nakamura Y, et al. Risk stratification using a combination of cardiac troponin T and brain natriuretic peptide in patients hospitalized for worsening chronic heart failure. *Am J Cardiol.* 2002;89:691–695.

15. Healey JS, Davies RF, Smith SJ, Davies RA, Ooi DS. Prognostic use of cardiac troponin T and troponin I in patients with heart failure. *Can J Cardiol.* 2003;19:383–386.

16. Perna ER, Macin SM, Canella JP, et al. Ongoing myocardial injury in stable severe heart failure: value of cardiac troponin T monitoring for high-risk patient identification. *Circulation.* 2004;110:2376–2382.

17. Ishii J, Cui W, Kitagawa F, et al. Prognostic value of combination of cardiac troponin T and B-type natriuretic peptide after initiation of treatment in patients with chronic heart failure. *Clin Chem.* 2003;49:2020–2026.

18. Bertinchant JP, Combes N, Polge A, et al. Prognostic value of cardiac troponin T in patients with both acute and chronic stable congestive heart failure: comparison with atrial natriuretic peptide, brain natriuretic peptide and plasma norepinephrine. *Clin Chim Acta.* 2005;352:143–153.

19. Peacock WF IV, De Marco T, Fonarow GC, et al. Cardiac troponin and outcome in acute heart failure. *N Engl J Med.* 2008;358:2117–2126.

20. Hudson MP, O'Connor CM, Gattis WA, et al. Implications of elevated cardiac troponin T in ambulatory patients with heart failure: a prospective analysis. *Am Heart J.* 2004;147:546–552.

21. Latini R, Masson S, Anand IS, et al. Prognostic value of very low plasma concentrations of troponin T in patients with stable chronic heart failure. *Circulation.* 2007;116:1242–1249.

22. Cohn JN, Tognoni G; Valsartan Heart Failure Trial Investigators. A randomized trial of the angiotensin-receptor blocker valsartan in chronic heart failure. *N Engl J Med.* 2001;345:1667–1675.

23. Logeart D, Beyne P, Cusson C, et al. Evidence of cardiac myolysis in severe nonischemic heart failure and the potential role of increased wall strain. *Am Heart J.* 2001;141:247–253.

24. Braunwald E. Biomarkers in heart failure. *N Engl J Med.* 2008;358: 2148–2159.

25. Del Carlo CH, Pereira-Barretto AC, Cassaro-Strunz C, Latorre Mdo R, Ramires JA. Serial measure of cardiac troponin T levels for

prediction of clinical events in decompensated heart failure. *J Card Fail.* 2004;10:43–48.

26. Capasso JM, Malhotra A, Li P, Zhang X, Scheuer J, Anversa P. Chronic nonocclusive coronary artery constriction impairs ventricular function, myocardial structure, and cardiac contractile protein enzyme activity in rats. *Circ Res.* 1992;70:148–162.
27. Olivetti G, Abbi R, Quaini F, et al. Apoptosis in the failing human heart. *N Engl J Med.* 1997;336:1131–1141.
28. Narula J, Pandey P, Arbustini E, et al. Apoptosis in heart failure: release of cytochrome c from mitochondria and activation of caspase-3 in human cardiomyopathy. *Proc Natl Acad Sci USA.* 1999;96: 8144–8149.
29. Sobel BE, LeWinter MM. Ingenuous interpretation of elevated blood levels of macromolecular markers of myocardial injury: a recipe for confusion. *J Am Coll Cardiol.* 2000;35:1355–1358.
30. Jeremias A, Gibson CM. Narrative review: alternative causes for elevated cardiac troponin levels when acute coronary syndromes are excluded. *Ann Intern Med.* 2005;142:786–791.
31. Thygesen K, Alpert JS, White HD, Joint ESC/ACCF/AHA/WHF Task Force for the Redefinition of Myocardial Infarction, et al. Universal definition of myocardial infarction. *Circulation.* 2007;116:2634–2653.
32. Goto T, Takase H, Toriyama T, et al. Circulating concentrations of cardiac proteins indicate the severity of congestive heart failure. *Heart.* 2003;89:1303–1307.
33. Arimoto T, Takeishi Y, Shiga R, et al. Prognostic value of elevated circulating heart-type fatty acid binding protein in patients with congestive heart failure. *J Card Fail.* 2005;11:56–60.
34. Niizeki T, Takeishi Y, Arimoto T, et al. Persistently increased serum concentration of heart-type fatty acid-binding protein predicts adverse clinical outcomes in patients with chronic heart failure. *Circ J.* 2008;72:109–114.
35. Niizeki T, Takeishi Y, Arimoto T, et al. Heart-type fatty acid-binding protein is more sensitive than troponin T to detect the ongoing myocardial damage in chronic heart failure patients. *J Card Fail.* 2007;13:120–127.
36. Setsuta K, Seino Y, Kitahara Y, et al. Elevated levels of both cardiomyocyte membrane and myofibril damage markers predict adverse out-

comes in patients with chronic heart failure. *Circ J.* 2008;72: 569–574.

37. Morrow DA, Cannon CP, Jesse RL, et al.; National Academy of Clinical Biochemistry. National Academy of Clinical Biochemistry Laboratory Medicine Practice Guidelines: Clinical characteristics and utilization of biochemical markers in acute coronary syndromes. *Circulation.* 2007;115:e356–375.
38. Sugiura T, Takase H, Toriyama T, Goto T, Ueda R, Dohi Y. Circulating levels of myocardial proteins predict future deterioration of congestive heart failure. *J Card Fail.* 2005;11:504–509.
39. Hansen MS, Stanton EB, Gawad Y; Canadian PROFILE investigators, et al. Relation of circulating cardiac myosin light chain 1 isoform in stable severe congestive heart failure to survival and treatment with flosequinan. *Am J Cardiol.* 2002;90:969–973.

8 ■ Necrosis Markers in Conditions Other than Acute Coronary Syndromes and Heart Failure

Walter E. Kelley, DO
Robert H. Christenson, PhD, DABCC, FACB

Introduction

Cardiovascular disease (CVD) accounts for over 800,000 deaths per year in the United States and is the most significant cause of mortality in the Western world. As a case in point, there were more than 6,000,000 hospitalizations attributed to CVD in the country in 2005, at an estimated cost of over $71 billion.[1]

The development of biomarkers has revolutionized the diagnosis, risk assessment, and management of acute coronary syndrome (ACS) and heart failure (HF) patients. In 2007, the National Academy of Clinical Biochemistry (NACB) developed guidelines for use of biomarkers in the diagnosis and management of ACS;[2] in this same year, an ESC/ACC/AHA/WHF task force redefined myocardial infarction based on biomarkers.[3] Both groups are united in establishing cardiac troponin as the preferred biomarker for ACS diagnosis and management. Further, compelling evidence has led to recommended diagnostic and prognostic cut points for cardiac troponin that are quite low, i.e., at the 99th percentile of a reference control population.[2,3] It is noteworthy that the NACB mentions CK-MB and myoglobin MYO measurements, but recommendations for these markers are unenthusiastic for use in ACS diagnosis and management. In the context of HF, evidence for the role of necrosis markers continues to develop, particularly for use in risk stratification. NACB guidelines for clinical utilization of biomarkers in HF list the following Class IIb recommendation:

"Troponin testing can identify patients with heart failure at increased risk beyond the setting of acute coronary syndromes."[4] As more evidence accumulates, it is anticipated that this recommendation will be more enthusiastic and expand to other clinical uses in the future.

Because cardiac necrosis biomarkers, in particular cardiac troponin (cTn), are clearly a cornerstone of ACS diagnosis and management and are evolving in the area of HF diagnosis, this testing is very common and is performed in a wide variety of patients. While CK-MB and MYO may be elevated in any number of clinical situations, the cardiac troponins are more specific[5,6] markers of cardiac injury. However, use of low cardiac troponin cut points leads to the potential for false positive results in non-ACS and non-HF etiologies. Although observation of the temporal pattern in cardiac troponin can improve ACS specificity and provide insight into the timing,[2,3] the practicing physician must have a working knowledge of clinical situations where cardiac troponin or other biomarkers may be elevated in etiologies other than ACS and HF to avoid unnecessary, costly interventions and delays in management decisions. As shown in Table 8–1, the list of non-ACS and non-HF etiologies that may be associated with elevated cardiac necrosis markers is long. The purpose of this chapter is to review these other elevations in necrosis biomarker elevations using the classification approach of acute disease, chronic disease, iatrogenic causes, and myocardial injury.

Acute Disease

Table 8–2 lists acute non-ACS and non-HF conditions that can show substantial increases in cTn and other cardiac biomarkers of necrosis.

Cardiac and Vascular

Acute Aortic Dissection

Acute aortic dissection (AAD) is characterized by separation of the layers within the wall of the aorta and is the most common

Table 8–1: Differential diagnosis of elevated troponin in non-ACS patients.

Acute Disease

Cardiac and Vascular

- Acute aortic dissection
- Apical ballooning syndrome
- Endocarditis
- Myocarditis
- Pericarditis
- Cerebrovascular accident
  - Ischemic stroke
  - Intracerebral hemorrhage
  - Subarachnoid hemorrhage
- Kawasaki disease
- Critical illness
  - Hypotension
  - Gastrointestinal bleeding
  - TTP

Respiratory

- Acute pulmonary embolism
- ARDS

Muscular Damage

- Rhabdomyolysis

Infectious

- Sepsis
- Viral illness

Other Acute Causes of Troponin Elevation

- Environmental exposure
  - Carbon monoxide
  - Hydrogen sulfide
  - Colchicine
- Acute complications of inherited disorders
  - Neurofibromatosis
  - Duchenne muscular dystrophy
  - Klippel-Feil syndrome
- Birth complications in infants
  - Extreme low birthweight
  - Preterm delivery

Chronic Disease

- ESRD (see Ch. 6)
- Heart failure (see Ch. 6)
- Cardiac infiltrative disorders
  - Amyloidosis
  - Sarcoidosis
  - Hemochromatosis
  - Scleroderma

Table 8–1: (Continued)

◦ Hypertension ◦ Diabetes ◦ Hypothyroidism **Iatrogenic** ◦ Invasive Procedures • PCI (see Ch. 9) • CABG (see Ch. 9) • Heart transplantation • Congenital defect repair • Radiofrequency catheter ablation • Lung resection ◦ Noninvasive Procedures • Cardioversion	◦ Pharmacologic sources • Chemotherapy • Other medications **Myocardial Injury** ◦ Blunt chest injury ◦ Endurance athletes ◦ Envenomation • Snake • Jellyfish • Scorpion • Centipede • Spider

disorder of the aorta requiring urgent surgical intervention, has a high mortality rate, and clinically may present with common risk factors to ACS.[7–9] Rapidly differentiating AAD from confounding conditions is paramount, both because rapid management is necessary to improve outcomes and given the potentially disastrous results of inappropriate treatment, for example, administration of thrombolytic therapy if AAD is misdiagnosed as ACS.[10]

According to a review of 82 patients[11] with AAD, 18% demonstrated positive cTn at presentation, which was associated with a three- to fourfold excess risk of delayed in-hospital diagnosis.[11] Additionally, in a study of 66 patients with the eventual diagnosis of AAD, elevated cTn occurred in seven patients (11%) and coronary compromise occurred as a consequence of aortic dissection in four patients (6%).[10] Overall, it appears that a minority of AAD

Table 8–2: Troponin elevation in the setting of acute noncoronary diseases.

DISEASE STATE	CITATIONS	COMMENT
Cardiac and Vascular		
Acute Aortic Dissection (AAD)	10, 11, 12, 13	AAD is frequently confused with ACS, leading to delayed diagnosis and significant bleeding due to inappropriate treatment with antithrombic agents. Troponin positivity, an ACS-like EKG, and dyspnea are clinical confounders. Elevated cTn in AAD is associated with long in-hospital diagnosis times. D-Dimer, along with troponin, may be useful tests for workup of AAD.
Apical Ballooning Syndrome	14[R], 15, 16, 138[R], 139[R], 140[R], 141, 142	While presentation (including elevated troponin) often mimics ACS, cardiac dysfunction resolves quickly and long-term prognosis is excellent.
Endocarditis	17, 18, 143	Patients with endocarditis and elevated cTn have an increased morbidity and mortality.
Myocarditis	19, 20, 21[R], 24[R], 44[R], 144[R], 145[R], 146[R], 147, 148, 149, 150[R*], 151[R*]	In all patients with suspected myocarditis, cTn should be measured to assess the presence and extent of myocardial cell damage and to aid in prognosis.
Pericarditis	22, 23, 145, 146	Perimyocarditis should be considered if myocardial infarction (MI) has been ruled out in a patient with dyspnea and chest discomfort, especially if the patient has a history of recent viral illness.

Table 8–2: (Continued)

Disease State	Citations	Comment
Cerebrovascular Accident • Ischemic Stroke • Intracerebral Hemorrhage • Subarachnoid Hemorrhage	27, 28[R], 29, 31, 32, 33, 34, 152 29, 36, 37, 153, 154 29, 38, 39, 40, 41	Cardiac troponin is increased in 15 to 20% of patients with stroke of ischemic, hemorrhagic or patients with subarachnoid hemorrhage subtype of stroke. Stroke patients with troponin increases are generally associated with poorer outcomes than similar patients without increases.
Kawasaki Disease	42, 43, 44[R], 45*, 155	While cTn elevation has been reported in KD, its role in diagnosis and monitoring of treatment effectiveness is still under investigation.
Critical Illness • Hypotension • Upper GI Bleeding • TTP	52[R], 53[R] 46[SR], 52, 48, 49, 50, 51, 156*, 54 6, 55, 56, 57, 58 59[R]	Cardiac troponin increases in critically-ill patients are associated with increased mortality and ICU length-of-stay. The underlying cause and clinical significance of elevated troponin in this population remains to be elucidated. Elevated cardiac troponin appears to confer prognostic importance similar to that in ACS patients. Frequency of cTn elevation is 43%, ranging from 12% to 85%.
Respiratory		
Pulmonary Embolism	63, 64, 65, 66, 67[R], 157[R], 158, 159, 160, 161, 162	cTn massive acute PE used most commonly in risk stratification with known PE; not a sensitive diagnostic tool. BNP may be elevated in CHF or other conditions that cause pulmonary hypertension. May help ID patients who will benefit from a more aggressive treatment.

Table 8–2: (Continued)

Disease State	Citations	Comment
Acute Respiratory Distress Syndrome	68, 163	Elevated cTn may be an important factor in morbidity and mortality in ARDS patients.
Muscular Damage		
Rhabdomyolysis	70, 71, 73, 74, 50, 164	Cross reactivity of newer cTn with skeletal muscle does not occur. The magnitude of cTn elevation in the setting of rhabdomyolysis is directly related to prognosis.
Infectious		
Sepsis	47, 75[R], 76, 77, 78, 79, 165[R], 166, 167	In the setting of sepsis, elevated cTn is associated with increased morbidity and mortality.
Acute Viral Infection	80, 81[SR], 82, 83, 168	Elevated cTn occurs in RSV and entrovirus infections and is an indicator of morbidity (both) and mortality (entrovirus).
Other Diseases (see Table 8–1 for a detailed list)	169, 170, 171, 172, 173, 174, 175, 176, 177	Reports of elevated cTn in preterm infants, hereditary syndromes, and environmental exposures have also been reported.

*Indicates a study demonstrating no correlation

[R]Indicates review article

[SR]Indicates systematic review

patients are cTn positive; in addition to the above studies, a review of 151 patients (76 control, 75 AAD) indicated that cTn was not increased in association with a diagnosis of AAD.[12] However, given consequences of misdiagnosis, AAD should be considered in suspected ACS patients, even if they are cTn positive. It is noteworthy that blood tests for risk stratification in suspected cases of AAD are being actively investigated; some of these tests include D-dimer, matrix metalloproteinases, smooth muscle myosin heavy chain, and soluble elastin fragments.[13]

Apical Ballooning Syndrome

Left ventricular apical ballooning (also termed Tako-Tsubo syndrome) is a stress cardiomyopathy that can mimic the abrupt onset of ACS-like chest pain; electrocardiographic changes can occur, including ST elevation changes. However, on angiogram, an absence of significant lesions is typical in left ventricular apical ballooning patients. The condition is usually related to increased stress, and is found mainly in elderly women.[14] cTn may be increased in about 75% of patients.[15] Left ventricular apical ballooning should be considered in the differential of patients presenting with suspected ACS, as it may account for 2% of hospital admissions in some populations.[16]

Endocarditis

Patients with endocarditis reportedly have a high prevalence of elevated cTn values; two recent studies indicated 65%[17] and 81%.[18] Patients with elevated cTn had worse outcomes that included death, abscess, and central nervous system events.[17] A combination of cTn and NT-proBNP measurements offered more prognostic information than either of the biomarkers alone.[18]

Myocarditis

Myocarditis is frequently mild; however, inflammation of the myocardium can lead to coronary artery thrombus, coronary ischemia, dilated cardiomyopathy, cardiac arrhythmias, and sudden death.

cTn and other necrosis biomarkers are frequently elevated in myocarditis and are useful for detecting myocardial injury. Several cardiac biomarkers have been evaluated in myocarditis patients; however, cTnI was superior.[19] For myocarditis diagnosis, cTn has a sensitivity of 53%, a specificity of 94%, a positive predictive value of 93%, and a negative predictive value of 56%.[20] Elevated cTn levels are prognostic and these measurements are recommended in all patients with suspected myocarditis to assess the presence and extent of myocardial cell damage.[21]

Pericarditis

An increase in cTn is observed frequently in those with pericarditis, and may suggest myopericarditis.[22] Pediatricians should be aware of postvaccination myopericarditis and its usually benign clinical course. Myopericarditis should be considered if myocardial infarction (MI) has been ruled out in a patient with dyspnea and chest discomfort, especially if the patient has a history of recent viral illness or vaccination.[23–24]

Cerebrovascular Accident

Stroke is defined as the rapid development of neurologic deficit resulting from disruption of the blood supply to the corresponding area of the brain.[25] Risk factors associated with stroke are similar to those for cardiovascular disease and include: ethnicity, transient ischemic attack (10% of patients who experience a TIA will suffer a stroke within 90 days), smoking, atrial fibrillation, age, hypertension, diabetes, physical inactivity, pregnancy/postpartum, and estrogen therapy.[26] Elevations in cTn have been reported in ischemic, intracerebral, and subarachnoid subtypes of stroke, even after patients with ischemic cardiac damage have been excluded.[27] In a review of the literature relating ischemic stroke and cTn, the majority of studies demonstrated an association with adverse outcomes,[28–31,27,32,33] while only a few reporting no association.[34,35] In a prospective study of 244 patients with acute ischemic stroke without demonstrable ischemic cardiac disease, elevated levels of cTnT (>0.03 μg/L) were observed in 10% of patients; univariate and multivariate analyses showed elevation of cTnT was significantly associated with mortality.[33] In a separate study that included 235 patients with intracerebral hemorrhage, cTnI measurements were independently associated with in-hospital mortality.[36] In a retrospective study of 110 patients with intracerebral hemorrhage, ten patients (9%) had abnormal serum cTnT levels; however, no correlation with early clinical outcomes was documented.[37] Retrospective[38] and prospective[39–41] studies have demonstrated a relationship between troponin elevation and adverse outcomes in subarachnoid hemorrhage, with between 17%[38] and 68%[39] of patients with subarachnoid hemorrhage and elevated troponin correlating with poor clinical outcomes, including death.[39,41]

Kawasaki Disease

Kawasaki disease (KD) produces irritation, high fever, and inflammation of the lymph nodes and other tissues and is the most common form of vasculitis that primarily affects children. Most children recover; however, myocarditis, pericardial effusion, congestive heart failure (CHF), conduction system abnormalities, and structural damage to the coronary arteries may occur in as many as 15% to 25% of cases.[42] Troponin is reportedly elevated in about 40% of KD patients.[43,44] Use of cTnI has been investigated for both the diagnosis of KD and the assessment of the effectiveness of intravenous immunoglobulin G (IgG) treatment. In one report, 16 of 18 patients with elevated cTn levels returned to normal with IV IgG treatment. Although these 16 had improvements in their clinical symptoms, it is not clear from the report that the two with no decrease had a worse outcome.[42] Interestingly, one paper stated that there was no correlation between cTnI measurements and myocarditis, even though there was a large difference between two KD groups and non-KD controls. However, the reported cTn levels were strikingly different; 0.11 ± 0.16 ng/mL for the KD patients and 0.04 ± 0.08ng/mL for the controls.[45] Thus, KD may have elevated cTn values, but it is not universal.

Critical Illness

Intensive care unit (ICU) patients may suffer from a number of high-risk disease states, including hypotension, infection (sepsis), arrhythmias, pulmonary embolism, increased intracranial pressure, and renal insufficiency.[46] According to a recent review, cTn elevations occur in 43% (interquartile range: 21% to 59%) of noncardiac ICU patients. This study indicated that ICU patients with elevated cTn most often did not have flow limiting coronary artery disease by stress echo or autopsy.[47] As indicated in Figure 8–1, elevated cTn levels are clearly associated with increased risk of in-hospital mortality with an odds ratio of approximately 2.5 (95% CI 1.9–3.4).[46] Clinical features that are common in the ICU setting will be discussed individually in the following paragraphs. Note that elevated cTn indicates myocardial injury, but not the mechanism of injury. Therefore, teasing out which clinical feature is the root cause for any cTn increase is complicated at best, and most probably impossible.

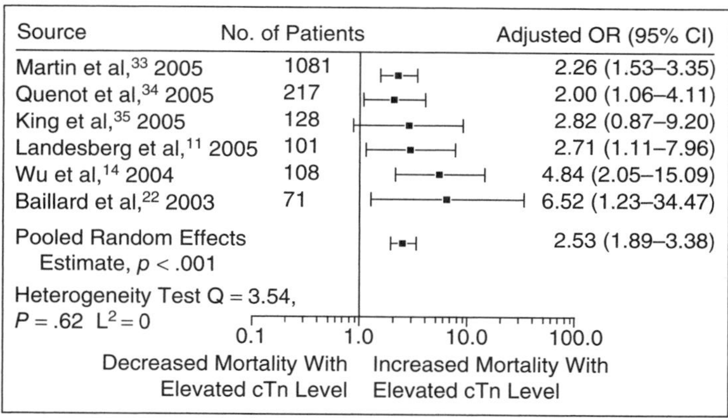

Source
No. of Patients
Adjusted OR (95% CI)
Martin et al,33 2005 1081 2.26 (1.53–3.35)
Quenot et al,34 2005 217 2.00 (1.06–4.11)
King et al,35 2005 128 2.82 (0.87–9.20)
Landesberg et al,11 2005 101 2.71 (1.11–7.96)
Wu et al,14 2004 108 4.84 (2.05–15.09)
Baillard et al,22 2003 71 6.52 (1.23–34.47)
Pooled Random Effects Estimate, p < .001 2.53 (1.89–3.38)
Heterogeneity Test Q = 3.54, P = .62 L2 = 0
0.1
1.0
10.0
100.0
Decreased Mortality With Elevated cTn Level
Increased Mortality With Elevated cTn Level

■ **Figure 8–1** Meta-analysis of 6 studies of critically ill patients demonstrating the association of mortality and elevated cTn. CI indicates confidence interval; OR, odds ratio.

From *Arch Intern Med.* 2006;166:2446–2454, with permission.

Hypotension may cause cardiac damage in critically-ill patients with noncardiac disease as shown by abnormal cTn levels, and it is likely that myocardial necrosis goes unnoticed on the ECG of many of these patients.[48] In one report, positive cTn measurements were found in 55% (6/11) of patients with systolic hypotension (<90 mm), whereas 17% (4/25) of nonhypotensive patients had no troponin increase. Also, patients with hypotension consistently have higher cTn levels than those without the condition.[49] In surgical ICU patients, hypotension was more frequently associated with patients (5/6 versus 2/11) who had subsequent increases in cTn.[50] Severity of hypotension is also related to cTn increase; the incidence of hypotension in patients requiring intravenous vasopressors increased from 21% with normal cTn, to 40% in an intermediate cTnI elevation group, to 55% in the high cTn group.[51] Troponin elevations were consistently associated with worse outcomes in hypotensive patients.[46,48–54]

Upper gastrointestinal (UGI) bleeding is a clinical feature that attributes substantially to morbidity, mortality, and excess length of stay in the ICU.[55] Up to 19% of UGI bleed patients have an increased cTn cardiac injury.[56] In patients for whom UGI bleeding is severe enough to require ICU admission, cTnT elevations are related to long-term but (interestingly) not short-term mortality.[57] cTn has been proposed as a possible means for screening ICU patients for cardiac damage, especially the elderly who are hemodynamically unstable.[56] Those patients with UGI and myocardial injury had longer hospital stays and required transfusion of more units of red blood cells (RBCs).[58]

Thrombotic thrombocytopenic purpura (TTP) results from a deficient activity of the enzyme ADAMTS13, which is responsible for cleaving large multimers of von Willebrand factor. This deficiency causes extensive microscopic clot formation in the small blood vessels throughout the body, including the heart.[59] An increased cTn occurs in approximately 40% of TTP patients,[59] and this proportion will likely increase with the advent of more sensitive assays and lower cut points.[60] Outcomes of patients with cTn increases are presumably worse than patients with no cTn increase because many of these patients suffer myocardial infarction.[59]

There is clearly a need for criteria for cardiac diagnoses and optimal management strategies in critically-ill patients with elevated cTn levels.[61] Indeed, it is logical to state that every elevated cTn level in ICU patients should be approached with caution and not be rigorously diagnosed or treated as MI.[62] Having said this, elevation of cTn in the ICU has prognostic meaning.[6]

Respiratory Diseases

Respiratory diseases including pulmonary embolism and acute respiratory distress syndrome (which may present with symptoms and signs similar to heart disease) are also associated with increased cTnI and adverse outcomes.

Acute Pulmonary Embolism

Pulmonary embolism (PE) is caused by the process of thromboembolism in which the pulmonary artery or one of its branches becomes occluded, usually from venous thrombus that becomes dislodged and embolizes to one of the lungs. Between 10%[63] and 50%[64] of PE patients are cTn positive. These troponin elevations are typically modest and appear to reflect the volume of myocardium injured. Troponin release has prognostic implications. Positive troponin was a significant predictor of an adverse hospital course in a multivariate analysis, which showed that patients with elevated cTn measurements were at significant risk of complicated course and fatal outcome.[64]

Three widely-available tests can be used to risk stratify patients with PE, including cTn, pulse oximetry, and the electrocardiogram; these may be used to risk stratify patients when formal echocardiography is not available.[63] Also, a PE scoring algorithm that includes cTn has been proposed.[65] Interestingly, elevated cTn levels do not appear to be associated with positive ventilation/perfusion scans.[66] cTn improves risk stratification in patients with PE and may aid in the identification of patients who would benefit from more aggressive therapy. cTn measurements in patients with massive acute PE are used most commonly in risk stratification; however, cTn is not an accurate diagnostic tool: cTn correlation with V/Q scans has a sensitivity of 32% and a specificity of 71%. However, cTn may be helpful in the management of PE patients by helping to identify high-risk patients who might benefit from aggressive treatment.[67]

Acute Respiratory Distress Syndrome

Acute respiratory distress syndrome (ARDS) is characterized by pulmonary and systemic inflammation and pulmonary endothelial and epithelial injury that cause alveolar filling and respiratory failure.[68] In this setting, hypotoxic vasoconstriction and thrombosis can occur and cause pulmonary hypertension, and, under these hypoxemic conditions, can result in right ventricular strain and myocardial injury.[69] Progression of disease worsens this situation and mechanical ventilation may raise intrathoracic pressures and further impact myocardial function.[68]

Myocardial injury in patients with ARDS has a high prevalence of elevated cardiac markers. In one study, 89 of 248 (35%) ARDS patients had elevated biomarkers. Although cTn's c-index was only 0.63 for predicting mortality, elevated values were significantly and independently associated with higher 60-day mortality and increased organ failure. Of note, this effect was most pronounced in lower severity illness. Occult myocardial injury may be an important factor in morbidity and mortality in ARDS patients.[68]

Muscular Damage

Rhabdomyolysis

Rhabdomyolysis is the rapid lysis of skeletal muscle tissue due to injury. The term is nonspecific and the muscle damage may be caused by physical (e.g., trauma), chemical, or biological factors. cTn in rhabdomyolysis patients may be increased, but is unrelated to the amount of skeletal muscle injured, renal insufficiency, and cardiovascular risk factors. Rather, the cTn elevation is related to the etiology of the rhabdomyolysis as evidenced by elevated cTnI levels in association with substance abuse, hypotension, and sepsis. However, the magnitude of the cTn increase is associated with prognosis.[70] The prevalence of cTn in emergency department patients with suspected rhabdomyolysis is reported as 17%[71] and 20%[70] in hospitalized patients. Early cTnT immunoassays showed substantial cross-reactivity with skeletal muscle troponin, and were a problem for evaluation of patients with rhabdomyolysis and/or renal insufficiency.[72] Newer redesigned cTn assays are far less susceptible to analytic interference than previous generations and patients with early posttraumatic rhabdomyolysis and second-generation cTnT and cTnI assays show similar results.[73] With the availability of cTn assays, discrimination between skeletal muscle and heart tissue injury is now possible.[50,74]

Infectious Processes

Sepsis

Bacterial sepsis is frequently associated with biochemical changes, such as high levels of TNF-alpha, IL-6, CRP, and systemic symptoms such as fever, chills, malaise, hypotension, and mental status changes. Reports indicate that approximately 50% of sepsis, severe sepsis, and septic shock patients admitted to intensive care units for non-ACS have elevated cTn that is not due to flow-limiting etiologies.[47,75,76]

Mechanistically, in sepsis, cTn release may result from a transient loss in membrane integrity or microvascular thrombotic injury. Myocardial dysfunction is a common complication in sepsis patients, and is accompanied by a poor prognosis.[75] This is particularly true of elderly patients with underlying cardiac disease.[77] Septic patients with elevated cTn are at increased risk of in-hospital mortality; in cTn positive patients, 63%[78] mortality and an 83%[79] death rate were reported; in contrast, these authors observed much lower mortality in cTn negative patients at 24% and 37%, respectively. Biochemical markers including cTn have emerged as possible tools for evaluation and quantification of cardiac dysfunction in sepsis patients. Other risk factors for elevated cTn were severity of underlying infection, renal insufficiency, and underlying cardiac disease; cTn elevation was a strong surrogate for mortality.[76]

The therapeutic implications of increased cTn in septic patients has not been elucidated; properly-designed studies are needed to evaluate the relationship between cTn's diagnostic use for assessing cardiac dysfunction and prognostic use for the guidance of the treatment of these patients.[58]

Viral Illness

Viral illness is another non-ACS condition that is occasionally associated with increased cTn. Myocarditis reportedly occurs in up to 10% of patients.[80] However, a more recent report that included 152 patients with acute viral influenza showed zero subjects with increased elevations in either cardiac troponin I or T.[80] In contrast, the prevalence of elevated cardiac troponin was 35 to 54% in very sick infants with serious respiratory syncytial virus (RSV) infection that required mechanical intervention.[81] In fact, it appears that myocardial involvement and cTn elevation are common in severe RSV lung disease, and are strongly associated with hypotension. In one study, 12 of 34 (35%) had elevated cTnT results; although there was no difference in the mortality endpoint in the study, the cTn positive patients had hypotension more frequently.[81] A preliminary study found that cTn was able to predict respiratory failure in children admitted with RSV. Of 25 children included, ten were positive for cTn; the ROC curve area was 0.939 (95% confidence interval = 0.82–1.0).[82]

cTn increases are evidently not strongly associated with adverse outcomes, such as death, according to reports of RSV infection.[81,82] However, in enterovirus 71-infected patients, cTn elevation was a bad prognostic sign. In one study that included 259 enterovirus 71-infected patients, 27 developed cardiopulmonary failure. Of these 27, eight died and five of six patients who died had the highest cardiac troponin levels.[83]

Other Acute Causes of Troponin Elevation

- Environmental exposure
  - Carbon monoxide
  - Hydrogen sulfide
  - Colchicine
- Acute complications of inherited disorders
  - Neurofibromatosis
  - Duchenne muscular dystrophy
  - Klippel-Feil syndrome
- Birth complications in infants
  - Extreme low birthweight
  - Preterm delivery

Chronic Diseases

Table 8–3 lists chronic conditions in which elevated cTn measurements have been reported.

Cardiac Infiltrative Diseases

Amyloidosis is a clinical disorder caused by extracellular deposition of insoluble abnormal fibrils, derived from aggregation of misfolded normally soluble proteins.[84] Cases with obvious cardiac association have a poor prognosis, with a median survival of six months, and 6% survival at three years.[85] Recent observational studies also suggest that the presence of detectable cTn in the serum of affected patients portends an adverse prognosis.[84,86] A retrospective assessment of 261 patients with newly-diagnosed systemic amyloidosis showed a median survival for patients with detectable cTnT and cTnI (6 and 8 months, respectively), which was worse than that for those with undetectable values (22 and 21 months, respectively), with cTnT providing a better predictor of survival than cTnI.[85] In a series of 50 consecutive patients with light-chain amyloidosis and 15 patients with hereditary amyloidosis, cTnT (0.105 ± 0.030 versus 0.019 ± 0.010 μg/L; $P < 0.05$) values were increased in patients with cardiac amyloidosis as compared to patients with light-chain amyloidosis, but no cardiac involvement.[87] Amyloid infiltration of the myocardium leads to elevation of cTnI and T

Table 8–3: Troponin elevation in chronic disease.

Disease	Citation(s)	Comment
End-stage renal disease	178	Please see Chapter 6, Interpretation of cardiac troponin elevation in patients with end-stage renal disease.
Heart failure	179	Please see Chapter 7, Necrosis marker testing in heart failure.
Cardiac Infiltrative Diseases		
Amyloidosis	84[SR], 85, 86[R], 87, 180, 181, 182	cTn elevation is related to mortality in patients with newly-diagnosed amyloidosis.
Other infiltrative/ inflammatory diseases	89, 90, 91, 92, 93	The significance of elevated cTn in other infiltrative/ inflammatory disorders (sarcoidosis, scleroderma, etc.) is not known.
Chronic systemic diseases		
Systemic hypertension	6, 77, 94	The significance of elevated cTn in relation to hypertension is still under investigation.
Pulmonary hypertension	95, 96	In the setting of PH, elevated troponin is associated with increased mortality.
Diabetes	97	The significance of elevated cTn in the setting of DM is not yet known.
Hypothyroidism	6	No reports of elevated cTn related to hypothyroidism have been published.

that is not related directly to cardiac hemodynamics or coronary anatomy.[88] While other infiltrative diseases, including hemochromatosis, sarcoidosis, scleroderma, and other inflammatory disorders, have been implicated as possible sources of elevated troponin,[6,89] published evidence is scarce.[89–93]

Chronic Systemic Diseases

Systemic hypertension has been cited as a potential source of troponin elevation in patients without overt ischemic cardiac disease.[6] When compared with cTnI-negative patients, cTnI-positive subjects tend to have a more frequent history of arterial hypertension.[77] However, in a retrospective study of 183 patients, no statistically significant difference in history of systemic hypertension ($p = 0.283$)[94] was demonstrated. In the setting of pulmonary hypertension, troponin T release persisting despite therapy is a poor prognostic sign,[95] acting as an independent marker of increased mortality risk.[96] In multivariable logistic regression analysis, left ventricular hypertrophy (LVH), HF, diabetes mellitus (DM), and chronic kidney disease (CKD) were independently associated with cTnT elevation. In the general population, cTnT elevation is rare in subjects without HF, LVH, CKD, or DM, suggesting that the upper limit of normal for the cTnT immunoassay should be <0.01 μg/L. Even though minimally increased cTnT may represent subclinical cardiac injury and have important clinical implications, a hypothesis that should be tested in longitudinal outcome studies.[97] Hypothyroidism has been suggested as a source of elevated cTn in non-ACS patients;[6] however, no published examples are available for review.

Iatrogenic

Table 8–4 lists iatrogenic causes of elevated cTn. Cardiac surgery and percutaneous coronary intervention are discussed elsewhere.

Table 8–4: Iatrogenic causes of troponin elevation.

Invasive Procedures	Citations	Comment
Percutaneous coronary intervention		Please see Chapter 9, Use of cardiac necrosis biomarkers following PCI or CABG.
Coronary arterial bypass grafting		Please see Chapter 9, Use of cardiac necrosis biomarkers following PCI or CABG.
Heart transplant	26[R], 44[R], 98, 99[R], 100, 101, 102, 103	Elevation in predonation circulating troponin is predictive of acute allograft rejection in heart transplantation.[103] In the setting of acute allograft rejection, the negative predictive value of troponin was 96.2%.[101] In the setting of CAV(chronic rejection), troponin correlates with both positive and negative EMB.[100]
Congenital defect repair	44[R], 104, 105	Elevated troponin prior to repair of congenital heart anomalies indicates poor prognosis. Postoperative troponin elevation correlates with significant complications.
Radiofrequency catheter ablation	107, 108, 109, 110	Troponin detects and quantifies the size of necrosis associated with RFCA.
Lung resection	111	Elevated troponin following lung resection is an independent risk factor for death.

Table 8–4: (Continued)

Noninvasive Procedures		
Cardioversion	112[*R], 113[+], 114[*], 115[*], 183[*R], 184[*], 185[+], 186[+], 187[+]	While a few studies have shown occasional increase in troponin (with rare significant increase) associated with cardioversion, most studies show no increase. Substantial elevations of troponin after cardioversion suggest the presence of myocardial injury from causes unrelated to cardioversion.
Pharmacologic Sources		
Chemotherapy	116[SR], 117[R], 118	Elevated troponin in the setting of HDCT predicts (up to 3 months in advance) the likelihood and severity of LV dysfunction. Persistent elevation (>1 month) is associated with an 85% likelihood of a major cardiac event within one year. A persistently negative troponin has a 99% negative predictive value for any cardiac complication. For a detailed list of potentially cardiotoxic chemotherapeutic agents, please see Dolci et al.[116]
Other medications	119, 120, 121, 122	Troponin is specific and sensitive for drug-related myocardial damage. Any increase in serum troponin above baseline is evidence of possible cardiac damage and warrants further investigation.

[*]No troponin elevation
[+]Positive correlation
[R]Indicates review article
[SR]Indicates systematic review

Invasive Procedures

Heart Transplantation

Cardiac allograft vasculopathy (CAV—commonly referred to as chronic rejection)[98] limits the long-term success of heart transplantation (HTx), with CAV being detectable by angiography in 8% of survivors within the first year, in 32% within the first five years, and in 43% within the first eight years of HTx. CAV and graft failure (most likely undetected CAV) are, in addition to malignancy, the most important causes of death in patients who survive the first year after HTx.[99] Endomyocardial biopsy (EMB) is the current diagnostic modality for assessment of CAV. In a study of 57 heart transplant patients, between one and twelve months post-op, both central and the corresponding peripheral cTnT concentrations demonstrated statistically significant correlation with endomyocardial biopsies, which were negative ($P = 0.001$) or positive ($P = 0.001$) for CAV.[100] In the setting of acute allograft rejection following HTx, the sensitivity and specificity of cTn for the detection of significant graft rejection were 80.4% and 61.8%, respectively, and the negative predictive value was 96.2%.[101] In a series of seven pediatric heart transplant recipients with a total of nine episodes of acute rejection, cTnT increased and remained elevated for at least one month, and the diagnostic power of a single cTnT measurement was not sufficient to replace endomyocardial biopsy.[102] The quality of the donor heart is an important prognostic factor in HTx. Some amount of myocardial dysfunction occurs in all brain-dead donors, and precludes heart donation in up to 20% of cases. Donor cardiac function is an important prognostic factor in the clinical outcome of HTx.[103] In a study of heart donors, a cTnI value >1.6 mg/L as a predictor of early graft failure had a specificity of 94%, and a cTnT value of >0.1 mg/L had a specificity of 99%. The odds ratio for the development of acute graft failure after heart transplantation was 42.7 for donors with cTnI >1.6 mg/L and 56.9 for donors with cTnT >0.1 mg/L. Significantly higher cTnI and cTnT values were found in peripheral blood at the time of explantation in donors of hearts with subsequently impaired graft function, demonstrating cTnI and cTnT as useful parameters for heart donor selection.[103] In the pediatric population, preoperative donor cTnI elevations have been shown to be predictive of early graft failure, which causes 25% of early mortality in infant heart transplant recipients. However, cTn measurement has not shown utility in assessing CAV in the pediatric HTx recipients.[44]

Repair of Congenital Heart Defect

The incidence of congenital heart disease (CHD) varies from about 4 in 1000 to 50 in 1000 live births, with the incidence of moderate and severe forms of CHD being about 6 per 1000 live births.[104] In a series of 73 elective corrections of cardiac defects, the prediction of severe postoperative complications showed a PPV of 100% and a NPV of 93% when cTnI values exceeded 35 μg/L, during the first 24 hours in the ICU.[105] Systematic review suggests that preoperative elevations in troponin preceding congenital heart defect repair are a poor prognostic sign.[44]

Radiofrequency Catheter Ablation

Atrial fibrillation, the most common arrhythmia encountered in clinical practice, is associated with significant morbidity and mortality.[106] Radiofrequency catheter ablation (RFCA) is a nonpharmacologic approach to treating tachyarrhythmia. However, RFCA inevitably causes some myocardial damage at the site where the catheter tip contacts tissue. Possible mechanisms of myocyte damage during RFCA include lipid membrane disruption, metabolic and structural protein inactivation, and denaturation, as well as nuclear damage.[107] In a study of 60 patients (with no underlying structural heart disease) undergoing RFCA, all were found to have increased post-procedure troponin, with all measurements exceeding the diagnostic threshold for AMI (>0.15 μg/L).[108] Investigation measuring ischemia-modified albumin has implied that myocardial necrosis associated with RFCA occurs without preceding ischaemia.[109] Monitoring of cTnI has been reported as the best way to detect and quantify the size of myocardial necrosis created by radiofrequency ablation.[110]

Lung Resection

In a study of 207 patients undergoing lung resection for primary lung cancer, 14 (7%) were identified with elevated serum cTn levels within 30 days of surgery, with nine (64%) having classical features of myocardial infarction. The median time to follow-up (interquartile range) was 22 (1 to 52) months, and the one- and five-year survival probabilities (95% CI) for patients without and with postoperative troponin elevation were 92% (85 to 96) versus 60% (31 to 80) and 61% (51 to 71) versus 18% (3 to 43), respectively ($p < 0.001$). Tumor stage and postoperative cTn elevation remained independent predictors of mortality in the final multivariable model. The acceleration factor for death of elevated cTn after adjusting for tumor stage was 9.19 (95% CI 3.75–22.54).[111]

Noninvasive Procedures

Cardioversion

Atrial fibrillation (AF), the most common chronic arrhythmia in the US, affects 2.2 million Americans and is present in eight to ten percent of those over 80 years old.[112] Although AF is commonly (and successfully) treated with direct current cardioversion (DCCV), concern for myocardial damage resulting from DDCV has been expressed, particularly in light of greater energies delivered to the myocardium as a consequence of biphasic devices. Table 8–4 details some of this data. In a study of 48 patients with persistent AF who underwent CV, all who received monophasic CV (45.2%) showed a significant increase in mean plasma cTnI concentration over 24 hours (0.23 ± 0.18 versus 0.41 ± 0.37 ng/mL, $P < 0.04$).[113] Conversely, in a randomized trial of 141 patients undergoing monophasic or biphasic DCCV for supraventricular tachycardia (SVT), no elevations in troponin were observed.[114] Substantial elevations of troponin after DCCV may therefore suggest the presence of myocardial injury from causes unrelated to the procedure, such as underlying structural heart disease.[115]

Pharmacologic Sources

Chemotherapy

The successful use of chemotherapeutic agents in the treatment of various malignancies has led to increased use and subsequent increases in reported cardiotoxicity.[116] Chemotherapy-related cardiotoxicity has been a known entity since 1967, is associated with many classes and individual therapeutic agents, and is often a significant limiting factor in treaetment.[117] In a cohort of 179 consecutive patients receiving high-dose chemotherapy (HDCT), cTnI > 0.08 μg/L occurred in 57 patients (32%) with echocardiographic monitoring revealing a mean decrease in LVEF of 18%, while the group of cTnI-negative patients had a mean decrease in LVEF of 2.5% ($P < 0.001$).[118] Systematic review of the available data for chemotherapy-related cardiotoxicity demonstrates the ability of cTn to predict clinically-significant left ventricular dysfunction at least three months in advance. Additionally, early increase in cTn concentrations predicts the degree and severity of future left ventricular dysfunction. Finally, persistence of an increased cTn one month after the last chemotherapy administration portends an 85% probability of major cardiac events within the first year of follow-up. However, a persistently negative cTn identifies patients who will likely never encounter cardiac complications, at least not within the first year after the end of chemotherapy (negative predictive value = 99%).[116]

Other Medications

Rare reports of elevated cTn resulting from medication (legal and illicit) administration have been published.[119–121] The conclusions of the Expert Working Group (EWG) on Biomarkers of Drug-Induced Cardiac Toxicity from the Center for Drug Evaluation and Research (CDER) of the U.S. Food and Drug Administration concerning drug-related cTn elevation (based on an exhaustive systematic review) have been published.[122]

Myocardial Injury

Table 8–5 lists mechanisms of myocardial injury which have been associated with elevated cTn.

Blunt Chest Injury

Although thoracic injury accounts for only 5–12% of the admissions to trauma centers, it may be associated with increased lethality.[123] The exact incidence of a cardiac contusion in patients with blunt chest trauma is unknown, however, the reported incidence ranges between 3–56% of patients with blunt chest injury (BCI).[124] The sensitivity of cTn for diagnosing BCI ranges from 68 (cTnI) to 100% (cTnI), while specificity ranges from 12.5% (cTnI) to 100% (cTnT). In the setting of BCI, the positive predictive value of troponin ranges from 20% (cTnI)–100% (cTnT) and the negative predictive value ranges from 74% (cTnT)–100% (cTnI).[125] No significant BCI-related complications occurred in patients with a normal ECG and normal serial measurements of cTnI, and the sensitivity of an abnormal ECG and elevated cTnI for clinically significant BCI was 100%.[125] It has been suggested that in the setting of BCI and an absence of other injuries or hemodynamic instability, patients with normal ECG and cTnI can be discharged. In the setting of BCI, elevated cTn may serve to identify patients at increased risk of mortality, however, the utility of cTn in predicting long-term BCI morbidity is undetermined.[126]

Endurance Athletes

Elevations in cardiac biomarkers in athletes after exercise may generate difficulties for clinicians in terms of differential diagnosis and may result in inappropriate consequences.[127] Of 105 asymptomatic finishers of competitive endurance events lasting several hours, increased blood concentrations of cTnT and I above the 99% upper reference values were found in 24 and 34 subjects, respectively. Within three months after the events, 21 cTn-positive participants underwent an extensive cardiac examination, which in all but one (critical coronary heart disease) revealed no signs of

Table 8–5: Troponin elevation in the setting of myocardial injury.

INJURY TYPE	CITATIONS	COMMENT
Blunt chest injury	44R, 50, 123R, 124R, 125R, 126R, 188R, 189, 190, 191, 192	In the setting of BCI and an absence of other injuries or hemodynamic instability, patients with normal ECG and troponin can be discharged. With a positive predictive value and sensitivity up to 100%, elevated troponin in the setting of BCI necessitates further testing.
Endurance athletes	127R, 128, 129R, 131R, 193R, 194	Exercise-related increases in cardiac troponins are only mild and of short duration. Significant troponin elevation in the setting of exercise warrants additional testing.
Envenomation • Snake • Jellyfish • Scorpion • Centipede • Spider	131, 132, 133 134, 195 131, 137 136 135	Troponin elevation resulting from biologic toxin exposure has been reported. Careful attention to the history and physical exam may elucidate this uncommon cause of elevated troponin.

[R]Indicates review article

persistent cardiac damage.[128] In a study, 34 endurance athletes with elevated cTn (marathon, 100-km run, mountain bike marathon; ranges of cTnT and cTnI: 0.01–0.56 and 0.08–1.93 μg/L, respectively) were evaluated a few months after the competitions. One athlete was diagnosed with left coronary artery main stem and descending artery stenosis, however no other athletes had cardiovascular abnormalities explaining the exercise-induced increases in cardiac troponins. An additional one hour of intensive and three hours of extensive standardized endurance exercise could not reproduce an increase in cardiac troponins in these athletes. This observation is consistent with a study which failed to reproduce exercise-induced cardiac troponin release in eight participants of the 2004 and 2005 London marathons.[127] A prospective study of 82 middle-aged marathon participants over the course of three annual marathons showed significant increases in MYO (38.4-fold at 4 hours post-race), CK-MB (4.9-fold and 13.5-fold at 4 and 24 hours post-race), and cTnI (6.5-fold at both 4 and 24 hours post-race). Repeating this study using a rapid quantitative fluorescence immunoassay, the elevations in myoglobin and CK-MB were confirmed (significantly elevated at 4 and 24 hours post-race). In contrast, there were no significant increases in cTnI or T at either time point.[129] Among a population of patients completing the Boston Marathon, concentrations of cTnT were associated with abnormalities of right ventricular size and function on echocardiography. As well, concentrations of cTnT were inversely proportional to the amount of premarathon training, suggesting that favorable cardiovascular adaptations to exercise may render the heart more resistant to exercise-related injury.[130]

In summary, exercise-related increases in cTns are clearly true positives. Given that these elevations are usually mild and of short duration, they likely reflect a reversible membrane leakage of cardiomyocytes with troponin release from the free cytosolic pool (not bound in the contractile apparatus).

Envenomation

Rare cases of biologic toxin-induced myocardial injury have been observed. AMI as a result of snake envenomation has been reported,[131] with sparse occurrences of non-AMI elevation of cTn related to snake envenomation.[132] In a prospective study of 45 patients who complained of snake bite, none were found to have increased cTn.[133] The mechanisms of myocardial damage resulting from snake envenomation are not known, but vasospasm (possibly as a result of mast cell degranulation), coagulation abnormalities, and direct myocardial toxicity have been implicated.[131] Envenomation by contact with *Cnidaria* spp. (jellyfish) occasionally results in Irukandji syndrome, characterized by back, chest, and abdominal pain, other nonspecific myalgias, nausea, vomiting, restlessness, localized piloerection and sweating, tachycardia, and hypertension. Elevation of cTnI has been reported in 22% of patients with Irukandji syndrome.[134] Arthropod envenomation, including bites from black widow spiders[135] and centipedes,[136] and stings from scorpions,[137] has been reported as a source of cTn elevation.

Conclusion

The cTns show excellent tissue specificity and are virtually a *sine qua non* for myocardial damage[5] and are established as the cornerstone for assessment of ACS and diagnosis of myocardial infarction.[2,3] Additionally, cTn has been shown to provide prognostic information in the setting of HF.[4] However, the pitfall of equating an elevated cTn with the exclusive diagnosis of ACS must be avoided. As with all aspects of medicine, a broad differential diagnosis must be considered, and appropriate diagnostic modalities must be employed to diagnose, predict risk, treat, and assess the effectiveness of each step. Acute and chronic diseases, iatrogenic causes, as well as myocardial injury, have all been related to elevated cTn outside of the context of ACS and HF. In some of these situations, cTn may aid in ruling a diagnosis in or out, however, it often is a clinical confounder. Evidence for cTn as a prognostic marker in most non-ACS and non-HF circumstances is also accumulating. It remains to the astute physician to interpret cTn as a dynamic marker of myocardial damage, using clinical acumen to determine the source and significance of any reported elevation of these versatile markers.

References

1. Rosamond W, Flegal K, Furie K, et al. Heart Disease and Stroke Statistics 2008 Update. A Report from the American Heart

Association Statistics Committee and Stroke Statistics Subcommittee. *Circulation.* 2008;117(4):e25–e146.

2. Morrow DA, Cannon CP, Jesse RL, et al. National Academy of Clinical Biochemistry Laboratory Medicine practice guidelines: clinical characteristics and utilization of biochemical markers in acute coronary syndromes. *Circulation.* 2007;115(13):e356–375.
3. Thygesen K, Alpert JS, White HD, et al. Universal definition of myocardial infarction. *Circulation.* 2007;116(22):2634–2653.
4. Tang WHW, Francis GS, Morrow DA, et al. National Academy of Clinical Biochemistry Laboratory Medicine practice guidelines: Clinical utilization of cardiac biomarker testing in heart failure. *Circulation.* 2007;116(5):e99–109.
5. Apple FS, Wu AHB, Jaffe AS. European Society of Cardiology and American College of Cardiology guidelines for redefinition of myocardial infarction: how to use existing assays clinically and for clinical trials. *Am Heart J.* 2002;144(6):981–986.
6. Babuin L, Jaffe AS. Troponin: the biomarker of choice for the detection of cardiac injury. *CMAJ.* 2005;173(10):1191–1202.
7. Hagan PG, Nienaber CA, Isselbacher EM, et al. The International Registry of Acute Aortic Dissection (IRAD): new insights into an old disease. *JAMA.* 2000;283(7):897–903.
8. Kamalakannan D, Rosman HS, Eagle KA. Acute aortic dissection. *Crit Care Clin.* 2007;23(4):vi, 779–800.
9. Barbetseas J, Alexopoulos N, Brili S, et al. Atherosclerosis of the aorta in patients with acute thoracic aortic dissection. *Circ J.* 2008;72(11):1773–1776.
10. Hansen MS, Nogareda GJ, Hutchison SJ. Frequency of and inappropriate treatment of misdiagnosis of acute aortic dissection. *Am J Cardiol.* 2007;99(6):852–856.
11. Rapezzi C, Longhi S, Graziosi M, et al. Risk factors for diagnostic delay in acute aortic dissection. *Am J Cardiol.* 2008;102(10):1399–1406.
12. Ohlmann P, Faure A, Morel O, et al. Diagnostic and prognostic value of circulating D-Dimers in patients with acute aortic dissection. *Crit Care Med.* 2006;34(5):1358–1364.
13. Mir MA. Aortic dissection—in pursuit of a serum marker. *Am J Emerg Med.* 2008;26(8):942–945.

14. Prasad A, Lerman A, Rihal CS. Apical ballooning syndrome (Tako-Tsubo or stress cardiomyopathy): a mimic of acute myocardial infarction. *Am Heart J.* 2008;155(3):408–417.
15. Hahn J, Gwon H, Park SW, et al. The clinical features of transient left ventricular nonapical ballooning syndrome: comparison with apical ballooning syndrome. *Am Heart J.* 2007;154(6):1166–1173.
16. Valbusa A, Abbadessa F, Giachero C, et al. Long-term follow-up of Tako-Tsubo-like syndrome: a retrospective study of 22 cases. *J Cardiovasc Med (Hagerstown).* 2008;9(8):805–809.
17. Purcell JB, Patel M, Khera A, et al. Relation of troponin elevation to outcome in patients with infective endocarditis. *Am J Cardiol.* 2008;101(10):1479–1481.
18. Kahveci G, Bayrak F, Mutlu B, et al. Prognostic value of N-terminal pro-B-type natriuretic peptide in patients with active infective endocarditis. *Am J Cardiol.* 2007;99(10):1429–1433.
19. Smith SC, Ladenson JH, Mason JW, Jaffe AS. Elevations of cardiac troponin I associated with myocarditis: experimental and clinical correlates. *Circulation.* 1997;95(1):163–168.
20. Lauer B, Niederau C, Kuhl U, et al. Cardiac troponin T in patients with clinically suspected myocarditis. *J Am Coll Cardiol.* 1997;30(5): 1354–1359.
21. Feldman AM, McNamara D. Myocarditis. *N Engl J Med.* 2000;343 (19):1388–1398.
22. Bonnefoy E, Godon P, Kirkorian G, et al. Serum cardiac troponin I and ST-segment elevation in patients with acute pericarditis. *Eur Heart J.* 2000;21(10):832–836.
23. Thanjan MT, Ramaswamy P, Lai WW, Lytrivi ID. Acute myopericarditis after multiple vaccinations in an adolescent: case report and review of the literature. *Pediatrics.* 2007;119(6):e1400–1403.
24. Cassimatis DC, Atwood JE, Engler RM, et al. Smallpox vaccination and myopericarditis: a clinical review. *J Am Coll Cardiol.* 2004;43(9): 1503–1510.
25. Grysiewicz RA, Thomas K, Pandey DK. Epidemiology of ischemic and hemorrhagic stroke: incidence, prevalence, mortality, and risk factors. *Neurol Clin.* 2008;26(4):871–895.
26. Thom T, Haase N, Rosamond W, et al. Heart disease and stroke statistics—2006 update: a report from the American Heart

Association Statistics Committee and Stroke Statistics Subcommittee. *Circulation.* 2006;113(6):e85–151.

27. Sandhu R, Aronow WS, Rajdev A, et al. Relation of cardiac troponin I levels with in-hospital mortality in patients with ischemic stroke, intracerebral hemorrhage, and subarachnoid hemorrhage. *Am J Cardiol.* 2008;102(5):632–634.
28. Jensen JK, Atar D, Mickley H. Mechanism of troponin elevations in patients with acute ischemic stroke. *Am J Cardiol.* 2007;99(6):867–870.
29. Apak I, Iltumur K, Tamam Y, Kaya N. Serum cardiac troponin T levels as an indicator of myocardial injury in ischemic and hemorrhagic stroke patients. *Tohoku J Exp Med.* 2005;205(2):93–101.
30. Iltumur K, Yavavli A, Karabulut A, et al. Elevated plasma N-terminal pro-brain natriuretic peptide levels in acute ischemic stroke. *Am Heart J.* 2006;151(5):1115–1122.
31. James P, Ellis CJ, Whitlock RM, et al. Relation between troponin T concentration and mortality in patients presenting with an acute stroke: observational study. *BMJ.* 2000;320(7248):1502–1504.
32. Di Angelantonio E, Fiorelli M, Toni D, et al. Prognostic significance of admission levels of troponin I in patients with acute ischaemic stroke. *J Neurol Neurosurg Psychiatry.* 2005;76(1):76–81.
33. Jensen JK, Kristensen SR, Bak S, et al. Frequency and significance of troponin T elevation in acute ischemic stroke. *Am J Cardiol.* 2007;99(1):108–112.
34. Ay H, Arsava EM, Saribas O. Creatine kinase-MB elevation after stroke is not cardiac in origin: comparison with troponin T levels. *Stroke.* 2002;33(1):286–289.
35. Etgen T, Baum H, Sander K, Sander D. Cardiac troponins and N-terminal pro-brain natriuretic peptide in acute ischemic stroke do not relate to clinical prognosis. *Stroke.* 2005;36(2):270–275.
36. Hays A, Diringer MN. Elevated troponin levels are associated with higher mortality following intracerebral hemorrhage. *Neurology.* 2006;66(9):1330–1334.
37. Maramattom BV, Manno EM, Fulgham JR, Jaffe AS, Wijdicks EFM. Clinical importance of cardiac troponin release and cardiac abnormalities in patients with supratentorial cerebral hemorrhages. *Mayo Clin Proc.* 2006;81(2):192–196.

38. Horowitz M, Willet D, Keffer J. The use of cardiac troponin-I (cTnI) to determine the incidence of myocardial ischemia and injury in patients with aneurysmal and presumed aneurysmal subarachnoid hemorrhage. *Acta Neurochirurgica.* 1998;140(1):87–93.

39. Naidech AM, Kreiter KT, Janjua N, et al. Cardiac troponin elevation, cardiovascular morbidity, and outcome after subarachnoid hemorrhage. *Circulation.* 2005;112(18):2851–2856.

40. Miss JC, Kopelnik A, Fisher LA, et al. Cardiac injury after subarachnoid hemorrhage is independent of the type of aneurysm therapy. *Neurosurgery.* 2004;55(6):1244–1250; discussion 1250–1251.

41. Tanabe M, Crago EA, Suffoletto MS, et al. Relation of elevation in cardiac troponin I to clinical severity, cardiac dysfunction, and pulmonary congestion in patients with subarachnoid hemorrhage. *Am J Cardiol.* 2008;102(11):1545–1550.

42. Kim M, Kim K. Elevation of Cardiac Troponin I in the Acute Stage of Kawasaki Disease. *Pediatr Cardiol.* 1999;20(3):184–188.

43. Kim M, Kim K. Changes in cardiac troponin I in Kawasaki disease before and after treatment with intravenous gammaglobulin. *Jpn Circ J.* 1998;62(7):479–482.

44. Kanaan UB, Chiang VW. Cardiac troponins in pediatrics. *Pediatr Emerg Care.* 2004;20(5):323–329.

45. Checchia P, Borensztajn J, Shulman S. Circulating cardiac troponin I levels in Kawasaki Disease. *Pediatr Cardiol.* 2001;22(2):102–106.

46. Lim W, Cook DJ, Griffith LE, Crowther MA, Devereaux PJ. Elevated cardiac troponin levels in critically ill patients: prevalence, incidence, and outcomes. *Am J Crit Care.* 2006;15(3):280–288.

47. Ammann P, Maggiorini M, Bertel O, et al. Troponin as a risk factor for mortality in critically ill patients without acute coronary syndromes. *J Am Coll Cardiol.* 2003;41(11):2004–2009.

48. Arlati S, Brenna S, Prencipe L, et al. Myocardial necrosis in ICU patients with acute non-cardiac disease: a prospective study. *Intensive Care Med.* 2000;26(1):31–37.

49. Noble JS, Reid AM, Jordan L, Glen A, Davidson J. Troponin I and myocardial injury in the ICU. *Br. J. Anaesth.* 1999;82(1):41–46.

50. Edouard AR, Benoist JF, Cosson C, et al. Circulating cardiac troponin I in trauma patients without cardiac contusion. *Intensive Care Med.* 1998;24(6):569–573.

51. Martin M, Mullenix P, Rhee P, et al. Troponin increases in the critically injured patient: mechanical trauma or physiologic stress? *J Trauma.* 2005;59(5):1086–1091.
52. Klein Gunnewiek JMT, van de Leur JJJPM. Elevated troponin T concentrations in critically ill patients. *Intensive Care Med.* 2003;29(12):2317–2322.
53. Lim W, Qushmaq I, Devereaux PJ, et al. Elevated cardiac troponin measurements in critically ill patients. *Arch Intern Med.* 2006;166(22): 2446–2454.
54. Grasselli G, Foti G, Patroniti N, et al. Extracorporeal cardiopulmonary support for cardiogenic shock caused by pheochromocytoma: a case report and literature review. *Anesthesiology.* 2008;108(5): 959–962.
55. Cook DJ, Griffith LE, Walter SD, et al. The attributable mortality and length of intensive care unit stay of clinically important gastrointestinal bleeding in critically ill patients. *Crit Care.* 2001;5(6):368–375.
56. Iser DM, Thompson AJV, Sia KK, Yeomans ND, Chen RYM. Prospective study of cardiac troponin I release in patients with upper gastrointestinal bleeding. *J Gastroenterol Hepatol.* 2008;23(6): 938–942.
57. Vasile V, Babuin L, Perez J, et al. Long-term prognostic significance of elevated cardiac troponin levels in critically ill patients with acute gastrointestinal bleeding. *Crit Care Med.* 2009;47:140–147.
58. Wu I, Yu F, Chou J, et al. Predictive risk factors for upper gastrointestinal bleeding with simultaneous myocardial injury. *Kaohsiung J Med Sci.* 2007;23(1):8–16.
59. Hawkins BM, Abu-Fadel M, Vesely SK, George JN. Clinical cardiac involvement in thrombotic thrombocytopenic purpura: a systematic review. *Transfusion.* 2008;48(2):382–392.
60. Sane DC, Owen J. Link between ADAMTS-13 and troponin levels? *Crit Care Med.* 2008;36(10):2959–2960; author reply 2960–2961.
61. Lim W, Holinski P, Devereaux PJ, et al. Detecting myocardial infarction in critical illness using screening troponin measurements and ECG recordings. *Crit Care.* 2008;12(2):R36.
62. Gunnewiek JMTK, Van Der Hoeven JG. Cardiac troponin elevations among critically ill patients. *Curr Opin Crit Care.* 2004;10(5): 342–346.

63. Kline JA, Hernandez-Nino J, Rose GA, Norton HJ, Camargo CA. Surrogate markers for adverse outcomes in normotensive patients with pulmonary embolism. *Crit Care Med.* 2006;34(11):2773–2780.

64. Pruszczyk P, Bochowicz A, Torbicki A, et al. Cardiac troponin T monitoring identifies high-risk group of normotensive patients with acute pulmonary embolism. *Chest.* 2003;123(6):1947–1952.

65. Ghanima W, Abdelnoor M, Holmen LO, Nielssen BE, Sandset PM. The association between the proximal extension of the clot and the severity of pulmonary embolism (PE): a proposal for a new radiological score for PE. *J Intern Med.* 2007;261(1):74–81.

66. Dieter RS, Ernst E, Ende DJ, Stein JH. Diagnostic utility of cardiac troponin-I levels in patients with suspected pulmonary embolism. *Angiology.* 2002;53(5):583–585.

67. Tapson VF. Acute pulmonary embolism. *N Engl J Med.* 2008;358(10): 1037–1052.

68. Bajwa EK, Boyce PD, Januzzi JL, et al. Biomarker evidence of myocardial cell injury is associated with mortality in acute respiratory distress syndrome. *Crit Care Med.* 2007;35(11):2484–2490.

69. Snow RL, Davies P, Pontoppidan H, Zapol WM, Reid L. Pulmonary vascular remodeling in adult respiratory distress syndrome. *Am Rev Respir Dis.* 1982;126(5):887–892.

70. Punukollu G, Gowda RM, Khan IA, et al. Elevated serum cardiac troponin I in rhabdomyolysis. *Int J Cardiol.* 2004;96(1):35–40.

71. Li SF, Zapata J, Tillem E. The prevalence of false-positive cardiac troponin I in ED patients with rhabdomyolysis. *Am J Emerg Med.* 2005;23(7):860–863.

72. Bhayana V, Gougoulias T, Cohoe S, Henderson AR. Discordance between results for serum troponin T and troponin I in renal disease. *Clin Chem.* 1995;41(2):312–317.

73. Lavoinne A, Hue G. Serum cardiac troponins I and T in early posttraumatic rhabdomyolysis. *Clin Chem.* 1998;44(3):667–668.

74. Benoist J, Cosson C, Mimoz O, Edouard A. Serum cardiac troponin I, creatine kinase (CK), and CK-MB in early posttraumatic rhabdomyolysis. *Clin Chem.* 1997;43(2):416–417.

75. Maeder M, Fehr T, Rickli H, Ammann P. Sepsis-associated myocardial dysfunction: diagnostic and prognostic impact of cardiac troponins and natriuretic peptides. *Chest.* 2006;129(5):1349–1366.

76. Kalla C, Raveh D, Algur N, et al. Incidence and significance of a positive troponin test in bacteremic patients without acute coronary syndrome. *Am J Med.* 2008;121(10):909–915.

77. ver Elst KM, Spapen HD, Nguyen DN, et al. Cardiac troponins I and T are biological markers of left ventricular dysfunction in septic shock. *Clin Chem.* 2000;46(5):650–657.

78. Spies C, Haude V, Overbeck M, et al. Serum cardiac troponin T as a prognostic marker in early sepsis. *Chest.* 1998;113(4):1055–1063.

79. Mehta NJ, Khan IA, Gupta V, et al. Cardiac troponin I predicts myocardial dysfunction and adverse outcome in septic shock. *Int J Cardiol.* 2004;95(1):13–17.

80. Greaves K, Oxford JS, Price CP, Clarke GH, Crake T. The prevalence of myocarditis and skeletal muscle injury during acute viral infection in adults: measurement of cardiac troponins I and T in 152 patients with acute influenza infection. *Arch Intern Med.* 2003;163(2): 165–168.

81. Eisenhut M. Extrapulmonary manifestations of severe respiratory syncytial virus infection—a systematic review. *Crit Care.* 2006;10(4): R107.

82. Moynihan JA, Brown L, Sehra R, Checchia PA. Cardiac troponin I as a predictor of respiratory failure in children hospitalized with respiratory syncytial virus (RSV) infections: a pilot study. *Am J Emerg Med.* 2003;21(6):479–482.

83. Hsia S, Wu C, Chang J, et al. Predictors of unfavorable outcomes in enterovirus 71-related cardiopulmonary failure in children. *Pediatr Infect Dis J.* 2005;24(4):331–334.

84. Selvanayagam JB, Hawkins PN, Paul B, Myerson SG, Neubauer S. Evaluation and management of the cardiac amyloidosis. *J Am Coll Cardiol.* 2007;50(22):2101–2110.

85. Dispenzieri A, Kyle RA, Gertz MA, et al. Survival in patients with primary systemic amyloidosis and raised serum cardiac troponins. *Lancet.* 2003;361(9371):1787–1789.

86. Shah KB, Inoue Y, Mehra MR. Amyloidosis and the heart: a comprehensive review. *Arch Intern Med.* 2006;166(17):1805–1813.

87. Kristen AV, Meyer FJ, Perz JB, et al. Risk stratification in cardiac amyloidosis: novel approaches. *Transplantation.* 2005;80(1 Suppl): S151–155.

88. Miller WL, Wright RS, McGregor CG, et al. Troponin levels in patients with amyloid cardiomyopathy undergoing cardiac transplantation. *Am J Cardiol.* 2001;88(7):813–815.

89. Martorell EA, Hong C, Rust DW, et al. A 32-year-old woman with arthralgias and severe hypotension. *Arthritis Rheum.* 2008;59(11): 1670–1675.

90. Yasutake H, Seino Y, Kashiwagi M, et al. Detection of cardiac sarcoidosis using cardiac markers and myocardial integrated backscatter. *Int J Cardiol.* 2005;102(2):259–268.

91. Ranque B, Authier F, Berezne A, Guillevin L, Mouthon L. Systemic sclerosis-associated myopathy. *Ann N Y Acad Sci.* 2007;1108: 268–282.

92. Al-mashaleh M, Bak H, Moore J, Manolios N, Englert H. Resolution of sclerodermatous myocarditis after autologous stem cell transplantation. *Ann Rheum Dis.* 2006;65(9):1247–1248.

93. Badsha H, Gunes B, Grossman J, Brahn E. Troponin I assessment of cardiac involvement in patients with connective tissue disease and an elevated creatine kinase MB isoform report of four cases and review of the literature. *J Clin Rheumatol.* 1997;3(3):131.

94. Carlson ER, Percy RF, Angiolillo DJ, Conetta DA. Prognostic significance of troponin T elevation in patients without chest pain. *Am J Cardiol.* 2008;102(6):668–671.

95. Torbicki A, Kurzyna M. Pulmonary arterial hypertension: evaluation of the newly diagnosed patient. *Semin Respir Crit Care Med.* 2005;26(4):372–378.

96. Torbicki A, Kurzyna M, Kuca P, et al. Detectable serum cardiac troponin T as a marker of poor prognosis among patients with chronic precapillary pulmonary hypertension. *Circulation.* 2003;108(7): 844–848.

97. Wallace TW, Abdullah SM, Drazner MH, et al. Prevalence and determinants of troponin T elevation in the general population. *Circulation.* 2006;113(16):1958–1965.

98. Stoica SC, Cafferty F, Pauriah M, et al. The cumulative effect of acute rejection on development of cardiac allograft vasculopathy. *J Heart Lung Transplant.* 2006;25(4):420–425.

99. Schmauss D, Weis M. Cardiac allograft vasculopathy: recent developments. *Circulation.* 2008;117(16):2131–2141.

100. Balduini A, Campana C, Ceresa M, et al. Utility of biochemical markers in the follow-up of heart transplant recipients. *Transplant Proc.* 2003;35(8):3075–3178.
101. Dengler TJ, Zimmermann R, Braun K, et al. Elevated serum concentrations of cardiac troponin T in acute allograft rejection after human heart transplantation. *J Am Coll Cardiol.* 1998;32(2):405–412.
102. Wåhlander H, Kjellström C, Holmgren D. Sustained elevated concentrations of cardiac troponin T during acute allograft rejection after heart transplantation in children. *Transplantation.* 2002;74(8):1130–1135.
103. Potapov EV, Ivanitskaia EA, Loebe M, et al. Value of cardiac troponin I and T for selection of heart donors and as predictors of early graft failure. *Transplantation.* 2001;71(10):1394–1400.
104. Hoffman JIE, Kaplan S. The incidence of congenital heart disease. *J Am Coll Cardiol.* 2002;39(12):1890–1900.
105. Immer FF, Stocker F, Seiler AM, et al. Troponin-I for prediction of early postoperative course after pediatric cardiac surgery. *J Am Coll Cardiol.* 1999;33(6):1719–1723.
106. Lubitz SA, Fischer A, Fuster V. Catheter ablation for atrial fibrillation. *BMJ.* 2008;336(7648):819–826.
107. Hirose H, Kato K, Suzuki O, et al. Diagnostic accuracy of cardiac markers for myocardial damage after radiofrequency catheter ablation. *J Interv Card Electrophysiol.* 2006;16(3):169–174.
108. Haegeli LM, Kotschet E, Byrne J, et al. Cardiac injury after percutaneous catheter ablation for atrial fibrillation. *Europace.* 2008;10(3):273–275.
109. Sbarouni E, Georgiadou P, Panagiotakos D, et al. Ischaemia modified albumin in radiofrequency catheter ablation. *Europace.* 2007;9(2):127–129.
110. Madrid AH, del Rey JM, Rubí J, et al. Biochemical markers and cardiac troponin I release after radiofrequency catheter ablation: Approach to size of necrosis. *Am Heart J.* 1998;136(6):948–955.
111. Lim E, Li Choy L, Flaks L, et al. Detected troponin elevation is associated with high early mortality after lung resection for cancer. *J Cardiothorac Surg.* 2006;1:37.
112. Joglar JA, Kowal RC. Electrical cardioversion of atrial fibrillation. *Cardiol Clin.* 2004;22(1):101–111.

113. Kosior DA, Opolski G, Tadeusiak W, et al. Serum troponin I and myoglobin after monophasic versus biphasic transthoracic shocks for cardioversion of persistent atrial fibrillation. *Pacing Clin Electrophysiol.* 2005;28 (Suppl 1):S128–132.

114. Skulec R, Belohlavek J, Kovarnik T, et al. Serum cardiac markers response to biphasic and monophasic electrical cardioversion for supraventricular tachyarrhythmia—a randomised study. *Resuscitation.* 2006;70(3):423–431.

115. Allan JJ, Feld RD, Russell AA, et al. Cardiac troponin I levels are normal or minimally elevated after transthoracic cardioversion. *J Am Coll Cardiol.* 1997;30(4):1052–1056.

116. Dolci A, Dominici R, Cardinale D, Sandri MT, Panteghini M. Biochemical markers for prediction of chemotherapy-induced cardiotoxicity: systematic review of the literature and recommendations for use. *Am J Clin Pathol.* 2008;130(5):688–695.

117. Pai VB, Nahata MC. Cardiotoxicity of chemotherapeutic agents: incidence, treatment and prevention. *Drug Saf.* 2000;22(4):263–302.

118. Sandri MT, Cardinale D, Zorzino L, et al. Minor increases in plasma troponin I predict decreased left ventricular ejection fraction after high-dose chemotherapy. *Clin Chem.* 2003;49(2):248–252.

119. Schechter E, Hoffman RS, Stajic M, et al. Pulmonary edema and respiratory failure associated with clenbuterol exposure. *Am J Emerg Med.* 2007;25(6):735.e1–3.

120. Putland M, Kerr D, Kelly A. Adverse events associated with the use of intravenous epinephrine in emergency department patients presenting with severe asthma. *Ann Emerg Med.* 2006;47(6):559–563.

121. Wolff B, Machill K, Schulzki I, Schumacher D, Werner D. Acute reversible cardiomyopathy with cardiogenic shock in a patient with Addisonian crisis: a case report. *International Journal of Cardiology.* 2007;116(2):e71–e73.

122. Wallace KB, Hausner E, Herman E, et al. Serum troponins as biomarkers of drug-induced cardiac toxicity. *Toxicol Pathol.* 32(1): 106–121.

123. Bliss D, Silen M. Pediatric thoracic trauma. *Crit Care Med.* 2002;30(11 Suppl):S409–415.

124. Sybrandy KC, Cramer MJM, Burgersdijk C. Diagnosing cardiac contusion: old wisdom and new insights. *Heart.* 2003;89(5):485–489.

125. Schultz JM, Trunkey DD. Blunt cardiac injury. *Crit Care Clin.* 2004;20(1):57–70.

126. Elie M. Blunt cardiac injury. *Mt Sinai J Med.* 2006;73(2):542–552.

127. Scharhag J, George K, Shave R, Urhausen A, Kindermann W. Exercise-associated increases in cardiac biomarkers. *Med Sci Sports Exerc.* 2008;40(8):1408–1415.

128. Urhausen A, Scharhag J, Herrmann M, Kindermann W. Clinical significance of increased cardiac troponins T and I in participants of ultra-endurance events. *Am J Cardiol.* 2004;94(5):696–698.

129. Sanchez LD, Corwell B, Berkoff D. Medical problems of marathon runners. *Am J Emerg Med.* 2006;24(5):608–615.

130. Neilan TG, Januzzi JL, Lee-Lewandrowski E, et al. Myocardial injury and ventricular dysfunction related to training levels among nonelite participants in the Boston Marathon. *Circulation.* 2006;114(22): 2325–2333.

131. Tsai S, Chu S, Hsu C, Cheng S, Yang S. Use and interpretation of cardiac troponins in the ED. *Am J Emerg Med.* 2008;26(3):331–341.

132. Lalloo DG, Trevett AJ, Nwokolo N, et al. Electrocardiographic abnormalities in patients bitten by taipans (Oxyuranus scutellatus canni) and other elapid snakes in Papua New Guinea. *Trans R Soc Trop Med Hyg.* 1997;91(1):53–56.

133. Açikalin A, Gökel Y, Kuvandik G, et al. The efficacy of low-dose antivenom therapy on morbidity and mortality in snakebite cases. *Am J Emerg Med.* 2008;26(4):402–407.

134. Huynh TT, Seymour J, Pereira P, et al. Severity of Irukandji syndrome and nematocyst identification from skin scrapings. *Med J Aust.* 2003;178(1):38–41.

135. Sari I, Zengin S, Davutoglu V, Yildirim C, Gunay N. Myocarditis after black widow spider envenomation. *Am J Emerg Med.* 2008;26(5): 630.e1–630.e3.

136. Yildiz A, Biçeroglu S, Yakut N, et al. Acute myocardial infarction in a young man caused by centipede sting. *Emerg Med J.* 2006;23(4):e30.

137. Meki AAM, Mohamed ZMM, Mohey El-deen HM. Significance of assessment of serum cardiac troponin I and interleukin-8 in scorpion envenomed children. *Toxicon.* 2003;41(2):129–137.

138. Buchholz S, Rudan G. Tako-tsubo syndrome on the rise: a review of the current literature. *Postgrad Med J.* 2007;83(978):261–264.

139. Dhar S, Koul D, Subramanian S, Bakhshi M. Transient apical ballooning: sheep in wolves' garb. *Cardiol Rev.* 2007;15(3):150–153.

140. Bybee KA, Prasad A. Stress-related cardiomyopathy syndromes. *Circulation.* 2008;118(4):397–409.

141. Reuss CS, Lester SJ, Hurst RT, et al. Isolated left ventricular basal ballooning phenotype of transient cardiomyopathy in young women. *Am J Cardiol.* 2007;99(10):1451–1453.

142. Azzarelli S, Galassi AR, Amico F, et al. Clinical features of transient left ventricular apical ballooning. *Am J Cardiol.* 2006;98(9): 1273–1276.

143. Barton T. Cunninghamella bertholletiae endocarditis: a case report and review of human cunninghamella infections. *Infectious diseases in clinical practice.* 2004;12(2):114–116.

144. Dennert R, Crijns HJ, Heymans S. Acute viral myocarditis. *Eur Heart J.* 2008;29(17);2073–2082.

145. Kruse RJ, Cantor CL. Pulmonary and cardiac infections in athletes. *Clin Sports Med.* 2007;26(3):361–382.

146. Oakley CM. Myocarditis, pericarditis and other pericardial diseases. *Heart.* 2000;84(4):449–454.

147. Skouri HN, Dec GW, Friedrich MG, Cooper LT. Noninvasive imaging in myocarditis. *J Am Coll Cardiol.* 2006;48(10):2085–2093.

148. Chang Y, Chao H, Hsia S, Yan D. Myocarditis presenting as gastritis in children. *Pediatr Emerg Care.* 2006;22(6):439–440.

149. Soongswang J, Durongpisitkul K, Nana A, et al. Cardiac troponin T: a marker in the diagnosis of acute myocarditis in children. *Pediatr. Cardiol.* 2005;26(1):45–49.

150. Kamblock J, Payot L, Iung B, et al. Does rheumatic myocarditis really exist? Systematic study with echocardiography and cardiac troponin I blood levels. *Eur Heart J.* 2003;24(9):855–862.

151. Bohn D, Benson L. Diagnosis and management of pediatric myocarditis. *Paediatr Drugs.* 2002;4(3):171–181.

152. Ay H, Koroshetz WJ, Benner T, et al. Neuroanatomic correlates of stroke-related myocardial injury. *Neurology.* 2006;66(9):1325–1329.

153. Mayer SA, Brun NC, Begtrup K, et al. Efficacy and safety of recombinant activated factor VII for acute intracerebral hemorrhage. *N Engl J Med.* 2008;358(20):2127–2137.

154. Sugg RM, Gonzales NR, Matherne DE, et al. Myocardial injury in patients with intracerebral hemorrhage treated with recombinant factor VIIa. *Neurology.* 2006;67(6):1053–1055.

155. Durall AL, Phillips JR, Weisse ME, Mullett CJ. Infantile Kawasaki disease and peripheral gangrene. *J Pediatr.* 2006;149(1):131–133.

156. Barasch E, Kaushik V, Gupta R, Ronen P, Hartwell B. Elevated cardiac troponin levels do not predict adverse outcomes in hospitalized patients without clinical manifestations of acute coronary syndromes. *Cardiology.* 2000;93(1–2):1–6.

157. Fromm RE. Cardiac troponins in the intensive care unit: common causes of increased levels and interpretation. *Crit Care Med.* 2007;35(2):584–588.

158. Aksay E, Yanturali S, Kiyan S. Can elevated troponin I levels predict complicated clinical course and inhospital mortality in patients with acute pulmonary embolism? *Am J Emerg Med.* 2007;25(2):138–143.

159. Tulevski II, ten Wolde M, van Veldhuisen DJ, et al. Combined utility of brain natriuretic peptide and cardiac troponin T may improve rapid triage and risk stratification in normotensive patients with pulmonary embolism. *Int J Cardiol.* 2007;116(2):161–166.

160. Hsu JT, Chu CM, Chang ST, et al. Prognostic role of right ventricular dilatation and troponin I elevation in acute pulmonary embolism. *Int Heart J.* 2006;47(5):775–781.

161. Kucher N, Wallmann D, Carone A, et al. Incremental prognostic value of troponin I and echocardiography in patients with acute pulmonary embolism. *Eur Heart J.* 2003;24(18):1651–1656.

162. Giannitsis E, Müller-Bardorff M, Kurowski V, et al. Independent prognostic value of cardiac troponin T in patients with confirmed pulmonary embolism. *Circulation.* 2000;102(2):211–217.

163. Christenson RH. What is the value of B-type natriuretic peptide testing for diagnosis, prognosis or monitoring of critically ill adult patients in intensive care? *Clin Chem Lab Med.* 2008;46(11):1524–1532.

164. Lofberg M, Tahtela R, Harkonen M, Somer H. Myosin heavy-chain fragments and cardiac troponins in the serum in rhabdomyolysis. Diagnostic specificity of new biochemical markers. *Arch Neurol.* 1995;52(12):1210–1214.

165. Favory R, Neviere R. Significance and interpretation of elevated troponin in septic patients. *Crit Care.* 2006;10(4):224.

166. Blum JA, Zellweger MJ, Burri C, Hatz C. Cardiac involvement in African and American trypanosomiasis. *Lancet Infect Dis.* 2008;8(10):631–641.

167. Quenot J, Le Teuff G, Quantin C, et al. Myocardial injury in critically ill patients: relation to increased cardiac troponin I and hospital mortality. *Chest.* 2005;128(4):2758–2764.

168. Eisenhut M, Sidaras D, Johnson R, Newland P, Thorburn K. Cardiac troponin T levels and myocardial involvement in children with severe respiratory syncytial virus lung disease. *Acta Paediatr.* 2004;93(7):887–890.

169. Schoeffler M, Wallet F, Robert M, et al. Élévation de troponine I à coronarographie normale chez un patient porteur d'une myopathie de Duchenne. *Annales Françaises d'Anesthésie et de Réanimation.* 2008;27(4):345–347.

170. El-Khuffash A, Davis PG, Walsh K, Molloy EJ. Cardiac troponin T and N-terminal-pro-B type natriuretic peptide reflect myocardial function in preterm infants. *J Perinatol.* 2008;28(7):482–486.

171. Cruz M, Bremmer Y, Porter B, et al. Cardiac troponin T and cardiac dysfunction in extremely low-birth-weight infants. *Pediatr Cardiol.* 2006;27(4):396–401.

172. Zhu B, Oritani S, Quan L, et al. Two suicide fatalities from sodium cyanide ingestion: differences in blood biochemistry. *Chudoku Kenkyu.* 2004;17(1):65–68.

173. Brvar M, Ploj T, Kozelj G, et al. Case report: fatal poisoning with Colchicum autumnale. *Crit Care.* 2004;8(1):R56–59.

174. Teksam O, Gumus P, Bayrakci B, Erdogan I, Kale G. 103: Acute cardiac effects of carbon monoxide poisoning in children. *Ann of Emerg Med.* 2008;51(4):502.

175. Yalamanchili C, Smith MD. Acute hydrogen sulfide toxicity due to sewer gas exposure. *Am J Emerg Med.* 2008;26(4):518.e5–518.e7.

176. Teoh DCA, Williams DL. Adult Klippel-Feil syndrome: haemodynamic instability in the prone position and postoperative respiratory failure. *Anaesth Intensive Care.* 2007;35(1):124–127.

177. Kanter RJ, Graham M, Fairbrother D, Smith SV. Sudden cardiac death in young children with neurofibromatosis type 1. *J Pediatr.* 2006;149(5):718–720.

178. Bozbas H, Yildirir A, Muderrisoglu H. Cardiac enzymes, renal failure and renal transplantation. *Clin Med Res.* 2006;4(1):79–84.

179. Potluri S, Ventura HO, Mulumudi M, Mehra MR. Cardiac troponin levels in heart failure. *Cardiol Rev.* 2004;12(1):21–25.

180. Kato T, Sato Y, Nagao K, et al. Serum cardiac troponin T in cardiac amyloidosis: serial observations in five patients. *Tohoku J Exp Med.* 2006;208(2):163–167.

181. Suhr OB, Anan I, Backman C, et al. Do troponin and B-natriuretic peptide detect cardiomyopathy in transthyretin amyloidosis? *J Intern Med.* 2008;263(3):294–301.

182. Cantwell RV, Aviles RJ, Bjornsson J, et al. Cardiac amyloidosis presenting with elevations of cardiac troponin I and angina pectoris. *Clin Cardiol.* 2002;25(1):33–37.

183. Gall NP, Murgatroyd FD. Electrical cardioversion for AF—the state of the art. *Pacing Clin Electrophysiol.* 2007;30(4):554–567.

184. Cemin R, Rauhe W, Marini M, Pescoller F, Pitscheider W. Serum troponin I level after external electrical direct current synchronized cardioversion in patients with normal or reduced ejection fraction: no evidence of myocytes injury. *Clin Cardiol.* 2005;28(10):467–470.

185. Zangrillo A, Landoni G, Crescenzi G, et al. A 20-joule electrical cardioversion applied directly to the heart elevates troponin I by at least 1.5 ng.mL–1. *Can J Anaesth.* 2005;52(3):336–337.

186. Boriani G, Biffi M, Cervi V, et al. Evaluation of myocardial injury following repeated internal atrial shocks by monitoring serum cardiac troponin I levels. *Chest.* 2000;118(2):342–347.

187. Piechota W, Gielerak G, Ryczek R, et al. Cardiac troponin I after external electrical cardioversion for atrial fibrillation as a marker of myocardial injury—a preliminary report. *Kardiol Pol.* 2007;65(6):664–669; discussion 670–671.

188. Baum VC. Cardiac trauma in children. *Paediatr Anaesth.* 2002;12(2):110–117.

189. Kaye P, O'Sullivan I. Myocardial contusion: emergency investigation and diagnosis. *Emerg Med J.* 2002;19(1):8–10.

190. Bertinchant JP, Polge A, Mohty D, et al. Evaluation of incidence, clinical significance, and prognostic value of circulating cardiac troponin I and T elevation in hemodynamically stable patients with

suspected myocardial contusion after blunt chest trauma. *J Trauma.* 2000;48(5):924–931.

191. Hirsch R, Landt Y, Porter S, et al. Cardiac troponin I in pediatrics: normal values and potential use in the assessment of cardiac injury. *J Pediatr.* 1997;130(6):872–877.
192. Maenza RL, Seaberg D, D'Amico F. A meta-analysis of blunt cardiac trauma: Ending myocardial confusion. *Am J Emerg Med.* 1996;14(3): 237–241.
193. Sanchez LD, Pereira J, Berkoff DJ. The evaluation of cardiac complaints in marathon runners. *J Emerg Med.* 2009;36(4):369–376.
194. Auer J, Punzengruber C, Berent R, Porodko M, Eber B. Elevated cardiac troponin I following heavy-resistance exercise in ostium secundum type-atrial septal defect. *Chest.* 2001;120(5):1752–1753.
195. McD Taylor D, Pereira P, Seymour J, Winkel KD. A sting from an unknown jellyfish species associated with persistent symptoms and raised troponin I levels. *Emerg Med (Fremantle).* 2002;14(2): 175–180.

9 ▪ Use of Cardiac Necrosis Biomarkers Following PCI or CABG

Evangelos Giannitsis, MD
Hugo A. Katus, MD

Introduction

Cardiac troponin I (cTnI) and T (cTnT) are highly sensitive and specific markers of myocardial damage and are regarded as the biochemical gold standard for the diagnosis of myocardial infarction in patients presenting with an acute coronary syndrome.[1] In suspected acute coronary syndrome, the use of cardiac enzymes, such as Creatine Kinase (CK) or CK-MB activities, is no longer recommended. For other purposes, such as assessment of perioperative risk, traditionally CK-MB was used for many years. Therefore, most information on the prognostic role of cardiac markers following cardiac procedures is available for CK-MB, and less so for cTn. Cardiac troponins have the advantage of being exclusively cardio-specific, thus giving a more reliable estimate of myocardial necrosis than CK-MB, which may be released after skeletal muscle damage as well.[2] Therefore, in patients undergoing noncardiac surgery, any increase in cTn above the 99th percentile should be considered as a perioperative myocardial infarction.

The problem is more complex in patients undergoing cardiac surgery with cardiopulmonary bypass (CPB) and after percutaneous coronary intervention (PCI) because an elevation of cardiac biomarkers occurs after virtually every cardiac surgery and in up to 10–69% of cases after elective PCI.[3] In this chapter, an overview is given on the utility of cardiac necrosis biomarkers following PCI and coronary artery bypass graft (CABG) surgery.

Cardiac Biomarkers Following Elective PCI

In an overview of 60 studies, Herrmann et al. showed that elevated levels of biomarkers after PCI are seen in up to 69% of patients.[3]

Table 9–1: Predictors of large troponin I elevations following PCI adapted after Nallamothu BK, et al.[18]

Clinical predictor	HR	95% CI	*P* value
Thrombus present	3.0	1.3–6.5	0.007
Abrupt vessel closure	8.0	2.3–27.9	0.001
No reflow	4.5	1.3–15.5	0.016
Perforation	6.4	1.1–37.0	0.04
Side branch occlusion	7.9	2.6–323.9	<0.001

HR = hazard ratio; CI = confidence interval

Average rates of periprocedural biomarker elevations were 23% for CK-MB and cTnT, and 27% for cTnI. The association between PCI and subsequent myonecrosis has been recognized for many years. It is also clear that delivery of a coronary stent, use of directional atherectomy, or rotablation causes higher rates of postprocedural cTn elevations than elective balloon angioplasty,[4] sometimes as high as 69%. Table 9–1 compiles factors that increase the propensity of PCI-related elevation of cardiac biomarkers, including: intervention of more complex lesion, multivessel disease; interventions on a saphenous vein graft; higher thrombotic burden or thrombus embolization; side branch occlusion; transient vessel closure; or other procedural complications, such as prolonged balloon inflation and severe dissection.[5–10] In principle, the reasons for CK-MB elevation are the same as for cTn elevations. However, due to the higher diagnostic sensitivity, the prevalence of elevated cTn is higher than the prevalence of CK-MB within the same study populations.[10,11]

Postprocedural Elevations and Outcomes

Many studies have demonstrated a consistent association between elevations of CK-MB and short- and long-term outcomes. The reason for this hazard is unclear. It has been speculated that cardiac marker release is a surrogate of coronary atheroma burden or complexity of the coronary lesion,[10] evolving left ventricular failure, and electrophysiologic destabilization due to microvascular dysfunction. Kugelmass et al.[9] showed that PCI complicated by a CK-MB increase of more than 5 times the upper limit of normal (ULN) was associated with higher mortality at two years. Abdelmeguid et al. confirmed this observation and found that even lower elevations of more than 1 to 2 times ULN were prognostically relevant.[6] This observation was supported by a cohort study on more than 8000 patients.[12] Ellis et al. demonstrated that CK-MB elevations to any level higher than reference range increased the risk of death after PCI, particularly elevations of more than 5 times higher than reference. A recent meta-analysis of seven studies with CK-MB measurements and survival outcomes on 23,230 subjects who underwent PCI ultimately demonstrated beyond doubt that any increase in CK-MB levels after PCI was associated with a small, but statistically and clinically significant, increase in the subsequent risk of death.[13]

Mechanistically, however, the cause of necrosis marker elevation following PCI remains unclear and is likely multifactorial. Using contrast-enhanced magnetic resonance imaging, Ricciardi et al. found an association between elevations of CK-MB and either side branch occlusion or embolization to the vascular bed, leading to myocardial necrosis.[14] All patients with CK-MB elevation had discrete hyperenhancement in the target vessel perfusion territory. Two different patterns of myonecrosis were prevalent in that study. In the first pattern (three patients), the necrotic tissue was immediately adjacent to the implanted stent, whereas the second pattern demonstrated that the necrotic tissue was located more distally in the myocardium subtended by the stented artery (six patients). Thus, the MRI data support two pathways by which myonecrosis occurs after successful PCI: incidental minor side-branch occlusion or microvascular obstruction from distal embolization of plaque contents, including platelets, thrombus, and/or atheroma (Figure 9–1).

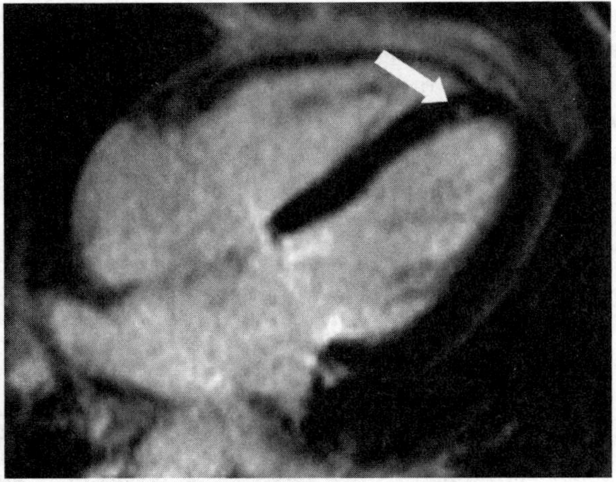

■ **Figure 9–1** Contrast-enhanced MRI scan showing discrete subendocardial late hyperenhancement located in the lateral wall (arrow) following elective PCI.

Troponin release is a more sensitive indicator of myocardial necrosis than elevations of CK-MB.[10,11] Accordingly, elevations of cardiac troponin have been reported following PCI in up to 69% of cases, depending on technique used.[3] The prognostic role of postprocedural elevation of cTn following elective PCI has been investigated less extensively, and studies investigating the association between postprocedural cTn concentration and outcomes are inconsistent. There are studies that have shown no significant relationship between cardiac troponin and long-term outcome.[11,15,16] In a study on 2873 patients undergoing PCI, Kini et al. demonstrated that a CK-MB elevation greater than 5 times normal, but not any level of cTnI, predicted mortality at 12 months.[10] In a study on 1129 patients undergoing elective PCI, Fuchs et al. found that a TnI elevation greater than three times the upper normal limit (>0.45 ng/ml) was a strong independent predictor of major in-hospital complications and was associated with lower procedural success, but not with an increased rate of later clinical events up to eight months.[15] Conversely, Ricciardi et al. demonstrated that a threefold elevation of TnI was independently predictive of future cardiac events for up to one year, primarily repeat revascularization in the first 30 days after the index PCI.[17] cTnI elevations were associated with procedural side branch occlusion and thrombus formation. In a study on 2796 consecutive cases of elective PCI, Nallamothu et al. demonstrated that troponin I elevations occurred often after PCI, with abnormal levels documented in 29% of patients, and large troponin I elevations (≥8x normal) in 6.5% of cases.[18] These large troponin I elevations (≥8x normal) were associated with decreased long-term survival, whereas smaller increases in troponin I were not associated with increased mortality. Many discrepancies may be explained by heterogeneity of study populations, different inclusion criteria, small numbers of patients, low rates of events, and different sensitivities and specificities of various cTn assays.

More recently, Prasad et al. investigated a mixed cohort of 5487 patients undergoing PCI for either stable coronary artery disease or acute coronary syndromes.[19] The authors found that 37% of all patients had preprocedural elevation of cTnT using the 99th percentile as the ULN. This percentage was surprisingly high given that CK-MB values prior to PCIs were in the normal range in the majority of patients with preprocedural cTnT values up to 0.1 ng/mL. These low-level preprocedural, but not postprocedural, elevations of cTnT were independently predictive of long-term adverse outcomes. In addition, CK-MB fraction elevation of more than five- to eightfold after PCI was extremely infrequent in patients with normal preprocedural cTnT. Consistently, Kizer and colleagues confirmed the predictive value on long-term adverse events associated with pre- but not postprocedural cTnT elevation in a small study with 212 patients.[20] However, a much less sensitive cutoff (>0.1 ng/mL) was used to diagnose myonecrosis. In the Evaluation of Drug Eluting Stents and Ischemic Events registry on 7592 patients undergoing elective PCI, Jeremias et al. found that baseline elevation of cTn was relatively common among patients with stable coronary artery disease and was an independent prognostic indicator of ischemic complications.[21] Of the 2382 patients who underwent PCI for stable coronary artery disease (CAD), 6% had a baseline cTn level above the ULN. These patients were found to have a 2.1-fold higher adjusted risk for the composite of death or MI at hospital discharge and a twofold higher adjusted risk at one year. Thus, preprocedural elevation of cTn may be more relevant than that of postprocedural. This hazard may be through the association of complex coronary anatomy, higher rates of intracoronary thrombus, difficult-to-treat lesions, and high-risk interventions with long-term outcomes associated with this preprocedural elevation.[22,23]

Diagnosis of PCI-Related MI

The diagnosis of periprocedural myocardial infarction following PCI is relatively straightforward, as the mechanism of PCI-related myocardial necrosis is ischemia. Consistently, Johansen et al. were able to demonstrate that the majority of cTnT elevations after PCI persisted for at least 96 hours, indicating ongoing release of cTnT from the contractile apparatus reflecting irreversible myocardial injury.[24] In contrast-enhanced cardiac MRI, areas of myocardial infarction were identified as the substrate of minor serum marker elevations.[14,25] Ricciardi et al. used contrast-enhanced MRI and demonstrated that even mild elevation of CK-MB levels after PCI is the result of discrete microinfarction.[14] All patients with CK-MB level elevations had discrete hyperenhancement in the target vessel perfusion territory.

There is currently no solid scientific basis for defining a biomarker threshold for the diagnosis of periprocedural myocardial infarction. In the universal definition of myocardial infarction, by arbitrary convention, it was suggested to label increases of more than three times the 99th percentile as PCI-related myocardial infarction.[1] Two subtypes are further distinguished according to whether a bare metal stent (BMS) or a drug-eluting stent (type

IVb) is being used to acknowledge different pathomechanisms of disease, e.g., restenosis with BMS, as opposed to subacute or late stent thrombosis with drug eluting stents.

Cardiac Biomarkers Following PCI in Patients with NSTE-ACS

Interpretation of postprocedural troponin elevation is problematic in patients with non-ST segment elevation acute coronary syndromes (NSTE-ACS) because it is difficult to demonstrate conclusively that postprocedural troponin release is only the result of the intervention, rather than a reflection of the acute disease itself. If cardiac troponin is elevated before the procedure and not stable for at least two samples 6 hours apart, there are insufficient data to recommend biomarker criteria for the diagnosis of periprocedural myocardial infarction.[26] If the values are stable or falling, criteria for reinfarction by further measurement of biomarkers together with ECG criteria can be applied.

With these caveats in mind, Fuchs et al. evaluated 132 patients with NSTE MI who underwent PCI more than 48 hours after admission.[27] Patients with TnI re-elevation had significantly higher in-hospital mortality (9.8% versus 0%; $P = 0.016$) and a higher 6-month cumulative death rate (24% versus 3.7%; $P = 0.001$) than those without re-elevation. In a prospective substudy of the SYMPHONY (Sibrafiban Versus Aspirin to Yield Maximum Protection from Ischemic Heart Events Post-acute Coronary Syndromes) and second SYMPHONY trials, which randomized patients with NSTE-ACS to receive aspirin or sibrafiban, biomarkers of myocardial damage were measured in 481 patients undergoing PCI.[28] Patients with postprocedural troponin elevation were at increased risk for death or MI at 90 days of follow-up (10.6% versus 4.2%; $P = 0.005$). In an analysis of 6164 patients from the GUSTO-IIb (Global Use of Strategies to Open Occluded Coronary Arteries IIb), PURSUIT (Platelet Glycoprotein IIb/IIIa in Unstable Angina: Receptor Suppression Using Integrilin Therapy), and PARAGON (Platelet IIb/IIIa Antagonism for the Reduction of

Acute Coronary Syndrome Events in a Global Organization Network International) A and B trials, undergoing PCI during the initial hospitalization to assess the impact of periprocedural CK-MB elevations on clinical outcomes, a significant relationship was found between peak CK-MB elevation after PCI and an increased risk of adverse outcomes.[29] The negative prognostic impact of periprocedural myocardial damage persisted after adjustment for angiographic and procedural factors. Previous angiography studies have shown that patients with NSTE-ACS and an elevated troponin level on presentation have more extensive coronary artery disease and more complex lesions, and more often demonstrate impaired thrombolysis in MI (TIMI) flow and thrombi at the site of a culprit lesion than those without elevated troponin levels.[22,23] Okamatsu et al.,[23] using coronary angioscopy, found the presence of a coronary thrombus to be the only independent factor that distinguished between troponin-positive and troponin-negative patients (88% versus 37%; $P < 0.0005$), even when the incidence of complex plaque was equally high in the two groups (64% versus 68%; $P = 0.77$). Furthermore, impaired tissue level perfusion was associated with biomarker release in patients with NSTE-ACS.[30,31]

Cardiac Biomarkers Following CABG

It has been demonstrated that patients undergoing cardiac surgery often release a significant amount of CK-MB and cTn in the absence of clear complication. Numerous factors can lead to periprocedural necrosis, including direct trauma due to sewing needles or manipulation of the heart, coronary dissection, global or regional ischemia, inadequate cardiac protection, reperfusion injury, and early graft or native vessel occlusion.[32,33] With transmural damage suggesting a graft or native vessel occlusion, concentrations of cTn or CK-MB are usually higher.[33] Nevertheless, a study using angiography to identify primary vessel occlusion found a substantial overlap between the values in patients with graft occlusion as compared to those without, thus limiting the role of CK-MB or cTn to define a primary vascular event by the biomarker result only.

The Prognostic Role of CK-MB Following CABG

The relationship between the magnitude of cardiac serum protein elevation and subsequent mortality after CABG is well established. Two large prospective trials evaluated the impact of the degree of CK-MB elevation on subsequent outcomes. In a trial of 2918 patients with high-risk features to develop myocardial necrosis,[34] after adjustment for ejection fraction, congestive heart failure, cerebrovascular disease, peripheral vascular disease, cardiac arrhythmias and the method of cardioplegia delivery, CK-MB remained a strong and independent predictor of mortality at six months. The optimal cutpoint for prediction of mortality at six months was found with CK-MB ratios between 5 to 10 times ULN, whereas CK-MB ratios above 10 times ULN predicted myocardial infarction. In another study, an elevation of CK-MB was seen in two-thirds of all patients whereas 38.1% had CK-MB within normal range.[32] An elevation of CK-MB greater than 1–3x ULN was found in 42.9%, greater than 3–5x ULN in 7.5%, and greater than 5x ULN in 11.5% of patients. Those with elevated CK-MB levels, particularly those with levels greater than five times normal, were at higher risk of death or myocardial infarction compared with those with normal or mild cardiac enzyme elevation. Another meta-analysis of four studies including 26,465 patients with NSTE ACS undergoing CABG within 30 days demonstrated that CK-MB was an independent predictor of 6-month mortality after adjustment for multiple confounders.[35]

Prognostic Role of Cardiac Troponins Following CABG

In contrast to the data pertaining to CK-MB, the studies assessing the prognostic utility of cardiac troponin levels after cardiac surgery have been relatively small with limited duration of follow-up. As cardiac troponin is commonly elevated, it is difficult to determine which degree of elevation is abnormal. Release of

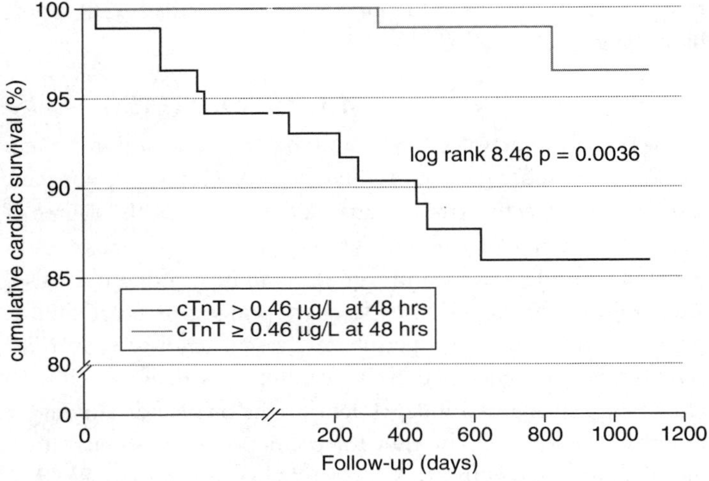

■ **Figure 9–2** Effect of the type of cardiac surgery on postoperative cTn release.

troponin is influenced by multiple variables, including the nature of the operation (Figure 9–2).

Therefore, a troponin level in the lowest quartile for valve surgery may have very different connotations if found in a patient after single-vessel CABG. Therefore, it is difficult to establish universally acceptable cutpoints for troponins, and prognostic data in most studies were related to percentiles. Still, data on the prognostic role of postoperative cTn elevation are controversial. However, an accumulating number of studies have conferred substantial evidence on the usefulness of cTn testing following CABG.[36–38] In a study of 224 consecutive patients undergoing a range of cardiac surgical procedures, Januzzi and colleagues have demonstrated that cardiac cTnT levels in the upper quintile were significant independent predictors of in-hospital complications.[36] In this study they also demonstrated that cTnT levels were superior for risk prediction to CK-MB. This superior prognostic performance regarding one-year outcome was later confirmed by the same authors in 136 patients who underwent isolated CABG.[37] A value of cTnT above 1.58 ng/ml from a specimen 18 to 24 hours after CABG was the strongest predictor of one-year mortality (5.45-fold higher risk, $P < 0.0001$), whereas CK-MB added no independent prognostic information.[36,37] Consistently, in a study published by Lehrke et al. on 204 patients undergoing a range of elective cardiac surgery who received serial blood sampling for seven consecutive days, a cTnT concentration of greater than 0.46 µg/L at 48 hours (determined using receiver operator characteristic curve analysis) after cardiac surgery (Figure 9–3) was an independent predictor of mortality.[33] Higher concentrations of cTnT were associated with new ECG changes, such as new Q-waves or new appearance of left bundle branch block, suggesting more extensive myocardial infarction. More recently, the prognostic role of cTn was confirmed in a large study enrolling 1365 patients. cTnI levels measured at 24 hours were independently predictive of

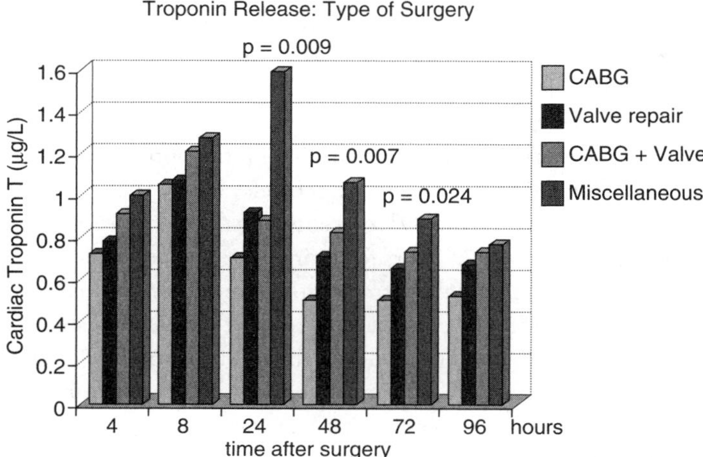

■ **Figure 9–3** Assocation between postoperative cTnT (>0.48 µg/L) increase and outcomes.

mortality at 30 days, one year, and three years.[38] The size of this trial allowed for adjustment with multiple confounders, thus establishing the prognostic role of cTn further. Whatever the various mechanisms for the postoperative cTn release in cardiac surgery may be, it has been shown that cTn elevation is an independent predictor of short- and long-term adverse outcome in cardiac surgical patients.

Biomarkers for Diagnosis of Perioperative Myocardial Infarction

Unlike the prognosis, very little information is available regarding the use of biomarkers for defining myocardial infarction in the setting of CABG. Recently, several small studies have evaluated patients with MRI after bypass surgery. These studies demonstrated that nearly 50% of post-CABG patients had late hyperenhancement on scans made six days after surgery.[39,40] In another MRI study, the magnitude of CK-MB elevation correlated positively with the infarct size.[41] More than half of the patients showed evidence of transmural or focal endocardial injury rather than patchy necrosis. These data support the hypothesis that the observed CK-MB elevations after CABG are likely not due only to cardiac manipulation or incomplete cardioplegia, but that isolated myocardial necrosis is also contributory.

The universal definition of myocardial infarction defines postoperative infarction following CABG by elevations of a cTn value more than five times the 99th percentile of the normal reference range during the first 72 hours following CABG; when patients are above this risk, a 5.45-fold increase in risk for adverse outcome is observed. This recommended cutoff may be problematically low unless combined with clinical variables. Myocardial infarction should only be considered when associated in conjunction with the appearance of new pathological Q-waves or new LBBB, an angiographically-documented new graft or native coronary artery occlusion, or imaging evidence of a new loss of viable myocardium. This recommendation is partly based on a previous consensus, which considered the adverse prognostic impact of biomarker elevation.[42]

Cardiac Biomarkers for Monitoring of Therapy and Outcomes

Patients with increased levels of cTn after CABG may merit more intensive monitoring during the index hospitalization and increased scrutiny for ischemic complications after discharge. As well, future efforts to "limit" release of cTn following surgery may be feasible: there is evidence that on-pump CABG is associated with higher cardiac enzyme release than off-pump CABG, and blood cardioplegia provides superior myocardial protection, as compared with crystalloid cardioplegia.[43] Thus, evaluation of postoperative cTn or CK-MB level after surgery may be useful to evaluate strategies and techniques to prevent or minimize myocardial necrosis.

References

1. Thygesen K, Alpert JS, White HD, et al., on behalf of the Joint ESC/ACCF/AHA/WHF Task Force for the redefinition of myocardial infarction. Universal definition of myocardial infarction. *Eur Heart J.* 2007;28:2525–2538.
2. Katus HA, Remppis A, Neumann FJ, et al. Diagnostic efficiency of troponin T measurements in acute myocardial infarction. *Circulation.* 1991;83:902–912.
3. Herrmann J. Peri-procedural myocardial injury: 2005 update. *Eur Heart J.* 2005;26:2493–2519.
4. Giannitsis E, von Lippa I, Müller Bardorff M, Wiegand U, Kübler W, Katus HA. Troponin T elevation after successful directional atherectomy. *Z Kardiol.* 2001;90:401–407.
5. Abbas SA, Glazier JJ, Wu AH, et al. Factors associated with the release of cardiac troponin T following percutaneous transluminal coronary angioplasty. *Clin Cardiol.* 1996;19:782–786.
6. Abdelmeguid AE, Topol EJ, Whitlow PL, et al. Significance of mild transient release of creatine kinase-MB fraction after percutaneous coronary interventions. *Circulation.* 1996;94:1528–1536.

7. Ravkilde J, Nissen H, Mickley H, et al. Cardiac troponin T and CK-MB mass release after visually successful percutaneous transluminal coronary angioplasty in stable angina pectoris. *Am Heart J.* 1994;127:13–20.
8. Karim MA, Shinn M, Oskarsson H, et al. Significance of cardiac troponin T release after percutaneous transluminal coronary angioplasty. *Am J Cardiol.* 1995;76:521–523.
9. Kugelmass AD, Cohen DJ, Moscucci M, et al. Elevation of the creatine kinase myocardial isoform following otherwise successful directional coronary atherectomy and stenting. *Am J Cardiol.* 1994;74:748–754.
10. Kini AS, Lee P, Marmur JD, et al. Correlation of postpercutaneous coronary intervention creatine kinase-MB and troponin I elevation in predicting mid-term mortality. *Am J Cardiol.* 2004;93:18–23.
11. Cavallini C, Savonitto S, Violini R, et al. Impact of the elevation of biochemical markers of myocardial damage on long-term mortality after percutaneous coronary intervention: results of the CK-MB and PCI study. *Eur Heart J.* 2005;26:1494–1498.
12. Ellis SG, Chew D, Chan A, et al. Death following creatine kinase-MB elevation after coronary intervention: identification of an early risk period: importance of creatine kinase-MB level, completeness of revascularization, ventricular function, and probable benefit of statin therapy. *Circulation.* 2002;106:1205–1210.
13. Ioannidis J, Karvouni E, Katritsis D. Mortality risk conferred by small elevations of creatine kinase-MB isoenzyme after percutaneous coronary intervention. *J Am Coll Cardiol.* 2003;42:1406–1411.
14. Ricciardi MJ, Wu E, Davidson CJ, et al. Visualization of discrete microinfarction after percutaneous coronary intervention associated with mild creatine kinase-MB elevation. *Circulation.* 2001;103:2780–2783.
15. Fuchs S, Kornowski R, Mehran R, et al. Prognostic value of cardiac troponin-I levels following catheter-based coronary interventions. *Am J Cardiol.* 2000;85:1077–1082.
16. Bertinchant JP, Polge A, Ledermann B, et al. Relation of minor cardiac troponin I elevation to late cardiac events after uncomplicated elective successful percutaneous transluminal coronary angioplasty for angina pectoris. *Am J Cardiol.* 1999;84:51–57.
17. Ricciardi MJ, Davidson CJ, Gubernikoff G, et al. Troponin I elevation and cardiac events after percutaneous coronary intervention. *Am Heart J.* 2003;145:522–528.

18. Nallamothu BK, Bates ER. Periprocedural myocardial infarction and mortality: causality versus association. *J Am Coll Cardiol.* 2003;42: 1412–1414.

19. Prasad A, Rihal CS, Lennon RJ, Singh M, Jaffe AS, Holmes DR Jr. Significance of periprocedural myonecrosis on outcomes after percutaneous coronary intervention: an analysis of preintervention and postintervention troponin T levels in 5487 patients. *Circ Cardiovasc Intervent.* In press.

20. Kizer JR, Muttrej MR, Matthai WH, et al. Role of cardiac troponin T in the long-term risk stratification of patients undergoing percutaneous coronary intervention. *Eur Heart J.* 2003;24:1314–1322.

21. Jeremias A, Kleiman NS, Nassif D, et al., for the EVENT Registry Investigators. Prevalence and prognostic significance of preprocedural cardiac troponin elevation among patients with stable coronary artery disease undergoing percutaneous coronary intervention: results from the Evaluation of Drug Eluting Stents and Ischemic Events Registry. *Circulation.* 2008;118:632–637.

22. Okamatsu K, Takano M, Sakai S et al. Elevated troponin T levels and lesion characteristics in non-ST-elevation acute coronary syndromes. *Circulation.* 2004;109:465–470.

23. Frey N, Dietz A, Kurowski V, et al. Angiographic correlates of a positive troponin T test in patients with unstable angina. *Crit Care Med.* 2001;29:1130–1136.

24. Johansen O, Brekke M, Stromme JH, et al. Myocardial damage during percutaneous transluminal coronary angioplasty as evidenced by troponin T measurements. *Eur Heart J.* 1998;19:112–117.

25. Selvanayagam JB, Porto I, Channon K, et al. Troponin elevation after percutaneous coronary intervention directly represents the extent of irreversible myocardial injury: insights from cardiovascular magnetic resonance imaging. *Circulation.* 2005;111:1027–1032.

26. Miller WL, Garratt KN, Burritt MF, Lennon RJ, Reeder GS, Jaffe AS. Baseline troponin level: key to understanding the importance of post-PCI troponin elevations. *Eur Heart J.* 2006;27:1061–1069.

27. Fuchs S, Gruberg L, Singh S, et al. Prognostic value of cardiac troponin I re-elevation following percutaneous coronary intervention in high-risk patients with acute coronary syndromes. *Am J Cardiol.* 2001;88:129–133.

28. Cantor WJ, Newby LK, Christenson RH, et al. Prognostic significance of elevated troponin I after percutaneous coronary intervention. *J Am Coll Cardiol.* 2002;39:1738–1744.

29. Roe MT, Mahaffey KW, Kilaru R, et al. Creatine kinase-MB elevation after percutaneous coronary intervention predicts adverse outcomes in patients with acute coronary syndromes. *Eur Heart J.* 2004;25: 313–321.

30. Wong GC, Morrow DA, Murphy S, et al. Elevations in troponin T and I are associated with abnormal tissue level perfusion: a TACTICS-TIMI 18 substudy. *Circulation.* 2002;106:202–207.

31. Bolognese L, Ducci K, Angioli P, et al. Elevations in troponin I after percutaneous coronary interventions are associated with abnormal tissue-level perfusion in high-risk patients with non-ST-segment-elevation acute coronary syndromes. *Circulation.* 2004;110:1592–1597.

32. Costa MA, Carere RG, Lichtenstein SV, et al. Incidence, predictors, and significance of abnormal cardiac enzyme rise in patients treated with bypass surgery in the arterial revascularization therapies study (ARTS). *Circulation.* 2001;104:2689–2693.

33. Lehrke S, Steen H, Sievers HH, et al. Cardiac troponin T for prediction of short- and long-term morbidity and mortality after elective open heart surgery. *Clin Chem.* 2004;50:1560–1567.

34. Klatte K, Chaitman BR, Theroux P, et al.; GUARDIAN Investigators (The GUARD during Ischemia Against Necrosis). Increased mortality after coronary artery bypass graft surgery is associated with increased levels of postoperative creatine kinase-myocardial band isoenzyme release: results from the GUARDIAN trial. *J Am Coll Cardiol.* 2001;38:1070–1077.

35. Mahaffey KW, Roe MT, Kilaru R, et al. Creatine kinase-MB elevation after coronary artery bypass grafting surgery in patients with non-ST-segment elevation acute coronary syndromes predict worse outcomes: results from four large clinical trials. *Eur Heart J.* 2007;28:425–432.

36. Januzzi JL, Lewandrowski K, MacGillivray TE, et al. A comparison of cardiac troponin T and creatine kinase-MB for patient evaluation after cardiac surgery. *J Am Coll Cardiol* 2002;39:1518–1523.

37. Kathiresan S, Servoss SJ, Newell JB, et al. Cardiac troponin T elevation after coronary artery bypass grafting is associated with increased one-year mortality. *Am J Cardiol.* 2004;94:879–881.

38. Croal BL, Hillis GS, Gibson PH, et al. Relationship between postoperative cardiac troponin I levels and outcome of cardiac surgery. *Circulation*. 2006;114:1468–1475.

39. Selvanayagam JB, Kardos A, Francis JM, et al. Value of delayed-enhancement cardiovascular magnetic resonance imaging in predicting myocardial viability after surgical revascularization. *Circulation*. 2004;110:1535–1541.

40. Selvanayagam JB, Petersen SE, Francis JM, et al. Effects of off-pump versus on-pump coronary surgery on reversible and irreversible myocardial injury: a randomized trial using cardiovascular magnetic resonance imaging and biochemical markers. *Circulation*. 2004;109:345–350.

41. Steuer J, Bjerner T, Duvernoy, et al. Visualisation and quantification of peri-operative myocardial infarction after coronary artery bypass surgery with contrast-enhanced magnetic resonance imaging. *Eur Heart J*. 2004;25:1293–1299.

42. Califf RM, Abdelmeguid AE, Kuntz RE, et al. Myonecrosis after revascularization procedures. *J Am Coll Cardiol*. 1998;31:241–251.

43. Guru V, Omura J, Alghamdi AA, Weisel R, Fremes SE. Is blood superior to crystalloid cardioplegia? A meta-analysis of randomized clinical trials. *Circulation*. 2006;114(1 Suppl):I331–I338.

10 ▪ Emerging Biomarkers in Acute Coronary Syndromes

Nitin K. Gupta, MD
James A. De Lemos, MD

Introduction

Cardiac troponins (cTn) play a pivotal role in modern diagnosis, risk assessment, and selection of therapy for patients with suspected acute coronary syndromes (ACS). Although troponins have appropriately emerged as the preferred biomarkers for use in ACS, they have several limitations. First, although they are very specific for cardiomyocyte necrosis, they are unable to differentiate ischemia from other mechanisms of injury. Second, troponins are only released when injury is irreversible. Therefore, they are unable to detect acutely ruptured atherosclerotic plaques, myocardium at risk for imminent ischemic injury, or ischemia without necrosis (i.e., unstable angina). Third, troponins alone fail to completely characterize risk among patients with ACS, likely because they do not account for pathophysiological processes beyond myocardial injury. Fourth, cTn release is often not detectable until 6–9 hours following injury, leading to delays in diagnosis and appropriate management, and potentially to unnecessary hospitalization for extended observation. Finally, the marker remains elevated for 7–14 days, rendering it inadequate to detect recurrent ischemic injury during this time period.

These limitations have contributed to interest in identifying additional biomarkers that may complement troponins for diagnosis and risk assessment in ACS. Such markers may detect early ischemia, acute myocardial wall stress, or the inflammatory processes involved in atherosclerosis, plaque rupture, or the early immune response to myocardial injury. These markers reflect specific pathological mechanisms involved in ACS, which may improve risk stratification and eventually could lead to a more individualized and targeted treatment algorithm for ACS patients.

Additionally, biomarkers of myocardial injury with more rapid kinetics than cTn may lead to earlier diagnoses, shorter observation periods, and recognition of recurrent ischemic injury.

The best studied biomarkers under consideration to complement troponins include the B-type natriuretic peptides (BNP, NT-proBNP) and C-reactive protein (CRP), which are discussed elsewhere. This chapter will focus on novel markers that reflect unique pathophysiological pathways involved in ACS. It should be noted at the outset that none of these markers is yet ready for clinical application. Clinicians should demand a very high level of evidence before considering any of these markers for incorporation into clinical practice (Table 10–1).[1]

GDF-15

Growth differentiation factor-15 (GDF-15) is a member of the transforming growth factor-β (TGF-β) family, and was first described as macrophage inhibitory cytokine 1 (MIC-1) because it is expressed by activated macrophages in response to various pro-inflammatory mediators (IL-1, macrophage colony stimulating factor, TNF-alpha). Since then it has also been described as placental bone morphogenetic protein (PLAB), placental transforming growth factor B (PTGF-B), and prostate-derived factor (PDF). Only recently was an *in vivo* function assigned to GDF-15, when Kempf et al. showed that GDF-15 expression and secretion is massively up-regulated by cardiomyocytes directly exposed to both transient and sustained ischemia. The protein appears to protect the myocardium from ischemia/reperfusion injury by promoting cellular survival and limiting the extent of infarction.[2]

Initial clinical evaluation of GDF-15 focused on atherosclerosis. In a small nested case-control analysis from the Women's Health Study, baseline GDF-15 levels were significantly higher among women who subsequently experienced myocardial infarction (MI), stroke, or cardiac death than among those free of such events through four years of follow-up.[3] Subsequent evaluation of GDF-15 has been performed almost exclusively by Wollert and his

Table 10–1: Evaluating novel biomarkers.

- **Can the clinician measure the biomarker?**
  - Accurate and reproducible analytical methods
  - Preanalytical issues (including stability) evaluated and manageable
  - Assay is accessible, cost effective, and provides high throughput and rapid turnaround
- **Does the biomarker add new information?**
  - Strong and consistent association between the biomarker and the outcome or disease of interest in multiple studies
  - Information adds to or improves upon existing tests
  - Decision limits are validated in more than one study
  - Evaluation includes data from community-based populations
- **Will the biomarker help the clinician to manage patients?**
  - Superior performance to existing diagnostic tests
  - Evidence that associated risk is modifiable with specific therapy
  - Evidence the biomarker-guided triage or monitoring enhances care

Adapted from Morrow DA, de Lemos JA. *Circulation.* 2007;115(8):949–952.

collaborators. Among 1682 patients with non-ST segment elevation acute coronary syndrome (NSTE-ACS) enrolled in the Global Use of Strategies to Open Occluded Arteries (GUSTO) IV trial, GDF-15 values measured upon presentation correlated with mortality at one year (1.7%, 5.6%, and 14.4% for GDF-15 levels <1200 ng/L, 1200–1800 ng/L, and >1800 ng/L, respectively).[4] These associations persisted after multivariable adjustment for clinical characteristics and various biomarkers, including cTnT, NT-proBNP, and CRP. The investigators extended these findings by demonstrating a role for GDF-15 in identifying NSTE-ACS individuals that benefit from invasive therapy[5] in the Fast

Table 10–2: Interaction between GDF-15 levels and benefit from invasive therapy in patients with non-ST elevation ACS at 2 years follow-up.

GDF-15 levels	Death or recurrent MI after conservative therapy [% (n)]	Death or recurrent MI after invasive therapy [% (n)]	Hazard ratio (95% CI)	*P* value
<1200	9.3 (37/400)	9.6 (40/416)	1.06 (0.68 to 1.65)	0.81
1200–1800	16.5 (65/394)	11.2 (42/376)	0.68 (0.46 to 1.00)	0.048
>1800	27.9 (67/240)	14.6 (37/253)	0.49 (0.33 to 0.73)	0.001

Adapted from Wollert et al. *Circulation*. 2007;116:1540–1548.

Revascularization during InStability in Coronary artery disease II (FRISC II) trial. A gradient of benefit was observed with invasive therapy according to GDF-15 tertiles. Risk of death or MI was reduced by greater than 50% among those with the highest levels and by approximately 32% among those with intermediate levels. In contrast, patients with the lowest GDF-15 levels did not derive benefit from the invasive strategy (Table 10–2).

The investigators subsequently showed that in a more heterogeneous population of 416 patients with acute chest pain without ST segment elevation, elevated GDF-15 levels were associated with an increased rate of death or MI at six months.[6] This finding was independent of clinical characteristics (age, gender, other cardiovascular disease [CVD] risk factors), peak cTnI level between 0–2 hours, and other biomarkers (NT-proBNP, CRP, cystatin C). This suggests that the risk stratification information provided by GDF-15 in ACS patients may extend to more heterogeneous populations. Although the data for GDF-15 are extremely promising, most studies have been performed by a single group of investigators. Confirmatory data by other groups would strengthen recommendations for use of GDF-15 levels in clinical practice. Currently, no commercially-available assay for GDF-15 exists, but efforts are underway to produce such a test.

ST2

ST2 is an interleukin (IL)-1 receptor family protein synthesized as both a membrane bound receptor (ST2L) and a soluble receptor (sST2).[7] In response to biomechanical stress, cardiac fibroblasts upregulate expression of both sST2 and its ligand (IL-33). Binding of IL-33 to ST2L initiates antihypertrophic signaling pathways in cardiomyocytes that appear to be cardioprotective, as targeted deletion of the ST2 gene in mice enhances cardiac hypertrophy and fibrosis, leading to left ventricular dysfunction and reduced survival.[8]

The functions of sST2 have not been completely elucidated, but it appears to function as a decoy receptor that competes with ST2L to bind IL-33, and thereby inhibits the cardioprotective effects of IL-33/ST2L signaling.[8] Preliminary studies identified sST2 (referred to as ST2 in clinical studies) elevation in the serum of mice and humans following acute myocardial infarction (AMI).[9] Subsequently, Shimpo et al. performed a larger evaluation of ST2 levels in 810 STEMI patients enrolled in the Thrombolysis in Myocardial Infarction (TIMI) 14 and 23 trials.[10] sST2 levels began to rise approximately three hours after presentation and peaked at 12–24 hours, with higher values observed among individuals with larger infarcts. Baseline sST2 levels were associated with a graded increase in the risk of death and worsening heart failure (HF) at 30 days, which persisted after adjustment of the model.

In a follow-up study from 1239 patients enrolled in the TIMI 28 trial, Sabatine et al. confirmed the associations between sST2 and death and heart failure events after STEMI.[11] In fully-adjusted multivariable analyses, each 1-SD increase in sST2 was associated with a 1.94-fold increase in the odds of cardiovascular (CV) death or HF at 30 days (95% CI [1.25, 3.03], $P < 0.003$). Because sST2

Table 10–3: Adjusted ORs (95% CIs) for cardiovascular death or MI at 30 days associated with NT-proBNP and sST2 levels.

		NT-proBNP		
		Quartile 1 & 2	Quartile 3	Quartile 4
ST2	Quartile 1 & 2	1.0 (reference)	0.72 (0.18–2.97)	1.99 (0.66–5.97)
	Quartile 3	1.14 (0.28–4.66)	1.32 (0.35–4.90)	2.98 (0.95–9.38)
	Quartile 4	2.24 (0.68–7.38)	5.62 (1.86–16.96)	6.58 (2.43–17.84)

Note: ORs adjusted for age, sex, DM, HTN, prior MI, prior CHF, infarct location, creatinine clearance, Killip class, lytic type and timing, and peak CK.
Adapted from Sabatine et al. *Circulation*. 2008;117(15):1936–1944.

is induced by mechanical strain, the investigators sought to determine whether the information provided by sST2 was redundant or complementary to NT-proBNP. In multivariable models containing both sST2 and NT-proBNP, both biomarkers provided independent and comparable prognostic information (Table 10–3); used together, the two biomarkers appeared to significantly improve risk stratification as assessed by the C statistic. In contrast to NT-proBNP, sST2 was not associated with variables related to chronic left ventricular wall stress, such as age, hypertension, prior MI, and prior congestive heart failure (CHF). However, sST2 was associated with peak CK, suggesting that sST2 may be more reflective of acute mechanical strain in the setting of MI, compared to NT-proBNP.

H-FABP

Heart-type fatty acid binding protein (H-FABP) is abundant in the cytosol of cardiomyocytes and is predominately responsible for intracellular translocation of long-chain fatty acids. Its small size (15 kDa) and location in the cytoplasm allow for quick release into the circulation in response to myocardial injury. H-FABP levels are detectable in blood 2–3 hours following initial injury, and they return to normal within 12–24 hours.[12] Its kinetics are similar to that of myoglobin; however H-FABP is approximately twentyfold more specific than myoglobin for cardiac muscle.

H-FABP is a more sensitive marker of cardiac injury than cTn, when measured within three hours of symptom onset;[13] this advantage disappears at later time points. Therefore, H-FABP has potential value in early detection of ACS, prior to detectable cTn elevation, and perhaps prior to irreversible cardiac injury. Additionally, it may allow for earlier risk stratification and more immediate management of ACS patients.

O'Donoghue et al. evaluated the prognostic value of H-FABP in 2287 ACS patients enrolled in the TIMI 16 trial. Elevated H-FABP levels were associated with increased risk of death, MI, or CHF at ten months (Hazard Ratio 2.6; 95% CI: [1.9, 3.5]), independent of established risk factors, cTnI, BNP, and myoglobin.[14] One important limitation of this study was the use of an older generation cTn assay that was less sensitive than current assays. However, Kilcullen et al. provided confirmatory data in 1448 patients with ACS by showing that elevated H-FABP levels were associated with a markedly increased risk of death independent of cTn, as determined by a newer generation, more sensitive assay.[15] H-FABP quartiles were strongly predictive of one year all-cause mortality (Figure 10–1), an association that persisted after adjustment for clinical variables included in the Global Registry of Acute Coronary Events risk score, as well as hs-CRP and cTnI. Interestingly, among unstable angina (UA) patients without elevated cTn, mortality was higher in individuals with elevated H-FABP (22.8% versus 2.1%; $P < 0.006$. Therefore, H-FABP may be another tool to identify previously unrecognized high-risk patients with persistently negative cTn values.

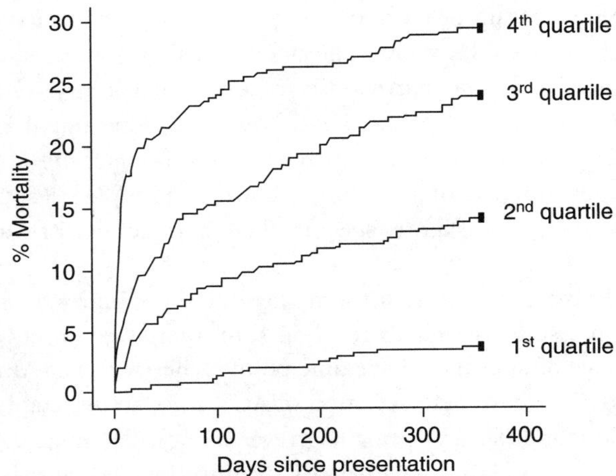

■ **Figure 10–1** Kaplan-Meier Curve According to H-FABP Quartiles. All cause mortality associated with H-FABP levels measured upon presentation in 1448 patients with suspected ACS.

Adapted from Kilcullen et al. *J Am Coll Cardiol.* 2007;50(21):2061–2067.

In addition to enhancing risk stratification and facilitating very early ACS diagnosis in the absence of an elevated cTn, H-FABP also has potential for detection of recurrent MI and determining success of reperfusion therapy.[16,17] Currently, a commercial whole blood assay for H-FABP is available and yields results in approximately 15 minutes. However, many questions remain about the pathophysiology underlying H-FABP elevation, as well as the utility of H-FABP measurements in clinical practice.

Inflammatory Markers

Inflammation plays a central role in ACS from atherogenesis to plaque progression, plaque rupture, thrombosis, and the immune response to ischemic cardiac injury. A number of protein and nucleotide products implicated in the inflammatory processes surrounding ACS have been investigated as potential biomarkers.

MPO

Myeloperoxidase (MPO) is a heme containing peroxidase that catalyzes hydrogen peroxide into various oxidizing agents, including hypochlorous acid, the active ingredient in commercial bleach. It is secreted upon leukocyte activation and degranulation and is the predominant component of neutrophil granules; it is also found in monocyte and macrophage granules.

In addition to its role in innate immunity, MPO is also involved in multiple stages of atherosclerosis. It contributes to foam cell production by stimulating low density lipoprotein oxidation and uptake by macrophages,[18] and it promotes endothelial dysfunction by consuming nitric oxide. Additionally, in post-mortem studies, ruptured, culprit plaques contain a higher concentration of MPO and MPO-modified products than nonruptured lesions.[19] MPO may promote disruption of atherosclerotic plaques by activating matrix metalloproteinases (MMPs), which leads to the destruction of the fibrous cap that protects the procoagulant core from the bloodstream.[20] Specifically, the MMP isoform located in macrophages closest to the fibrous cap is uniquely activated by MPO oxidation.[21] Finally, individuals with total or subtotal MPO deficiencies appear to be protected from cardiovascular disease,[22] and those with promoter region polymorphisms associated with decreased MPO expression have less angiographic evidence of coronary artery disease, fewer MIs, and a reduced incidence of cardiac death.[23]

MPO's possible role in plaque destabilization makes it a candidate marker for evaluation of patients with suspected ACS. Elevation of MPO may signify plaque rupture in advance of evidence of cardiac necrosis, allowing for earlier diagnosis of ACS and better targeting of therapy.

In a recent case control study, MPO levels were significantly higher among individuals with ACS than those with normal coronary angiograms or stable coronary artery disease (CAD).[24] Several larger, prospective observational studies have reported associations between MPO and various clinical outcomes. Brennan et al.

evaluated the diagnostic and prognostic value of MPO in 604 patients who presented to the emergency department with chest pain.[25] When compared to CK-MB, CRP, and cTnT, MPO provided similar discrimination for ACS, as determined using the area under the receiver operating characteristic (ROC) curve. MPO levels measured upon presentation were associated with a significantly increased risk of death, MI, and revascularization at 30 days and six months. The association persisted among the 462 patients who were cTn negative throughout their 16-hour monitoring period (Figure 10–2). This highlights the potential value of MPO as any early marker of plaque instability among patients with suspected ACS and negative cTn levels.

In a substudy from the c7E3 Fab Antiplatelet Therapy in Unstable Angina (CAPTURE) trial of patients with ACS randomized to abciximab or placebo, Baldus et al. demonstrated that MPO levels greater than 350 ug/L were associated with an HR of 2.25 [95% CI

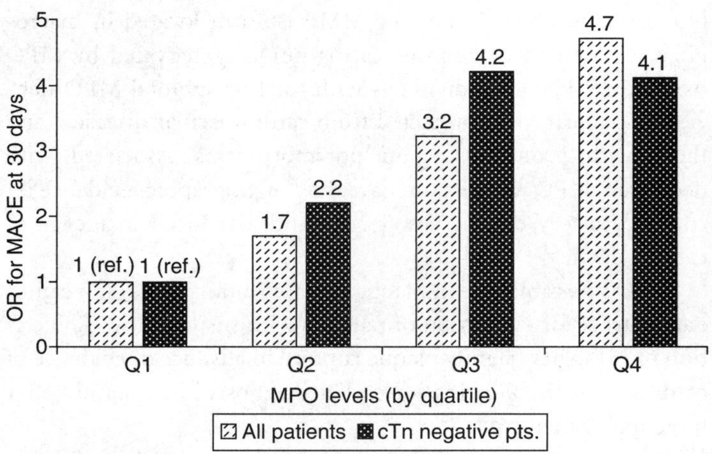

■ **Figure 10–2** Odds ratio (OR) for Major Adverse Cardiac Events (MACE) associated with MPO Quartiles (in all patients and in those with persistently negative cTnT).

Adapted from Brennan et al. *N Engl J Med.* 2003;349:1595–1604.

1.32–3.82] for death or MI at six months.[26] This association was also independent of cTn levels, but no incremental benefit from abciximab was reported among individuals with elevated MPO levels.

Although the FDA has approved an assay for MPO based on the promising data above, several important limitations merit comment. First, the level of evidence to support this biomarker is only modest; more consistent data from larger studies are needed to validate the associations reported to date. In particular, additional studies are needed to confirm that MPO is useful for distinguishing ACS from other causes of chest pain. MPO, like other inflammatory markers, is elevated in a variety of inflammatory conditions and infections, which may confound its use both in research and in practice. Therefore, future studies should include typical heterogeneous emergency department populations rather than highly-selected individuals with clear ACS. Moreover, no studies have yet demonstrated that elevated MPO levels identify individuals who benefit from specific therapies in ACS. If MPO levels are elevated due to plaque rupture, it is possible that such individuals may benefit from early invasive therapies, even in the absence of cTn elevations. However, this hypothesis has not been proven. Finally, because MPO likely plays a pathogenic role in CAD, therapeutics that target MPO may slow the progression of atherosclerosis and stabilize existing plaques.

MCP-1

Monocyte chemoattractant protein-1 (MCP-1) is a CC family chemokine produced by monocytes, vascular smooth muscle cells, and endothelial cells. It mediates proinflammatory effects by binding to the CCR2 receptor in monocytes, T lymphocytes, natural killer cells, and basophils.[27] MCP-1 is involved in the initiation, progression, and destabilization of atherosclerosic disease, as well as in a harmful postinfarction inflammatory response. Oxidized LDL up-regulates endothelial cell synthesis of MCP-1.[28] This contributes to atherogenesis by causing subendothelial recruitment and activation of monocytes, as well as initiation of foam cell formation.[29] Progression of atherosclerotic disease is also promoted by MCP-1, which stimulates smooth muscle cell proliferation and plaque neovascularization.[30] Additionally, MCP-1 may play a role in plaque instability by stimulating MMP synthesis which leads to fibrous cap degradation, and by up-regulating tissue factor expression which has procoagulant effects.[31] Finally, MCP-1 is involved in postinfarct inflammation. Initially, it promotes wound healing by recruiting macrophages to clear dead cells and debris. However, the continued activity of MCP-1 results in adverse ventricular remodeling.[32] Therefore, in ACS, MCP-1 may be a marker of increased atherosclerotic burden and possibly adverse cardiac remodeling.

Several observational studies have evaluated plasma levels of MCP-1 in ACS patients. In a substudy of the TIMI 16 trial, baseline MCP-1 levels largely overlapped with normal values, suggesting that this biomarker is not useful as a diagnostic test for ACS. MCP-1 was positively associated with older age, female gender, hypertension, diabetes, prior cardiovascular disease, CHF, renal insufficiency, and BNP, but not with cTnI, CRP, body-mass index, smoking status, or ejection fraction. Baseline MCP-1 levels were significantly associated with increased risk of death or MI at ten months, following adjustment for known ACS risk factors (4th quartile versus 1st quartile, HR 1.53, [95% CI 1.09, 2.14], $P = 0.01$).[33]

In a follow-up study of 4497 ACS patients randomized to either early high-dose statin therapy or delayed low-dose statin therapy in the A to Z trial, MCP-1 was measured at admission, at four months, and at 12 months.[34] In contrast to prior small studies, no effect of statin therapy was seen on MCP-1 levels. However, MCP-1 levels greater than 238 pg/ml measured at admission were associated with an increased risk of mortality through two years of follow-up after adjustment for known predictors of poor outcome, including various clinical characteristics, LDL-C, CRP, and BNP (HR 2.16, [95% CI 1.54, 3.02], $P < 0.0001$). MCP-1 levels greater than 238 pg/ml obtained at four months were also associated with increased risk of mortality at two years in multivariable analysis (HR 1.76, [95% CI 1.12–2.76], *P* = 0.009). Furthermore, a multi-marker panel composed of MCP-1, CRP, and BNP predicted a stepwise sevenfold increase in mortality correlating with the number of elevated markers at baseline and at four months (Figure 10–3). In aggregate, these data suggest that MCP-1 will not be useful in the initial diagnosis of ACS; however, it may be valuable for long-term risk stratification. Specifically, it may identify individuals at increased risk independent of LDL-C, CRP, BNP and

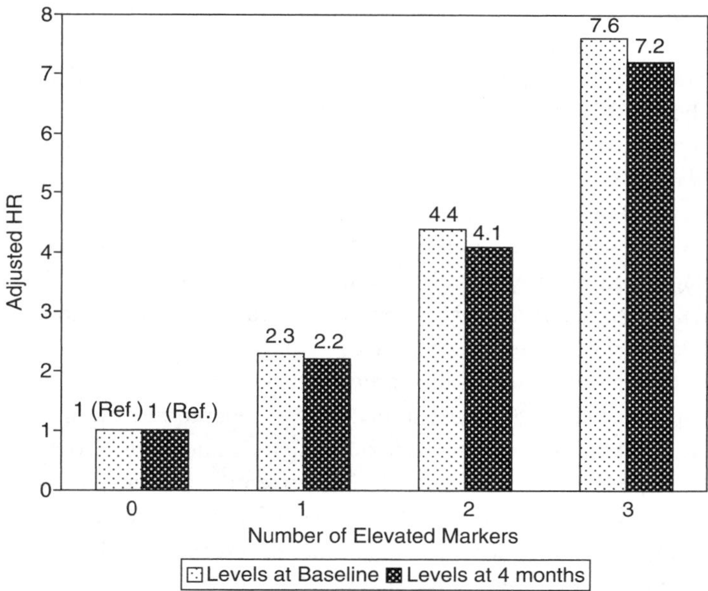

■ **Figure 10–3** Multiple-Biomarker Panel including MCP-1 for Risk Prediction After ACS. Hazard ratios (HR) for death through 2 years predicted by biomarker panel of MCP-1, BNP, and CRP at baseline and 4 months.

Adapted from de Lemos et al. *J Am Coll Cardiol.* 2007;50(22):2117–2124.

other clinical characteristics. However, this study did not find that the elevated risk in such individuals was modified by early high-dose statin therapy.

Neopterin

Neopterin is small pteridine derivative produced by monocytes and macrophages as a by-product of guanosine triphosphate (GTP) degradation. Neopterin has been implicated both in atherogenesis, by recruiting inflammatory cells into the vascular wall via induction of cellular adhesion molecules on the surface of endothelial cells, and in thrombosis, by increasing tissue factor production.[35] Circulating levels of neopterin appear to reflect macrophage activity, and have been used as a marker of cellular immunity in various inflammatory, infectious, and malignant diseases, as well as following organ transplantation.[36] Levels also have been shown to be elevated in patients with CAD.[37] Small studies have reported that neopterin is more strongly associated with complex plaques compared to stable plaques, and that its levels are more elevated in ACS compared to stable CAD.[38,39]

The value of neopterin in risk stratification was suggested by data from 3946 ACS patients randomized to high-dose or standard-dose statin therapy as part of the TIMI-22 trial.[40] Following the initial ACS event, neopterin levels measured within seven days, at four months, and at the end of the study appeared to be relatively stable, suggesting that, like MCP-1, neopterin measured in ACS may reflect the chronic, rather than the acute, state. Neopterin levels greater than12.11 nmol/L (75th percentile) measured at baseline and at four months were associated with increased risk of death or nonfatal ACS compared to levels less than 12.11 nmol/L, independent of known risk factors (HR at baseline 1.33, [95% CI 1.09 to 1.63], $P = 0.006$; and at four months 1.60 [95% CI 1.21 to 2.11], $P = 0.001$). Interestingly, neopterin levels were associated with increased risk even in patients with LDL less than 70 mg/dL and CRP less than 2 mg/L. Furthermore, patients with elevated neopterin levels seemed to derive incremental benefit from high-dose statin therapy compared to standard-dose statin therapy independent of clinical factors, LDL, and CRP. Although intriguing, this post-hoc finding requires validation and much more work is needed before the clinical utility of neopterin is established.

Osteoprotogerin

Osteoprotogerin (OPG) is a glycoprotein belonging to the tumor necrosis factor (TNF) receptor family that is produced by a variety of cells types, including osteoblasts, vascular smooth muscle cells, and endothelial cells. It functions as a decoy receptor for receptor activator of nuclear factor kappa-B ligand (RANKL) and TNF-related apoptosis-inducing ligand (TRAIL), and has been linked to the calcification and inflammatory processes involved in atherosclerosis. It is unclear whether OPG promotes atherosclerosis or is released as a compensatory defense mechanism in the setting of vascular disease.

Observational data suggest that serum OPG is a marker of atherosclerotic burden. OPG is elevated in patients with CAD, and its levels correlate with the extent of disease, as determined by angiography or calcium scanning.[41,42] Also, OPG levels measured at admission are elevated in NSTE-ACS patients, compared to those with stable angina.[43] Among 724 ACS patients, OPG levels predicted mortality and heart failure at long term follow-up independent of left ventricular function, cTnI, CRP, BNP (HR for death 1.4 [95% CI 1.2–1.7], $P < 0.0001$; and for HF 1.6, [95% CI 1.2–2.1], $P < 0.001$).[44] A better understanding of the role of OPG in atherosclerosis and ACS may help to determine possible treatment strategies that may benefit individuals with elevated OPG levels.

Conclusion

Considerable investigative efforts have focused on identifying novel biomarkers that may serve in a complementary role to troponins (Table 10–4), by addressing limitations of troponins and identifying additional individuals at high risk for complications.

Table 10–4: Emerging ACS biomarkers.

Biomarker	Pathological association to ACS	Outcomes predicted by biomarker (prospectively)	Therapies associated with benefit in subgroups with elevated biomarker levels	Clinically-available commercial assay
GDF-15	Early ischemia	Death;[4,6] MI[6]	PCI	No
ST2	Acute myocardial strain	Death;[10] CV death;[11] heart failure[10,11]	None	No
H-FABP	Myocardial injury	Death;[14 15] MI;[14] heart failure[14]	None	Yes
MPO	Plaque rupture/ instability	Death;[25,26] MI; [25,26] need for revascularization[25]	None	Yes
MCP-1	Monocyte infiltration into atheroma	Death;[33,34] MI[33]	None	No
Neopterin	Monocyte/ macrophage activity	Death;[40] ACS[40]	Intensive statin therapy	Yes
OPG	Measure of RANK/ RANKL activity	Death;[44] heart failure[44]	None	No

The stages of development of the biomarkers reviewed in this chapter vary substantially and some appear more promising than others (Table 10–4). Ultimately, the choice of which markers—if any—to add to troponin will depend on the additive diagnostic and prognostic utility from these novel markers, as well as their value for selecting specific therapies.

References

1. Morrow DA, de Lemos JA. Benchmarks for the assessment of novel cardiovascular biomarkers. *Circulation.* 2007;115(8):949–952.
2. Kempf T, Eden M, Strelau J, et al. The transforming growth factor-beta superfamily member growth-differentiation factor-15 protects the heart from ischemia/reperfusion injury. *Circ Res.* 2006;98(3): 351–360.
3. Brown DA, Breit SN, Buring J, et al. Concentration in plasma of macrophage inhibitory cytokine-1 and risk of cardiovascular events in women: a nested case-control study. *Lancet.* 2002;359:2159–2163.
4. Wollert KC, Kempf T, Peter T, et al. Prognostic value of growth-differentiation factor-15 in patients with non–ST-segment elevation acute coronary syndrome. *Circulation.* 2007;115:962–971.
5. Wollert KC, Kempf T, Lagerqvist B, et al. Growth-differentiation factor-15 for risk stratification and selection of an invasive treatment strategy in non-ST-elevation acute coronary syndrome. *Circulation.* 2007;116:1540–1548.
6. Eggers KM, Kempf T, Allhoff T, Lindahl B, Wallentin L, Wollert KC. Growth-differentiation factor-15 for early risk stratification in patients with acute chest pain. *Eur Heart J.* 2008. Epub July 29, 2008.
7. Bergers G, Reikerstorfer A, Braselmann S, Graninger P, Busslinger M. Alternative promoter usage of the Fos-responsive gene Fit generates mRNA isoforms coding for either secreted or membrane bound proteins related to the IL-1 receptor. *EMBO J.* 1994;13:1176–1188.
8. Sanada S, Hakuno D, Higgins LJ, Schreiter ER, McKenzie AN, Lee RT. IL-33 and ST2 comprise a critical biomechanically induced and cardioprotective signaling system. *J Clin Invest.* 2007;117: 1538–1549.
9. Weinberg EO, Shimpo M, De Keulenaer GW, et al. Expression and regulation of ST2, an interleukin-1 receptor family member, in

cardiomyocytes and myocardial infarction. *Circulation.* 2002;106: 2961–2966.

10. Shimpo M, Morrow DA, Weinberg EO, et al. Serum levels of the interleukin-1 receptor family member ST2 predict mortality and clinical outcome in acute myocardial infarction. *Circulation.* 2004; 109:2186–2190.
11. Sabatine MS, Morrow DA, Higgins LJ, et al. Complementary roles for biomarkers of biomechanical strain ST2 and N-terminal prohormone B-type natriuretic peptide in patients with ST-elevation myocardial infarction. *Circulation.* 2008;117(15):1936–1944.
12. Tanaka T, Hirota Y, Sohmiya K, Nishimura S, Kawamura K. Serum and urinary human heart fatty acid-binding protein in acute myocardial infarction. *Clin Biochem.* 1991;24:195–201.
13. Seino Y, Tomita Y, Takano T, Ohbayashi K; Tokyo Rapid-Test Office Cardiologists (Tokyo-ROC) Study. Office cardiologists cooperative study on whole blood rapid panel tests in patients with suspicious acute myocardial infarction: comparison between heart-type fatty acid-binding protein and troponin T tests. *Circ J.* 2004;68: 144–148.
14. O'Donoghue M, de Lemos JA, Morrow DA, et al. Prognostic utility of heart-type fatty acid binding protein in patients with acute coronary syndromes. *Circulation.* 2006;114:550–557.
15. Kilcullen N, Viswanathan K, Das R, et al.; EMMACE-2 Investigators. Heart-type fatty acid-binding protein predicts long-term mortality after acute coronary syndrome and identifies high-risk patients across the range of troponin values. *J Am Coll Cardiol.* 2007;50(21): 2061–2067.
16. de Lemos JA, Antman EM, Morrow DA, et al. Heart-type fatty acid binding protein as a marker of reperfusion after thrombolytic therapy. *Clin Chim Acta.* 2000;298(1–2):85–97.
17. de Groot MJ, Muijtjens AM, Simoons ML, Hermens WT, Glatz JF. Assessment of coronary reperfusion in patients with myocardial infarction using fatty acid binding protein concentrations in plasma. *Heart.* 2001;85(3):278–285.
18. Steinberg D, Parthasarathy S, Carew TE, Khoo JC, Witztum JL. Beyond cholesterol: modifications of low-density lipoprotein that increase its atherogenicity. *N Engl J Med.* 1989;320:915–924.

19. Sugiyama S, Okada Y, Sukhova GK, Virmani R, Heinecke JW, Libby P. Macrophage myeloperoxidase regulation by granulocyte macrophage colony-stimulating factor in human atherosclerosis and implications in acute coronary syndromes. *Am J Pathol.* 2001;158: 879–891.

20. Halpert I, Roby JD, Sires UI, et al. Matrilysin is expressed by lipid-laden macrophages at sites of potential rupture in atherosclerotic lesions and localizes to areas of versican deposition, a proteoglycan substrate for the enzyme. *Proc. Natl. Acad. Sci.* 1996;93: 9748–9753.

21. Fu X, Kassim SY, Parks WC, Heinecke JW. Hypochlorous acid oxygenates the cysteine switch domain of pro-matrilysin (MMP-7). A mechanism for matrix metalloproteinase activation and atherosclerotic plaque rupture by myeloperoxidase. *J Biol Chem.* 2001;276: 41279–41287.

22. Kutter D, Devaquet P, Vanderstocken G, Paulus JM, Marchal V, Gothot A. Consequences of total and subtotal myeloperoxidase deficiency: risk or benefit? *Acta Haematol.* 2000;104:10–15.

23. Nikpoor B, Turecki G, Fournier C, Theroux P, Rouleau GA. A functional myeloperoxidase polymorphic variant is associated with coronary artery disease in French-Canadians. *Am Heart J.* 2001;142: 336–339.

24. Ndrepepa G, Braun S, Mehilli J, von Beckerath N, Schömig A, Kastrati A. Myeloperoxidase level in patients with stable coronary artery disease and acute coronary syndromes. *Eur J Clin Invest.* 2008;38(2): 90–96.

25. Brennan ML, Penn MS, Van Lente F, et al. Prognostic value of myeloperoxidase in patients with chest pain. *N Engl J Med.* 2003;349: 1595–1604.

26. Baldus S, Heeschen C, Meinertz T, et al. Myeloperoxidase serum levels predict risk in patients with acute coronary syndromes. *Circulation.* 2003;108:1440–1445.

27. Rollins BJ. Chemokines. *Blood.* 1997;90:909–992.

28. Cushing SD, Berliner JA, Valente AJ, et al. Minimally modified low density lipoprotein induces monocyte chemotactic protein 1 in human endothelial cells and smooth muscle cells. *Proc. Natl. Acad. Sci.* 1990;87:5134–5138.

29. Tabata T, Mine S, Kawahara C, Okada Y, Tanaka Y. Monocyte chemoattractant protein-1 induces scavenger receptor expression and monocyte differentiation into foam cells. *Biochem Biophys Res Commun.* 2003;305(2):380–385.

30. Frangogiannis NG. The prognostic value of monocyte chemoattractant protein-1/CCL2 in acute coronary syndromes. *J Am Coll Cardiol.* 2007;50(22):2125–2127.

31. Schecter AD, Rollins BJ, Zhang YJ, et al. Tissue factor is induced by monocyte chemoattractant protein-1 in human aortic smooth muscle and THP-1 cells. *J Biol Chem.* 1997;272:28568–28573.

32. Dewald O, Zymek P, Winkelmann K, et al. CCL2/monocyte chemoattractant protein-1 regulates inflammatory responses critical to healing myocardial infarcts. *Circ Res.* 2005;96:881–889.

33. de Lemos JA, Morrow DA, Sabatine MS, et al. Association between plasma levels of monocyte chemoattractant protein-1 and long-term clinical outcomes in patients with acute coronary syndromes. *Circulation.* 2003;107(5):690–695.

34. de Lemos JA, Morrow DA, Blazing MA, et al. Serial measurement of monocyte chemoattractant protein-1 after acute coronary syndromes: results from the A to Z trial. *J Am Coll Cardiol.* 2007;50(22): 2117–2124.

35. Cirillo P, Pacileo M, De Rosa S, et al. Neopterin induces proatherothrombotic phenotype in human coronary endothelial cells. *Thromb Haemost.* 2006;4:2248–2255.

36. Fuchs D, Weiss G, Reibnegger G, Wachter H. The role of neopterin as a monitor of cellular immune activation in transplantation, inflammatory, infectious, and malignant diseases. *Crit Rev Clin Lab Sci.* 1992;29:307–341.

37. Avanzas P, Arroyo-Espliguero R, Quiles J, Roy D, Kaski JC. Elevated serum neopterin predicts future adverse cardiac in patients with chronic stable angina pectoris. *Eur Heart J.* 2005;26:457–463.

38. García-Moll X, Coccolo F, Cole D, Kaski JC. Serum neopterin and complex stenosis morphology in patients with unstable angina. *J Am Coll Cardiol.* 2000;35:956–962.

39. Schumacher M, Halwachs G, Tatzber F, et al. Increased neopterin in patients with chronic and acute coronary syndromes. *J Am Coll Cardiol.* 1997;30:703–707.

40. Ray KK, Morrow DA, Sabatine MS, et al. Long-term prognostic value of neopterin: a novel marker of monocyte activation in patients with acute coronary syndrome. *Circulation*. 2007;115(24):3071–3078.

41. Jono S, Ikari Y, Shioi A, et al. Serum osteoprotegerin levels are associated with the presence and severity of coronary artery disease. *Circulation*. 2002;106(10):1192–1194.

42. Abedin M, Omland T, Ueland T, et al. Relation of osteoprotegerin to coronary calcium and aortic plaque (from the Dallas Heart Study). *Am J Cardiol*. 2007;99(4):513–518.

43. Palazzuoli A, Ascione R, Gallotta M, et al. Osteoprotegerin and B-type natriuretic peptide in acute coronary syndromes with preserved systolic function: relation to coronary artery disease extension. *Int J Cardiol*. 2008. Epub August 15, 2008.

44. Omland T, Ueland T, Jansson AM, et al. Circulating osteoprotegerin levels and long-term prognosis in patients with acute coronary syndromes. *J Am Coll Cardiol*. 2008;51(6):627–633.

11 ■ Ischemia Markers

W. Frank Peacock, MD, FACEP

Introduction

Although the science of necrosis markers—notably including the troponins—has moved forwards at a remarkable pace, a marker specifically identifying coronary ischemia remains elusive. This chapter will consider why a marker of ischemia would be of importance, what markers exist currently for this application, and potential future markers for ischemia detection.

Why Do We Need an Ischemia Marker?

To answer this question, we must first discuss what currently occurs in the medical care delivery system today. In the United States, cardiovascular disease (CVD), defined as acute coronary syndrome (ACS) and acute ischemic stroke (AIS), are of great importance: 79 million US adults (1 of every 3) suffer from either affliction, and a CVD death occurs every 2.8 seconds.[1]

Pathophysiology

Patients presenting with a suspected ACS may appear in the acute care environment anywhere along a continuum of absolutely no cardiac disease mimicking a cardiovascular event, extending to acute myocardial ischemia manifested as unstable angina (UA). This may progress through a continuum of non-ST segment elevation myocardial infarction (NSTEMI), and culminate with ST segment elevation myocardial infarction (STEMI) (Figure 11–1); the earlier the presentation the greater the opportunity of salvage, but the more difficult it is to detect potential injury as currently no ischemia marker is in general usage. Indeed, our current diagnostics are predominantly oriented toward the terminal events in the ACS cascade, after necrosis has already occurred. Newer diagnostic approaches focus on events that potentially precede the

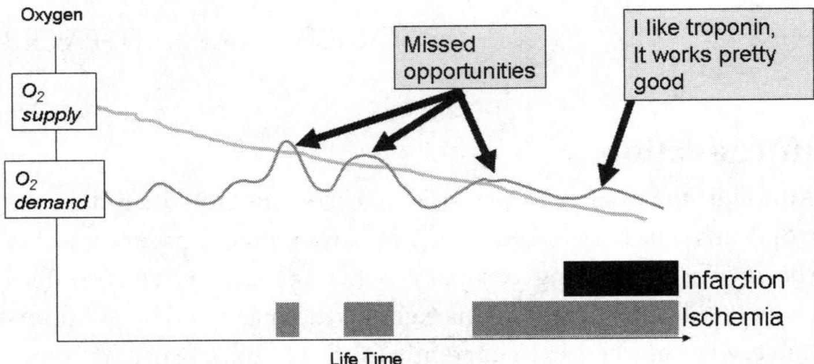

■ **Figure 11–1** What is ischemia?

occurrence of myocellular necrosis—during the period before cellular injury is irreversible—and offer the hope of improved diagnostic and prognostic accuracy.

Focus of Ischemia Markers: Emergency Department Application

Chest pain is one of the most common presentations in hospital emergency departments (EDs)—there were an estimated 11.2 million ED chest pain visits in 2008. This is a challenge as our diagnostic tools are limited and the risks are high. Patients discharged in the throes of impending ACS suffer disproportionate morbidity and mortality, and with missed MI representing opportunity lost for patients. While some presentations are clearly low risk, some may result in short-term mortality and assigning patients to the appropriate risk group is difficult. In patients presenting with suspected myocardial ischemia, 12-lead ECG diagnosed STEMI identifies the highest risk cohort, but occurs in only 3% of all chest pain patients.[2] Unfortunately, the majority of ACS presentations fall into the gray zone where unclear risk drives a number of testing strategies.

As recently as ten years ago, emergency physicians made admission and discharge decisions based solely on clinical grounds. It is now recognized that basing admission and discharge decisions solely on clinical grounds is inaccurate. Some three million patients with chest pain are discharged from the ED each year, and 40,000 of these people will ultimately suffer acute myocardial infarction (AMI). This group accounts for 20–39% of malpractice dollars awarded in litigation cases settled in emergency medicine.[3–5] Triaging patients into risk categories is performed clinically, after obtaining a patient's initial history, physical, and electrocardiogram (ECG), and represents the most challenging part of the evaluation of a patient presenting with a suspected ACS. While technology exists to rapidly and objectively identify those acute presentations at highest risk of adverse outcomes (e.g., STEMI, NSTEMI), it is only a minority of patients that will ultimately receive these diagnoses.[6]

History and Risk Factors

Chest pain is the typical presentation of ACS. Induced by exertion or stress, it usually resolves with several minutes of rest. While the patient's descriptions are variable, they are commonly termed as pressure, tightness, stabbing, burning, or sharp pain. Other associated symptoms include: nausea, vomiting, diaphoresis, dyspnea, palpitations, and fatigue. The most common anginal equivalent symptom is isolated new onset or worsening exertional dyspnea.[7,8] Unfortunately, only 18% of patients diagnosed with ACS are preceded by chronic angina.[9]

Typical symptoms may increase the likelihood of ACS, but atypical symptoms cannot exclude it. In one study of patients ultimately proven to have an ACS, 13% had pleuritic chest pain and 7% had pain reproducible by palpation.[10] In another analysis of 1996 AMIs, only 87% of men and 80% of women presented with chest pain.[11,12] Atypical symptoms at presentation are more common in women, the elderly, and diabetics.

Traditional cardiac risk factors for the prediction of coronary artery disease are limited for predicting an ACS.[13–16] These issues notwithstanding, about 90% of coronary heart disease (CHD) patients have at least one risk factor,[17] greater than 90% of CHD events occur in patients with at least one risk factor, and 8% of CHD events occur in people with only borderline levels of multiple risk factors.[18]

Physical Examination

The physical exam is very insensitive and poorly specific for any ACS diagnosis, but may identify characteristics that place a patient at higher risk for untoward outcome. Although nonspecific, abnormal vital signs increase adverse ACS outcome risk, as do findings of acute heart failure or new murmurs. While the physical exam must always be performed, its greatest utility may be in providing data to suggest an alternative diagnosis.

Electrocardiogram

After history and physical exam, patients presenting to the ED with acute chest pain typically have a 12-lead ECG performed within ten minutes. Unfortunately, the overwhelming majority of 12-lead ECGs done in the ED for acute presentations are nondiagnostic,[2,19] providing a diagnosis in only about 5% of ED patients with suspected ACS.[20] Despite a low sensitivity for diagnosing AMI and UA,[21] ST-segment elevation remains the diagnostic criterion for administering fibrinolytic therapy[22] and triggering early invasive reperfusion strategies. Other limitations include that ECG is a static image of a single 12-second period of cardiac activity, has poor visualization in certain areas of the myocardium,[23,24] and occasionally its waveforms are difficult to interpret.[25] Studies of continuous ST-segment trend monitoring or 80-lead ECG have suggested these modalities may be of greater value than standard ECG,[26–31] however their use presents challenges in lower risk groups and have not found wide acceptance.

The Role of Necrosis Markers in Chest Pain Evaluation

While CK-MB is useful, it has largely been replaced by the troponins for evaluating chest pain. Adding rapid-turnaround troponin assays does help identify high-risk patients, but suffers from a critical sensitivity deficit, and data would suggest that first-draw troponins simply cannot exclude an ACS. In one ED study of low-risk patients,[32] troponin had a specificity and sensitivity of 99.2%, and 9.5%, respectively, for predicting acute adverse events. Therefore, a marker that excluded ischemia, rather than myocellular death, would allow the physician to focus on other reasons for the patient's presentation. Although an event marker (e.g., necrosis) is helpful, in the "clinical value" hierarchy, this isn't optimal. Better yet would be a marker indicating an adverse event is about to occur.

To address the inability to exclude ACS, chest pain centers (CPCs) have been proposed, and the Society of Chest Pain was formed to ensure appropriate quality processes. In an optimal circumstance, CPCs appear to improve outcomes,[33] but with variable cost-effectiveness,[34,35] given the need to observe many patients who ultimately do not have a cardiac diagnosis; clearly, the healthcare system cannot sustain this type of approach—the need for ischemia markers is clear.

Serum Ischemia Markers

At the time of publication, only a limited number of cardiac ischemia markers are available to the practitioner in the acute care environment.

Ischemia-Modified Albumin

Oxidative stress and other poorly described physiological processes occurring in the setting of myocardial ischemia cause modifications to circulating albumin. The resulting changes, termed "ischemia modified albumin" (IMA), result in a diminished capacity for binding transition metals—specifically cobalt.[36] This has resulted in the development of the albumin cobalt binding (ACB) test for measurement of IMA as reflective of the presence or absence of myocardial ischemia. Studies have demonstrated a very rapid rise of IMA following induced myocardial ischemia, which resolves over the next 6–12 hours, suggesting that within the appropriate time periods this marker may correlate with the presence of ischemia. Confounders to IMA that have been described include: stroke, end-stage renal disease, severe cirrhosis, and end-stage cancers. While these predominantly represent other expected causes of ischemia, it is unlikely that the use of IMA will generate specific testing results. Its greatest use may be in the exclusion of potential ischemic syndromes. As such, the ACB test for IMA was FDA-cleared as a serum biomarker of cardiac ischemia and risk stratification tool in suspected ACS in the following manner: discharge of patients may be considered if the ECG is nondiagnostic for ischemia, the cardiac troponin is negative, and the IMA test is also negative.

A meta-analysis of over 1000 patients, including all studies evaluating the sensitivity and negative predictive value (NPV) of IMA in ED-suspected ACS patients, was performed by Peacock, et al.[37] The authors reported that considering the combined results of an ECG nondiagnostic for acute myocardial ischemia, a negative cardiac troponin, and a negative IMA test performed within six hours of chest pain provided a sensitivity of 94.4% and a NPV of 97.1% for ACS (Figure 11–2) and that the sensitivity and NPV for longer-term outcomes were 89.2% and 94.5%, respectively.[37] These results compared favorably to a smaller cohort undergoing serial ECG and marker testing, followed by resting myocardial perfusion imaging. No evaluation of the specificity or positive predictive value was included in this analysis, suggesting that its primary use was as an agent to assist in ED discharge, rather than to confirm an ACS diagnosis.

Although the clinical evidence for IMA suggests promise for use in ruling out ACS and early risk stratification in the ED, several

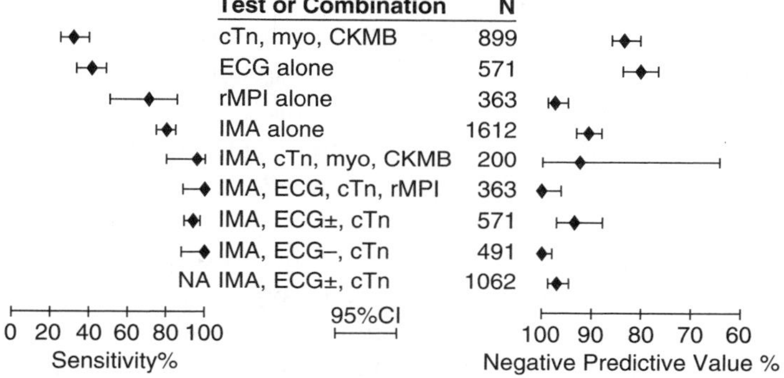

■ **Figure 11–2** Sensitivity and negative predictive value for acute coronary syndrome diagnosis using various strategies at emergency department admission.

unexplained issues regarding its utilization persist. For example, positive IMA results have not been demonstrated to discriminate between unstable angina and cardiac necrosis. Thus, the interpretation of a positive IMA result is unclear. Furthermore, markedly-elevated IMA levels have been reported, but the appropriate evaluation in this scenario has yet to be defined.

Myeloperoxidase

Myeloperoxidase (MPO) is a white blood cell enzyme known to catalyze the *in vivo* production of hypochlorite (bleach) from chloride and hydrogen peroxide. It is stored in the azurophilic granules of polymorphonuclear neutrophils and macrophages. The hypochlorite product of MPO is potentially a physiological asset as the enzyme is released during the inflammatory response, presumably because hypochlorite's highly caustic properties are essential for resolving infections and in clearing damaged tissue after injury. In fact, patients deficient in MPO suffer greater numbers of severe infections and inflammatory conditions. Thus, MPO increases are not necessarily indicative of myocardial ischemia, as they are also increased in infectious, inflammatory, and infiltrative disease processes. Like IMA, MPO may have limited specificity, but provides a sensitivity value that is clinically relevant.

Mechanistically, MPO may also contribute to the development of coronary artery disease as its hypochlorite end product is involved in oxidizing low density lipoprotein, and it may be an active agent in destabilizing coronary plaque by collagen degradation. This is particularly problematic if it occurs at the vulnerable plaque shoulder where plaque erosion may result in increased susceptibility of plaque rupture. Thus, MPO may actually be associated with the cause of ACS.

Several studies have demonstrated that ACS patients with increased serum MPO are at increased risk of short- and long-term adverse outcomes.[38–40] One study conducted in the ED environment, but limited by an excessive ACS rate not reflective of most ED populations, showed that the odds of major adverse cardiac events at 30 and 180 days increased with each quartile increase in MPO levels (Figure 11–3). Importantly, this increase in risk was 4.4-fold higher in patients with an elevated MPO, despite having undetectable cardiac troponin levels.[40]

There is currently only one MPO assay with FDA clearance as an aid for risk stratification in suspected ACS. Therefore, when comparing MPO levels from experimental MPO assays which are not standardized (some measure the enzymatic activity while others use immunoassay technology to determine protein levels), caution must be exercised.

B-Type Natriuretic Peptide and N-Terminal proBNP

B-type natriuretic peptide (BNP) is an active cardiac hormone with powerful physiological effects that include natriuresis, vasodilation, and inhibition of the renin-angiotensin-aldosterone system.[41] Any ventricular stress is an important stimulus for BNP synthesis and release,[42] which is accompanied by the release of its

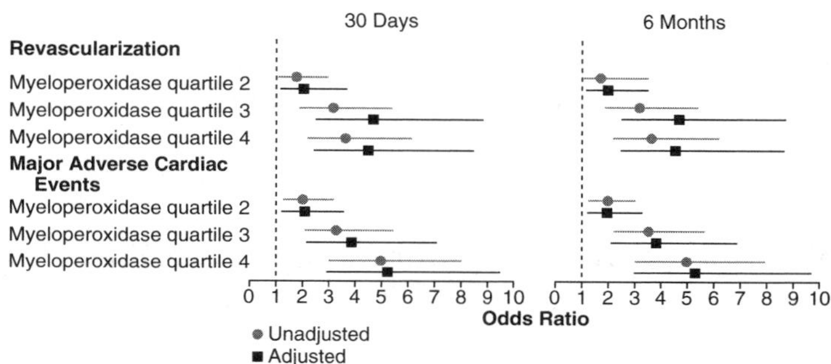

■ **Figure 11–3** Outcomes in Troponin negative patients stratified by quartile of MPO.

Source: Baldus S, Heeschen C, Meinertz T, Zeiher AM, Eiserich JP, Münzel T et al. Myeloperoxidase serum levels predict risk in patients with acute coronary syndromes. *Circulation* 2003;108:1440–1445.

inert cometabolite amino-terminal proBNP (NT-proBNP). Released from cardiac myocytes in response to hemodynamic and ventricular wall stress, levels of these proteins are proportional to the severity of myocardial strain.[43] In the setting of myocardial ischemia, one of the earliest results is impairment of ventricular relaxation, which leads to ventricular dysfunction that precedes even angina chest pain and ECG ST-segment deviation. This pathophysiology, and a strong association between BNP and NT-proBNP levels with mortality in patients with unstable angina, supports the premise that cardiac ischemia may cause elevated natriuretic peptide levels even without irreversible necrosis.[44] Several studies have demonstrated a strong relationship between BNP or NT-proBNP and outcomes in patients with ACS without evidence of necrosis.[45,46]

In patients with AMI, elevated natriuretic peptides predict a greater probability of death or heart failure, independent of other prognostic variables.[45,47,48] In general, BNP concentrations rise rapidly, peaking at approximately 24 hours post infarction, and reflect the probability of the development of future heart failure. When measured about 40 hours after presentation, a significant association between BNP increases and mortality is observed.[49] It is clinically relevant that natriuretic peptides identify patients without systolic dysfunction or signs of heart failure who are at higher risk of death and post-AMI heart failure, thus providing prognostic data complementary to cardiac troponin.[45]

Emerging Markers: Choline and Unesterified Fatty Acids

Although not yet clinically available, both whole blood choline and unesterified free fatty acids have promise for the diagnostic evaluation of patients with coronary ischemia, but without myocardial necrosis. The origin of both markers remains unclear, but a metabolic alteration within myocytes (from aerobic to anaerobic metabolism) is suspected. Both markers have been shown to be elevated among patients with coronary ischemia, but negative necrosis markers,[50,51] and may provide prognostic information. Larger studies of choline and unesterified free fatty acids as markers of coronary ischemia are awaited.

References

1. Rosamond W, Flegal K, Friday G, et al. Heart disease and stroke statistics—2007 update. *Circulation.* 2007;e69–e171.
2. Pope JH, Aufderheide TP, Ruthazer R, et al. Missed diagnoses of acute cardiac ischemia in the emergency department. *New Engl J Med.* 2000;342(16):1163–1170.
3. Braunwald E, Jones RH, Mark DB, et al. Diagnosing and managing unstable angina. Agency for Health Care Policy and Research. *Circulation.* 1994;90(1):613–622.
4. McCarthy BD, Beshansky JR, D'Agostino RB, Selker HP. Missed diagnoses of acute myocardial infarction in the emergency department: results from a multicenter study. *Ann Emerg Med.* 1993;22(3): 579–582.
5. Rosamond W, Flegal K, Furie K, et al. Heart disease and stroke statistics—2008 update: a report from the American Heart Association Statistics Committee and Stroke Statistics Subcommittee. *Circulation.* 2008;117(4):e25–e146.

6. Storrow AB, Gibler WB. Chest pain centers: diagnosis of acute coronary syndromes. *Ann Emerg Med.* 2000;35(5):449–461.
7. Anderson JL, Adams CD, Antman EM, et al. ACC/AHA 2007 guidelines for the management of patients with unstable angina/non ST-elevation myocardial infarction: a report of the American College of Cardiology/American Heart Association Task Force on Practice Guidelines (Writing Committee to Revise the 2002 Guidelines for the Management of Patients With Unstable Angina/Non ST-Elevation Myocardial Infarction). *Circulation.* 2007;116(7):e148–e304.
8. Brogan GX. Risk stratification for patients with non-ST-segment elevation acute coronary syndromes in the emergency department. Emergency Medicine Cardiac Research and Education Group. 2007; 6:1–10.
9. Rosamond W, Flegal K, Furie K, et al. Heart disease and stroke statistics—2008 update: a report from the American Heart Association Statistics Committee and Stroke Statistics Subcommittee. *Circulation.* 2008;117(4):e25–e146.
10. Lee TH, Cook EF, Weisberg M, Sargent RK, Wilson C, Goldman L. Acute chest pain in the emergency room. Identification and examination of low-risk patients. *Arch Int Med.* 1985;145(1):65–69.
11. Goodacre SW, Locker T, Morris F, Campbell S. How useful are clinical features in the diagnosis of acute, undifferentiated chest pain? *Acad Emerg Med.* 2002;9(3):203–208.
12. Goodacre SW, Angelini K, Arnold J, Revill S, Morris F. Clinical predictors of acute coronary syndromes in patients with undifferentiated chest pain. *QJM* 2003;96(12):893–898.
13. Jayes RL Jr, Beshansky JR, D'Agostino RB, Selker HP. Do patients' coronary risk factor reports predict acute cardiac ischemia in the emergency department? A multicenter study. *J Clin Epidemiol.* 1992; 45(6):621–626.
14. Selker HP, Griffith JL, D'Agostino RB. A tool for judging coronary care unit admission appropriateness, valid for both real-time and retrospective use. A time-insensitive predictive instrument (TIPI) for acute cardiac ischemia: a multicenter study. *Med Care.* 1991;29(7): 610–627.
15. Tintinalli JE, Kelen GD, Stapcyzynski JS. *Emergency Medicine: A Comprehensive Study Guide.* 6th ed. New York: McGraw-Hill Companies, Inc.; 2004.

16. Han JH, Lindsell CJ, Storrow AB, et al. The role of cardiac risk factor burden in diagnosing acute coronary syndromes in the emergency department setting. *Ann Emerg Med.* 2007;49(2):52 e1, 145–152.

17. Greenland P, Knoll MD, Stamler J, et al. Major risk factors as antecedents of fatal and nonfatal coronary heart disease events. *JAMA.* 2003;290(7):891–897.

18. Vasan RS, Sullivan LM, Wilson PW, et al. Relative importance of borderline and elevated levels of coronary heart disease risk factors. *Ann Intern Med.* 2005;142(6):393–402.

19. Gibler WB, Lewis LM, Erb RE, et al. Early detection of acute myocardial infarction in patients presenting with chest pain and nondiagnostic ECGs: serial CK-MB sampling in the emergency department. *Ann Emerg Med.* 1990;19(12):1359–1366.

20. Lee TH, Rouan GW, Weisberg MC, et al. Sensitivity of routine clinical criteria for diagnosing myocardial infarction within 24 hours of hospitalization. *Ann Intern Med.* 1987;106(2):181–186.

21. Goldman L, Cook EF, Brand DA, et al. A computer protocol to predict myocardial infarction in emergency department patients with chest pain. *N Engl J Med.* 1988;318(13):797–803.

22. Selker HP, Zalenski RJ, Antman EM, et al. An evaluation of technologies for identifying acute cardiac ischemia in the emergency department: a report from a National Heart Attack Alert Program Working Group. *Ann Emerg Med.* 1997;29(1):13–87.

23. Rude RE, Poole WK, Muller JE, et al. Electrocardiographic and clinical criteria for recognition of acute myocardial infarction based on analysis of 3,697 patients. *Am J Cardiol.* 1983;52(8):936–942.

24. Wrenn KD. Protocols in the emergency room evaluation of chest pain: do they fail to diagnose lateral wall myocardial infarction. *J Gen Intern Med.* 1987;2(1):66–67.

25. Lee TH, Rouan GW, Weisberg MC, et al. Clinical characteristics and natural history of patients with acute myocardial infarction sent home from the emergency room. *Am J Cardiol.* 1987;60(4):219–224.

26. Fesmire FM. A rapid protocol to identify and exclude acute myocardial infarction: continuous 12-lead ECG monitoring with 2-hour delta CK-MB. *Am J Emerg Med.* 2000;18(6):698–702.

27. Fesmire FM, Decker WW, Diercks DB, et al. Clinical policy: critical issues in the evaluation and management of adult patients with

non-ST-segment elevation acute coronary syndromes. *Ann Emerg Med.* 2006;48(3):270–301.

28. Fesmire FM, Hughes AD, Fody EP, et al. The Erlanger chest pain evaluation protocol: a one-year experience with serial 12-lead ECG monitoring, two-hour delta serum marker measurements, and selective nuclear stress testing to identify and exclude acute coronary syndromes. *Ann Emerg Med.* 2002;40(6):584–594.
29. Menown IBA, Allen J, Anderson JM, Adgey AAJ. ST segment depression only on initial 12-lead ECG: early diagnosis of acute myocardial infarction. *Eur Heart J.* 2001;22:218–227.
30. Menown IBA, Allen J, Anderson JM, Adgey AA. Early diagnosis of right ventricular or posterior infarction associated with inferior wall left ventricular acute myocardial infarction. *Am J Cardiol.* 2000; 85:934–938.
31. Ornato JP, Menown IBA, Riddell JW, et al. 80-lead body map detects acute ST segment elevation myocardial infarction missed by standard 12-lead electrocardiography. *J Am Coll Cardiol.* 2002;vol:39–332.
32. Peacock WF, Emerman CL, McErlean ES, et al. Prediction of short- and long-term outcomes by troponin-T in low-risk patients evaluated for acute coronary syndromes. Ann Emerg Med. 2000;35(3): 213–220.
33. Kugelmass AD, Anderson AL, Brown PP, et al. Does having a chest pain center impact the treatment and survival of acute myocardial infarction patients? *Circulation.* 2004;110(17):111–409, #1932.
34. Mitchell AM, Garvey JL, Chandra A, et al. Prospective multicenter study of quantitative pretest probability assessment to exclude acute coronary syndrome for patients evaluated in emergency department chest pain units. *Ann Emerg Med.* 2006;47:438–447.
35. Reilly BM, Evans AT, Schaider JJ, et al. Triage of patients with chest pain in the emergency department: a comparative study of physicians' decisions. *Am J Med.* 2002;112:95–103.
36. Bar-Or D, Lau E, Winkler JV. A novel assay for cobalt-albumin binding and its potential as a marker for myocardial ischemia—a preliminary report. *J Emerg Med.* 2000;19:311–315.
37. Peacock F, Morris DL, Anwaruddin S, Christenson RH, Collinson PO, Goodacre SW, et al. Meta-analysis of ischemia-modified albumin to rule out acute coronary syndromes in the emergency department. *Am Heart J.* 2006;152:253–262.

38. Apple FS, Wu AH, Mair J, Ravkilde J, Panteghini M, Tate J, et al. Future biomarkers for detection of ischemia and risk stratification in acute coronary syndrome. *Clin Chem*. 2005;51:810–824.

39. Baldus S, Heeschen C, Meinertz T, Zeiher AM, Eiserich JP, Münzel T, et al. Myeloperoxidase serum levels predict risk in patients with acute coronary syndromes. *Circulation*. 2003;108:1440–1445.

40. Brennan ML, Penn MS, Van Lente F, Nambi V, Shishehbor MH, Aviles RJ, et al. Prognostic value of myeloperoxidase in patients with chest pain. *N Engl J Med*. 2003;349:1595–1604.

41. Azzazy HM, Christenson RH. B-type natriuretic peptide: physiologic role and assay characteristics. *Heart Fail Rev*. 2003;8:315–320.

42. Tateishi J, Masutani M, Ohyanagi M, Iwasaki T. Transient increase in plasma brain (B-type) natriuretic peptide after percutaneous transluminal coronary angioplasty. *Clin Cardiol*. 2000;23:776–780.

43. de Lemos JA, McGuire DK, Drazner MH. B-type natriuretic peptide in cardiovascular disease. *Lancet*. 2003;362:316–322.

44. de Lemos JA, Morrow DA. Brain natriuretic peptide measurement in acute coronary syndromes: ready for clinical application? *Circulation*. 2002;106:2868–2870.

45. Morrow DA, Cannon CP, Jesse RL, et al. National Academy of Clinical Biochemistry Laboratory Medicine Practice Guidelines: Clinical characteristics and utilization of biochemical markers in acute coronary syndromes. *Circulation*. 2007;115:e356–e375.

46. Omland T, de Lemos JA, Morrow DA, Antman EM, Cannon CP, Hall C, et al. Prognostic value of N-terminal pro-atrial and pro-brain natriuretic peptide in patients with acute coronary syndromes: A TIMI 11B substudy. *Am J Cardiol*. 2002;89:463–465.

47. Arakawa N, Nakamura M, Aoki H, Hiramori K. Plasma brain natriuretic peptide concentrations predict survival after acute myocardial infarction. *J Am Coll Cardiol*. 1996;27:1656–1661.

48. Richards AM, Nicholls MG, Yandle TG, Frampton C, Espiner EA, Turner JG, et al. Plasma N-terminal pro-brain natriuretic peptide and adrenomedullin: new neurohormonal predictors of left ventricular function and prognosis after myocardial infarction. *Circulation*. 1998;97:1921–1929.

49. de Lemos JA, Morrow DA, Bentley JH, Omland T, Sabatine MS, McCabe CH, et al. The prognostic value of B-type natriuretic peptide

in patients with acute coronary syndromes. *N Engl J Med*. 2001;345: 1014–1021.

50. Azzazy HM, Pelsers MM, Christenson RH. Unbound free fatty acids and heart-type fatty acid-binding protein: diagnostic assays and clinical applications. *Clin Chem*. 2006;52(1):19–29.
51. Danne O, Lueders C, Storm C, Frei U, Mockel M. Whole blood choline and plasma choline in acute coronary syndromes: prognostic and pathophysiological implications. *Clin Chim Acta*. 2007;383(1–2): 103–109.

Section II

Inflammatory Markers

12 ■ Inflammation and Inflammatory Markers in Cardiovascular Disease: From Bench to Bedside

Elena Ladich, MD
Naima Carter-Monroe, MD
Frank Kolodgie, PhD
Renu Virmani, MD

Introduction

Evidence that inflammation contributes to the natural history of atherosclerosis from earliest fatty streaks to plaque rupture is well established. The cellular components of atherosclerosis, in particular inflammatory cells and their mediators, are now identified as biological determinants responsible for local complications and acute clinical events. The Framingham Heart Study first established the concept of risk factor analysis for coronary heart disease in 1961 where hyperlipidemia, smoking, diabetes, hypertension, family history, age, and sex were identified. This scheme was further modified in 1998 as risk categories (age, cholesterol, etc.) were assigned a point scale of very low, low, moderate, high, and very high risk with estimated risks for coronary heart disease over a ten-year period based on the Framingham experience in men and women 30 to 74 years old at baseline.[1] Despite its utility, this modified scheme falls short of predictive values for patients identified with intermediate risk scores requiring screening based on visualization of the actual plaque.

Consistent with this notion, atherosclerosis is a focal disease where lesions are most common at branch points at sites of low shear in contrast to high shear areas, the latter being resistant to plaque formation. Early lesion development is marked by lipid retention within a proteoglycan-rich neointima with activation of endothelial adhesion molecules allowing the attachment and diapedesis of monocytes. The initial step of monocyte invasion of the neointima cannot be overemphasized because inflammatory macrophages play a significant role throughout all phases of atherosclerosis progression.[2] Given that further improvements in risk prediction have occurred by the assessment of inflammatory biomarkers such as C-reactive protein (CRP), homocystine, and lipoprotein associated phospholipase A_2 ($LpPLA_2$), assessment of systemic inflammatory status has become important in overall risk stratification.[3–5] This chapter will focus on discussion of the natural history of atherosclerosis plaque progression in human disease, as well as highlight some of the newer risk factors associated with high-risk plaque prone to rupture.

Natural History of Atherosclerotic Plaques

Adaptive Intimal Thickening and Intimal Xanthomas

Early atherosclerotic lesions consist of two distinct nonatherosclerotic intimal lesions referred to as adaptive intimal thickening and intimal xanthoma ("fatty streak"). There is substantial evidence that while some human lesions may begin as intimal xanthomas, the most likely precursor lesion leading to the majority of obstructive lesions is likely the adaptive intimal thickening. As shown by the Pathobiologic Determinants of Atherosclerosis in Youth (PDAY) studies, sites where fatty streaks in young individuals are commonly seen, such as thoracic aorta and mid-right coronary arteries, are not associated with progression in older individuals. Also, intimal thickening in children occurs in similar locations to those of the more advanced lesions in adults and is thought to be a precursor to coronary obstructive lesions. These intimal masses consist mainly of smooth muscle cells (SMCs) in a proteoglycan-rich matrix (Figure 12–1).

Observations from experimental models and autopsy studies in young human subjects suggest that monocyte adherence to the endothelial surface and transmigration into the intima occur as the earliest events in the development of atherosclerotic lesions.[6] We

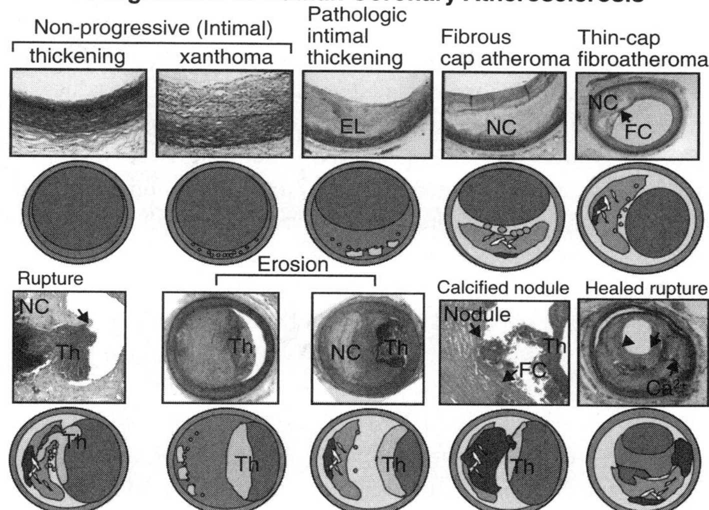

■ **Figure 12–1 Spectrum of representative coronary lesion morphologies seen in our sudden coronary death population forming the basis for our modified AHA descriptive classification. See Plate 2 for color image.**

The two non-progressive lesions are intimal thickening, and intimal xanthomas (foam cell collections known as fatty streaks, AHA type II). Pathologic intimal thickening (AHA type III transitional lesions) marks the first of the progressive plaques since they are the assumed precursors to more advanced fibroatheromas. Thin-cap fibroatheromas (TCFAs) are considered precursors to plaque rupture. Essentially missing from the AHA consensus classification are two alternative entities that give rise to coronary thrombosis, namely erosion and the calcified nodule. Erosions can occur on a substrate of pathologic intimal thickening or fibroatheroma while calcified nodules (a minor but viable mechanism of thrombosis) depict eruptive fragments of calcium that protrude into the lumen causing a thrombotic event. Lastly, healed plaque ruptures are lesions with generally smaller necrotic cores and focal areas of calcification where the surface generally shows areas of healing rich in proteoglycans. Multiple healed plaque ruptures are thought responsible for progressive luminal narrowing.

Reproduced with permission from Virmani et al., *Arterioscler Thromb and Vasc Biol.* 2000;2:1262.

believe the lesion of adaptive intimal thickening is characterized by retention of modified lipoproteins within the proteoglycan-rich matrix in the intima. Witzum et al. has shown that modification of these lipoproteins is associated with up-regulation of adhesion molecular expression, such as vascular adhesion molecule 1 (VCAM-1) and intercellular adhesion molecule-1 (ICAM-1) on the endothelial cells. VCAM-1 binds monocytes and lymphocytes to the endothelium, the first step in invasion through the vascular wall. The initiation of adhesion increases the expression of selectins, which facilitates the rolling of monocytes followed by firm attachment by endothelial integrins.[7] LDL oxidation, a critical step in atherosclerosis development, has been shown to occur through induction of lipoxygenases, myeloperoxidases (MPOs), inducible nitric oxide synthase, and NADPH oxidase. Oxidized LDL is a potent chemoattractant and induces the secretion of macrophage-chemotactic protein 1 (MCP-1) by endothelial cells. Macrophages phagocytose lipid deposited in the intima through several receptors, including scavenger receptor A and CD36, can bind a broad spectrum of ligands, including modified lipoproteins, native lipoproteins, and anionic phospholipids, many of which facilitate intimal cholesterol accumulation and "foam cell" formation. The lipid-laden macrophages (foam cells) secrete proinflammatory cytokines that amplify the local inflammatory response in the nascent atherosclerotic lesion, including matrix metalloproteinases (MMPs), tissue factor, and growth factors.[8]

Pathologic Intimal Thickening

One current theory holds that pathologic intimal thickening (PIT) is the earliest of the progressive plaques. According to this theory, the transition between early lesions of atherosclerosis and the more advanced fibroatheroma is characterized by the invasion of extracellular lipid pools by macrophages. As a result, lipid pools form in regions of the proteoglycan-rich matrix devoid of smooth muscle cells. A variable number of T lymphocytes are also observed at this stage, but a true necrotic core is absent. Areas of lipid pools may also contain free cholesterol appearing as cholesterol clefts on paraffin-stained sections. Accumulated free cholesterol may be observed to varying degrees in early fibroatheromas, but is more prominent in late fibroatheromas with a well-defined necrotic core. By contrast, very few B lymphocytes are found within the developing plaque and are restricted mostly to the adventitia. It has been proposed that the presence of macrophages in lesions of PIT are at a more advanced stage of atherosclerotic development.[9]

Although the precise origin of the "lipid pool" is debatable, studies suggest that the loss of smooth muscle cells (death by apoptosis) may be involved as their remnant basement membranes can be visualized by periodic acid Schiff (PAS) staining and show microcalcification. In addition, the confirmation of lipids by oil red O staining is highly suggestive of a lipid retention process facilitated by select proteoglycans and oxidation, which may lead to activation of factors responsible for apoptosis. Kockx et al. have shown that matrix vesicles are BAX-immunoreactive cytoplasmic remnants of fragmented, necrotic plaque-based smooth muscle cells.[10]

Progression to Complex Atherosclerotic Lesions

Fibroatheroma

The fibrous cap atheroma is the first of the advanced lesions of coronary atherosclerosis by the American Heart Association classification scheme (Table 12–1). Its defining feature is the presence of a lipid-rich necrotic core encapsulated by collagen-rich fibrous tissue (Figure 12–1). The fibrous cap atheroma may result in significant luminal narrowing and is also prone to complications of surface disruption, thrombosis, and calcification. The origin and development of the core is fundamental to understanding the progression of coronary artery disease. The fibrous cap consists of collagen, smooth muscle cells, and proteoglycan with varying degrees of inflammatory cells—mostly macrophages and

Table 12–1: Modified AHA consensus classification based on morphologic descriptions.

	Description	Thrombosis
Nonatherosclerotic intimal lesions		
Intimal thickening	Normal accumulation of SMCs in the intima in the absence of lipid or macrophage foam cells	Absent
Intimal xanthoma	Superficial accumulation of foam cells without a necrotic core or fibrous cap. Based on animal and human data, such lesions usually regress.	Absent
Progressive atherosclerotic lesions		
Pathologic intimal thickening	SMC-rich plaque with proteoglycan matrix and focal accumulation of extracellular lipid	Absent
Fibrous cap atheroma	Early necrosis–focal macrophage infiltration into areas of lipid pools with an overlying fibrous cap Late necrosis–loss of matrix and extensive cellular debris with an overlying fibrous cap	Absent
Thin cap fibroatheroma	A thin fibrous cap (<65 μm) infiltrated by macrophages and lymphocytes with rare or absence of SMCs and relatively large underlying necrotic core. Intraplaque hemorrhage/fibrin may be present	Absent
Lesions with acute thrombi		
Plaque rupture	Fibroatheroma with fibrous cap disruption; the luminal thrombus communicates with the underlying necrotic core.	Occlusive or nonocclusive

Table 12–1: (Continued)

	Description	Thrombosis
Plaque erosion	Plaque composition, as above; no communication of the thrombus with the necrotic core. Can occur on a plaque substrate of pathologic intimal thickening or fibroatheroma	Usually nonocclusive
Calcified nodule	Eruptive (shedding) of calcified nodules with an underlying fibrocalcific plaque with minimal or absence of necrosis	Usually nonocclusive
Lesions with healed thrombi		
Fibrotic (without calcification)	Collagen-rich plaque with significant luminal stenosis.	Absent
Fibrocalcific (± necrotic core)	Lesions may contain large areas of calcification with few inflammatory cells and minimal or absence of necrosis. These lesions may represent healed erosions or ruptures.	

Source: Virmani et al., Lessons from sudden coronary death: a comprehensive morphological classification scheme for atherosclerotic lesions. *Arterioscler Thromb and Vasc Biol*; 2000;20:1262–1275.

lymphocytes. The thickness of the fibrous cap distinguishes the fibroatheroma (relatively thick) from the thin fibrous cap atheroma (classic "vulnerable" plaque).

Recognition of early necrosis is identified by macrophage infiltration within lipid pools associated with a substantial increase in free cholesterol and breakdown of extracellular matrix, presumably by MMPs. The majority of macrophages within areas of necrosis display features consistent with apoptotic cell death. Accumulated free cholesterol appears as empty clefts by routine histologic staining and is another distinguishing feature of late necrotic core. The production of free cholesterol in macrophages is in part regulated by a re-esterification process involving acyl coenzyme A: acylcholesterol transferase, or ACAT1.[11] Manipulating the activity of expression of ACAT1 in culture or animal models favors necrotic core formation. This, together with the death of macrophages in the setting of defective phagocytic clearance of apoptotic cells, is thought to contribute to the development of late plaque necrosis. Ultimately, the size of the necrotic core is a strong predictor of lesion vulnerability.[12]

Thin-Cap Fibroatheroma ("Vulnerable Plaque") and Plaque Rupture

The thin-cap atheroma is thought to be a precursor lesion to plaque rupture and is characterized by a necrotic core (~25% of plaque area) overlaid by a thin fibrous cap (<65 μm), which is heavily infiltrated by macrophages and T lymphocytes (Figure 12–2).[13] The density of macrophages at the site of rupture is typically very high, although in some cases macrophages may be sparse. However, because plaque rupture for 76% of fatal coronary events is associated with thrombi in sudden coronary death patients, identification of the thin-cap atheroma is critical. A common mechanism of disruption of the fibrous cap atheroma occurs via the thinning or weakening of the fibrous cap resulting in fissures and ruptures.

Plaque rupture is defined as an area of fibrous cap disruption in which the overlying thrombus is in contact with the underlying necrotic core. The fibrous cap is composed of type I collagen with varying degrees of macrophages and lymphocytes and very few, if any, alpha-actin positive smooth muscle cells. The luminal thrombus is platelet-rich at the rupture site. Plaque ruptures are most prevalent in the proximal coronary artery near branch points and are frequently found in the proximal left anterior descending coronary artery, followed by the right and left circumflex coronary arteries.

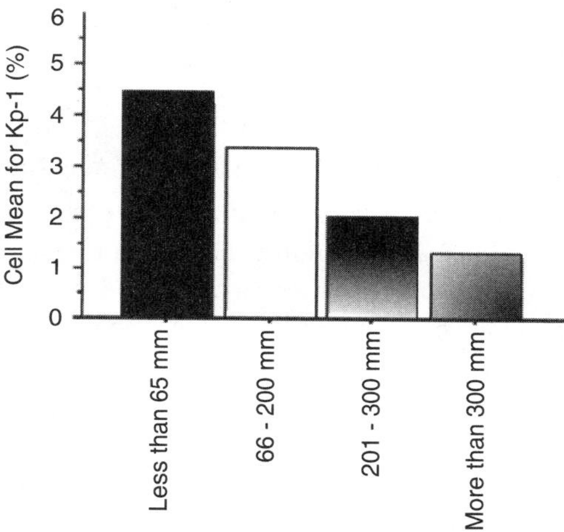

■ **Figure 12–2** **Bar graphs showing the relationship of fibrous cap thickness and macrophage infiltration.**

Cap thickness stratified into quartiles is shown on the x-axis where the extreme left bar represents vulnerable plaques. There is an increasing progression of fibrous cap macrophages with thinner caps.

The major pathobiologic determinants of plaque rupture include expression of factors that weaken the fibrous cap, such as MMPs, enzymes (e.g., MPOs produced by inflammatory cells),[14] high shear regions,[14,15] stress points, macrophage calcification, and iron deposition.[16] Recent data are also beginning to emerge that demonstrate critical differences in gene expression between stable and unstable atherosclerotic plaques. In one of these studies, differential expression of 18 genes associated with lesion instability included the metalloproteinase (ADAMDEC1), retinoic acid receptor responder-1, cysteine protease legumain (a potential activator of MMPs) and cathepsins.[17] Recently, kinesin family member variant 6 (KIF6) has been associated with a higher risk of coronary disease and myocardial infarction (MI)[18] and the carriers of 719Arg, a polymorphism in KIF6, receive a significantly greater benefit from intensive statin therapy than do noncarriers.[19]

Necrotic Core Expansion and the Risk for Plaque Rupture

Expansion of the necrotic core is an important pathogenic process contributing to plaque vulnerability. The presenting inflammatory stimuli for macrophage recruitment into lipid pools are poorly understood along with the respective signaling pathways for subsequent apoptotic cell death and necrosis. Recent studies[20,21] point towards the involvement of the endoplasmic reticulum (ER) stress pathway or so-called unfolded protein response (UPR) as the primary mechanisms of macrophage cell death in plaques. This pathway promotes the death of macrophages—the resultant accumulation of dead macrophages coupled with defective phagocytic clearance has been cited as one of the principal factors causing necrotic core expansion (Figure 12–3).

Emerging data are beginning to unravel candidate molecules involved in phagocytic clearance of apoptotic cells by professional scavengers. Mild fat globule-EGF factor 8 (Mfge8 or lactadherin) has been identified as a potential bridging factor among apoptosis, phagocytic clearance, and secondary necrosis.[22] In this study, LDL receptor-deficient mice subjected to medullar aplasia by radiation were given bone marrow–derived cells from Mfege8-deficient mice leading to substantial accumulation of apoptotic debris within the developing lesion. Accumulated apoptotic material was associated with a marked acceleration of atherosclerosis accompanied by decreased anti-inflammatory (IL-10) production by protective T-cells. In addition to lactadherin, other putative molecules in plaques potentially linked to efferocytosis and defective clearance of apoptotic debris include Fas ligand and transglutaminase-2 (TG2).[23,24] These correlative studies provide potential explanations for necrotic core expansion and lesion progression.

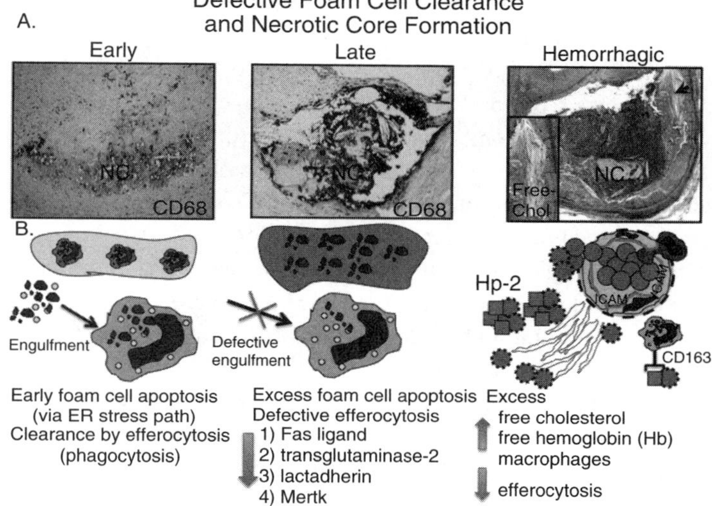

■ Figure 12–3 **Putative mechanism(s) of necrotic core formation in humans, in part, guided by mouse models of atherosclerosis. See Plate 3 for color image.**

Panel A shows representative micrographs of human coronary plaques illustrating early, late, and hemorrhagic necrosis. Early necrosis is marked by the infiltration of CD68-positive macrophages within lipid pools whereas late necrosis is represented by increased macrophage death, cell lysis, and loss of extracellular matrix. Hemorrhagic necrosis is accompanied by accumulated free-cholesterol (Free-Chol, arrow), presumably derived from erythrocyte membranes, and is thought to lead to the relatively rapid expansion of the necrotic core. Panel B is a diagrammatic representation of necrotic core formation, highlighted by defective efferocytosis (phagocytosis). The bulk of literature describing pathways of cell death, defective clearance, and mediators of efferocytosis is derived from mouse models of atherosclerosis. Abbreviations: Mertk = Mer receptor tyrosine kinase, FAS = apoptosis stimulating fragment, HP-2 = haptoglobin protein type 2 allele.

Intraplaque Hemorrhage and Necrotic Core Expansion

Data from our laboratory provide evidence that repeated intraplaque hemorrhage is a contributing factor to necrotic core expansion because red blood cells are a rich source of free cholesterol, which is an important constituent of ruptured plaques (Figure 12–3).[25] The red blood cells are enriched with lipid constituting 40% of their weight and a free cholesterol content within membranes exceeding all other cell types.[26] More importantly, excess membrane cholesterol can phase separate and form immiscible membrane domains consisting of pure cholesterol arranged in a tail-to-tail orientation favoring crystal formation.[27] The expression of glycophorin-A (a protein exclusive to red blood cell membranes) within the necrotic cores of advanced coronary atheroma is strongly positive while its presence in plaques with early necrosis or pathological intimal thickening remains absent or low.[28] It is our belief that intraplaque hemorrhage likely occurs from leaky vasa vasorum that infiltrate the plaque as the lesion thickness increases.[29] Therefore, intraplaque hemorrhage, together with the death of macrophages in the setting of defective phagocytic clearance of apoptotic cells, is thought to contribute to the development of necrotic core in advance stage plaques.

Inflammation and Causation of Occlusive Thrombi in Plaque Rupture

Mononuclear cells and their tissue counterpart, the macrophage, are critical to the atherosclerosis process (Figures 12–4 and 12–5). Macrophages elaborate many cytokines that regulate the function of various cells involved in the initiation, progression, and complications of atherosclerosis. Macrophages express receptors that recognize molecular patterns foreign to the body, like bacterial pathogens. These receptors include the various scavenger receptors as stated above, as well as Toll-like receptors (TLRs), which are now being identified in many cardiovascular diseases. TLRs activate the proinflammatory transcription factor nuclear factor kappa B

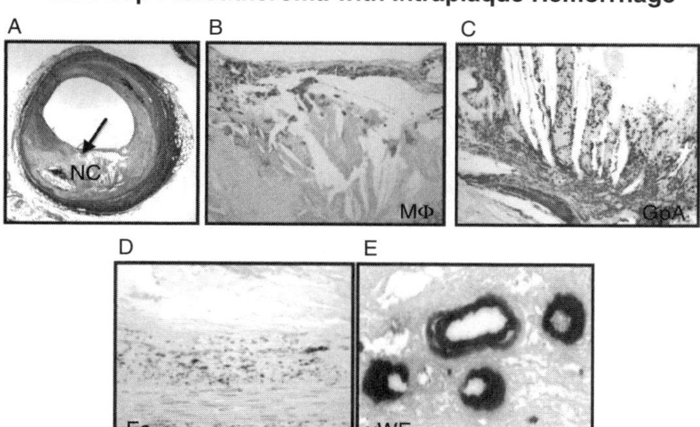

■ **Figure 12–4 Representative thin-cap fibroatheroma selectively stained for macrophages, glycophorin A, iron and von Willebrand factor. See Plate 4 for color image.**

Panel A, thin-cap fibroatheroma identified by the thin fibrous cap (arrow) and relatively larger necrotic core (NC); section stained by Movat pentachrome. Panel B, immunostaining against CD68 showing extensive macrophage infiltration (MF) in the peri-core and fibrous cap area. Panel C, extensive accumulation of red blood cell membranes in the necrotic core is shown by specific glycophorin A staining (GpA). Panel D, accumulated iron is also found in macrophages surrounding the necrotic core. Panel E, immunostaining against von Willebrand factor-related antigen shows diffuse staining of intraplaque microvessels near shoulder regions suggesting endothelial leakage.

Modified from Kolodgie FD et al. *N Engl J Med* 2003;349:2316–25.

(NF-κβ) on endothelial cells and macrophages and the mitogen-activated protein kinase (MAPK) pathway resulting in the production of cytokines that augment local inflammation and smooth muscle cell proliferation. TLR-4 has been identified as the signaling receptor for endotoxins and is expressed by macrophages

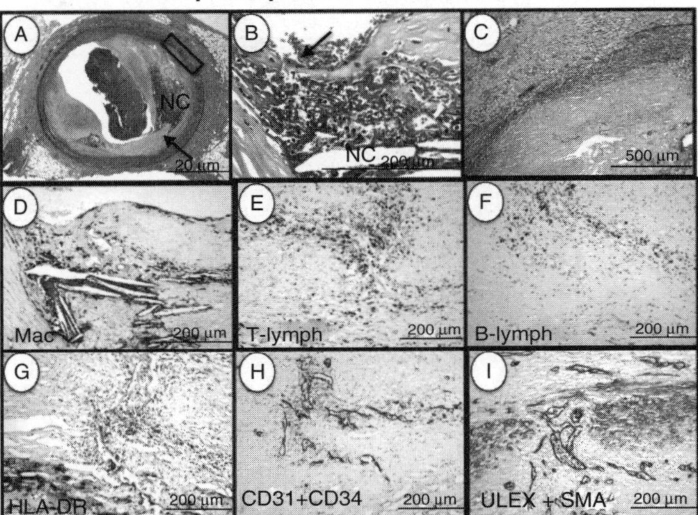

■ Figure 12–5 Plaque rupture and inflammation. See Plate 5 for color image.

Left main coronary artery with plaque rupture and luminal thrombus (A). Note high power view of the ruptured thin fibrous cap (arrow) with an underlying necrotic core (NC) in B. C. Shows the media adventitial border boxed in A with medial destruction and chronic inflammation. D. Shows the cap rupture site stained for macrophages (Mac). E, F, and G serial sections in the pericore region shown in A by an arrow stained for T and B-lymphocytes and G is stained for HLA-DR, respectively. H. Shows an areas of medial destruction highlighting angiogenesis by CD 31 + CD34 stain whereas section I is double stained by both ULEX (endothelial marker) and a-smooth muscle actin (SMA) stain, for smooth muscle cells showing focal destruction of the media.

in murine and human lipid-rich atherosclerotic plaques.[30] In vitro studies have shown basal expression of TLR-4 by macrophages with up-regulation by oxidized LDL.[30] The uptake of oxidized LDL transforms macrophages into foam cells that proliferate in the presence of MCP-1 and macrophage colony-stimulating factor

(MCSF) and play a critical role in the formation of the atherosclerotic plaque.

The groups of Edington, Nemerson, and Wilcox pointed to the expression of tissue factor in plaque macrophages as a likely instigator of thrombosis when these cells come into contact with circulating coagulation factors.[31] It was proposed that tissue factor released by leukocytes or by platelet-leukocyte aggregates (PLA) may trigger the extrinsic coagulation cascade through generation of thrombin thereby promoting platelet activation. It is now thought that circulating monocytes, rather than plaque macrophages, support the development of acute thrombi in unstable coronary plaques.[32]

There is evidence that MPO is involved in plaque rupture and thrombosis. MPO, released by activated granulocytes and in the atherosclerotic lesion by monocytes, can serve as a biomarker of risk for acute coronary events. MPO binds to the extracellular matrix and converts chloride ion to hypochlorous acid (HOCL) thereby promoting breakdown of the fibrous cap.[33] Moreover, the ability of MPO to reduce nitric oxide (NO) enhances the thrombogenicity of the endothelial surface via the expression of various prothrombotic factors and proinflammatory molecules. In addition, MPO-derived lipid oxidation products embedded in an atheroma will activate endothelial cells, promoting the surface expression of P-selectin, favoring platelet adhesion. Finally, incubation of endothelial cells with low doses of MPO, or MPO-expressing macrophages, results in increase expression and activity of tissue factor.

MPO also plays a role in thrombus maturation. Preliminary data from our laboratory suggest that monocyte infiltration of the thrombus correlates with the severity and physical length of the occlusion given that greater densities of CD68-positive macrophages, MPO-positive monocytes, and neutrophils were found more often in occlusive than nonocclusive thrombi.[34] Similarly, the total length of the thrombus showed a positive correlation with the density of macrophages and MPO-positive cells within the thrombus. In the disrupted fibrous caps, the density of MPO-positive cells and macrophages was greater in occlusive than nonocclusive thrombi, respectively, although this association was not found for neutrophils.

Extracellular Matrix Degradation and Lesion Development

Over the last decade, much interest has focused on the role of matrix metalloproteinases (MMPs) as the main cause of fibrous cap disruption in plaque rupture. Fibrillar collagen, especially type I, provides most of the tensile strength to the fibrous cap and certain proinflammatory cytokines, such as interferon (IFN)-γ, inhibit collagen synthesis by smooth muscle cells. Macrophages produce MMPs, which are zinc-dependent endopeptidases that possess catalytic activity. MMPs-1, 8, and 13 provide the initial proteolytic nick in the collagen chain, while the gelatinases MMP-2 and 9 attack type IV collagen (a nonfibrillar collagen), a prominent component of the subendothelial basement membrane.[35] It has been shown that atheromatous, rather than fibrous plaques, preferentially exhibit type I collagen cleavage occurring at sites that are rich in macrophages expressing both MMP-1 and 13. The artery also possesses endogenous antagonists to MMPs, the tissue inhibitors of metalloproteinases (TIMPS), although evidence for collagenolysis *in situ* indicates excess active forms of interstitial collagenases over the TIMPS in human atherosclerotic plaques.[36] Other proteinases capable of degrading extracellular matrix include the cathepsin family and inhibitor cystatin C. These possess potent elastolytic activity and have been implicated more with matrix remodeling and migration of cells. While elastolysis may be more important in aneurysm formation, collagenolysis may be a major determinant of plaque rupture.

The Role of Apoptosis and Plaque Rupture

Apoptosis may also play a critical role in the development of plaque rupture[37] and smooth muscle cell apoptosis has been observed in both progression and regression of the atherosclerotic plaque. Plaque rupture sites typically show very few smooth muscle cells, which are required for synthesis of extracellular matrix proteins and maintenance of the fibrous cap. Invitro studies have shown that various mediators secreted by macrophages and T-lymphocytes including: IFN-γ, FasL, TNF-α, IL-1 and reactive oxygen species, can promote smooth muscle cell apoptosis. The upstream effectors can activate caspases causing mitochondrial dysfunction and death via the release of cytochrome c. Apoptosis is thought to account for the decrease in smooth muscle cells seen in thin-cap fibroatheroma and ruptured plaques.

In advanced atherosclerotic plaques, macrophage apoptosis is frequently observed and we have shown excessive macrophage cell death at sites of plaque rupture.[37] Although our results show an association between macrophage apoptosis and plaque rupture, it is unresolved whether apoptosis triggers the primary event. Invitro studies have suggested that oxidized LDL is capable of inducing macrophage apoptosis. In addition to smooth muscle cells, IFN-γ has also been shown to induce apoptotic cell death of THP-1 macrophages. Moreover, IFN-γ, while inducing apoptosis in macrophages, also leads to overexpression of MCP-1, which may further promote an inflammatory response. IFN-γ regulates the mRNA expression of proapoptotic molecules like TNF-α and caspase-8 and treatment with TNF-α antibodies completely neutralizes the inhibition of DNA synthesis, as well as apoptosis of macrophages induced by IFN-γ. Our lab has also demonstrated caspase-1 cleavage in plaque ruptures, but not in stable plaques.[37] Immunohistochemical studies showed caspase-1 localized to rupture sites heavily infiltrated by macrophages, although reactivity for caspase-3 in these areas was weak.

The precise etiology of macrophage apoptosis at rupture sites is speculative; experimental evidence suggests that dissolution of extracellular matrix, as occurs in the fibrous cap, may threaten cell survival. This process termed "anoikis" is defined as a process of programmed cell death induced by the loss of cell/matrix interactions. Active proteases, such as elastase and cathepsin G, secreted directly by polymorphonuclear leukocytes; chymases and tryptase by mast cells; granzymes by lymphocytes; or those generated from circulating zymogens may promote matrix degradation.[6]

Alternatively, thin-cap fibroatheromas may form *de novo* and protease activation accompanies all stages of atherosclerosis, including plaque rupture. This possibility is suggested by the finding that ruptured lesions in some cases form at superficial sites (e.g., close to the lumen) and that leaky vasa vasorum or plaque fissures are responsible for intraplaque hemorrhage, which induces excessive macrophage infiltration.

Healed Lesions

Healed lesions represent a distinct category of atherosclerotic disease. These consist of healed plaque ruptures (HPRs), erosions, and total occlusions. HPRs in the coronary vasculature are characterized by a disrupted fibrous cap with a surrounding repair reaction.[38] The matrix within the healed rupture lesions may consist of a proteoglycan-rich mass or a collagen-rich scar, depending on the phase of healing. Lesions with HPRs may exhibit multilayering of their lipid and necrotic core, suggestive of previous episodes of thrombosis. It is speculated that repeated fibrous-cap rupture and thrombosis can incite plaque progression. Autopsy studies have shown that repeated plaque ruptures that heal result in a significant increase in plaque burden and luminal narrowing occurring in the absence of cardiac symptoms. Burke et al. reported in sudden death cases that patients who died with acute plaque rupture and those with healed MI had the highest frequency of healed plaque ruptures (75% and 80%, respectively).[39]

It has been shown that plaque progression beyond 50% cross-sectional luminal narrowing likely occurs secondary to repeated episodes of plaque disruption and mural thrombus formation, ultimately forming a fibrotic lesion characterized by distinct layers of dense collagen. Early, healed lesions are rich in proteoglycans, which are eventually replaced by type I collagen. In our laboratory, 61% of hearts from sudden coronary death victims show HPRs.

This incidence is highest in stable plaques (80% HPRs), followed by acute plaque ruptures (75% HPRs), and plaque erosions (9% HPRs).[39] Multiple healed ruptures with layering were common in segments with acute and healed ruptures and the percent cross-sectional luminal narrowing was dependent on the number of healed repair sites. Libby et al. performed studies of collagen synthesis by vascular smooth muscle cells and showed that multiple mediators released at sites of thrombosis, which could augment procollagen gene expression and protein production.[40] For example, platelet-derived growth factor (PDGF) and in particular TGF-β, both constituents of platelets released upon activation, increase interstitial collagen synthesis by vascular smooth muscle cells. In addition, elaboration of PDGF and generation of thrombin also likely recruit SMCs by migration and proliferation, providing more cells capable of producing proteoglycans and collagen.

Erosion

While plaque rupture is the most common cause of coronary thrombosis, acute coronary syndromes may occur in the absence of rupture. In fact, thrombi may occur as a result of three different events: plaque rupture, plaque erosion, or, rarely, a calcified nodule. Plaque erosion is characterized by an absence of the endothelium at the site of erosion, with exposed intima composed of smooth muscle cells and proteoglycans, and typically minimal inflammation (Figure 12–1). In a series of 20 patients who died with acute MI, van der Wal et al. found plaque ruptures in 60% of lesions with thrombi, while the remaining 40% showed "superficial erosion." The term "erosion" was chosen because the luminal surface beneath the thrombus lacked endothelial cells.[41] In these lesions, the thrombus was confined to the most luminal portion of the plaque and there was an absence of ruptures following serial sectioning of these lesions.[42]

In addition, we studied nearly 100 cases of sudden coronary death and found that 60% of all thrombi could be attributed to plaque rupture and 40% to erosions.[42] Notably, 69% of coronary thrombi in erosions occurred in patients less than 50 years of age and with a far greater frequency in women than in men. Both clinical and morphologic differences are widely apparent between ruptures and erosion. Morphologically, major differences exist in the cellular composition ruptured versus erosion lesions. Unlike the prominent fibrous-cap inflammation described in ruptures, eroded surfaces contain few macrophages (rupture 100% versus erosion 50%, $P < 0.0001$) and T-lymphocytes (rupture 75% versus erosion 32%, $P < 0.004$).[42] Cell activation, indicated by HLA-DR staining, was identified in macrophages and T-cells in 89% of plaque ruptures and in 36% of plaque erosions ($P = 0.0002$). The SMCs near the erosion site appear "activated," often displaying bizarre shapes with hyperchromatic nuclei and prominent nucleoli. The incidence of calcification was also less common in erosion than in ruptures.

The lack of inflammation in eroded plaques reported by our laboratory conflicts with reports from other researchers. In the original paper by van der Wal et al., plaque erosions identified in eight of 20 patients who had died of acute MI were divided into different morphologic subtypes consisting of lipid-rich plaques without a substantial fibrous cap (n = 2), solid fibrous caps with an underlying atheroma (n = 3), and fibrous plaques (n = 3).[41] The inflammatory cells (macrophages and T-lymphocytes) were the predominant cell types in all erosion cases with lipid-rich plaques with or without an overlying fibrous cap, and in two of the three lesions with fibrous plaque, one case showed a mixture of both macrophages, T-cells, and SMCs/collagen. Another laboratory reported on a small series of culprit plaques and found an increased number of MPO-expressing macrophages in both ruptures (n = 8) and erosions (n = 7) relative to fibroatheromas or atheromatous plaques.[33] Perhaps one explanation for these variant observations may be the difficulty in separating true lesional macrophages from those residing in the thrombus. Finally, a small subset of erosions actually displays a relatively high degree of inflammation, but this is fairly atypical in our experience. The lack of an inflammatory response in plaque erosion raises the question of whether these lesions truly represent an atherosclerotic process.

Inflammatory Biomarkers and Unstable Coronary Syndromes

A biomarker for cardiovascular disease should reflect important pathophysiological processes in atherogenesis and plaque destabilization with the goal of enhancing stratification of at-risk patients where various treatment strategies can be matched to the appropriate level of risk. Conceptually, the failure of candidate biomarkers to predict cardiovascular events has been attributed to their inability to represent a multicomplex disease or they were proven indicators of epiphenomena independent of the disease itself.[43] Consistent with these observations, the prototypical marker CRP does not play a direct pathogenic role, but represents a potential downstream clinical indicator based on its ability to predict upstream inflammatory activity. Regardless, potential biomarkers that are more reflective of systemic inflammation and not necessarily vascular inflammation may fail because they will incur a high rate of false-positives.

Lipid-related biomarkers, specifically LDL-C, represent the prototypical biomarkers of coronary artery disease. Despite the significance of cholesterol in acute coronary syndromes, however, many individuals who experience MI have cholesterol concentrations at or below recommended levels.[44,45] Notwithstanding, patients receiving pharmacotherapy for dyslipidemia, who have LDL levels at currently mandated targets or below, still remain at risk for MI.[46] Indeed, having a marker that may identify plaques that rupture potentially meets an important unmet clinical need because greater than 66% of all MIs occur in coronary arteries with greater than 50% stenosis on coronary angiography.[47] Thus, the apparent divergence of clinical risk associated with traditional lipid biomarkers and adverse outcome highlights the necessity for improving the ability to predict cardiovascular events. Recent work has focused on whether plasma markers of inflammation can noninvasively diagnose and prognosticate coronary artery disease (CAD) and other forms of atherosclerosis. Inflammatory biomarkers, or "acute-phase reactant proteins," namely CRP, fibrinogen, serum amyloid (SAA) and other less notable proteins, such as type II secretory phospholipase A_2 (sPLA2-II),[48] have been recently studied. Indeed, acute phase reactants increase greatly during systemic inflammatory conditions, such as sepsis, rheumatoid arthritis, or inflammatory bowel disease. In addition to CRP, other inflammatory biomarkers of recent clinical interest include: IL-6, IL-3, IL-8, M-CSF, and soluble CD40 ligand.[49–54]

The biology of CRP contributes to the human innate immune system response representing a stable plasma biomarker reflective of low-grade systemic inflammation. It is produced predominantly by hepatocytes as an acute phase reactant, which is transcriptionally driven by IL-6, with synergistic enhancement by IL-1.[55] Recent data, however, have challenged the view that the liver exclusively produces CRP where transcriptional polymerase chain reaction data suggest that smooth muscle cells, endothelial cells, and macrophages[56–58] are also capable of producing CRP. Aside from cells themselves, CRP is also produced in atherosclerotic plaques[59,60] where, according to several independent studies, it is involved in atherothrombosis and plaque vulnerability by mediating the expression of adhesion molecules, induction of nitric oxide, altered complement function, uptake of oxidized LDL, matrix degradation, and inhibition of intrinsic fibrinolysis.[61] More recently, CRP has been identified in human high-risk coronary plaques of the carotid reflecting an active proinflammatory stage where local synthesis of CRP could be involved in plaque neovascularization and increased intraplaque hemorrhage.[62,63]

The introduction of high-sensitivity immunoassays for CRP in the mid-nineties expanded the notion that values of CRP, in a range that was previously considered normal, were now capable of predicting future events.[64] In large epidemiologic studies carried out in individuals without history of prior cardiovascular disease, a single CRP measure is a strong predictor of future cardiovascular risk.[65] It has also been shown that CRP has an additive value across all levels of lipid screening, even after adjustment for age, smoking, blood pressure, obesity, and diabetes.[66] More recently, however, the clinical value of CRP as a risk predictor for CAD has come under scrutiny. Given the fact that elevations in CRP are caused by inflammation and tissue damage, it has a low specificity and thus a high rate of false positives in predicting future cardiovascular events. A published meta-analysis of 22 population-based prospective studies, with a mean follow-up of 12 years and 7068 cardiovascular events,[67] showed that odds ratios for cardiovascular events after correction for other established risk factors were only 1.6, suggesting that CRP only marginally adds to the predictive values of established risk factors for coronary heart disease.

In a recent autopsy study from our laboratory, serum levels of hs-CRP were significantly elevated in patients dying suddenly of plaque rupture, erosion, or stable plaque relative to control patients where death was attributed to noncoronary causes independent of age, body mass index, and smoking (control hs-CRP 1.4 micrograms/dl[67] versus sudden death 2.7 micrograms/dl, $P < 0.0001$). Moreover, high serum hs-CRP from sudden death victims showed a positive correlation with its recognition by immunostaining of plaques and as a predictor of high-risk thin-cap fibroatheromas.[68] Accumulated CRP was localized mainly to the necrotic core and surrounding macrophages where its strongest expression was found in patients with high serum CRP levels. Although an association of CRP with plaque burden and acute thrombosis was observed, this relationship was lessened when the covariates glycohemoglobin and HDL cholesterol were considered.

Lipoprotein-Associated Phospholipase A2 (Lp-PLA2) and Cardiovascular Disease Risk

Another potentially important biomarker of inflammation receiving clinical attention of late in relation to atherosclerosis and its adverse outcomes is lipoprotein-associated phospholipase A2

(Lp-PLA$_2$), a unique phospholipase that circulates primarily bound to low-density lipoprotein.[69] A number of recent publications support the role of Lp-PLA$_2$ as a cardiovascular risk marker independent of and in addition to traditional risk factors.[70] Functionally, Lp-PLA$_2$ is an enzyme capable of specifically hydrolyzing oxidized phospholipids with breakdown products of oxidized free fatty acids and lysophosphatidylcholine. These mediators in turn potentially stimulate endothelial adhesion molecules and cytokines leading to recruitment of monocytes into the intima. In a recent study, Lavi et al. collected blood samples simultaneously from the left main coronary artery and coronary sinus and demonstrated a net increase in Lp-PLA$_2$ levels as blood traverses arterial segments in the coronary vascular bed with significant atherosclerotic disease relative to control nondiseased segments (0% angiographic stenosis).[71] Although inconclusive, these data suggest that activated cells, such as macrophages, are capable of producing Lp-PLA$_2$. Further support for this argument comes from immunohistochemical studies of Lp-PLA$_2$ in coronary plaques from sudden coronary death victims from our laboratory.[72] Using a specific monoclonal antibody, immunostaining against Lp-PLA$_2$ in early plaque was minimal, whereas rupture-prone and ruptured plaques showed intense staining for Lp-PLA$_2$. Abundant reaction products were found in necrotic cores, both within macrophages and extracellularly; and in fibrous caps, in particular thin-fibrous caps. Further transcriptional studies of Lp-PLA$_2$ messenger RNA expression have shown that lesional macrophages are a potential source of Lp-PLA$_2$ production.[73]

Evidence of Lp-PLA2 as a Clinical Biomarker of Cardiovascular Risk

Recent evidence suggests that Lp-PLA$_2$ is an independent cardiovascular risk marker and an additive risk factor for cardiovascular mortality.[74] Currently, there are over 25 collective prospective epidemiologic studies investigating the association of Lp-PLA$_2$ with future coronary artery disease events and stroke. In the

Atherosclerosis Risk in Communities (ARIC) study involving an apparently healthy middle-aged population, elevated Lp-PLA_2 significantly raised the area under the curve (AUC) score for the risk of coronary events when 18 other novel cardiac markers, including CRP, did not.[75] Reminiscent of clinical studies showing elevated hs-CRP, increased levels of circulating Lp-PLA_2 approximately doubles the risk for first and recurrent cardiovascular events. Moreover, reported complementarities of Lp-PLA_2 and CRP in predicting the future risk of cardiovascular events are noted in the ARIC study, where individuals with increased levels of both markers were three times more likely to experience a coronary event compared to those with lower levels.[76] Considering approximately 80% of circulating Lp-PLA_2 is bound to LDL particles, lipid-modifying treatments proven to lower primary and secondary cardiovascular events including statins, niacin, fenofibrate, omega-3 fatty acids, and ezetimibe, coincidentally lower Lp-PLA_2.[77]

Although the clinical value of Lp-PLA_2 as an inflammatory biomarker capable of predicting future coronary events is becoming increasingly apparent, less is known of whether specific targeting of Lp-PLA_2 can actually modify the plaque. The answer to this important question may lie in two complementary studies reported in diabetic and hypercholesterolemic swine[78] and 330 patients with angiographically-documented coronary disease[79] using darapladib, an oral inhibitor Lp-PLA_2. In the swine, darapladib markedly inhibited plasma and lesion Lp-PLA_2 activity and reduced lesional lysophosphatidylcholine content. Further, transcriptional analysis of coronary samples showed that darapladib exerted a general anti-inflammatory action thereby reducing the expression of 24 genes associated with macrophage and T-cell function. In patients, 12 months of darapladib treatment resulted in a 59% decrease in Lp-PLA_2 activity and despite similar lesion burden, the placebo group showed a progressive increase in necrotic core volume, while no changes in necrotic core expansion were observed for patients receiving the Lp-PLA_2 oral inhibitor.

Taken together, these observations implicate a causative role for Lp-PLA_2 in coronary lesion progression involving the activation of inflammatory cells where its inhibition could decrease a phenotypic hallmark of lesion instability, namely necrotic core development.

Hyperhomocysteinemia and Unstable Coronary Syndromes

Hyperhomocysteinemia is a rare inborn error of metabolism that is a result of cystathionine beta-synthase deficiency and results in a high plasma homocysteine concentration and premature mortality from thromboembolism. Modest elevations of total homocysteine between 10 and 100 micromol/L are due to variations in vitamin B intake and genetic factors, especially 5,10-methylenetetrahydrofolate reductase (MTHFR C677T) gene polymorphism. There has been a link between modest elevations of total homocysteine with acute MI, stroke, aortic atherosclerosis, and mortality in patients with known coronary artery disease.[80]

In our studies of men dying suddenly with severe coronary atherosclerosis, plasma homocysteine levels were significantly higher compared to deaths attributed to noncoronary causes. Autopsy patients with severe coronary disease without thrombosis had the highest serum homocysteine levels (15.6 micromol/L) compared to those with thrombi (10.8) and controls (9.8 micromol/L; $P = 0.007$). Moreover, homocysteine levels in the upper tertile (>15 micromol/L) were associated with sudden death without acute or organized thrombus (odds ratio 3.8, $P = 0.03$) independent of age and other risk factors; the coexistence of diabetes increased the association (odds ratio 25.1, $P = 0.009$, versus lowest tertile < 8.5 micromol/L).[81] A recent study called PREDICT (Prospective Evaluation of *Diabetic Ischaemic Heart Disease* by Computed *Tomography*) showed age as a major factor influencing the coronary artery calcification seen in type II diabetes with weaker contributions from waist-hip ratio, but no association with homocysteine.[82]

References

1. Wilson PW, D'Agostino RB, Levy D, Belanger AM, Silbershatz H, Kannel WB. Prediction of coronary heart disease using risk factor categories. *Circulation.* 1998;97(18):1837–1847.

2. Berliner JA, Navab M, Fogelman AM, et al. Atherosclerosis: basic mechanisms. Oxidation, inflammation, and genetics. *Circulation.* 1995;91(9):2488–2496.

3. Genest JJ Jr, McNamara JR, Upson B, et al. Prevalence of familial hyperhomocyst(e)inemia in men with premature coronary artery disease. *Arterioscler Thromb.* 1991;11(5):1129–1136.

4. Ridker PM, Rifai N, Rose L, Buring JE, Cook NR. Comparison of C-reactive protein and low-density lipoprotein cholesterol levels in the prediction of first cardiovascular events. *N Engl J Med.* 2002;347(20):1557–1565.

5. Weintraub HS. Identifying the vulnerable patient with rupture-prone plaque. *Am J Cardiol.* 2008;101(12A):3F–10F.

6. Libby P. Inflammation in atherosclerosis. *Nature.* 2002;420(6917): 868–874.

7. Libby P. Changing concepts of atherogenesis. *J Intern Med.* 2000; 247(3):349–358.

8. Newby AC. Metalloproteinase expression in monocytes and macrophages and its relationship to atherosclerotic plaque instability. *Arterioscler Thromb Vasc Biol.* 2008;28(12):2108–2114.

9. Nakashima Y, Fujii H, Sumiyoshi S, Wight TN, Sueishi K. Early human atherosclerosis: accumulation of lipid and proteoglycans in intimal thickenings followed by macrophage infiltration. *Arterioscler Thromb Vasc Biol.* 2007;27(5):1159–1165.

10. Kockx MM, De Meyer GR, Muhring J, Jacob W, Bult H, Herman AG. Apoptosis and related proteins in different stages of human atherosclerotic plaques. *Circulation.* 1998;97(23):2307–2315.

11. Tabas I. Cholesterol and phospholipid metabolism in macrophages. *Biochim Biophys Acta.* 2000;1529(1–3):164–174.

12. Virmani R, Kolodgie FD, Burke AP, Farb A, Schwartz SM. Lessons from sudden coronary death: a comprehensive morphological classification scheme for atherosclerotic lesions. *Arterioscler Thromb Vasc Biol.* 2000;20(5):1262–1275.

13. Burke AP, Farb A, Malcom GT, Liang YH, Smialek J, Virmani R. Coronary risk factors and plaque morphology in men with coronary disease who died suddenly. *N Engl J Med.* 1997;336(18):1276–1282.
14. Hazen SL. Myeloperoxidase and plaque vulnerability. *Arterioscler Thromb Vasc Biol.* 2004;24(7):1143–1146.
15. Gijsen FJ, Wentzel JJ, Thury A, et al. Strain distribution over plaques in human coronary arteries relates to shear stress. *Am J Physiol Heart Circ Physiol.* 2008;295(4):1608–1614.
16. Vengrenyuk Y, Carlier S, Xanthos S, et al. A hypothesis for vulnerable plaque rupture due to stress-induced debonding around cellular microcalcifications in thin fibrous caps. *Proc Natl Acad Sci U S A.* 2006;103(40):14678–14683.
17. Papaspyridonos M, Smith A, Burnand KG, et al. Novel candidate genes in unstable areas of human atherosclerotic plaques. *Arterioscler Thromb Vasc Biol.* 2006;26(8):1837–1844.
18. Shiffman D, Chasman DI, Zee RY, et al. A kinesin family member 6 variant is associated with coronary heart disease in the Women's Health Study. *J Am Coll Cardiol.* 2008;51(4):444–448.
19. Iakoubova OA, Sabatine MS, Rowland CM, et al. Polymorphism in KIF6 gene and benefit from statins after acute coronary syndromes: results from the PROVE IT-TIMI 22 study. *J Am Coll Cardiol.* 2008;51(4):449–455.
20. Feng B, Yao PM, Li Y, et al. The endoplasmic reticulum is the site of cholesterol-induced cytotoxicity in macrophages. *Nat Cell Biol.* 2003; 5(9):781–792.
21. Myoishi M, Hao H, Minamino T, et al. Increased endoplasmic reticulum stress in atherosclerotic plaques associated with acute coronary syndrome. *Circulation.* 2007;116(11):1226–1233.
22. Ait-Oufella H, Kinugawa K, Zoll J, et al. Lactadherin deficiency leads to apoptotic cell accumulation and accelerated atherosclerosis in mice. *Circulation.* 2007;115(16):2168–2177.
23. Aprahamian T, Rifkin I, Bonegio R, et al. Impaired clearance of apoptotic cells promotes synergy between atherogenesis and autoimmune disease. *J Exp Med.* 2004;199(8):1121–1131.
24. Boisvert WA, Rose DM, Boullier A, et al. Leukocyte transglutaminase 2 expression limits atherosclerotic lesion size. *Arterioscler Thromb Vasc Biol.* 2006;26(3):563–569.

25. Virmani R, Kolodgie FD, Burke AP, et al. Atherosclerotic plaque progression and vulnerability to rupture: angiogenesis as a source of intraplaque hemorrhage. *Arterioscler Thromb Vasc Biol.* 2005;25(10): 2054–2061.

26. Yeagle PL. Cholesterol and the cell membrane. *Biochim Biophys Acta.* 1985;822(3–4):267–287.

27. Tulenko TN, Chen M, Mason PE, Mason RP. Physical effects of cholesterol on arterial smooth muscle membranes: evidence of immiscible cholesterol domains and alterations in bilayer width during atherogenesis. *J Lipid Res.* 1998;39(5):947–956.

28. Kolodgie FD, Gold HK, Burke AP, et al. Intraplaque hemorrhage and progression of coronary atheroma. *N Engl J Med.* 2003;349(24): 2316–2325.

29. Kolodgie FD, Narula J, Yuan C, Burke AP, Finn AV, Virmani R. Elimination of neoangiogenesis for plaque stabilization: is there a role for local drug therapy? *J Am Coll Cardiol.* 2007;49(21):2093–2101.

30. Xu XH, Shah PK, Faure E, et al. Toll-like receptor-4 is expressed by macrophages in murine and human lipid-rich atherosclerotic plaques and upregulated by oxidized LDL. *Circulation.* 2001;104(25): 3103–3108.

31. Bogdanov VY, Balasubramanian V, Hathcock J, Vele O, Lieb M, Nemerson Y. Alternatively spliced human tissue factor: a circulating, soluble, thrombogenic protein. *Nat Med.* 2003;9(4):458–462.

32. Rauch U, Nemerson Y. Tissue factor, the blood, and the arterial wall. *Trends Cardiovasc Med.* 2000;10(4):139–143.

33. Sugiyama S, Okada Y, Sukhova GK, Virmani R, Heinecke JW, Libby P. Macrophage myeloperoxidase regulation by granulocyte macrophage colony-stimulating factor in human atherosclerosis and implications in acute coronary syndromes. *Am J Pathol.* 2001;158(3): 879–891.

34. Burke AP, Kolodgie FD, Farb A, Weber DK. Role of circulating myeloperoxidase positive monocytes and neutrophils in occlusive coronary thrombi. *J Am Coll Cardiol.* 2002;39:256A.

35. Galis ZS, Muszynski M, Sukhova GK, et al. Cytokine-stimulated human vascular smooth muscle cells synthesize a complement of enzymes required for extracellular matrix digestion. *Circ Res.* 1994; 75(1):181–189.

36. Sukhova GK, Schonbeck U, Rabkin E, et al. Evidence for increased collagenolysis by interstitial collagenases-1 and -3 in vulnerable human atheromatous plaques. *Circulation.* 1999;99(19):2503–2509.

37. Kolodgie FD, Narula J, Guillo P, Virmani R. Apoptosis in human atherosclerotic plaques. *Apoptosis.* 1999;4(1):5–10.

38. Mann J, Davies MJ. Mechanisms of progression in native coronary artery disease: role of healed plaque disruption. *Heart.* 1999;82(3): 265–268.

39. Burke AP, Kolodgie FD, Farb A, et al. Healed plaque ruptures and sudden coronary death: evidence that subclinical rupture has a role in plaque progression. *Circulation.* 2001;103(7):934–940.

40. Amento EP, Ehsani N, Palmer H, Libby P. Cytokines and growth factors positively and negatively regulate interstitial collagen gene expression in human vascular smooth muscle cells. *Arterioscler Thromb.* 1991;11(5):1223–1230.

41. van der Wal AC, Becker AE, van der Loos CM, Das PK. Site of intimal rupture or erosion of thrombosed coronary atherosclerotic plaques is characterized by an inflammatory process irrespective of the dominant plaque morphology. *Circulation.* 1994;89(1):36–44.

42. Farb A, Burke AP, Tang AL, et al. Coronary plaque erosion without rupture into a lipid core. A frequent cause of coronary thrombosis in sudden coronary death. *Circulation.* 1996;93(7):1354–1363.

43. Aukrust P, Halvorsen B, Yndestad A, et al. Chemokines and cardiovascular risk. *Arterioscler Thromb Vasc Biol.* 2008;28(11):1909–1919.

44. Hansson GK. Inflammation, atherosclerosis, and coronary artery disease. *N Engl J Med.* 2005;352(16):1685–1695.

45. Packard RR, Libby P. Inflammation in atherosclerosis: from vascular biology to biomarker discovery and risk prediction. *Clin Chem.* 2008;54(1):24–38.

46. Libby P, Aikawa M. Stabilization of atherosclerotic plaques: new mechanisms and clinical targets. *Nat Med.* 2002;8(11):1257–1262.

47. Falk E, Shah PK, Fuster V. Coronary plaque disruption. *Circulation.* 1995;92(3):657–671.

48. Koenig W, Khuseyinova N. Lipoprotein-associated and secretory phospholipase A2 in cardiovascular disease: the epidemiological evidence. *Cardiovasc Drugs Ther.* 2009;23(1):85–92.

49. Casas JP, Shah T, Hingorani AD, Danesh J, Pepys MB. C-reactive protein and coronary heart disease: a critical review. *J Intern Med.* 2008;264(4):295–314.

50. Ikonomidis I, Stamatelopoulos K, Lekakis J, Vamvakou GD, Kremastinos DT. Inflammatory and non-invasive vascular markers: the multimarker approach for risk stratification in coronary artery disease. *Atherosclerosis.* 2008;199(1):3–11.

51. Inoue T, Komoda H, Nonaka M, Kameda M, Uchida T, Node K. Interleukin-8 as an independent predictor of long-term clinical outcome in patients with coronary artery disease. *Int J Cardiol.* 2008;124(3):319–325.

52. Oren H, Erbay AR, Balci M, Cehreli S. Role of novel biomarkers of inflammation in patients with stable coronary heart disease. *Angiology.* 2007;58(2):148–155.

53. Ridker PM, Rifai N, Stampfer MJ, Hennekens CH. Plasma concentration of interleukin-6 and the risk of future myocardial infarction among apparently healthy men. *Circulation.* 2000;101(15): 1767–1772.

54. Tan J, Hua Q, Gao J, Fan ZX. Clinical implications of elevated serum interleukin-6, soluble CD40 ligand, metalloproteinase-9, and tissue inhibitor of metalloproteinase-1 in patients with acute ST-segment elevation myocardial infarction. *Clin Cardiol.* 2008;31(9):413–418.

55. Du Clos TW. Function of C-reactive protein. *Ann Med.* 2000;32(4): 274–278.

56. Calabro P, Willerson JT, Yeh ET. Inflammatory cytokines stimulated C-reactive protein production by human coronary artery smooth muscle cells. *Circulation.* 2003;108(16):1930–1932.

57. Dong Q, Wright JR. Expression of C-reactive protein by alveolar macrophages. *J Immunol.* 1996;156(12):4815–4820.

58. Venugopal SK, Devaraj S, Jialal I. Macrophage conditioned medium induces the expression of C-reactive protein in human aortic endothelial cells: potential for paracrine/autocrine effects. *Am J Pathol.* 2005;166(4):1265–1271.

59. Kobayashi S, Inoue N, Ohashi Y, et al. Interaction of oxidative stress and inflammatory response in coronary plaque instability: important role of C-reactive protein. *Arterioscler Thromb Vasc Biol.* 2003;23(8): 1398–1404.

60. Yasojima K, Schwab C, McGeer EG, McGeer PL. Generation of C-reactive protein and complement components in atherosclerotic plaques. *Am J Pathol.* 2001;158(3):1039–1051.

61. Devaraj S, Singh U, Jialal I. The evolving role of C-reactive protein in atherothrombosis. *Clin Chem.* 2009;55(2):229–238.

62. Krupinski J, Turu MM, Martinez-Gonzalez J, et al. Endogenous expression of C-reactive protein is increased in active (ulcerated noncomplicated) human carotid artery plaques. *Stroke.* 2006;37(5): 1200–1204.

63. Slevin M, Matou-Nasri S, Turu M, et al. Modified C-reactive protein is expressed by stroke neovessels and is a potent activator of angiogenesis in vitro. *Brain Pathol.* 2009;Jan 19 Epub ahead of print.

64. Lowe GD, Pepys MB. C-reactive protein and cardiovascular disease: weighing the evidence. *Curr Atheroscler Rep.* 2006;8(5):421–428.

65. Blake GJ, Ridker PM. Novel clinical markers of vascular wall inflammation. *Circ Res.* 2001;89(9):763–771.

66. Ridker PM, Rifai N, Cook NR, Bradwin G, Buring JE. Non-HDL cholesterol, apolipoproteins A-I and B100, standard lipid measures, lipid ratios, and CRP as risk factors for cardiovascular disease in women. *JAMA.* 2005;294(3):326–333.

67. Danesh J, Wheeler JG, Hirschfield GM, et al. C-reactive protein and other circulating markers of inflammation in the prediction of coronary heart disease. *N Engl J Med.* 2004;350(14):1387–1397.

68. Burke AP, Tracy RP, Kolodgie F, et al. Elevated C-reactive protein values and atherosclerosis in sudden coronary death: association with different pathologies. *Circulation.* 2002;105(17):2019–2023.

69. Zalewski A, Macphee C. Role of lipoprotein-associated phospholipase A2 in atherosclerosis: biology, epidemiology, and possible therapeutic target. *Arterioscler Thromb Vasc Biol.* 2005;25(5):923–931.

70. Macphee C, Benson GM, Shi Y, Zalewski A. Lipoprotein-associated phospholipase A2: a novel marker of cardiovascular risk and potential therapeutic target. *Expert Opin Investig Drugs.* 2005;14(6):671–679.

71. Lavi S, McConnell JP, Rihal CS, et al. Local production of lipoprotein-associated phospholipase A2 and lysophosphatidylcholine in the coronary circulation: association with early coronary atherosclerosis and endothelial dysfunction in humans. *Circulation.* 2007;115(21): 2715–2721.

72. Kolodgie FD, Burke AP, Skorija KS, et al. Lipoprotein-associated phospholipase A2 protein expression in the natural progression of human coronary atherosclerosis. *Arterioscler Thromb Vasc Biol.* 2006;26(11):2523–2529.

73. Hakkinen T, Luoma JS, Hiltunen MO, et al. Lipoprotein-associated phospholipase A(2), platelet-activating factor acetylhydrolase, is expressed by macrophages in human and rabbit atherosclerotic lesions. *Arterioscler Thromb Vasc Biol.* 1999;19(12):2909–2917.

74. Carlquist JF, Muhlestein JB, Anderson JL. Lipoprotein-associated phospholipase A2: a new biomarker for cardiovascular risk assessment and potential therapeutic target. *Expert Rev Mol Diagn.* 2007;7(5):511–517.

75. Folsom AR, Chambless LE, Ballantyne CM, et al. An assessment of incremental coronary risk prediction using C-reactive protein and other novel risk markers: the atherosclerosis risk in communities study. *Arch Intern Med.* 2006;166(13):1368–1373.

76. Ballantyne CM, Hoogeveen RC, Bang H, et al. Lipoprotein-associated phospholipase A2, high-sensitivity C-reactive protein, and risk for incident coronary heart disease in middle-aged men and women in the Atherosclerosis Risk in Communities (ARIC) study. *Circulation.* 2004;109(7):837–842.

77. Corson MA, Jones PH, Davidson MH. Review of the evidence for the clinical utility of lipoprotein-associated phospholipase A2 as a cardiovascular risk marker. *Am J Cardiol.* 2008;101(12A):41F–50F.

78. Wilensky RL, Shi Y, Mohler ER 3rd, et al. Inhibition of lipoprotein-associated phospholipase A2 reduces complex coronary atherosclerotic plaque development. *Nat Med.* 2008;14(10):1059–1066.

79. Serruys PW, Garcia-Garcia HM, Buszman P, et al. Effects of the direct lipoprotein-associated phospholipase A(2) inhibitor darapladib on human coronary atherosclerotic plaque. *Circulation.* 2008;118(11): 1172–1182.

80. Zoungas S, McGrath BP, Branley P, et al. Cardiovascular morbidity and mortality in the Atherosclerosis and Folic Acid Supplementation Trial (ASFAST) in chronic renal failure: a multicenter, randomized, controlled trial. *J Am Coll Cardiol.* 2006;47(6):1108–1116.

81. Burke AP, Fonseca V, Kolodgie F, Zieske A, Fink L, Virmani R. Increased serum homocysteine and sudden death resulting from

coronary atherosclerosis with fibrous plaques. *Arterioscler Thromb Vasc Biol.* 2002;22(11):1936–1941.

82. Godsland IF, Elkeles RS, Feher MD, et al. Coronary calcification, homocysteine, C-reactive protein and the metabolic syndrome in Type 2 diabetes: the Prospective Evaluation of Diabetic Ischaemic Heart Disease by Coronary Tomography (PREDICT) Study. *Diabet Med.* 2006;23(11):1192–1200.

13 ▪ Inflammation in the Development and Complications of Coronary Artery Disease

Tariq Ahmad, MD
Paul Ridker, MD

Dr. Ahmad is supported by a T32 Training Grant from the NHLBI. Dr. Ridker is listed as a coinventor on patients held by the Brigham and Women's Hospital that relate to the use of inflammatory biomarkers in cardiovascular disease and diabetes.

Introduction

This chapter reviews the epidemiological and practical criteria for inflammatory biomarkers as predictors of coronary risk, specifically as they pertain to primary and secondary prevention in cardiology and heart failure. Because high sensitivity C-reactive protein (hsCRP) is by far the best characterized inflammatory marker for clinical use in primary and secondary prevention (Figure 13–3), we primarily focus on its characteristics and use in the clinical arena and then describe potential promising biomarkers for predicting vascular risk in cardiovascular disease. The topic of inflammation and acute coronary syndromes, as well as heart failure is more thoroughly discussed elsewhere in the text.

Inflammation in Cardiovascular Disease

Deciphering the process by which stable atherosclerotic plaques become vulnerable, rupture, and subsequently lead to acute vascular ischemia is a major issue in cardiovascular research. At the core of our understanding of how this process occurs is a change in our appreciation of atherosclerosis as not merely a progressive lipid storage disease, but also as a complex process characterized by endothelial dysfunction and inflammation. From the initial recruitment of inflammatory cells to the diseased endothelium to eventual rupture of a vulnerable plaque, inflammation and hyperlipidemia work in tandem to promote atherosclerosis. Stable plaques are characterized by a predominance of smooth muscle cells and few inflammatory cells, whereas unstable plaques are characterized by accumulations of inflammatory cells. As atherosclerotic disease progresses, the inflammatory environment eventually overwhelms the plaque's capacity for repair, resulting in fissure and erosion of the fibrous cap, and subsequent plaque rupture.[1] Inflammatory signals promote thrombogenicity of the atheroma via effects on tissue factor and various other mediators of coagulation. This results in thrombus formation, tissue ischemia, and eventual infarction.[2] As ischemic heart disease progresses to heart failure, the chronic activation of inflammatory mediators continues to exert deleterious effects on the heart and the circulation, contributing to further progression of myocardial dysfunction.[3] Thus, from plaque inception to rupture and subsequently to progressive deterioration of cardiac function, inflammation plays a central role in atherosclerotic cardiovascular disease (Figure 13–1).

Inflammatory Markers in Primary Prevention

Among the approximately 800,000 people[4] within the United States who suffer annually from myocardial infarction or stroke, roughly half have average or even low lipid levels and 15 to 20 percent do not exhibit any of the traditional Framingham coronary risk factors, such as hypertension, hyperlipidemia, smoking, or diabetes.[5,6] This suggests that traditional coronary risk factors do not identify a substantive portion of apparently healthy men and women who are at a risk for acute coronary syndrome (ACS) or acute stroke.[7] This discrepancy has been termed the 'detection gap'[8] and may be due at least in part to the exclusion from traditional risk algorithms of biomarkers that are now widely accepted as important contributors to cardiovascular disease.

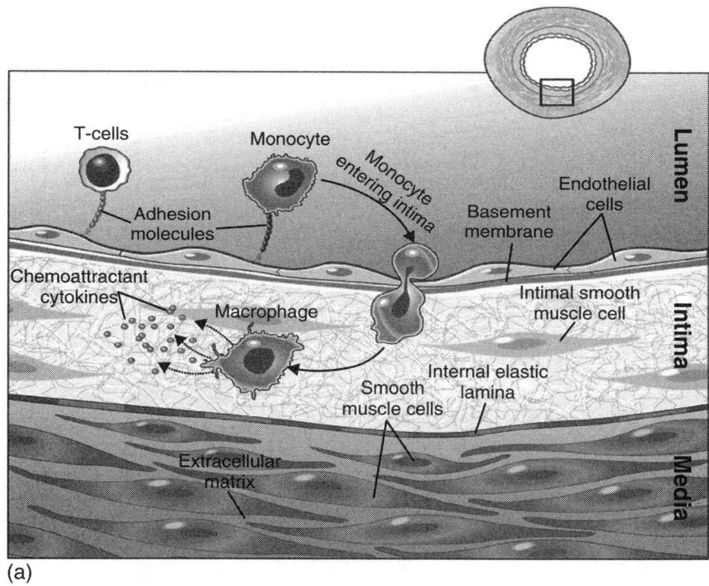

■ **Figure 13–1** Mechanisms of plaque formation and rupture (A) Transition from the normal artery wall to an atherosclerotic lesion: Molecules associated with risk factors stimulate inflammatory stress and induce the expression of adhesion molecules for leukocytes and chemoattractants that draw leukocytes into the intimal layer. (B) Formation of the plaque: Mononuclear phagocytes ingest ox-LDL through scavenger receptors to form foam cells. Macrophages in the lesions release chemoattractant cytokines, proinflammatory mediators, and small lipid molecules such as leukotrienes and prostaglandins, as well as reactive oxygen species. (C) Maturation of the atherosclerotic plaque: Proinflammatory mediators released from activated white cells, endothelial cells, and smooth muscle cells (SMCs) potentiate cell death. SMCs disappear and fewer remain to renew the extracellular matrix in the plaque's fibrous cap. (D) The thrombotic complications of atherosclerosis. Finally, the plaque's fibrous cap ruptures, either from mechanical causes or superficial erosion of the endothelial cells caused by desquamation and endothelial apoptosis. This permits blood and its coagulation factors to contact tissue factor, activate the clotting cascade, and form a thrombus. **See Plate 6 for color image.**

Source: Libby, P. and P.M. Ridker. Inflammation and atherothrombosis from population biology and bench research to clinical practice. *J Am Coll Cardiol.* 2006; 48(9 Suppl):A33–46.

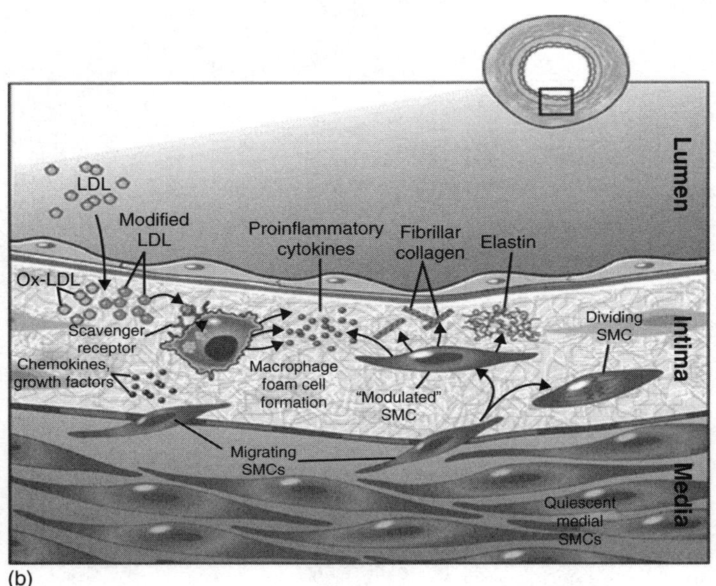

(b)

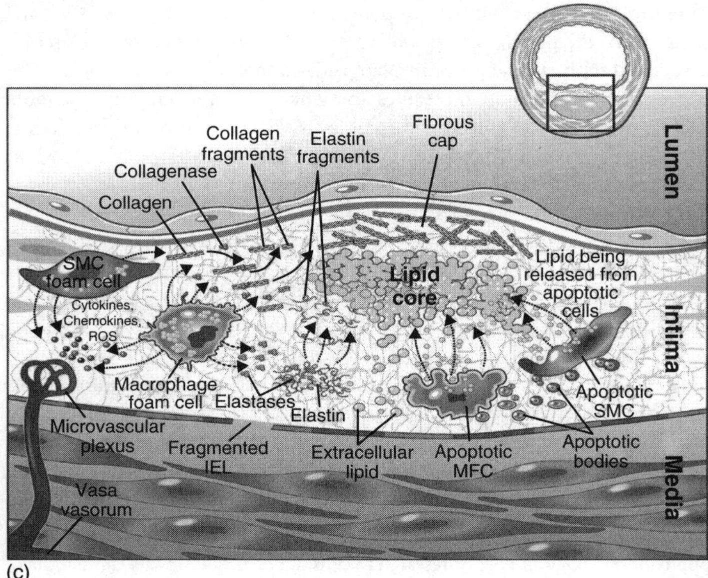

(c)

■ **Figure 13–1 (Continued)**

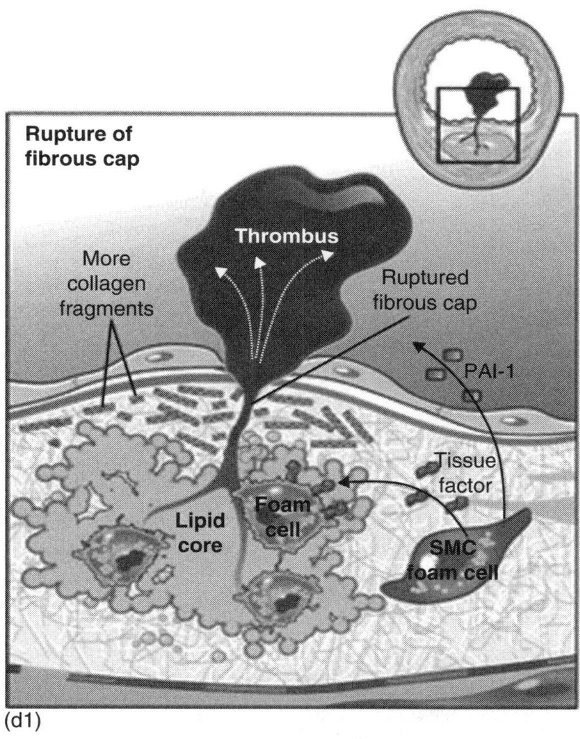

■ **Figure 13–1 (Continued)**

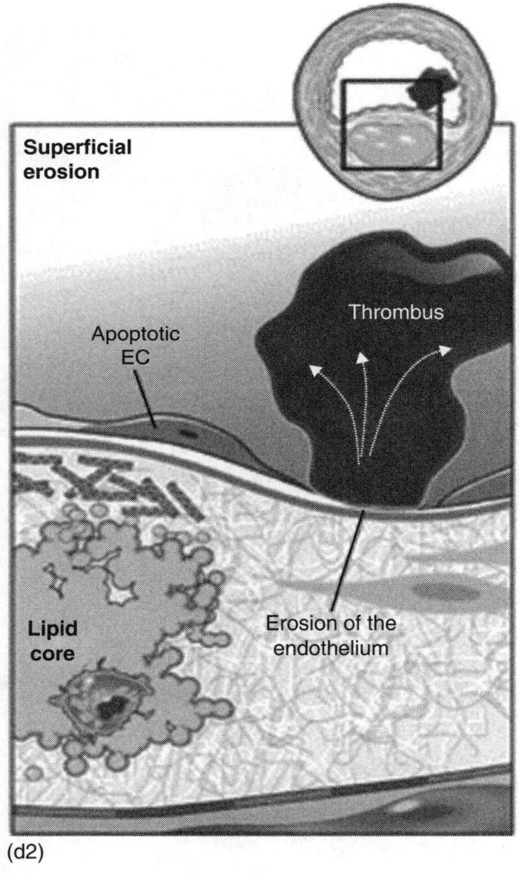

■ **Figure 13–1 (Continued)**

A review of the role of various inflammatory markers in atherosclerosis is presented in Figure 13–2.[9] The first wave of inflammatory cytokines that are released arise from either vascular (atheroma) or extravascular (chronic infection or visceral fat) sources. These cytokines include TNF-α and IL-1β and cause the

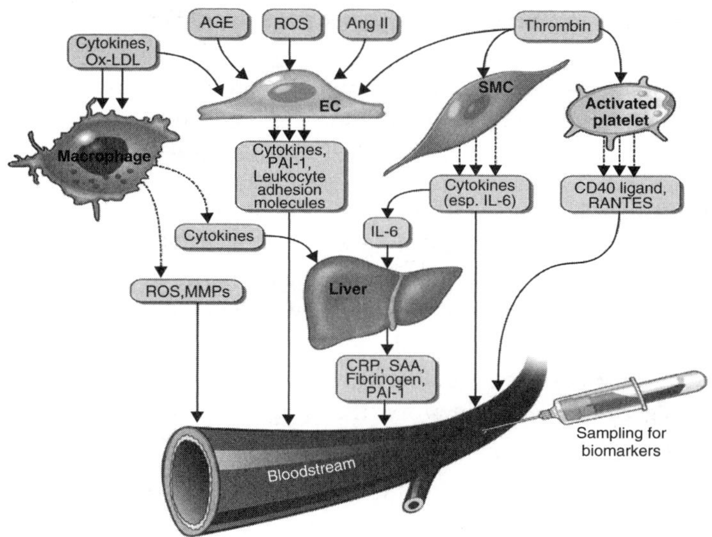

■ **Figure 13–2** The inflammatory hypothesis: The primary proinflammatory risk factors depicted on the top of this diagram activate the various cell types prominent in the atherosclerotic plaque, including the macrophage, endothelial cells (EC), smooth muscle cells (SMC), and, in complicated lesions, the activated platelet. These various cell types in turn secrete inflammatory mediators and reactive oxygen species (ROS). The primary proinflammatory cytokines, including interleukin-1 (IL-1) and TNF-α, can stimulate large amounts of IL-6 production by intrinsic vascular wall cells. IL-6 functions as a messenger and acts on the liver to elicit the acute-phase response. The acute-phase reactants include C-reactive protein (CRP), serum amyloid A (SAA), fibrinogen, and plasminogen activator inhibitor-1. **See Plate 7 for color image.**

Source: Libby, P. and P.M. Ridker. Inflammation and atherothrombosis from population biology and bench research to clinical practice. *J Am Coll Cardiol.* 2006; 48(9 Suppl):A33–46.

production and release of IL-6 by vascular endothelium and smooth muscle cells. IL-6 is a mediator of the hepatic acute-phase response and induces production of fibrinogen, PAI-1, serum amyloid A (SAA), and C-reactive protein (CRP). These biomarkers are released into peripheral blood and can be measured by venipuncture.

Although biomarkers of inflammation are an attractive metric for coronary artery risk stratification, they must fulfill the following criteria before they can gain widespread clinical applicability:[10]

- Standardized, reproducible, and cost-effective biomarker assays with quick turnaround times must be available and the test results must be easy to interpret in a primary care setting.
- Prospective studies must demonstrate consistently that the biomarker predicts future risk.
- Addition of the biomarker to existing risk prediction algorithms must improve the prognostic accuracy of the algorithm.

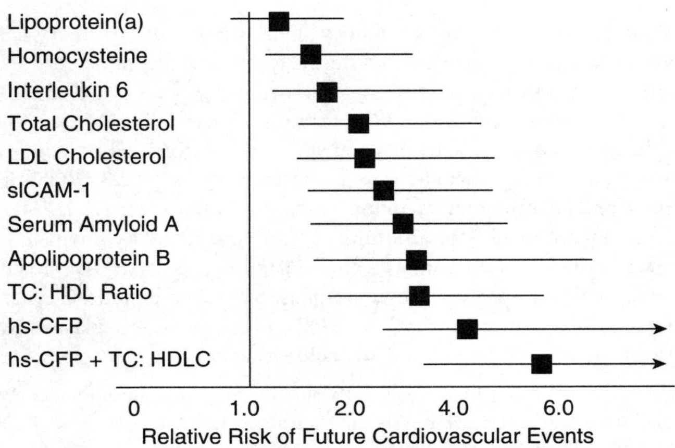

■ **Figure 13–3** Relative risks of future myocardial infarctions in apparently healthy women according to baseline characteristics of risk detection markers.

Source: Libby, P. and P.M. Ridker. Inflammation and atherothrombosis from population biology and bench research to clinical practice. *J Am Coll Cardiol.* 2006;48(9 Suppl):A33–46.

CRP in Primary Prevention

A large step forward was taken when assays with sufficient refinement to detect subtle differences in CRP concentrations were developed. These "high sensitivity" CRP (hsCRP) assays have proven quite important: studies in vascular biology have found hsCRP to be a reliable marker of endothelial inflammation, and to have the greatest relevance to clinical care among inflammatory markers. Numerous prospective epidemiological studies (Figure 13–4) have demonstrated a strong linear relationship of hsCRP to

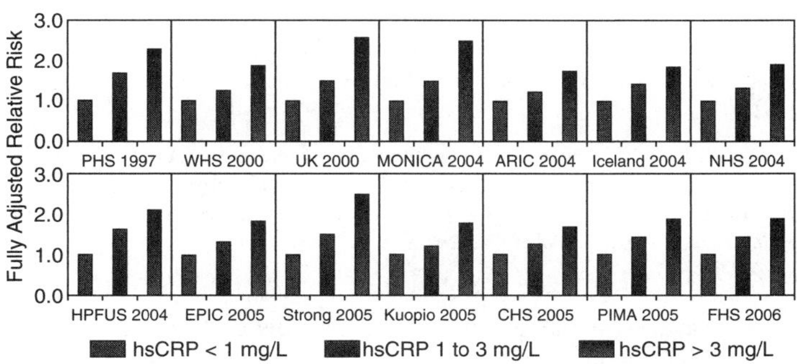

■ **Figure 13–4** Independent Impact of hsCRP on Cardiovascular Risk. Multivariate adjusted relative risks of future cardiovascular events according to baseline levels of high sensitivity C-reactive protein (hsCRP) <1 mg/l, 1 to 3 mg/l, and >3 mg/l in 14 major prospective cohort studies. ARIC = Atherosclerosis Risk in Communities study; CHS = Cardiovascular Health Study; EPIC = Evaluation for Prevention of Ischemic Complications-Norfolk study; FHS = Framingham Heart Study; HPFUS = Health Professionals Follow-Up Study; Iceland = Reykjavik Heart Study data; Kuopio = Kuopio Heart Study; MONICA = Monitoring Trends and Development in Cardiovascular Disease study; NHS = Nurses Health Study; PHS = Physicians Health Study; PIMA = Pima Indian study; Strong = Strong Heart Study; UK = British general practice cohort; WHS = Women's Health Study.

Source: Libby, P. and P.M. Ridker. Inflammation and atherothrombosis from population biology and bench research to clinical practice. *J Am Coll Cardiol.* 2006;48(9 Suppl):A33–46.

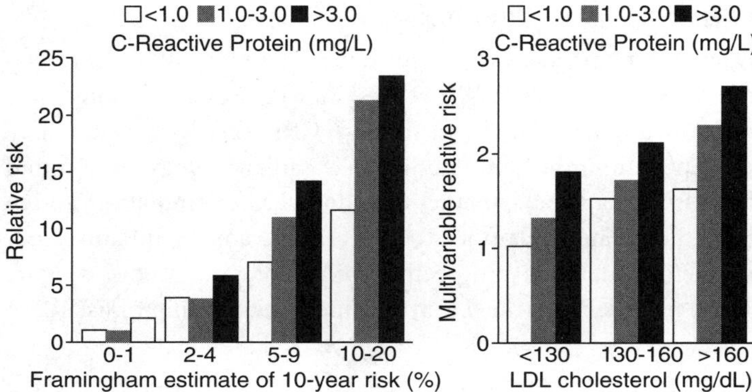

■ **Figure 13–5** hsCRP adds prognostic information on vascular risk at all levels of LDL-C (right) and at all levels of the Framingham Risk Score (left).

Source: Ridker, P.M. Rosuvastatin in the primary prevention of cardiovascular disease among patients with low levels of low-density lipoprotein cholesterol and elevated high-sensitivity C-reactive protein: Rationale and design of the JUPITER trial. *Circulation.* 2003;108(19):2292–2297.

future cardiovascular events[11–31], independent of traditional risk factors such as age, smoking, diabetes, and hyperlipidemia. These findings are consistent in both men and women, at all age levels, with up to two decades of follow-up. The magnitude of the predictive accuracy of hsCRP has been shown to be comparable or superior to that of LDL (low-density lipoprotein) level[11,12] and at least as large as that associated with hypertension.[13] Importantly, hsCRP adds prognostic value to all values of LDL cholesterol and across a full range of Framingham risk scores (Figure 13–5). Vascular risk has been found to be higher in individuals with elevated hsCRP and low LDL than in those with low hsCRP and high LDL.

Mechanisms and Analytic Issues

CRP is a pentraxin, one of a family of proteins that are composed of five identical and noncovalently-bound protein subunits. It is one of the earliest acute phase proteins to be released after activa-

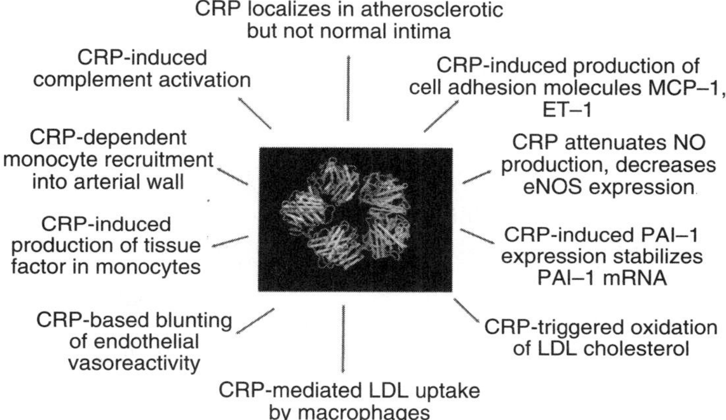

■ **Figure 13–6** Potential mechanisms relating CRP to development and progression of atherothrombosis.

Source: Ridker, P.M. Rosuvastatin in the primary prevention of cardiovascular disease among patients with low levels of low-density lipoprotein cholesterol and elevated high-sensitivity C-reactive protein: Rationale and design of the JUPITER trial. *Circulation.* 2003;108(19):2292–2297.

tion of the inflammatory response and is thought to play a fundamental role in innate immunity by binding to polysaccharides of infectious agents and activating the classic complement system.[14] It is synthesized by hepatocytes in response to tissue injury or infection, induced by cytokines such as IL-6, IL-1β, and TNF-α. While a robust predictor of risk, it remains uncertain as to whether or not CRP itself plays a direct role in atherothrombosis. Several potential mechanisms by which CRP might directly promote atherogenesis are outlined in Figure 13–6. Ongoing experimental studies with direct CRP inhibitors are needed to resolve this issue.

hsCRP levels increase mildly with age,[15] likely due to age-related obesity. These levels are unaffected by intra-individual circadian variation or dietary intake and can be measured at any time of the day. Year-to-year, and even decade-to-decade, variability in hsCRP measurements are similar to those of cholesterol.[13] Several environmental factors and medications modestly influence hsCRP concentrations. For example, hsCRP levels correlate negatively with cardiopulmonary fitness[16] and positively with weight.[17] Increased and decreased hsCRP levels are associated with increases in smoking[18] and moderate alcohol levels,[19] respectively. Certain medications can also influence hsCRP concentrations: hormone replacement therapy except droloxifene[20,21] increases hsCRP and statins consistently show reduction in levels of hsCRP.[22–24]

The American Heart Association (AHA) and the Centers for Disease Control (CDC) have endorsed the use of hsCRP as a marker of vascular risk and[25] multiple commercial assays of hsCRP exist that have been standardized for consistency, with results being reported in mg/L.[25]

Clinical Applications

The AHA/CDC guidelines issued in 2003 recommend that hsCRP levels be interpreted as a component of global risk and only in the context of other risk factors. In general, hsCRP levels less than 1 mg/L, 1 mg/L to 3 mg/L, and greater than 3 mg/L represent lower, average, and higher relative risks, given other risk factors.[25] When hsCRP levels are greater than 5 mg/L, they should be rechecked in 2–3 weeks and the lower of these values used for vascular risk prediction. As transient increases in hsCRP may occur, the lowest values available for a given patient are probably best used for this purpose. For most patients, only one measurement of hsCRP is required. hsCRP levels should be used in conjunction with traditional markers of risk; it is important to note that although hsCRP levels predict risk across the population spectrum, they are likely most useful in risk stratification among intermediate risk patients, that is, those with ten-year event rates are predicted to be between 5% and 20%. This is evident in a recent analysis where the use of hsCRP and family history were included in risk prediction models for women and men. Known as the Reynolds Risk Score (available online at http://www.reynoldsriskscore.org), the addition of hsCRP and family history correctly reclassify global risk into clinically-relevant higher or lower risk categories in approximately 20% of men and women.[26,27]

Elevated levels of hsCRP positively correlate with several markers of metabolic syndrome, such as insulin sensitivity, endothelial dysfunction, and hypofibrinolysis.[28–30] Increased levels are also associated with increased vascular risk amongst those with metabolic syndrome and diabetes (Figure 13–7).[31–33] Furthermore, elevated levels of hsCRP in apparently healthy individuals correlate with increased risk of developing type 2 diabetes mellitus,

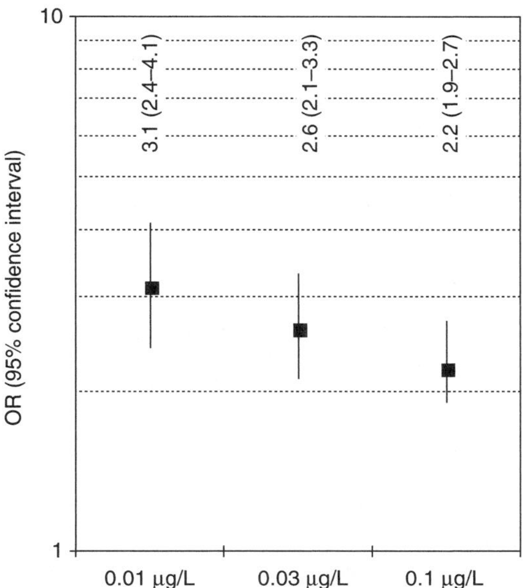

■ **Figure 13–7** Cardiovascular event-free survival according to baseline levels of hsCRP among individuals with metabolic syndrome (adapted from).

Source: Ridker, P.M., et al. C-reactive protein, the metabolic syndrome, and risk of incident cardiovascular events: an 8-year follow-up of 14 719 initially healthy American women. *Circulation.* 2003;107(3):391–397.

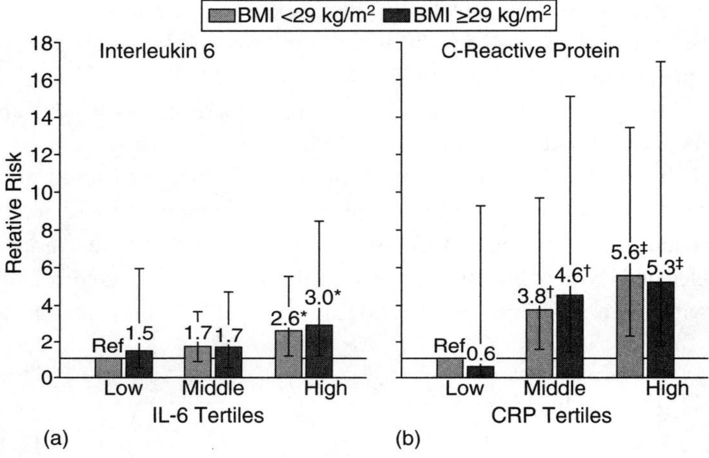

■ **Figure 13–8** Relative risk of type 2 diabetes mellitus in women according to baseline levels of interleukin 6, C-reactive protein, and body mass index.

Source: Pradhan, A.D., et al. C-reactive protein, interleukin 6, and risk of developing type 2 diabetes mellitus. JAMA. 2001;286(3):327–334.

independently of risk factors such as obesity (Figure 13–8).[34–39] These observations, along with basic research into the inflammatory mechanisms of both diabetes and vascular dysfunction, provide evidence that insulin resistance and atherosclerosis share a common inflammatory basis.

Weight reduction, smoking cessation, increased physical activity, and dietary modification reduce vascular risk and lower hsCRP levels.[18,40–43] Statins reduce the levels in a manner that appears to be independent of the magnitude of LDL cholesterol reduction.[44–47] Data from several primary and secondary prevention trials have shown that the benefit of statin therapy extends beyond patients with increased LDL cholesterol; in fact, apparently healthy individuals with low levels of LDL-C, but high levels of hsCRP, are at higher absolute risk of future vascular events than are those with high levels of LDL-C, but low levels of hsCRP.[22,23,48] These observations led to the hypothesis that statin therapy may benefit patients whose LDL-C profiles are within the normal range, but who have increased levels of hsCRP. Achieving low LDL-C and hsCRP levels with statin therapy has been shown to improve outcomes in the arena of secondary prevention in the A-to-Z and TIMI 22 trials[49,50] and in intravascular ultrasound studies on plaque progression.[51]

The Justification for the Use of Statin in Prevention: an Intervention Trial Evaluating Rosuvastatin (JUPITER) trial was designed to test whether long-term treatment with rosuvastatin would reduce the rate of first major cardiovascular death, stroke, myocardial infarction, hospitalization for unstable angina, or arterial revascularization among individuals with LDL-C levels less than 130 mg/dl, who were at high vascular risk by virtue of having hsCRP levels greater than 2 mg/L.[52] Conducted among 17,802 men and women in 26 countries, the JUPITER trial was terminated early due to a 54% reduction in myocardial infarction, a 48% reduction in stroke, a 47% reduction in bypass surgery or angioplasty, and a 20% reduction in all cause mortality (Figure 13–9).[53] Perhaps most striking, despite evaluating a low LDL-C population, the Number Needed to Treat (NNT) within JUPITER after five years of therapy was projected to be only 25, a value smaller than that observed in prior primary prevention statin trials that alternatively targeted individuals with overt hyperlipidemia. JUPITER also demonstrated highly significant effects for women and minority populations who traditionally have been excluded from such studies. Further, in a subgroup of JUPITER that had elevated hsCRP levels and no major ATP-III risk factors, similar large event reductions were observed. Preliminary JUPITER analysis also suggests that achieving low levels of both LDL-C and hsCRP are important to maximize the benefits of statin therapy.

In addition to statins, several other medications routinely administered to patients with risk factors for cardiovascular disease decrease hsCRP levels; however, their role in the prevention of cardiovascular disease has yet to be determined.[54] Intriguingly, a

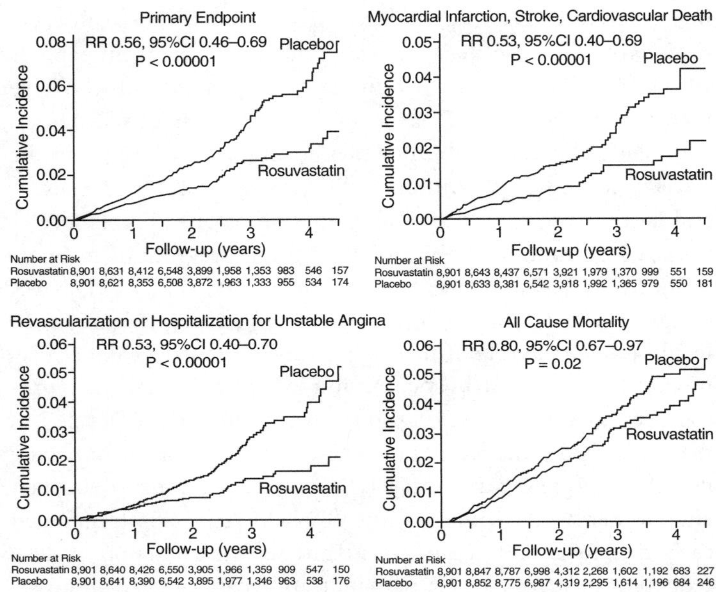

■ **Figure 13–9** Cumulative incidence of cardiovascular events among patients with normal cholesterol but elevated hsCRP, as a function of treatment allocation in the JUPITER study.

Source: Morrow, D.A., et al. Clinical relevance of C-reactive protein during follow-up of patients with acute coronary syndromes in the Aggrastat-to-Zocor Trial. *Circulation.* 2006;114(4): p. 281–288. and Ridker, P.M., et al. C-reactive protein levels and outcomes after statin therapy. *N Engl J Med.* 2005;352(1):20–28.

recent trial showed that valsartan reduced hsCRP levels independently of its effects on blood pressure, raising the possibility that angiotensin receptor blockage may have anti-inflammatory effects.[55] Aspirin therapy has inconsistent effects on hsCRP levels,[56,57] but aspirin's beneficial effect for primary prevention has been mainly seen in patients with elevated hsCRP levels.[11] Hormone replacement therapy tends to increase hsCRP levels. Interestingly, the Women's Health Initiative (WHI) study showed that vascular events at a given level of hsCRP were similar in women on HRT and women not on HRT.[58] To date, only statin therapy has been shown to reduce vascular event rates among those with elevated hsCRP; thus, in addition to lifestyle interventions, maximizing statin regimens should be the first line of pharmacologic intervention for those with elevated hsCRP.

Other Inflammatory Markers

Several other markers of inflammation appear promising in predicting vascular risk. These include: acute phase reactants like fibrinogen; serum amyloid A (SAA); cytokines, such as interleukin-6; cell adhesion molecules, such as sICAM-1; P-selectin, or the mediator CD40 ligand; as well as markers of leukocyte activation, such as myeloperoxidase. Other inflammatory markers associated with lipid oxidation, such as lipoprotein-associated phospholipase A_2 (Lp-PLA$_2$) and pregnancy-associated plasma protein A (PAPP-A) could also be relevant. These markers are not commonly used in clinical settings because of analytical issues, marginal ability to predict risk in broad populations, or lack of information regarding benefits of reduction in biomarker levels. Their use may expand with further studies and in the future they may provide new therapeutic targets.

Fibrinogen and Fibrin D-Dimer

Fibrinogen is an acute phase reactant, as well as a crucial component of the fibinolytic cascade made by the liver in response to several cytokines. It appears to be a marker for inflammation, while concurrently promoting atherothrombosis by altering the hemodynamic properties of blood or enhancing interactions between thrombin and platelets, thus leading to increased intravascular fibrin deposition and thrombosis. Elevated levels of plasma fibrinogen associate positively with most of the known risk factors for cardiovascular disease. Several prospective studies and a recent meta-analysis have also shown that elevated plasma fibrinogen levels are an independent predictor for increased risk of coronary artery disease, stroke, and peripheral vascular disease.[59]

Fibrinogen and hsCRP are also additive in their ability to predict risk, although the effect of hsCRP appears to be somewhat larger. Epidemiological evidence has also shown that D-dimer levels predict recurrent events after myocardial infarctions and are also predictive of poor outcomes in troponin-negative ACS.[60]

At this time, the role of fibrinogen in preventive cardiology and D-dimer elevations in arterial thrombosis is limited due to suboptimal assay standardization, lack of definitive data, and disappointing outcomes from trials that evaluated the benefits of fibrinogen reduction.[61,62]

Lipoprotein-Associated Phospholipase A_2 (Lp-PLA_2)

Discussed in greater detail elsewhere, Lp-PLA_2 is an acute phase reactant and one of a family of phospholipase enzymes. It is upregulated in the atherosclerotic vessel wall where it hydrolyzes phospholipids and contributes to the production of oxidized LDL and foam cells. In the core of the vulnerable plaque, Lp-PLA_2 hydrolyzes oxidized phospholipids into oxidized lipid products that stimulate adhesion molecule expression and release of cytokines, which recruit more leukocytes to the lesion.[63]

Studies showing the relationship between elevated levels of Lp-PLA_2 and increased risk for subsequent coronary events in primary and secondary prevention settings have been generally, but not always, positive. Some studies have shown statistically significant risk ratios after controlling for traditional risk factors and currently known biomarkers,[64–66] whereas in other studies this relationship disappears after similar adjustments.[67,68] Of note, results from the MONICA (Monitoring of Trends and Determinants in Cardiovascular Disease), which was a prospective study of initially healthy middle-aged men who were followed for 14 years, showed that increased Lp-PLA_2 levels were independently related to first-ever events (HR 1.21; 95% CI: 1.01–1.45). The majority of studies have been done on healthy individuals and data regarding the use of Lp-PLA_2 are limited in patients with established coronary artery disease.[69] Some studies have also suggested that using Lp-PLA_2 in conjunction with hsCRP could provide prognostication of future events better than use of the individual marker.[65,68]

Pregnancy-Associated Plasma Protein A (PAPP-A)

PAPP-A is one of the matrix metalloproteinases (MMPs) that degrades the extracellular matrix of the arterial wall and contributes to plaque instability. It activates the insulin-like growth factor-1, a mediator of atherosclerosis, implying a mechanism that results in plaque vulnerability.[70] Plaque investigations of patients who died from ACS showed that PAPP-A was highly expressed in the ruptured or vulnerable plaques, but minimally expressed in the stable plaques.[71] Its role in prognostication has been most fruitful in settings of troponin-negative ACS and chronic angina.[71–73] The use of this biomarker in the clinical setting will require assay standardization and clinical validation in larger cohorts.

Serum Amyloid A (SAA)

Serum amyloid A is a group of three related apolipoproteins that are activated during the acute phase response. It likely works on HDL (high-density lipoprotein) to convert into a higher density particle that has diminished antiatherosclerotic effects and may promote foam cell formation. SAA levels increase during a myocardial infarction and can be predictive of 14-day mortality after unstable angina or non-ST segment elevation myocardial infarction.[74] Epidemiologic data for SAA largely parallel that of hsCRP.[75] Elevated levels are predictive of cardiovascular outcomes when checked at discharge levels, but not at two months.[76,77]

References

1. Libby P. Current concepts of the pathogenesis of the acute coronary syndromes. *Circulation.* 2001;104(3):365–372.
2. Libby P, Ridker PM, Maseri A. Inflammation and atherosclerosis. *Circulation.* 2002;105(9):1135–1143.
3. Braunwald E. Biomarkers in heart failure. *N Engl J Med.* 2008; 358(20):2148–2159.

4. Thom T, Haase N, Rosamond W, et al. Heart disease and stroke statistics—2006 update: a report from the American Heart Association Statistics Committee and Stroke Statistics Subcommittee. *Circulation.* 2006;113(6):e85–e151.
5. Kannel WB, Dawber TR, Kagan A, Revotskie N, Stokes J 3rd. Factors of risk in the development of coronary heart disease—six year follow-up experience. The Framingham Study. *Ann Intern Med.* 1961; 55:33–50.
6. Khot UN, Khot MB, Bajzer CT, et al. Prevalence of conventional risk factors in patients with coronary heart disease. *JAMA.* 2003;290(7): 898–904.
7. Ajani UA, Ford ES. Has the risk for coronary heart disease changed among U.S. adults? *J Am Coll Cardiol.* 2006;48(6):1177–1182.
8. Pasternak RC, Abrams J, Greenland P, Smaha LA, Wilson PW, Houston-Miller N. 34th Bethesda Conference: Task force #1—Identification of coronary heart disease risk: is there a detection gap? *J Am Coll Cardiol.* 2003;41(11):1863–1874.
9. Libby P, Ridker PM. Novel inflammatory markers of coronary risk: theory versus practice. *Circulation.* 1999;100(11):1148–1150.
10. Vasan, RS. Biomarkers of cardiovascular disease: molecular basis and practical considerations. *Circulation.* 2006;113(19):2335–2362.
11. Ridker PM, Cushman M, Stampfer MJ, Tracy RP, Hennekens CH. Inflammation, aspirin, and the risk of cardiovascular disease in apparently healthy men. *N Engl J Med.* 1997;336(14):973–979.
12. Boekholdt SM, Hack CE, Sandhu MS, et al. C-reactive protein levels and coronary artery disease incidence and mortality in apparently healthy men and women: the EPIC-Norfolk prospective population study 1993–2003. *Atherosclerosis.* 2006;187(2):415–422.
13. Danesh J, Wheeler JG, Hirschfield GM, et al. C-reactive protein and other circulating markers of inflammation in the prediction of coronary heart disease. *N Engl J Med.* 2004;350(14):1387–1397.
14. Pepys MB, Hirschfield GM, Tennent GA, et al. Targeting C-reactive protein for the treatment of cardiovascular disease. *Nature.* 2006; 440(7088):1217–1221.
15. Hutchinson WL, Koenig W, Frohlich M, Sund M, Lowe GD, Pepys MB. Immunoradiometric assay of circulating C-reactive protein: age-related values in the adult general population. *Clin Chem.* 2000; 46(7):934–938.

16. Church TS, Barlow CE, Earnest CP, Kampert JB, Priest EL, Blair SN. Associations between cardiorespiratory fitness and C-reactive protein in men. *Arterioscler Thromb Vasc Biol.* 2002;22(11):1869–1876.
17. Ford ES. Body mass index, diabetes, and C-reactive protein among U.S. adults. *Diabetes Care.* 1999;22(12):1971–1977.
18. Bermudez EA, Rifai N, Buring JE, Manson JE, Ridker PM. Relation between markers of systemic vascular inflammation and smoking in women. *Am J Cardiol.* 2002;89(9):1117–1119.
19. Albert MA, Glynn RJ, Ridker PM. Alcohol consumption and plasma concentration of C-reactive protein. *Circulation.* 2003;107(3):443–447.
20. Ridker PM, Hennekens CH, Rifai N, Buring JE, Manson JE. Hormone replacement therapy and increased plasma concentration of C-reactive protein. *Circulation.* 1999;100(7):713–716.
21. Herrington DM, Brosnihan KB, Pusser BE, et al. Differential effects of E and droloxifene on C-reactive protein and other markers of inflammation in healthy postmenopausal women. *J Clin Endocrinol Metab.* 2001;86(9):4216–4222.
22. Ridker PM, Rifai N, Pfeffer MA, et al. Inflammation, pravastatin, and the risk of coronary events after myocardial infarction in patients with average cholesterol levels. Cholesterol and Recurrent Events (CARE) Investigators. *Circulation.* 1998;98(9):839–844.
23. Ridker PM, Rifai N, Clearfield M, et al. Measurement of C-reactive protein for the targeting of statin therapy in the primary prevention of acute coronary events. *N Engl J Med.* 2001;344(26):1959–1965.
24. Jialal I, Stein D, Balis D, Grundy SM, Adams-Huet B, Devaraj, S. Effect of hydroxymethyl glutaryl coenzyme a reductase inhibitor therapy on high sensitive C-reactive protein levels. *Circulation.* 2001;103(15):1933–1935.
25. Pearson TA, Mensah GA, Alexander RW, et al. Markers of inflammation and cardiovascular disease: application to clinical and public health practice. A statement for healthcare professionals from the Centers for Disease Control and Prevention and the American Heart Association. *Circulation.* 2003;107(3):499–511.
26. Ridker PM, Buring JE, Rifai N, Cook NR. Development and validation of improved algorithms for the assessment of global cardiovascular risk in women: the Reynolds Risk Score. *JAMA.* 2007;297(6):611–619.

27. Ridker PM, Paynter NP, Rifai N, Gaziano JM, Cook NR. C-reactive protein and parental history improve global cardiovascular risk prediction: the Reynolds Risk Score for men. *Circulation*. 2008; 118(22):2243–2251.

28. Frohlich M, Imhof A, Berg G, et al. Association between C-reactive protein and features of the metabolic syndrome: a population-based study. *Diabetes Care*. 2000;23(12):1835–1839.

29. Festa A, D'Agostino R Jr, Howard G, Mykkanen L, Tracy RP, Haffner SM. Chronic subclinical inflammation as part of the insulin resistance syndrome: the Insulin Resistance Atherosclerosis Study (IRAS). *Circulation*. 2000;102(1):42–47.

30. Stehouwer CD, Gall MA, Twisk JW, Knudsen E, Emeis JJ, Parving HH. Increased urinary albumin excretion, endothelial dysfunction, and chronic low-grade inflammation in type 2 diabetes: progressive, interrelated, and independently associated with risk of death. *Diabetes*. 2002;51(4):1157–1165.

31. Ridker PM, Buring JE, Cook NR, Rifai N. C-reactive protein, the metabolic syndrome, and risk of incident cardiovascular events: an 8-year follow-up of 14,719 initially healthy American women. *Circulation*. 2003;107(3):391–397.

32. Sattar N, Gaw A, Scherbakova O, et al. Metabolic syndrome with and without C-reactive protein as a predictor of coronary heart disease and diabetes in the West of Scotland Coronary Prevention Study. *Circulation*. 2003;108(4):414–419.

33. Schulze MB, Rimm EB, Li T, Rifai N, Stampfer MJ, Hu FB. C-reactive protein and incident cardiovascular events among men with diabetes. *Diabetes Care*. 2004;27(4):889–994.

34. Pradhan AD, Manson JE, Rifai N, Buring JE, Ridker PM. C-reactive protein, interleukin 6, and risk of developing type 2 diabetes mellitus. *JAMA*. 2001;286(3):327–334.

35. Freeman DJ, Norrie J, Caslake MJ, et al. C-reactive protein is an independent predictor of risk for the development of diabetes in the West of Scotland Coronary Prevention Study. *Diabetes*. 2002;51(5): 1596–1600.

36. Doi Y, Kiyohara Y, Kubo M, et al. Elevated C-reactive protein is a predictor of the development of diabetes in a general Japanese population: the Hisayama Study. *Diabetes Care*. 2005;28(10):2497–2500.

37. Festa A, D'Agostino R Jr, Tracy RP, Haffner SM. Elevated levels of acute-phase proteins and plasminogen activator inhibitor-1 predict the development of type 2 diabetes: the Insulin Resistance Atherosclerosis Study. *Diabetes.* 2002;51(4):1131–1137.
38. Laaksonen DE, Niskanen L, Nyyssonen K, et al. C-reactive protein and the development of the metabolic syndrome and diabetes in middle-aged men. *Diabetologia.* 2004;47(8):1403–1410.
39. Hu FB, Meigs JB, Li TY, Rifai N, Manson JE. Inflammatory markers and risk of developing type 2 diabetes in women. *Diabetes.* 2004;53(3):693–700.
40. Esposito K, Pontillo A, Di Palo C, et al. Effect of weight loss and lifestyle changes on vascular inflammatory markers in obese women: a randomized trial. *JAMA.* 2003;289(14):1799–1804.
41. Mora S, Lee IM, Buring JE, Ridker PM. Association of physical activity and body mass index with novel and traditional cardiovascular biomarkers in women. *JAMA.* 2006;295(12):1412–1419.
42. Tchernof A, Nolan A, Sites CK, Ades PA, Poehlman ET. Weight loss reduces C-reactive protein levels in obese postmenopausal women. *Circulation.* 2002;105(5):564–569.
43. Wannamethee SG, Lowe GD, Whincup PH, Rumley A, Walker M, Lennon L. Physical activity and hemostatic and inflammatory variables in elderly men. *Circulation.* 2002;105(15):1785–1790.
44. Ridker PM, Rifai N, Pfeffer MA, Sacks F, Braunwald E. Long-term effects of pravastatin on plasma concentration of C-reactive protein. The Cholesterol and Recurrent Events (CARE) Investigators. *Circulation.* 1999;100(3):230–235.
45. Crisby M, Nordin-Fredriksson G, Shah PK, Yano J, Zhu J, Nilsson J. Pravastatin treatment increases collagen content and decreases lipid content, inflammation, metalloproteinases, and cell death in human carotid plaques: implications for plaque stabilization. *Circulation.* 2001;103(7):926–933.
46. Williams JK, Sukhova GK, Herrington DM, Libby P. Pravastatin has cholesterol-lowering independent effects on the artery wall of atherosclerotic monkeys. *J Am Coll Cardiol.* 1998;31(3):684–691.
47. Bustos C, Hernandez-Presa MA, Ortego M, et al. HMG-CoA reductase inhibition by atorvastatin reduces neointimal inflammation in a rabbit model of atherosclerosis. *J Am Coll Cardiol.* 1998;32(7):2057–2064.

48. Ridker PM, Rifai N, Rose L, Buring JE, Cook NR. Comparison of C-reactive protein and low-density lipoprotein cholesterol levels in the prediction of first cardiovascular events. *N Engl J Med.* 2002; 347:1557–1565.
49. Morrow DA, de Lemos JA, Sabatine MS, et al. Clinical relevance of C-reactive protein during follow-up of patients with acute coronary syndromes in the Aggrastat-to-Zocor Trial. *Circulation.* 2006;114(4): 281–288.
50. Ridker PM, Cannon CP, Morrow D, et al. C-reactive protein levels and outcomes after statin therapy. *N Engl J Med.* 2005;352(1): 20–28.
51. Nissen SE, Tuzcu EM, Schoenhagen P, et al. Statin therapy, LDL cholesterol, C-reactive protein, and coronary artery disease. *N Engl J Med.* 2005;352(1):29–38.
52. Ridker PM. Rosuvastatin in the primary prevention of cardiovascular disease among patients with low levels of low-density lipoprotein cholesterol and elevated high-sensitivity C-reactive protein: Rationale and design of the JUPITER trial. *Circulation.* 2003;108(19): 2292–2297.
53. Ridker PM, Danielson E, Fonseca FA, et al. Rosuvastatin to prevent vascular events in men and women with elevated C-reactive protein. *N Engl J Med.* 2008;359(21):2195–2207.
54. Prasad K. C-reactive protein (CRP)-lowering agents. *Cardiovasc Drug Rev.* 2006;24(1):33–50.
55. Ridker PM, Danielson E, Rifai N, Glynn RJ. Valsartan, blood pressure reduction, and C-reactive protein: primary report of the Val-MARC trial. *Hypertension.* 2006;48(1):73–79.
56. Ikonomidis I, Andreotti F, Economou E, Stefanadis C, Toutouzas P, Nihoyannopoulos P. Increased proinflammatory cytokines in patients with chronic stable angina and their reduction by aspirin. *Circulation.* 1999;100(8):793–798.
57. Feldman M, Jialal I, Devaraj S, Cryer B. Effects of low-dose aspirin on serum C-reactive protein and thromboxane B2 concentrations: a placebo-controlled study using a highly sensitive C-reactive protein assay. *J Am Coll Cardiol.* 2001;37(8):2036–2041.
58. Pradhan AD, Manson JE, Rossouw JE, et al. Inflammatory biomarkers, hormone replacement therapy, and incident coronary heart

disease: prospective analysis from the Women's Health Initiative observational study. *JAMA*. 2002;288(8):980–987.

59. Danesh J, Lewington S, Thompson SG, et al. Plasma fibrinogen level and the risk of major cardiovascular diseases and nonvascular mortality: an individual participant meta-analysis. *JAMA*. 2005;294(14): 1799–1809.

60. Menown IB, Mathew TP, Gracey HM, et al. Prediction of recurrent events by D-Dimer and inflammatory markers in patients with normal cardiac troponin I (PREDICT) study. *Am Heart J*. 2003;145(6): 986–992.

61. Meade T, Zuhrie R, Cook C, Cooper J. Bezafibrate in men with lower extremity arterial disease: randomised controlled trial. *BMJ*. 2002;325(7373):1139.

62. Tanne D, Benderly M, Goldbourt U, et al. A prospective study of plasma fibrinogen levels and the risk of stroke among participants in the bezafibrate infarction prevention study. *Am J Med*. 2001;111(6): 457–463.

63. Lerman A, McConnell JP. Lipoprotein-associated phospholipase A2: a risk marker or a risk factor? *Am J Cardiol*. 2008;101(12A): 11F–22F.

64. Packard CJ, O'Reilly DS, Caslake MJ, et al. Lipoprotein-associated phospholipase A2 as an independent predictor of coronary heart disease. West of Scotland Coronary Prevention Study Group. *N Engl J Med*. 2000;343(16):1148–1155.

65. Koenig W, Khuseyinova N, Lowel H, Trischler G, Meisinger C. Lipoprotein-associated phospholipase A2 adds to risk prediction of incident coronary events by C-reactive protein in apparently healthy middle-aged men from the general population: results from the 14-year follow-up of a large cohort from southern Germany. *Circulation*. 2004;110(14):1903–1908.

66. Oei HH, van der Meer IM, Hofman A, et al. Lipoprotein-associated phospholipase A2 activity is associated with risk of coronary heart disease and ischemic stroke: the Rotterdam Study. *Circulation*. 2005;111(5):570–575.

67. Blake GJ, Dada N, Fox JC, Manson JE, Ridker PM. A prospective evaluation of lipoprotein-associated phospholipase A(2) levels and the risk of future cardiovascular events in women. *J Am Coll Cardiol*. 2001;38(5):1302–1306.

68. Ballantyne CM, Hoogeveen RC, Bang H, et al. Lipoprotein-associated phospholipase A2, high-sensitivity C-reactive protein, and risk for incident coronary heart disease in middle-aged men and women in the Atherosclerosis Risk in Communities (ARIC) study. *Circulation.* 2004;109(7):837–842.

69. Sabatine MS, Morrow DA, O'Donoghue M, et al. Prognostic utility of lipoprotein-associated phospholipase A2 for cardiovascular outcomes in patients with stable coronary artery disease. *Arterioscler Thromb Vasc Biol.* 2007;27(11):2463–2469.

70. Lawrence JB, Oxvig C, Overgaard MT, et al. The insulin-like growth factor (IGF)-dependent IGF binding protein-4 protease secreted by human fibroblasts is pregnancy-associated plasma protein-A. *Proc Natl Acad Sci U S A.* 1999;96(6):3149–3153.

71. Bayes-Genis A, Conover CA, Overgaard MT, et al. Pregnancy-associated plasma protein A as a marker of acute coronary syndromes. *N Engl J Med.* 2001;345(14):1022–1029.

72. Heeschen C, Dimmeler S, Hamm CW, Fichtlscherer S, Simoons ML, Zeiher AM. Pregnancy-associated plasma protein-A levels in patients with acute coronary syndromes: comparison with markers of systemic inflammation, platelet activation, and myocardial necrosis. *J Am Coll Cardiol.* 2005;45(2):229–237.

73. Lund J, Qin QP, Ilva T, et al. Circulating pregnancy-associated plasma protein a predicts outcome in patients with acute coronary syndrome but no troponin I elevation. *Circulation.* 2003;108(16):1924–1926.

74. Morrow DA, Rifai N, Antman EM, et al. Serum amyloid A predicts early mortality in acute coronary syndromes: A TIMI 11A substudy. *J Am Coll Cardiol.* 2000;35(2):358–362.

75. Armstrong EJ, Morrow DA, Sabatine MS. Inflammatory biomarkers in acute coronary syndromes: part II: acute-phase reactants and biomarkers of endothelial cell activation. *Circulation.* 2006;113(7): e152–e155.

76. Biasucci LM, Liuzzo G, Grillo RL, et al. Elevated levels of C-reactive protein at discharge in patients with unstable angina predict recurrent instability. *Circulation.* 1999;99(7):855–860.

77. Harb TS, Zareba W, Moss AJ, et al. Association of C-reactive protein and serum amyloid A with recurrent coronary events in stable patients after healing of acute myocardial infarction. *Am J Cardiol.* 2002;89(2):216–221.

14 ■ Role of Inflammatory Marker Testing in Acute Coronary Syndromes

Luigi M. Biasucci, MD
Milena Leo, MD

Introduction

Acute coronary syndromes (ACS) are frequent and life-threatening conditions, which, despite the many advancements in diagnostic and therapeutic tools, still have elusive characteristics that may represent clinical challenges for the physician. Diagnosis of ACS is one of the trickiest diagnoses in emergency departments, as patients presenting with chest pain of suspected cardiac origin, but normal EKG and troponin levels, are difficult to characterize and the decision process may be expensive and time-consuming. There are still unnecessary admissions, carrying considerable costs, but also late or missed diagnoses with erroneous discharges, carrying considerable risk to the patients. In addition, short- and long-term prediction of risk in patients with ACS is a challenging clinical problem: despite diagnostic and therapeutic advances, the rate of event recurrence is still relatively high (in the range of 14% to 16% at six months) and not completely explained by risk algorithms. Correct and prompt diagnosis and risk assessment of patients with ACS are crucial in guiding treatment and improving outcome. Biochemical markers, therefore, are very important for a more accurate diagnosis and prognostic stratification of patients with suspected or proven ACS. This has led to an explosion of research in the field; recently, much interest has been focused on biomarkers of inflammation because of the pathophysiological link between inflammation and plaque destabilization.

A Brief Pathophysiological Reappraisal

Inflammation is not only the basis of atherosclerosis,[1] but it also represents one of the primary mechanisms leading to plaque rupture and thrombus formation. Proinflammatory cytokines, released by inflammatory cells as neutrophils, lymphocytes and monocytes, and by resident macrophages, may induce endothelial activation, plaque rupture, and a procoagulant state.

The growing evidence of the important role of inflammatory processes in plaque instability has led to the study and use of inflammatory cells and proteins as prognostic markers in patients with ACS. Inflammatory biomarkers currently studied include (Figure 14–1):

- Acute-phase reactants
  - C-reactive protein (CRP)
  - serum amyloid A (SAA)
- Cytokines
  - interleukins (IL6, IL18, IL10)
  - monocyte chemotactic protein (MCP-1)
  - tumor necrosis factor-alpha (TNFα)
- Cellular adhesion molecules
  - Soluble intercellular adhesion molecule (sICAM)
  - Soluble vascular cell adhesion molecule (sVCAM)
  - sSelectins
- Markers of plaque destabilization and rupture
  - myeloperoxidase (MPO)
  - matrix metalloproteinases (MMPs)
  - placental growth factor (PlGF)
  - pregnancy-associated plasma protein (PAPP-A)
  - soluble CD40 ligand (sCD40L)

Preliminary Considerations

A massive number of inflammatory biomarkers have been proposed so far. Although some of them have a reasonable link with a clinical use, most have only a speculative interest. To be clinically relevant, a cardiovascular marker should be biologically plausible; measurable at a reasonable cost with rapid, high quality assays (accurate, reproducible, standardized); and especially, it should have an incremental clinical value on top of already existing

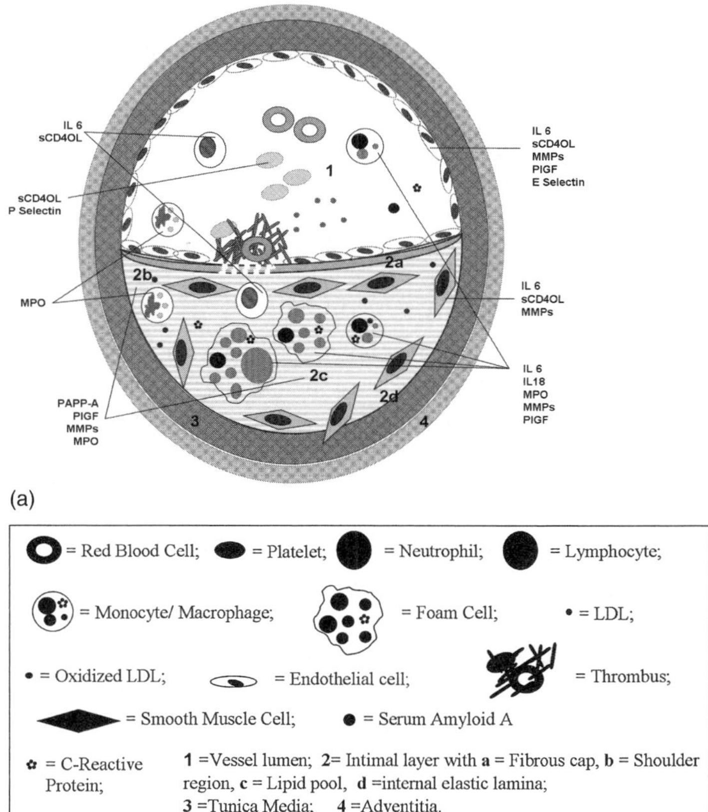

(b)

■ **Figure 14–1** The different inflammatory molecules, and endothelial, plaque, and hemostatic system cells involved in plaque and endothelial activation and thrombus formation. Inflammatory cells and mediators, that in turn may also represent markers of activation of the inflammatory cascade, are responsible for endothelial activation and plaque rupture and cooperate with platelets and haemostatic protein for the final thrombus formation.

biomarkers. All inflammatory biomarkers are important research tools, but the clinical utility of most of them is limited by their lack of additional information regarding troponin and natriuretic peptides, unfavorable biological profile, high cost, low availability, and a lack of a standardized assay. In this chapter, we will describe the clinical role, for some of the more studied inflammatory biomarkers, with the aim of giving a critical overview of their potential, indications, and limitations.

Acute Phase Reactants

Acute phase reactants are inflammatory proteins, mostly produced in the liver, of which levels increase sharply after an inflammatory or infective stimulus. As any stimulus (damage, trauma, oxidation, infection) may induce such a reaction, these proteins are nonspecific, but because of their sensitivity, they are very useful in detecting and monitoring an established process, such as an ACS. These proteins are also relatively easy to measure with robust methods and have good pre-analytical performances. For the reasons described above, in ACS their levels are much greater than in primary prevention and tend to return to pre-acute event levels in a few days; persistence of elevated levels after discharge has been associated with an increased risk.

C-Reactive Protein (CRP)

C-reactive protein (CRP) is the prototypic acute phase response protein and plays a pivotal role in inflammatory processes. As inflammation is a recognized key component of atherosclerosis,[1] much interest has been focused on CRP during the last 15 years. Although a number of inflammatory mediators are of potential clinical interest, CRP is the inflammatory marker most extensively assessed in prognostic studies[2] and the only one recommended in guidelines.[3] This is due in part to pre-analytical and analytical reasons, such as the availability of high-sensitivity (hs), relatively low-cost, assays for its measurement, and in part to its biological profile that makes this protein an almost perfect marker of inflammation (it has a half-life of 19 hours and is not consumed during the reaction as are other inflammatory proteins like fibrinogen). Because of its high sensitivity and the ability to rise several times above the normal levels (up to one thousandfold) after an inflammatory stimulus, CRP has been widely used since its discovery in 1930 by Tillet and Francis[4] to monitor inflammatory and infectious diseases and, more recently, ischemic heart disease (IHD).[5] However, because of its high sensitivity but very low specificity and because it increases following any inflammatory stimulus, CRP cannot be recommended for diagnostic purposes. It has been extensively studied in IHD, either for the prediction of incident myocardial infarction (MI), coronary heart disease (CHD), and death (primary prevention) or for the prediction of recurrent events in patients with manifest atherosclerotic disease (secondary prevention).

CRP and Diagnosis of ACS

CRP should not be considered for diagnostic purposes. In the past, it has been shown consistently that low levels of CRP (<3 mg/L), when associated with low levels of troponin, have an important negative predictive value, with no death after six months[6–8]. However, the development of high-sensitivity troponins and the use of natriuretic peptides have reduced the interest in this use of CRP. No paper has demonstrated a clinically useful association of CRP levels in emergency department diagnoses of ACS.

CRP and Secondary Prevention

The prognostic role of CRP in unstable angina and MI was first described in 1994 for short-term cardiovascular complications[9] and later confirmed for long-term adverse events (Figure 14–2 and Figure 14–3).[10]

Most of the more recent data confirm that in secondary prevention CRP is independently associated with risk of death for up to five years.[11] In particular, large studies involving thousands of patients have shown a significant association between CRP levels and risk of death in patients with unstable angina/non-ST

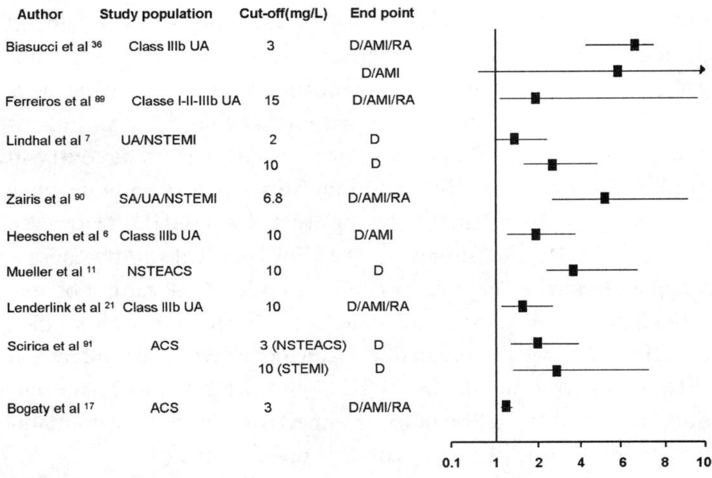

Author
Study population
Cut-off(mg/L)
End point
Biasucci et al 36
Class IIIb UA
3
D/AMI/RA
D/AMI
Ferreiros et al 89
Classe I-II-IIIb UA
15
D/AMI/RA
Lindhal et al 7
UA/NSTEMI
2
D
10
D
Zairis et al 90
SA/UA/NSTEMI
6.8
D/AMI/RA
Heeschen et al 6
Class IIIb UA
10
D/AMI
Mueller et al 11
NSTEACS
10
D
Lenderlink et al 21
Class IIIb UA
10
D/AMI/RA
Scirica et al 91
ACS
3 (NSTEACS)
D
10 (STEMI)
D
Bogaty et al 17
ACS
3
D/AMI/RA
0.1
1
2
4
6
8
10

■ **Figure 14–2** Overview of the studies analyzing the intermediate to long term prognostic value of CRP levels in ACS. The figure shows the relative risks (RR) and relative 95% confidence interval (CI) in studies in consideration of the population studied, end-point analyzed, and cut-off (not meta-analysis). UA = Unstable Angina; NSTEMI = Non-ST-segment Elevation Myocardial Infarction; STEMI = ST-segment Elevation Myocardial Infarction; SA = Stable Angina; NSTEACS = Non-ST-segment Elevation Acute Coronary Syndromes; D = Death; AMI = Acute Myocardial Infarction; RA = Recurrent Angina.

Updated from Biasucci LM, Abbate A, and Liuzzo G in Wu *Cardiac Markers*, 2nd edition, Humana Press, Totowa, NJ. 2003.

elevation MI (NSTEMI). Intriguingly, CRP levels predicted events either in medically and in invasively- or surgically-treated patients and its levels provided incremental information on top of the TIMI risk score and of other biomarkers as amino-terminal pro-B type natriuretic peptide (NT-proBNP) and troponins.[12] The lack of association between CRP and the extent and progression of atherosclerotic lesions[13,14] that have been observed by several investigators suggest that CRP in ACS is not a marker of atherosclerosis, but it seems to be linked to plaque destabilization. Apparently, this

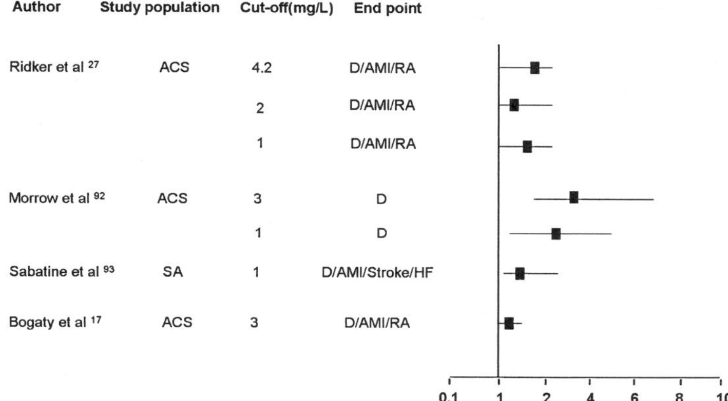

Author
Study population
Cut-off(mg/L)
End point
Ridker et al 27
ACS
4.2
D/AMI/RA
2
D/AMI/RA
1
D/AMI/RA
Morrow et al 92
ACS
3
D
1
D
Sabatine et al 93
SA
1
D/AMI/Stroke/HF
Bogaty et al 17
ACS
3
D/AMI/RA
0.1
1
2
4
6
8
10

■ **Figure 14–3** Overview of the studies analyzing the long-term prognostic value of CRP levels in stable angina or stabilized ACS. The figure shows the relative risks (RR) and relative 95% confidence interval (CI) in studies in consideration of the population studied, end-point analyzed, and cutoff (not meta-analysis). Legend: SA = Stable Angina; ACS = Acute Coronary Syndromes; D = Death; AMI = Acute Myocardial Infarction; RA = Recurrent Angina; HF = Heart Failure.

Updated from Biasucci LM, Abbate A, and Liuzzo G in Wu *Cardiac Markers*. 2nd edition, 2003.

observation is in contrast with the strong evidence that in the case of ACS, CRP is associated with risk of death, but only weakly with the risk of new MI. However, no data are available on whether cardiac death in these cases was due to fatal MI. The observation that CRP increases myocardial tissue damage after infarction by colocalizing with complement may explain this finding.[15]

As in many studies, different cutoff values or analysis of data by tertiles or quartiles have been used. In 2003, the Centers for Disease Control and the American Heart Association[16] sponsored an expert panel that proposed a cutoff level of 10 mg/L in the acute phase of ACS and a cutoff of 3 mg/L in the follow-up. Recently, Bogaty et al.[17] have found only a weak association between CRP and events after ACS, however the authors have analyzed the whole spectrum of the syndrome from accelerating angina to ST-elevation MI, including patients with infectious and inflammatory diseases, and furthermore used a cutoff (3 mg/L) which is too low for ACS, according to the AHA/CDC scientific statement.[16] CRP has been shown[18,19] to have a significant predictive value also for the occurrence of restenosis after percutaneous coronary intervention (PCI) and of ventricular tachycardia/fibrillation in patients with implantable cardioverter-defibrillators (ICD) for primary prevention after myocardial infarction.[20]

CRP and Medical Therapy

To be truly useful, a biomarker should be able to identify a therapeutic imperative for patients with elevated levels. In a recent ACS study, CRP was neither found to be of help in identifying an invasive treatment,[21] nor was it associated with improvement after treatment with a glycoprotein (GP) IIb-IIIa antagonist (Figure 14–4).[22] On the other hand, treatments associated with reduced mortality in ACS are associated with a reduction in CRP, which

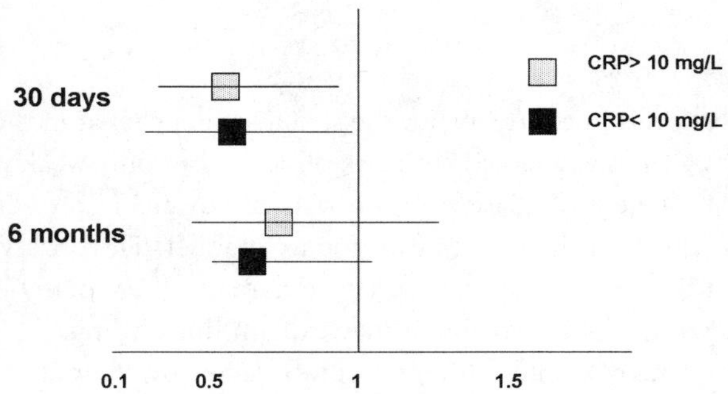

■ **Figure 14–4** CRP levels are not useful in predicting which group of patients take advantage of treatment with abcximab in ACS. Above: 30 days follow-up, no differences were found in outcome between patients with CRP >10 mg/L (above) or <10 mg/L treated with abicximab. Below: 6 months follow-up, similar results.

Modified from Heeschen et al.[22]

raises the question of whether monitoring of therapy might be accomplished with serial measurements of this marker. Aspirin, clopidogrel, GP IIb/IIIa inhibitors, and statins appear to simultaneously lower cardiac risk and CRP levels, and are most effective in patients with high CRP.[23–26]

The CRP lowering effect is of particular significance with statins. Several studies have shown that aggressive lipid lowering leads to a marked improvement in clinical outcome only when both low-density lipoprotein (LDL) and CRP levels are lowered. In the TIMI-22 study,[27] the lower event rate was achieved only when LDL was reduced below 70 mg/L and CRP was reduced below 2 mg/L. In another trial,[28] the possibility that high doses of statins could reduce or reverse progression of atherosclerosis was assessed by intravascular ultrasound. In these patients, a reduction in plaque volume was only observed when both LDL and CRP levels were lowered below the median. With the presentation and publication of the JUPITER study,[29,30] interest in the use of CRP for lipid management will grow. This study has tested the hypothesis of whether subjects with normal LDL levels (<130 mg/dl) who were not candidates for statin therapy based on NCEP III guidelines,[31] might still benefit from statin treatment if their CRP was mildly increased (>2 mg/L). The study was prematurely terminated by the Data Safety Monitoring Board on April 30, 2008, because of superiority of rosuvastatin over placebo on a combined cardiovascular endpoint. Although designed for primary prevention, the Justification for Use of Statins in Prevention: an Intervention Trial Evaluating Rosuvastatin (JUPITER) trial reinforces the hypothesis that CRP is an effective tool with which to guide therapy with statins, even in patients with ACS.

In smaller studies, angiotensin converting enzyme-inhibitors and angiotensin receptor blockers have also been shown to reduce CRP levels.[32] Pepys et al.[33] recently reported that a small molecule, called 1,6 bis(phosphocholine) hexane, that binds and inhibits human CRP, reduces the size of MI in a rat model. Whether this molecule might also be useful in the prevention of ACS is currently unknown. It is also unknown whether a strategy aimed at reaching very low CRP levels (<1 mg/L) by increasing dosage of statins or other drugs may represent the gold standard of medical therapy for ACS patients, however this possibility seems highly likely (Table 14–1).

Serum Amyloid A

Serum amyloid A is another acute-phase reactant that has been recently proposed as a marker of risk in ischemic heart disease. SAA, as CRP, is routinely used as an inflammatory marker. These proteins usually respond in parallel to a given stimulus; however, the magnitude of the SAA response has been found to be greater than that of CRP.[34] During acute MI, SAA levels were found to increase within 24 hours and peak within three days after the onset of chest pain.[35]

Despite parallels with CRP, associations between SAA and outcomes are variable. In one study, SAA was not associated with long-term risk[10] and was only marginally associated with long-term risk by Biasucci et al.[36] A TIMI 11A substudy found that elevated levels of SAA, like CRP levels, predicted risk of 14-day mortality in patients with unstable angina or NSTEMI.[37] Patients with elevated SAA at discharge after hospitalization for ACS were more likely to be readmitted and/or have recurrent angina within one year.[36] In contrast, measurement of SAA two months after MI in the Thrombogenic Factors and Recurrent Coronary Events (THROMBO) Study showed no significant association between SAA and risk of recurrent cardiovascular events over two years.[38] Johnson et al.[39] recently found that SAA levels, but not CRP levels, were related to the severity of coronary artery disease (CAD) in women, as assessed by coronary angiography. Both had a similar association with events, possibly suggesting a different role of these acute-phase proteins in the pathogenesis of atherosclerosis, but not in prediction of events. In a more recent study[40] enrolling 277 patients with NSTE-ACS, elevated SAA levels were found to be associated with adverse 30-day outcomes in these patients, irrespective of the presence or absence of elevated CRP levels, while

Table 14–1: Potential therapeutic applications of inflammatory biomarkers in ACS patients undergoing PCI or ICD implantation, on the basis of current evidence.

Treatment	Biomarker
Statins	♦ Reduce **CRP** levels. **CRP as additional target for tailoring lipid lowering therapy with statins**: ideal hsCRP levels <1 mg/L ♦ Reduce **MPO** levels ♦ Reduce **sCD40L** levels
ACE-inhibitors ARBs	♦ Reduce **CRP** levels in patients with high CRP levels, useful treatment independent of the presence of other risk factors
Aspirin Clopidogrel	♦ Reduce **CRP** levels
GP IIb/IIIa antagonists	♦ Reduce **CRP** levels ♦ Reduce **sCD40L** levels: in patients with elevated sCD40L levels, greater benefit from early antiplatelet therapy with GPIIb/IIIa antagonists
Early revascularization	♦ Major benefit from early invasive strategy in patients with elevated **IL6** levels ♦ Major benefit from early invasive strategy in patients with elevated **sCD40L** levels
Outcome after PCI	♦ Preprocedural **CRP** levels predict late restenosis and instability and death after PCI
ICD implantation after AMI	♦ **CRP** levels predict occurrence of ventricular tachycardia/fibrillation in patients with ICD after AMI

Notes: AMI = Acute Myocardial Infarction; ARBs = Angiotensin Receptor Blockers; CRP = C-Reactive Protein; ICD = Implantable Cardioverter Defibrillator; MPO = myeloperoxidase; PCI = Percutaneous Coronary Intervention; sCD40L = soluble CD40 Ligand.

elevated CRP levels with normal SAA levels were not associated with adverse outcomes at 30 days. While these results are intriguing, information from SAA levels is largely redundant to that of CRP. Because the incremental value of SAA is still unknown, the routine use of it in cases of ACS is not recommended.

Cytokines

IL-6

IL-6 is a ubiquitous cytokine, promoting hepatic production of acute-phase reactants, including CRP[41]; it is also expressed at the shoulder region of atherosclerotic plaques and may increase plaque instability.[42] Several prospective studies have consistently shown that baseline levels of IL-6 are powerful predictors of future CV in apparently healthy asymptomatic subjects.[43,44] IL-6 levels are higher in patients with unstable angina (UA) compared with those with stable angina.[45] In the FRISC-II ([Fragmin] and/or early revascularization during instability in coronary artery disease) study,[46] elevated IL-6 levels (>5 ng/L) were associated with higher 6- and 12-month mortality and were additive to and independent of cardiac troponin T status and of CRP levels. In the same study, elevated IL-6 levels, but not those of CRP, also identified a subgroup of patients who derived the greatest mortality benefit from an early invasive strategy. Biasucci et al.[47] have observed that among patients with unstable angina, increases in IL-6 (and IL-1RA) levels 48 hours after admission, compared with the admission value, are associated with increased in-hospital morbidity and mortality similar to acute inflammatory and septic disease.

The large circadian variations in IL-6 levels with a relatively short half-life, a lack of confirmatory studies and of large-volume and low-cost methods of measurement, limit the inclusion of this biomarker in clinical routine.

IL-18

IL-18 is a pleiotropic proinflammatory cytokine and a potent mediator of atherosclerotic plaque growth and destabilization[48];

however, the clinical evidence for this biomarker in cross-sectional studies is controversial. Two studies[49,50] assessed the prognostic value of elevated IL-18 levels for future cardiovascular events in apparently healthy subjects, however, the evidence associating this cytokine with ACS is not unequivocal. Blankenberg et al.[51] found that increased IL-18 levels were independently associated with future cardiovascular death during a 3.9-year follow-up, both in stable and unstable angina patients with angiographically-confirmed coronary artery disease; although independent from CRP, its prognostic value was similar to that of CRP. In a more recent study,[52] IL-18 levels were not found to be predictive of outcome in 1288 patients with coronary artery disease prospectively followed during a median period of 5.9 years. The available data may suggest that IL-18 is associated with future risk of death/MI in primary, but not in secondary, prevention.

Markers of Plaque Destabilization and Rupture

Myeloperoxidase (MPO)

Covered in several chapters within this textbook, myeloperoxidase (MPO) is a well-known enzyme, mainly released by activated neutrophils, characterized by powerful pro-oxidative and proinflammatory properties.[53] Recently, MPO has been proposed as a useful risk marker and diagnostic tool in acute coronary syndromes and in patients admitted to emergency rooms for chest pain. The association between MPO and CAD was first observed by Biasucci et al.,[54] who found that circulating neutrophils in patients with acute myocardial infarction (AMI) and UA had a low MPO content—indicating their activation—as compared with those patients with chronic stable angina and variant angina. The lack of neutrophil activation in patients with variant angina and after stress test suggested that MPO was prevalently a marker of instability and not simply a marker of oxidative stress and damage due to ischemia. Zhang et al.[55] have recently found higher blood and leukocyte MPO activity in patients with CAD compared with angiographically-verified normal controls; moreover, this increase was independently associated with the presence of CAD. Ndrepepa et al.[56] have observed a progressive increase of MPO levels from stable CAD to non-ST-segment elevation ACS and to acute MI. Kubala[57] has also found stable plasma MPO levels in patients with stable CAD, suggesting that systemic release of MPO (i.e., elevation) is not a feature of asymptomatic CAD, but probably a marker of instability. These studies consistently demonstrate that CAD is associated with increased levels of MPO and that a gradient exists toward higher levels of MPO in more active forms of disease.

For MPO, as for all novel biomarkers, a key point is the amount of additional information provided. The additional clinical value of MPO has been evaluated in several trials. In a study of ACS subjects, MPO mass concentration was measured in 1090 patients with ACS: elevated MPO levels were associated with a statistically significant increase in the risk of death or MI. Intriguingly, the predictive value of MPO was independent of those for C-reactive protein and troponin.[58] In a study of 604 consecutive initially troponin-negative patients presenting to the emergency department with chest pain, Brennan et al.[59] demonstrated a progressive increase in odds ratios for major adverse events at 30 days and 6 months with each quartile increase in MPO concentration. They also demonstrated a direct relationship between MPO values on admission with subsequent acute MI diagnosis, again in patients with an initially negative troponin (Table 14–2).

In the TIMI 18 trial,[60] conducted on 1524 patients with ACS, MPO was found to predict recurrent ischemic events at 30 days follow-up, adding incremental information to BNP and cardiac troponin I. Several studies have also demonstrated the value of MPO in predicting long-term outcomes[61–63] up to five years. Importantly, in these studies the MPO predictive value was independent from ejection fraction, BNP, and troponin levels.

Thus, MPO is a promising biomarker: elevated plasma MPO levels may be a marker of unstable angina preceding myocardial necrosis, and therefore, a predictor of vulnerable plaque. MPO

Table 14–2: Features of proposed novel biomarkers in ACS (on a scale from – to ++++).

	Available, Low Cost, Standardized Assay?	Additional Diagnostic Value?	Additional Prognostic Value?	Additional Therapeutic Value?	Convincing Prospective Studies?	Recommended by NACB Guidelines?
CRP	++++	+/–	++++	+++	++++	Yes (classIIa, level A)
SAA	+	–	+/–	–	++	No
IL 6	–	–	++	+	++	No
IL 18	–	–	+/–	–	+	No
MPO	++	+	++	+	++	No
MMPs	–	–	+/–	+	+/–	No
sCD40L	–	–	+	+	++	No
PAPP-A	–	+	++	–	+	No

Notes: The table summarizes the characteristics of the inflammatory biomarkers treated in the chapter. CRP = C-Reactive Protein; SAA = Serum Amyloid A; IL 6 = interleukin 6; IL 18 = interleukin 18, MPO = myeloperoxidase; MMPs = Matrix metalloproteinases; sCD40L = soluble CD40 Ligand; PAPP-A = Pregnancy-Associated Plasma Protein A; NACB = National Academy of Clinical Biochemistry (Laboratory).

may be useful in triage in the emergency department for early ACS diagnosis and short-term risk assessment, in particular in patients with negative troponin levels. Furthermore, statin therapy has been found to reduce circulating MPO levels, suggesting that like CRP, MPO might be used for monitoring the efficacy of therapy.[64] Several problems, however, preclude a large scale clinical use of MPO. Large prospective studies are lacking; MPO specificity is unknown (but as a marker of neutrophil activation, it is expected to be low); the preanalytical phase is critical; and samples must be taken in tubes containing EDTA only and quickly processed. Furthermore, methods of standardization have not been established and different cutoffs have been used in the different studies, making the applicability of this study difficult in everyday practice. An issue has been raised recently that might impact on the reliability of MPO assessment in ACS: heparin seems to unbind MPO from endothelial cells and endothelium.[65]

Soluble CD40 Ligand (sCD40L)

Circulating sCD40L is a glycoprotein largely derived from activated platelets with a wide array of proatherogenic and prothrombotic functions in vitro and in vivo, in particular, CD40L may induce lymphocyte activation and synthesis of tissue factor in monocytes.[66] Up-regulation of the CD40L-CD40 system may play a pathogenic role in triggering ACS. Increased sCD40L levels were found in patients with AMI and UA.[67] Cipollone et al.[68] found that increased sCD40L levels in patients undergoing PCI were associated with late restenosis after PCI. In a study of patients with non-ST segment elevation ACS,[69] elevated sCD40L levels identified a subgroup of patients who were at increased risk of death or nonfatal MI at 6 months who had benefited from early antiplatelet therapy with abciximab. Another study[70] demonstrated the utility of early statin therapy in high-risk ACS patients with elevated sCD40L levels. A nested case-control study from the TIMI 16 trial[71] showed that patients who experienced death, MI, or congestive heart failure had significantly higher levels of sCD40L than did matched controls and that sCD40L prognostic value was independent of cardiac troponin I or CRP. Data from the FRISC trial[72] confirmed that sCD40L levels are related to outcome and can identify a subgroup of patients having particularly benefited from antithrombotic and early invasive treatment. In the TIMI 18 trial,[60] however, in patients with ACS, an elevated concentration of sCD40L was only associated with a modest trend towards higher risk of recurrent ischemic events at 30 days follow-up, although this might be due to the use of GPIIb/IIIa receptor antagonists in all patients. More recently, sCD40L was not found to be associated with risk of events in a large cohort from the TIMI16 study.[73] This observation, with the recent reports of Weber[74] and Ivandic[75] on the large variability of sCD40L measurement due to preanalytical problems (platelet activation, sample preparation, use of heparin), have markedly reduced the first enthusiasm about the use of sCD40L in diagnosing ACS.

Matrix Metalloproteinases (MMPs)

Matrix metalloproteinases (MMPs) are zinc-dependent endopeptidases, highly expressed in macrophage-rich areas of the atherosclerotic plaque (especially at the shoulder region of the cap); MMPs may promote weakening of the fibrous cap and subsequent destabilization of plaque.[76] Several cross-sectional studies have demonstrated significantly increased levels of MMPs (in particular MMP-1, MMP-2 and MMP-9), in patients with ACS compared with healthy controls or in patients with more advanced CAD.[77,78] The time course of elevation is controversial: some groups found a late elevation—7 to 14 days after the acute event; others found a rapid rise and fall of MMP-9 within the first week after ACS. Although many small pathophysiological studies have positively assessed the role of MMPs in ACS, little data exist on the association between MMP levels in ACS and cardiovascular outcomes. In a study[79] of 24 patients with ACS, elevation of MMP-1 levels at 7 and 14 days after ACS predicted a worse left ventricular ejection fraction. In Blankenberg's study,[80] which enrolled 1227 patients with angiographically-confirmed CAD, but not definite ACS, increased concentrations of MMP-9 were associated with future cardiovascular death. Interestingly, in this study, as in others, high concentrations of the endogenous tissue inhibitors of metalloproteinase-1 (TIMP) were also predictive of future cardiovascular events.

Pregnancy-Associated Plasma Protein A (PAPP-A)

Pregnancy-associated plasma protein A is a zinc-binding metalloproteinase, expressed in the shoulder regions and in the extracellular matrix of ruptured and eroded plaques. It activates the IGF pathway, thus contributing to plaque progression and destabilization.[81] Several studies have investigated PAPP-A as a potential marker of cardiovascular risk. Bayes-Genis et al.[82] described increased circulating PAPP-A levels in patients with UA and MI compared with controls. In another study,[83] PAPP-A levels were able to detect unstable ACS in patients presenting for coronary angiography—even in patients with negative troponin. Furthermore, in a series of 136 patients presenting to the emergency department for suspected ACS, PAPP-A levels independently predicted ischemic cardiac events and the need for revascularization during 6-month follow-up.[84] Within the CAPTURE trial,[85] PAPP-A levels indicated increased risk of death and MI in both troponin negative and troponin positive patients. Similarly, in patients with STEMI,[86] PAPP-A levels were increased and predicted a 12-month risk of death and recurrent nonfatal MI. In addition, PAPP-A and its endogenous inhibitor, the proform of eosinophil major basic protein (proMBP), were related to complex angiographic stenosis morphology in patients with stable CAD; additionally, PAPP-A was prospectively associated with future death and ACS in such patients. Finally, PAPP-A appears to be a marker of cardiovascular risk also in asymptomatic hyperlipidemic individuals, showing a correlation with the degree of echogenicity of carotid atherosclerotic plaques.[87] However, there are not consistent data on its reduction level by statin treatment.

Additional and larger studies are needed to clarify if PAPP-A provides incremental risk stratification information to the clinician. Moreover, because PAPP-A exists in at least two isoforms, new assays—specifically for ACS-related isoforms of PAPP-A—should be developed.

References

1. Ross R. Atherosclerosis—an inflammatory disease. *N Engl J Med.* 1999;340:115–126.
2. Biasucci LM, Liuzzo G, Colizzi C, Rizzello V. Clinical use of C-reactive protein for the prognostic stratification of patients with ischemic heart disease. *Ital Heart J.* 2001;2:164–171.
3. Morrow DA, Cannon CP, Jesse RL, et al. National Academy of Clinical Biochemistry Laboratory Medicine Practice Guidelines: clinical characteristics and utilization of biochemical markers in acute coronary syndromes. *Circulation.* 2007;115(13):e356–e375.
4. Tillett WS, Francis T. Serologic reactions in pneumonia with a non-protein somatic fraction of pneumococcus. *J Exp Med.* 1930;52: 561–571.
5. Biasucci LM; CDC; AHA. CDC/AHA Workshop on Markers of Inflammation and Cardiovascular Disease: Application to Clinical and Public Health Practice: clinical use of inflammatory markers in patients with cardiovascular diseases: a background paper. *Circulation.* 2004;110(25):e560–e567.
6. Heeschen C, Hamm CW, Bruemmer J, Simoons ML. Predictive value of C-reactive protein and troponin T in patients with unstable angina: a comparative analysis. CAPTURE Investigators. Chimeric c7E3 Antiplatelet Therapy in Unstable Angina Refractory to Standard Treatment Trial. *J Am Coll Cardiol.* 2000;35(6):1535–1542.
7. Lindhal B, Toss H, Siegbahn A, et al. Markers of myocardial damage and inflammation in relation to long-term mortality in unstable coronary artery disease. *N Engl J Med.* 2000;343:1139–1147.
8. Rebuzzi AG, Quaranta G, Liuzzo G, et al. Incremental prognostic value of serum levels of troponin T and C-reactive protein on admission in patients with unstable angina pectoris. *Am J Cardiol.* 1998;82(6):715–719.

9. Liuzzo G, Biasucci LM, Gallimore JR, et al. The prognostic value of C-reactive protein and serum amyloid A protein in severe unstable angina. *N Engl J Med.* 1994;331(7):417–424.

10. Haverkate F, Thompson SG, Pyke SD, Gallimore JR, Pepys MB. Production of C-reactive protein and risk of coronary events in stable and unstable angina. European Concerted Action on Thrombosis and Disabilities Angina Pectoris Study Group. *Lancet.* 1997;349(9050): 462–466.

11. Mueller C, Buettner HJ, Hodgson JM, et al. Inflammation and long-term mortality after non-ST elevation acute coronary syndrome treated with a very early invasive strategy in 1,042 consecutive patients. *Circulation.* 2002;105:1412–1415.

12. Sabatine MS, Morrow DA, Cannon CP, et al. Relationship between baseline white blood cell count and degree of coronary artery disease and mortality in patients with acute coronary syndromes: a TACTICS-TIMI 18 (Treat Angina with Aggrastat and determine Cost of Therapy with an Invasive or Conservative Strategy—Thrombolysis in Myocardial Infarction 18 trial) substudy. *J Am Coll Cardiol.* 2002; 40(10):1761–1768.

13. Zebrack JS, Muhlestein JB, Horne BD, Anderson JL. Intermountain Heart Collaboration Study Group. C-reactive protein and angiographic coronary artery disease: independent and additive predictors of risk in subjects with angina. *J Am Coll Cardiol.* 2002;39:632–637.

14. Niccoli G, Biasucci LM, Biscione C, et al. Independent prognostic value of C-reactive protein and coronary artery disease extent in patients affected by unstable angina. *Atherosclerosis.* 2008;196(2): 779–785.

15. Lagrand WK, Niessen HW, Wolbink GJ, et al. C-reactive protein colocalizes with complement in human hearts during acute myocardial infarction. *Circulation.* 1997;95(1):97–103.

16. Pearson TA, Mensah GA, Alexander RW, et al. Markers of inflammation and cardiovascular disease: application to clinical and public health practice: a statement for healthcare professionals from the Centers for Disease Control and Prevention and the American Heart Association. *Circulation.* 2003;107:499–511.

17. Bogaty P, Boyer L, Simard S, et al. Clinical utility of C-reactive protein measured at admission, hospital discharge, and 1 month later to predict outcome in patients with acute coronary disease. The RISCA

(recurrence and inflammation in the acute coronary syndromes) study. *J Am Coll Cardiol.* 2008;51(24):2339–2346.

18. Buffon A, Liuzzo G, Biasucci LM, et al. Preprocedural serum levels of C-reactive protein predict early complications and late restenosis after coronary angioplasty. *J Am Coll Cardiol.* 1999;34(5):1512–1521.
19. Versaci F, Gaspardone A, Tomai F, et al. Immunosuppressive Therapy for the Prevention of Restenosis after Coronary Artery Stent Implantation Study. Immunosuppressive Therapy for the Prevention of Restenosis after Coronary Artery Stent Implantation (IMPRESS Study). *J Am Coll Cardiol.* 2002;40(11):1935–1942.
20. Bellocci F, Biasucci LM, Gensini GF, et al. Prognostic role of post-infarction C-reactive protein in patients undergoing implantation of cardioverter-defibrillators: design of the C-reactive protein Assessment after Myocardial Infarction to Guide Implantation of Defibrillator (CAMI GUIDE) study. *J Cardiovasc Med (Hagerstown).* 2007;8(4):293–299.
21. Lenderink T, Boersma E, Heeschen C, et al. CAPTURE Investigators. Elevated troponin T and C-reactive protein predict impaired outcome for 4 years in patients with refractory unstable angina, and troponin T predicts benefit of treatment with abciximab in combination with PTCA. *Eur Heart J.* 2003;24(1):77–85.
22. Heeschen C, Hamm CW, Bruemmer J, Simoons ML. Predictive value of C-reactive protein and troponin T in patients with unstable angina: a comparative analysis. CAPTURE Investigators. Chimeric c7E3 Antiplatelet Therapy in Unstable Angina Refractory to Standard Treatment Trial. *J Am Coll Cardiol.* 2000;35(6):1535–1542.
23. Kennon S, Price CP, Mills PG, et al. The effect of aspirin on C-reactive protein as a marker of risk in unstable angina. *J Am Coll Cardiol.* 2001;37:1266–1270.
24. Chew DP, Bhatt DL, Robbins MA, et al. Effect of clopidogrel added to aspirin before percutaneous coronary intervention on the risk associated with C-reactive protein. *Am J Cardiol.* 2001;88(6):672–674.
25. Lincoff AM, Kereiakes DJ, Mascelli MA, et al. Abciximab depresses the rise in levels of circulating inflammatory markers after percutaneous coronary revascularization. *Circulation.* 2001;104:163–167.
26. Jialal I, Stein D, Balis D, et al. Effect of hydroxymethyl glutaryl coenzyme A reductase inhibitor therapy on high sensitive C-reactive protein levels. *Circulation.* 2001;103:1933–1935.

27. Ridker PM, Cannon CP, Morrow D, et al. Pravastatin or Atorvastatin Evaluation and Infection Therapy—Thrombolysis in Myocardial Infarction 22 (PROVE IT-TIMI 22) Investigators. C-reactive protein levels and outcomes after statin therapy. *N Engl J Med.* 2005;352(1): 20–28.
28. Nissen SE, Tuzcu EM, Schoenhagen P, et al. Reversal of Atherosclerosis with Aggressive Lipid Lowering (REVERSAL) Investigators. Statin therapy, LDL cholesterol, C-reactive protein, and coronary artery disease. *N Engl J Med.* 2005;352(1):29–38.
29. Ridker PM; JUPITER Study Group. Rosuvastatin in the primary prevention of cardiovascular disease among patients with low levels of low-density lipoprotein cholesterol and elevated high-sensitivity C-reactive protein: rationale and design of the JUPITER trial. *Circulation.* 2003;108(19):2292–2297.
30. Ridker PM, Fonseca FA, Genest J, et al. JUPITER Trial Study Group. Baseline characteristics of participants in the JUPITER trial, a randomized placebo-controlled primary prevention trial of statin therapy among individuals with low low-density lipoprotein cholesterol and elevated high-sensitivity C-reactive protein. *Am J Cardiol.* 2007; 100(11):1659–1664.
31. NCEP ATP-III; Expert panel on Detection, Evaluation, and Treatment of High Blood Cholesterol in Adults. Executive Summary of the Third Report of the National Cholesterol Program (NCEP) Expert Panel on Detection, Evaluation, and Treatment of High Blood Cholesterol in Adults. *JAMA.* 2001;285:2486–2497.
32. Prasad K. C-reactive protein (CRP)-lowering agents. *Cardiovasc Drug Rev.* 2006;24(1):33–50. Review.
33. Pepys MB, Hirschfield GM, Tennent GA, et al. Targeting C-reactive protein for the treatment of cardiovascular disease. *Nature.* 2006;440: 1217–1221.
34. Nakayama T, Sonoda S, Urano T, Yamada T, Okada M. Monitoring both serum amyloid protein A and C-reactive protein as inflammatory markers in infectious diseases. *Clin Chem.* 1993;39:293–297.
35. Shainkin-Kestenbaum R, Winikoff Y, Cristal N. Serum amyloid A concentrations during the course of acute ischaemic heart disease. *J Clin Pathol.* 1986;39:635–637.
36. Biasucci LM, Liuzzo G, Grillo RL, et al. Elevated levels of C-reactive protein at discharge in patients with unstable angina predict recurrent instability. *Circulation.* 1999;99:855–860.

37. Morrow D, Rifai N, Antman E, et al. Serum amyloid A predicts early mortality in acute coronary syndromes: a TIMI 11A substudy. *J Am Coll Cardiol.* 2000;35:358–362.

38. Harb T, Zareba W, Moss A, et al. Association of C-reactive protein and serum amyloid A with recurrent coronary events in stable patients after healing of acute myocardial infarction. *Am J Cardiol.* 2002; 89:216–221.

39. Johnson BD, Kip KE, Marroquin OC, et al. Serum amyloid A as a predictor of coronary artery disease and cardiovascular outcome in women: the National Heart, Lung, and Blood Institute-sponsored Women's Ischemia Syndrome Evaluation (WISE). *Circulation.* 2004; 109:726–732.

40. Kosuge M, Ebina T, Ishikawa T, et al. Serum amyloid A is a better predictor of clinical outcomes than C-reactive protein in non-ST-segment elevation acute coronary syndromes. *Circ J.* 2007;71(2): 186–190.

41. Woods A, Brull D, Humphries S, Montgomery H. Genetics of inflammation and risk of coronary artery disease: the central role of interleukin-6. *Eur Heart J.* 2000;21:1574–1583.

42. Schieffer B, Schieffer E, Hilfiker-Kleiner D, et al. Expression of angiotensin II and interleukin 6 in human coronary atherosclerotic plaques. *Circulation.* 2000;101:1372–1378.

43. Ridker PM, Rifai N, Stampfer MJ, Hennekens CH. Plasma concentration of interleukin-6 and the risk of future myocardial infarction among apparently healthy men. *Circulation.* 2000;101:1767–1772.

44. Volpato S, Guralnik JM, Ferrucci L, et al. Cardiovascular disease, interleukin-6, and risk of mortality in older women: the women's health and aging study. *Circulation.* 2001;103:947–953.

45. Biasucci L, Vitelli A, Liuzzo G, et al. Elevated levels of interleukin-6 in unstable angina. *Circulation.* 1996;94:874–877.

46. Lindmark E, Diderholm E, Wallentin L, Siegbahn A. Relationship between interleukin 6 and mortality in patients with unstable coronary artery disease. *JAMA.* 2001;286:2107–2113.

47. Biasucci L, Liuzzo G, Fantuzzi G, et al. Increasing levels of interleukin (IL)-1Ra and IL-6 during the first 2 days of hospitalization in unstable angina are associated with increased risk of in-hospital coronary events. *Circulation.* 1999;99:2079–2084.

48. Mallat Z, Corbaz A, Scoazec A, et al. Expression of interleukin-18 in human atherosclerotic plaques and relation to plaque instability. *Circulation.* 2001;104:1598–1603.
49. Blankenberg S, Luc G, Ducimetiere P, et al. PRIME Study Group Interleukin-18 and the risk of coronary heart disease in European men: the Prospective Epidemiological Study of Myocardial Infarction (PRIME). *Circulation.* 2003;108:2453–2459.
50. Koenig W, Khuseyinova N, Baumert J, et al. Increased concentrations of C-reactive protein and IL-6 but not IL-18 are independently associated with incident coronary events in middle-aged men and women: results from the MONICA/KORA Augsburg case-cohort study, 1984–2002. *Arterioscler Thromb Vasc Biol.* 2006;26(12):2745–2751.
51. Blankenberg S, Tiret L, Bickel C, et al. AtheroGene Investigators. Interleukin-18 is a strong predictor of cardiovascular death in stable and unstable angina. *Circulation.* 2002;106:24–30.
52. Tiret L, Godefroy T, Lubos E, et al. AtheroGene Investigators. Genetic analysis of the interleukin-18 system highlights the role of the interleukin-18 gene in cardiovascular disease. *Circulation.* 2005;112: 643–650.
53. Nicholls SJ, Hazen SL. Myeloperoxidase and cardiovascular disease. *Arterioscler Thromb Vasc Biol.* 2005;25:1102–1111.
54. Biasucci LM, D'Onofrio G, Liuzzo G, et al. Intracellular neutrophil myeloperoxidase is reduced in unstable angina and acute myocardial infarction, but its reduction is not related to ischemia. *J Am Coll Cardiol.* 1996;27(3):611–616.
55. Zhang R, Brennan ML, Fu X, et al. Association between myeloperoxidase levels and risk of coronary artery disease. *JAMA.* 2001;286(17): 2136–2142.
56. Ndrepepa G, Braun S, Mehilli J, von Beckerath N, Schömig A, Kastrati A. Myeloperoxidase level in patients with stable coronary artery disease and acute coronary syndromes. *Eur J Clin Invest.* 2008;38(2): 90–96.
57. Kubala L, Lu G, Baldus S, Berglund L, Eiserich JP. Plasma levels of myeloperoxidase are not elevated in patients with stable coronary artery disease. *Clin Chim Acta.* 2008;394(1–2):59–62.
58. Baldus S, Heeschen C, Meinertz T, et al. CAPTURE Investigators. Myeloperoxidase serum levels predict risk in patients with acute coronary syndromes. *Circulation.* 2003;108:1440–1445.

59. Brennan ML, Penn MS, Van Lente F, et al. Prognostic value of myeloperoxidase in patients with chest pain. *N Engl J Med.* 2003;349: 1595–1604.

60. Morrow DA, Sabatine MS, Brennan ML, et al. Concurrent evaluation of novel cardiac biomarkers in acute coronary syndrome: myeloperoxidase and soluble CD40 ligand and the risk of recurrent ischaemic events in TACTICS-TIMI 18. *Eur Heart J.* 2008;29(9):1096–1102.

61. Li S-H, Xing Y-W, Li Z-Z, Bai S-G, Wang J. Clinical implications of relationship between myeloperoxidase and acute coronary syndromes. *Zhonghua Xin Xue Guan Bing Za Zhi.* 2007;35(3):241–244.

62. Cavusoglu E, Ruwende C, Eng C, et al. Usefulness of baseline plasma myeloperoxidase levels as an independent predictor of myocardial infarction at two years in patients presenting with acute coronary syndrome. *Am J Cardiol.* 2007;99(10):1364–1368.

63. Mocatta TJ, Pilbrow AP, Cameron VA, et al. Plasma concentrations of myeloperoxidase predict mortality after myocardial infarction. *J Am Coll Cardiol.* 2007;49(20):1993–2000.

64. Zhou T, Zhou SH, Qi SS, Shen XQ, Zeng GF, Zhou HN. The effect of atorvastatin on serum myeloperoxidase and CRP levels in patients with acute coronary syndrome. *Clin Chim Acta.* 2006;368(1–2): 168–172.

65. Baldus S, Rudolph V, Roiss M, et al. Heparins increase endothelial nitric oxide bioavailability by liberating vessel-immobilized myeloperoxidase. *Circulation.* 2006;113(15):1871–1878.

66. Schonbeck U, Libby P. CD40 signaling and plaque instability. *Circ Res.* 2001;89:1092–1103.

67. Garlichs CD, Eskafi S, Raaz D, et al. Patients with acute coronary syndromes express enhanced CD40 ligand/CD154 on platelets. *Heart.* 2001;86:649–655.

68. Cipollone F, Ferri C, Desideri G, et al. Preprocedural level of soluble CD40L is predictive of enhanced inflammatory response and restenosis after coronary angioplasty. *Circulation.* 2003;108:2776–2782.

69. Heeschen C, Dimmeler S, Hamm CW, et al. CAPTURE Study Investigators. Soluble CD40 ligand in acute coronary syndromes. *N Engl J Med.* 2003;348:1104–1111.

70. Kinlay S, Schwartz GG, Olsson AG, et al. Myocardial Ischemia Reduction with Aggressive Cholesterol Lowering (MIRACL) Study

Investigators. Effect of atorvastatin on risk of recurrent cardiovascular events after an acute coronary syndrome associated with high soluble CD40 ligand in the Myocardial Ischemia Reduction with Aggressive Cholesterol Lowering (MIRACL) Study. *Circulation.* 2004;110:386–391.

71. Varo N, de Lemos JA, Libby P, et al. Soluble CD40L: risk prediction after acute coronary syndromes. *Circulation.* 2003;108(9): 1049–1052.

72. Malarstig A, Lindahl B, Wallentin L, Siegbahn A. Soluble CD40L levels are regulated by the -3459 A > G polymorphism and predict myocardial infarction and the efficacy of antithrombotic treatment in non-ST elevation acute coronary syndrome. *Arterioscler Thromb Vasc Biol.* 2006;26:1667–1673.

73. Olenchock BA, Wiviott SD, Murphy SA, et al. Lack of association between soluble CD40L and risk in a large cohort of patients with acute coronary syndrome in OPUS TIMI-16. *J Thromb Thrombolysis.* 2007;26:79–84.

74. Weber M, Rabenau B, Stanisch M, et al. Influence of sample type on soluble CD40 ligand assessment in patients with acute coronary syndromes. *Thromb Res.* 2007;120(6):811–814.

75. Ivandic BT, Spanuth E, Haase D, Lestin HG, Katus HA. Increased plasma concentrations of soluble CD40 ligand in acute coronary syndrome depend on in vitro platelet activation. *Clin Chem.* 2007;53(7): 1231–1234.

76. Galis ZS, Sukhova GK, Lark MW, Libby P. Increased expression of matrix metalloproteinases and matrix degrading activity in vulnerable regions of human atherosclerotic plaques. *J Clin Invest.* 1994;94: 2493–2503.

77. Inokubo Y, Hanada H, Ishizaka H, Fukushi T, Kamada T, Okumura K. Plasma levels of matrix metalloproteinase-9 and tissue inhibitor of metalloproteinase-1 are increased in the coronary circulation in patients with acute coronary syndrome. *Am Heart J.* 2001;141: 211–217.

78. Kai H, Ikeda H, Yasukawa H, et al. Peripheral blood levels of matrix metalloproteases-2 and -9 are elevated in patients with acute coronary syndromes. *J Am Coll Cardiol.* 1998;32:368–372.

79. Soejima H, Ogawa H, Sakamoto T, et al. Increased serum matrix metalloproteinase-1 concentration predicts advanced left ventricular

remodeling in patients with acute myocardial infarction. *Circ J.* 2003;67(4):301–304.

80. Blankenberg S, Rupprecht HJ, Poirier O, et al. AtheroGene Investigators. Plasma concentrations and genetic variation of matrix metalloproteinase 9 and prognosis of patients with cardiovascular disease. *Circulation.* 2003;107:1579–1585.
81. Bayes-Genis A, Conover CA, Schwartz RS. The insulin-like growth factor axis: a review of atherosclerosis and restenosis. *Circ Res.* 2000;86:125–130.
82. Bayes-Genis A, Conover CA, Overgaard MT, et al. Pregnancy-associated plasma protein A as a marker of acute coronary syndromes. *N Engl J Med.* 2001;345:1022–1029.
83. Elesber AA, Lerman A, Denktas AE, et al. Pregnancy associated plasma protein-A and risk stratification of patients presenting with chest pain in the emergency department. *Int J Cardiol.* 2007;117(3):365–369.
84. Lund J, Qin QP, Ilva T, et al. Circulating pregnancy-associated plasma protein A predicts outcome in patients with acute coronary syndrome but no troponin I elevation. *Circulation.* 2003;108:1924–1926.
85. Heeschen C, Dimmeler S, Hamm CW, et al. CAPTURE Study Investigators. Pregnancy-associated plasma protein-A levels in patients with acute coronary syndromes: comparison with markers of systemic inflammation, platelet activation, and myocardial necrosis. *J Am Coll Cardiol.* 2005;45:229–237.
86. Lund J, Qin QP, Ilva T, et al. Pregnancy-associated plasma protein A: a biomarker in acute ST-elevation myocardial infarction (STEMI). *Ann Med.* 2006;38:221–228.
87. Stulc T, Malbohan I, Malik J, Fialova L, Soukupova J, Ceska R. Increased levels of pregnancy-associated plasma protein-A in patients with hypercholesterolemia: the effect of atorvastatin treatment. *Am Heart J.* 2003;146:e21.

15 ■ Role of Inflammatory Biomarkers in Heart Failure

Biykem Bozkurt, MD
Anita Deswal, MD, MPH
Douglas L. Mann, MD

The views expressed in the article are those of the authors and do not necessarily represent the views of the Department of Veterans Affairs.

ACKNOWLEDGEMENTS

Dr. Bozkurt is a recipient of a Merit Entry Level grant support from Veterans Affairs Medical Research Service (MRS). Dr. Deswal was recipient of an Advanced Career Development Award (# 612 A) from the Veterans Affairs Cooperative Studies Program at the time of this work. This research was supported by grants HL58081, HL42250, HL073017 and UO-1HL084890-01 from the National Institutes of Health.

Introduction

Chronic heart failure (HF) is characterized by an ongoing inflammatory response that correlates with HF disease severity and prognosis. The link between HF and inflammation was formally recognized and reported in 1990 by Levine et al.,[1] who noted that levels of an inflammatory cytokine, tumor necrosis factor (TNF), were elevated in the setting of HF. Since this first report, a number of studies have shown that in addition to TNF, other pro-inflammatory cytokines and chemokines are also involved in cardiac depression and the progression of HF (Table 15–1).[2–7] In this chapter, we will review the implications of inflammatory biomarkers in HF, with emphasis on inflammatory biomarkers that correlate with disease severity, prognosis, and clinical outcomes in HF.

Table 15–1: Peripheral levels of cytokines and cytokine receptors in heart failure.

	Cytokines					Cytokine Receptors				
	TNF-α	IL-1	IL-2	IL-6	IFN-γ	sTNFR1	sTNFR2	IL-1RA	sST-2	IL-6R
Levine[1]	+	nd	nd	nd	nd	nd	nd	nd	nd	nd
McMurray[32]	+	nd	nd	nd	nd	nd	nd	nd	nd	nd
Dutka[11]	+	nd	nd	nd	nd	nd	nd	nd	nd	nd
Wiedermann[18]	+	–	nd	+	–	nd	nd	nd	nd	nd
Katz[12]	+	–	+	nd	nd	nd	nd	nd	nd	nd
Matsumori[10]	+	–	–	–	–	nd	nd	nd	nd	nd
Ferrari[19]	+	nd	nd	nd	nd	+	+	nd	nd	nd
Torre-Amione[6]	+	nd	nd	nd	nd	+	+	nd	nd	nd
Torre-Amione[5]	+	nd	nd	+	nd	nd	nd	nd	nd	nd
Milani[92]	+	nd	nd	nd	nd	+	nd	+	nd	nd
Munger[20]	–	–	nd	+	nd	nd	nd	nd	nd	Nd
Testa[30]	+	+	–	+	nd	nd	+	+	nd	+
Anker[93]	+	nd	nd	nd	nd	nd	nd	nd	nd	nd
MacGowan[21]	+	nd	nd	+	nd	nd	nd	nd	nd	nd
Mohler[41]	+	nd	nd	+	nd	nd	nd	nd	nd	nd
Nishigaki[94]	+	nd	nd	+	nd	nd	nd	nd	nd	nd
Anker[17]	+	nd	nd	nd	nd	+	+	nd	nd	nd
Tsutamoto[24]	+	nd	nd	+	nd	nd	nd	nd	nd	nd
Aukrust[13]	+	nd	nd	+	nd	+	+	nd	nd	–
Dibbs[25]	+	nd	nd	+	nd	nd	nd	nd	nd	–
Rauchhaus[26]	+	nd	nd	+	nd	+	+	nd	nd	nd
Deswal[34]	+	nd	nd	+	nd	+	+	nd	nd	nd
Weinberg[14]	nd	nd	nd	nd	nd	nd	nd	nd	+	nd

Note 1: (nd): not done, (+): levels elevated, (–) levels not elevated; TNF-α: Tumor necrosis factor alpha; IL-1: Interleukin-1; IL-2: Interleukin-2; IL-6: Interleukin-6; IFN-γ: Interferon gamma; sTNFR1: Soluble TNF receptor R1; sTNFR2: Soluble TNF receptor R2; IL-1RA: IL-1 receptor antagonist; sST2: Soluble ST2—member of IL-1 receptor family; IL-6R: IL-6 receptor.

Note 2: See end of chapter text for references a–c above.

Overview of Cytokines Involved in Heart Failure

The term *cytokine* is applied to a group of relatively small molecular weight protein molecules (generally 15–30 Kda), which are secreted by cells in response to a variety of stimuli. Classically, cytokines are thought to be secreted by "producer cells" and act in an autocrine, juxtacrine, or paracrine fashion to influence the biological behavior of neighboring "target cells."[8] The group of cytokines that is responsible for initiating both the primary host response to a bacterial infection, as well as the repair of tissue following injury, has been termed "pro-inflammatory cytokines." Thus far, two major classes of cytokines have been identified in HF: vasoconstrictor cytokines, such as endothelin; and vasodepressor pro-inflammatory cytokines, such as TNF, interleukin (IL)-6, and IL-1.[4] These inflammatory mediators are now known to be expressed by all nucleated cell types residing in the myocardium, including the cardiac myocyte, suggesting that these molecules may do more than simply orchestrate inflammatory responses in the heart.[9] Peripheral-circulating, as well as intracardiac levels of these cytokines, are elevated in patients with HF.[4,6,10–12] Table 15–1 provides a summary of the studies that examined circulating levels of cytokines and cytokine receptors in patients with HF. As shown in the table, most of these studies have consistently described elevated levels of TNF in HF and a number of studies have demonstrated elevated levels of IL-6. However, fewer studies have examined and have not consistently found elevated levels of IL-1, IL-2, IL-18, and IFN-γ in HF.

The pro-inflammatory cytokine response is controlled by a series of immunoregulatory molecules, termed the "anti-inflammatory" cytokines. These cytokines act in concert with specific cytokine inhibitors and soluble cytokine receptors to regulate the human immune response. Their physiologic role in inflammation and pathologic role in HF is being increasingly recognized.[3] Major anti-inflammatory cytokines include: interleukin-1 receptor antagonist (IL-1ra), IL-10, IL-11, and IL-13. Specific cytokine receptors for IL-1, TNF, and IL-18 also function as pro-inflammatory cytokine inhibitors. Hence, in several inflammatory disorders the potential pathogenic effect of inflammatory cytokines will depend on the balance in the cytokine network, particularly on the levels of counteracting anti-inflammatory mediators. For example, patients with severe HF were found to have decreased levels of transforming growth factor β-1 and inadequately raised levels of IL-10 in relation to the elevated TNF concentrations, and these abnormalities in the cytokine network were most pronounced in patients with the most severe HF.[13]

There has been considerable recent interest in ST2, a member of the IL-1 receptor family and a protein secreted by cultured myocytes subjected to mechanical strain.[14] The protein product of ST2 encodes a membrane receptor of the IL-1 receptor family and a truncated soluble receptor (sST2) that can be detected in human serum. The transmembrane form of ST2 is thought to play a role in modulating responses of T helper type 2 cells, whereas the soluble form of ST2 is up-regulated in growth-stimulated fibroblasts. Infusion of sST2 appears to dampen inflammatory responses by suppressing the production of the inflammatory cytokines IL-6 and IL-12. Interruption of the ST2 gene results in progressive myocardial fibrosis and hypertrophy in experimental models. Despite the potential role played by ST2 in inflammation, significant parallels between ST2 and natriuretic peptides exist: the ST2 gene is markedly up-regulated in states of myocyte stretch, similar to the induction of the B-type natriuretic peptide (BNP) gene, and in analogy to the phenotype seen in BNP-deficient mice, mice deficient in ST2 develop dilated and hypertrophied left ventricles, lower ejection fractions, and reduced survival. This raises the possibility for a pluripotent role for ST2, representing a bridge between inflammatory and neurohormonal systems. The ligand for ST2 was recently identified as IL-33, a product released by endothelial cells, fibroblasts, and myocytes in response to stretch.[15] Similar to ST2, IL-33 has been suggested to play at least a dual role, acting as a pro-inflammatory cytokine, as well as an intracellular nuclear factor with transcriptional regulatory properties. ST2 might act as a soluble decoy receptor for IL-33, mitigating the effects of excessive IL-33 exposure and therefore mediating the interaction between cardiac myocytes, fibroblasts, and possibly endothelial cells.[16]

Cytokine Levels Are Elevated and Correlate with Disease Severity in Heart Failure

Circulating levels of TNF, IL-6, and IL-18 are elevated in patients with HF (Table 15–2).[6,10–12,15,17–29,30,32] Because they were initially identified in patients with cardiac cachexia[31,32] and edematous decompensation,[33] these cytokines were thought to be expressed only in patients with end-stage HF. However, as reported in several studies,[3,6,10–13,27,34,35,44,48] pro-inflammatory molecules are activated starting at earlier phases of HF (i.e., New York Heart Association [NYHA] functional class II HF)[6] or asymptomatic left ventricular dysfunction,[27] and continue to rise in direct relation to worsening NYHA functional class[6,24,34,36] (Figure 15–1) regardless of the etiology of HF.[3,6,20,30]

In addition to the inflammatory cytokines, circulating levels of cytokine receptors are elevated in HF. These include the soluble TNF receptors (sTNFR1 and sTNFR2),[19,22,37–39] and soluble transmembrane glycoprotein 130 (one of the receptors for IL-6 family), which are increased in HF in close relation to functional class.[13,27,39,40] Of note, even though IL-6 and glycoprotein 130 levels are elevated, soluble IL-6 receptor (IL-6R) levels are not increased in HF patients (Table 15–2).[13,25] Levels of sST2 are significantly higher in patients with advanced chronic HF, as well as acute decompensated HF compared with control subjects.[14,16] Similar to the above-mentioned neutralizing soluble receptor levels, IL-1 receptor antagonist levels are also elevated in patients with HF.[13,22,30] Although HF patients have enhanced expression of anti-inflammatory cytokine IL-10 compared to the normal population,[22] in patients with severe HF, the levels of transforming growth factor-beta 1 are decreased and IL-10 levels in relation to the elevated TNF concentrations are considered inadequately raised.[27]

TABLE 15–2: **Role of inflammatory biomarkers in heart failure.**

	TNF-α	IL-6	IL-18	sTNF-R1	sTNF-R2	IL-1 RA	sST2	IL-10	Chemokines (MCP-1)	CRP	ESR	Myeloperoxidase, galectin-3	Leukocyte subsets (Lymphopenia, Monocytosis)
Levels are elevated in HF	+++	++	+	++	++	+	+	+	+	++	++	++	+
Supporting references	1, 5, 6, 10–13, 17–21, 24–26, 30, 32, 34, 35, 41, a–c	22, 27, 40	23	19, 37, 38	22, 38	22	14, 16	22	3	71, 73, 74	76, 79	86, 87, 89	85
Levels correlate with disease severity	+++	+++	n/d	++	++	+	n/d	n/d	+	++	n/d	+	n/d
Supporting references	1, 5, 11, 13, 27, 30–32, 34	5, 20, 24, 27, 28, 30, 34, 40		28, 30, 34, 39	30, 34, 28, 39	30			3	71, 74		86	
Levels correlate with prognosis and HF outcomes	+++	+++	n/d	++	++	n/d	+	n/d	n/d	++	+	+	+

Supporting references	19, 24, 26, 34, 35, 41–44	24, 41–44		26, 34	26, 34		14, 16, 95				43, 73–75	76, 79§	87		84, 85
Levels predict development of HF in asymptomatic patients	++	++	n/d	n/d	n/d	n/d		n/d	n/d		++	n/d	n/d		n/d
Supporting references	27	27									27				
Levels change with HF therapy	+++	+++	n/d	++	++	n/d		++	n/d		+	n/d	n/d		n/d
Supporting references	47, 48, 51, 52, 54, 55, 57, 58	42, 47, 50, 56		22, 58	22, 51, 54, 57, 58			22, 52, 54			64, 96				

Note 1: TNF-α: Tumor necrosis factor alpha; IL-6: Interleukin-6; IL-18: Interleukin-18; sTNFR1: Soluble TNF receptor R1; sTNFR2: Soluble TNF receptor R2; IL-1RA: IL-1 receptor antagonist; sST2: Soluble ST2—member of IL-1 receptor family; IL-10: Interleukin-10; MCP-1: Monocyte chemo-attractant protein-1; CRP: C-reactive protein; ESR: Erythrocyte sedimentation rate, HF: Heart failure.

Note 2: See end of chapter text for references a–e above.

+++Supported by large number of studies and more than one large-scale clinical trial

++Supported by several studies and/or small-scale clinical trials and/or one large-scale clinical trial

+Supported by one small study or one small clinical trial

n/d: No data available

§One study suggested that elevated levels were associated with increased mortality,[76] the other study suggested that elevated levels were associated with better prognosis.[79]

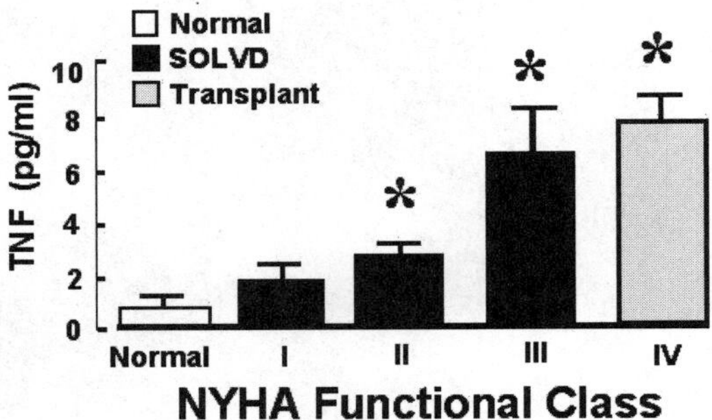

■ **Figure 15–1** TNF-a levels in patients with class I to IV HF. Compared with age-matched control subjects (open bar), there was a progressive increase in serum TNF-α levels in direct relation to decreasing functional classification. The solid bars denote values for patients enrolled in Studies of Left Ventricular Dysfunction (SOLVD); the shaded bar denotes values for NYHA class IV patients who were undergoing cardiac transplantation. *Significantly different from normal.

Reproduced from Seta Y, Shan K, Bozkurt B, Oral H, Mann DL. Basic mechanisms in heart failure: the cytokine hypothesis. *J Card Fail.* 1996;2:243–249, by permission of Churchill Livingstone ©1996.

Therefore, the balance is tipped towards enhanced expression of pro-inflammatory cytokines compared to anti-inflammatory cytokines in the HF population.

Pro-Inflammatory Cytokines Predict Poor Prognosis in Heart Failure

In addition to correlating with disease severity (i.e. with worsening functional class), elevated blood levels of pro-inflammatory cytokines correlate with increased mortality in patients with HF. Circulating levels of TNF,[26,34] IL-6,[41,24,34,41–44] and TNF soluble receptors (sTNFR1 and sTNFR2),[26,34] have been reported to predict poorer survival. As shown in Figure 15–2A, data on 384 patients with moderate to severe HF in the placebo arm of the Vesnarinone Trial (VEST) have demonstrated that there is decline in survival as a function of increasing TNF levels, with the worst survival in

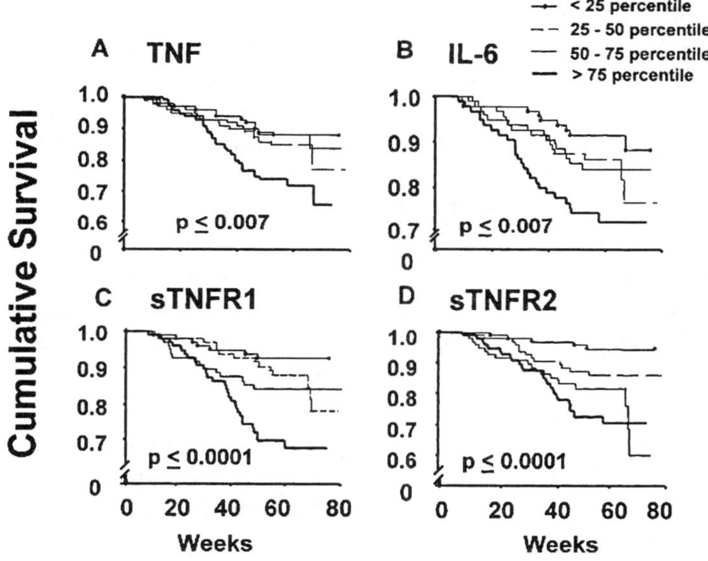

■ **Figure 15–2** Kaplan-Meier survival analysis. The circulating levels of TNF (A), IL-6 (B), sTNFR1 (C), and sTNFR2 (D) were examined in relation to patient survival during follow-up (mean duration 55 weeks; maximum duration 78 weeks). For this analysis, the circulating levels of cytokines and cytokine receptors were arbitrarily divided into quartiles.

Reproduced with permission from Deswal A, Petersen NJ, Feldman AM, Young JB, White BG, Mann DL. Cytokines and cytokine receptors in advanced heart failure: an analysis of the cytokine database from the Vesnarinone Trial (VEST). *Circulation.* 2001;103:2055–2059, by permission of the American Heart Association ©2001.

patients with TNF levels greater than the 75th percentile.[34] Similar findings were observed with circulating levels of IL-6 (Figure 15–2B) and levels of soluble TNF receptors types 1 and 2 (Figure 15–2C and D). When each cytokine and/or cytokine receptor was separately entered into a multivariate Cox proportional hazards model (that included age, sex, etiology of HF, NYHA class, ejection fraction, and serum sodium), TNF, IL-6, sTNFR1, and sTNFR2 remained significant independent predictors of mortality, along with NYHA class and ejection fraction. However, when all the cytokines and receptors were entered into the model together, only sTNFR2 remained a significant predictor of mortality.[34] Of interest, in another study of 37 patients with HF and 26 age-matched control subjects, the circulating levels of sTNFR2 also appeared to be the most powerful predictor of mortality.[19] In a larger study of 152 patients with HF, Rauchhaus et al., however, reported that sTNF-R1 was the strongest and most accurate prognosticator, as the receiver operating characteristic area under the curve for sTNF-R1 was greater than for sTNF-R2 at 6, 12, and 18 months (all $P < 0.05$).[26] Most studies have evaluated patients with HF and depressed ejection, but a recent community-based study demonstrated that higher TNF levels were independently associated with a greater risk of mortality—even in patients with HF and preserved ejection fraction.[35] Although these clinical studies cannot address whether elevated circulating levels of cytokines and cytokine receptors represent an epiphenomenon that is associated with—but not causally related to—worsening disease severity and outcomes, the preponderance of data support that pro-inflammatory cytokines, TNF and IL-6, contribute to further progression of HF and worse outcomes.

It has also been suggested that sST2 levels may correlate with prognosis. A study by Weinberg demonstrated that an increase in ST2 levels over a two-week period was a significant predictor of mortality or need for transplantation independent of BNP or Pro-atrial natriuretic peptide (ANP) in patients with advanced chronic HF.[14] In addition, recent studies have shown that increased sST2 plasma concentrations in patients presenting with acute decompensated HF were independently and strongly associated with one-year mortality.[21,45]

Inflammatory Cytokines as Markers for Monitoring Response to Therapy in Heart Failure

There have been several studies examining the changes in levels of inflammatory cytokines during standard therapy for HF. Some of these changes can be attributed to direct interaction of the medications used, such as the interaction between neurohormonal antagonists and the pro-inflammatory cytokines.[46,47] Clinical studies have shown that treatment with angiotensin receptor antagonists can lead to significant reductions in circulating levels of TNF and/or cell adhesion molecules in patients with HF.[48] Beta-adrenergic blockade has also been shown to prevent the expression of inflammatory mediators in postinfarction animal models,[49] and results in significant reductions in pro-inflammatory cytokine levels in clinical studies with HF patients.[22,50–55] Compared to angiotensin receptor blockers and beta blockers, the effect of angiotensin converting enzyme (ACE) inhibitors on inflammatory cytokines is not as clear. In a study by Gage et al., TNF production was significantly lower in patients receiving ACE inhibitors and there was a trend toward lower levels of serum IL-6 in patients receiving both ACE inhibitors and beta blockers.[52] Again, in the same study, the ratios of interferon gamma to IL-10 levels were lower in patients receiving a combination of beta blocker and ACE inhibitor therapy. In an animal infarct model, use of ACE inhibitors over 28 days resulted in reduction of cardiac cytokine expression.[47] Contrarily, in a clinical study by Gullestad and colleagues, treatment with ACE inhibitors over 34 weeks resulted in a rise in the peripheral levels of chemokines, cell adhesion molecules, and pro-inflammatory cytokines, except for IL-6.[56] There is little information regarding inflammatory cytokines and other medications used in the treatment of HF. Mohler et al. demonstrated that treatment with the long-acting dihydropyridine calcium antagonist, amlodipine, over 26 weeks lowered plasma IL-6 levels in patients with HF.[41] Other studies have noted that optimization of background standard therapy of HF with diuretics, ACE inhibitors, beta blockers, and digoxin can result in significant reductions in circulating levels of TNF and IL-6.[42] Physical training reduces plasma levels of TNF, IL-6, sTNFR1, sTNFR2, and sIL-6R in patients with HF.[57,58] Furthermore, in patients with advanced HF, mechanical circulatory support with ventricular assist devices results in markedly-reduced myocardial expression of TNF after several weeks of support.[59,60]

These studies suggest that there are important interactions among the renin-angiotensin and adrenergic systems, and pro-inflammatory cytokines; and many of the conventional therapies for HF may work, at least in part, through the modulation of pro-inflammatory cytokines. Nevertheless, it should be noted despite these temporal parallel changes in the levels of cytokines with optimal HF therapy, we currently do not have data from large-scale trials on the changes in inflammatory biomarkers over time correlating with morbidity and mortality in HF patients. Furthermore, the sensitivity, specificity, and negative and positive predictive values of inflammatory biomarkers for response to therapy for HF are not known and whether any of the inflammatory markers provide additional information over and above established variables remains to be shown.[25]

Pro-Inflammatory Cytokines as Predictors for Development of Heart Failure in Asymptomatic Patients

Elevated levels of IL-6 and TNF have been reported in patients with left ventricular dysfunction in the absence of clinical symptoms of HF,[5,61] but only recently was the predictive role of pro-inflammatory cytokines for development of HF in asymptomatic patients described. In a subgroup of 732 elderly Framingham Heart Study subjects without prior HF, Vasan and colleagues reported that baseline levels of IL-6 and spontaneous production of TNF by peripheral blood mononuclear cells (PMBC) were predictive of development of HF in the next five years.[27] After adjustment for established risk factors, including the occurrence of myocardial infarction during follow-up, the investigators found that the risk of developing HF increased approximately 1.6-fold to 1.7-fold per tertile increment in PBMC TNF and IL-6 levels, respectively. Subjects with elevated serum IL-6 and PBMC TNF greater than median values, as well as CRP greater than or equal to 5 mg/dL, had a 4.1-fold risk for developing HF. The study population consisted of predominantly elderly, white subjects (67% female) with a high prevalence of hypertension (~70%), atrial fibrillation (~7%), and preexisting cardiovascular disease without prior documented myocardial infarction. It is important to point out that in this study there was no assessment of left ventricular function at baseline. Elevated inflammatory markers in this study may have identified patients with vascular disease at risk for myocardial infarction[62,63] or patients with preexisting subclinical left ventricular dysfunction.[64] Without a baseline assessment of ventricular function, it is not possible to determine whether elevated levels of IL-6, TNF, and CRP predict the de novo development of cardiomyopathy versus the transition from subclinical left ventricular dysfunction to overt HF.

Chemokines

Chemokines are potent pro-inflammatory and immune modulators. Chemokines regulate several biological processes such as chemotaxis, activation and migration of leukocytes to areas of inflammation, collagen turnover, angiogenesis, and apoptosis.[3] TNF and other pro-inflammatory cytokines, such as IL-1β and IL-6 or interferon-γ, are known to induce these chemotactic polypeptides.[65] Potent chemokines, such as macrophage chemoattractant protein-1 (MCP-1) and macrophage inflammatory protein-1alpha (MIP-1α), not only can attract the monocytes and the lymphocytes, but also can modulate other functions of these cells, e.g., generation of reactive oxygen species.[3] MCP-1 has been reported to be up-regulated in experimental models of HF with pressure or volume-overload.[66,67] Furthermore, transgenic overexpression of MCP-1 in the myocardium has been shown to result in myocarditis and subsequent development of HF in experimental models.[68] Similar to the pro-inflammatory cytokines, the failing human heart expresses chemokine and chemokine receptors.[69] Increased expression of chemokines, e.g., MCP-1, has recently been described in clinical HF.[3] Aukrust and colleagues reported that HF patients had significantly elevated levels of all chemokines with the highest levels in patients in New York Heart Association functional class IV. In this study, MCP-1 and MIP-1α levels significantly and inversely correlated with left ventricular ejection fraction. Further studies on cells isolated from peripheral blood of these patients suggest that platelets, CD3+ lymphocytes, and in particular, monocytes, may contribute to the elevated chemokine levels in HF.[3]

C-Reactive Protein

C-reactive protein (CRP) is a phylogenetically highly-conserved plasma protein that participates in the systemic response to inflammation.[70] It is exclusively produced in the liver and its plasma concentration increases during inflammatory states, a characteristic that has long been employed for clinical purposes. With recent recognition of its diagnostic and prognostic role in ischemic heart disease and acute coronary syndromes, CRP has gained attention as a laboratory marker for standard testing. As will be reviewed in the following paragraph, CRP has been described to correlate with disease severity and prognosis in patients with HF.

The first observation of raised concentrations of CRP in HF was published in 1990. In this study, the serum concentration of CRP was higher than normal in 70% of the HF patients and the concentration was directly related to the severity of HF and the stage of decompensation.[71] Subsequently, another group measured CRP values in 188 patients with idiopathic dilated cardiomyopathy and left ventricular ejection fraction less than 40%.[72] Those patients who died during a follow-up period of five years had significantly higher CRP concentrations than those who survived (1.05 +/− 1.37 versus 0.49 +/− 1.04 mg/dL, $P < 0.05$). Sixty-two percent of the patients with CRP greater than 1.0 mg/dL died within five years. Similarly, Milo et al. reported that in 30 patients admitted with acute HF, CRP levels were elevated in nonischemic as well as ischemic patients, compared to controls.[73] In another study of 76 patients hospitalized for HF, the mean CRP level was found to be significantly higher in patients with HF compared to a control group (3.94 +/− 5.87 versus 0.84 +/− 1 mg/dL). CRP levels were increased in relation to NYHA class and the HF patients with elevated CRP levels (>0.9 mg/dL) were at greater risk of hospitalization during the 18 month follow-up period compared to patients with normal CRP levels.[74] Similarly, Cesari et al. reported that among elderly patients, for every one standard deviation increase in CRP, the risk of HF events increased by 48%.[75] These studies underline the association of CRP with disease severity and prognosis in HF patients.

Recently, Vasan and colleagues reported the role of CRP in the prediction of HF development. They examined CRP as an antecedent to HF among elderly subjects enrolled in the Framingham Heart Study. Elevated CRP (serum CRP level ≥5 mg/dL) was associated with a 2.8-fold increased risk of development of HF during a follow-up period of approximately five years compared to subjects with normal CRP levels.[27] Given the association of CRP to atherosclerotic coronary events, it should be noted that in the studies by Vasan et al.[27] and Cesari et al.,[75] the subjects were free of ischemic heart disease at the time of entry; however, the outcomes included both ischemic and nonischemic HF events.

Lastly, it is important to note that use of ACE inhibitors and beta blockers has been associated with lower levels of CRP in HF patients.[64] At the present time, despite its clear associations with HF disease severity and outcomes, it is not clear whether CRP is merely a marker of inflammation with no particular role in the development of HF or whether it is involved in the pathogenesis and progression of HF. It is also not clear whether it can be used as a biomarker for monitoring success of therapy for HF.

Erythrocyte Sedimentation Rate (ESR)

Erythrocyte sedimentation rate has been of particular interest in HF due to its low cost, easy applicability, and reproducibility. However, clinical studies—which are historically separated from each other by decades—have yielded controversial results on the role of the ESR in HF. Based on the potential misinterpretation of the results in a single report published in 1936, physicians have long believed that the erythrocyte sedimentation rate is low in patients with HF.[76–78] To reevaluate this concept in the modern era, Haber et al. measured the ESR in 242 HF patients and reported that the ESR was low (<5 mm per hour) in only 10% of the patients, but was increased (>25 mm per hour) in 50% of subjects. Surprisingly, patients with low or normal sedimentation rates (≤25 mm per hour) had more severe hemodynamic abnormalities, worse NYHA functional class symptoms, and worse one-year survival rates compared with patients with elevated ESR.[76] Subsequently, in 2001, Sharma and colleagues studied ESR in relation to plasma levels of inflammatory cytokines and mortality in 159 HF patients.[79] ESR ranged from 1 to 96 mm/h (median 14 mm/h) and, similar to the study by Haber et al.,[76] only 16% of the patients in this study had an ESR less than 5 mm/h; in addition, ESR correlated with TNF, sTNFR1, sTNFR2 and IL-6 levels. However, contrary to the findings in Haber's study, high ESR levels indicated a poor prognosis, which was independent of age, NYHA class, ejection fraction, and peak oxygen consumption (Figure 15–3).

Peripheral Leukocyte Subsets

Despite the wealth of information available on the role of inflammation in HF, relatively little has been published on the prognostic role of white blood cells or the leukocyte subsets in this setting. For patients presenting with acute myocardial infarction, elevated leukocyte count,[80,81] or relative neutrophilia (>65%), on admission has been associated with subsequent development of HF.[82] Similarly, peripheral monocytosis 24 hours after the onset of myocardial infarction has been associated with the development of left ventricular (LV) dysfunction and LV aneurysm.[83]

In a study of 211 heart failure patients referred for cardiac transplantation,[84] survival rates were significantly lower for patients with a relatively low percent lymphocyte count. In this study, multivariate analysis showed that NYHA class and percent lymphocyte count were independent predictors of survival.[84] The

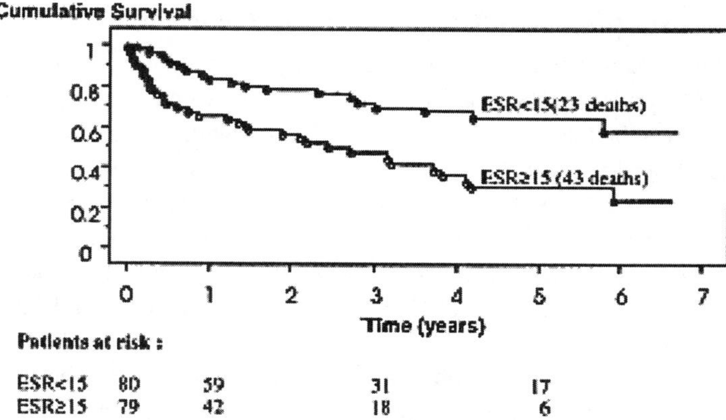

■ **Figure 15–3** Kaplan-Meier survival plot for 159 patients with chronic heart failure. Patients were sub-grouped according to erythrocyte sedimentation rate (ESR). The group of patients with high ESR (≥15 mm/h) had an impaired survival compared with patients with ESR <15 mm/h (RR 2.62, 95% CI 1.58–4.36, $P < 0.0001$).

Reproduced with permission from Sharma R, Rauchhaus M, Ponikowski PP, Varney S, Poole-Wilson PA, Mann DL et al. The relationship of the erythrocyte sedimentation rate to inflammatory cytokines and survival in patients with chronic heart failure treated with angiotensin-converting enzyme inhibitors. *J Am Coll Cardiol.* 2000;36(2):523–528, by permission of the American College of Cardiology and Elsevier Science Inc. ©2000.

authors hypothesized that the physiological stress suffered by patients with HF may result in an increased production of cortisol and a shift in the leukocyte differential toward a decreased percentage of lymphocytes. Similarly, in 861 elderly patients enrolled in the Chronic HF Italian Study, Aconfora and colleagues[85] reported that 38% of the patients had a relative lymphocyte count of ≤ 20%. The 3-year all-cause mortality in patients with HF and a relative lymphocyte count was 64% compared with 40% in patients with a normal relative lymphocyte count ($P < .0001$). Thus, these studies suggest that a low relative lymphocyte count is an independent marker of poor prognosis in patients with HF.

Neutrophil and Macrophage Activation

Biomarkers characterizing activation of polymorphonuclear neutrophils or macrophages have been implicated as prognostic markers in HF.[86–88] Myeloperoxidase, a peroxidase enzyme most abundantly present in neutrophil granulocytes which gets released into the plasma with activation of neutrophils, has been reported to be elevated in heart failure patients with LV dysfunction with ischemic or nonischemic cardiomyopathy; it has also been associated with an increased likelihood of more advanced HF and reported to be predictive of increased adverse clinical outcomes.[86,89] Similarly, cardiac macrophages have been demonstrated to be activated at an early stage in failure-prone, hypertrophied hearts and that these activated cardiac macrophages produce galectin-3, a substance that has been reported to contribute to cardiac contractile dysfunction[88] and may be prognostically meaningful in HF.[87]

Use of Inflammatory Biomarkers in the Management of Patients with HF

Although the development of clinical practice guidelines and disease management strategies for patients with HF has resulted in dramatic overall improvements in patient care and outcomes, the day-to-day management of individual patients with HF remains challenging. This is partly due to the fact that HF management is quite complex and involves numerous therapies, including—but not limited to—lifestyle modification with diet and exercise, use of defibrillator or pacing devices, antiremodeling surgery, and medications that need to be up-titrated to clinically proven doses. Furthermore, there may be race-, gender-, and age-specific differences in the way patients respond to these therapies. Thus, there is a need for useful biomarkers to help individualize management strategies and guide appropriate selection, timing, and/or dosing of therapies in patients with HF.[90] Data from large-scale well-designed clinical trials provide evidence that changes in neurohormonal levels over time are associated with changes in morbidity and mortality in HF patients,[91] however, at the present time, it is not clear whether clinicians should use changes in levels of these biomarkers, such as plasma norepinephrine levels and/or BNP, to guide HF management.[90] Furthermore, we currently do not have similar data from large-scale trials on the changes in inflammatory biomarkers over time correlating with morbidity and mortality in HF patients. Much more information is necessary before the use of inflammatory markers will become a standard of practice in treatment of HF. For example, assays will need to be standardized and better information regarding the degree of natural variability of these markers in patients with HF will need to be gathered.[25] However, it is likely that multimarker strategies that combine inflammatory biomarkers may ultimately prove beneficial in guiding HF therapy in the future.

Conclusion

Inflammatory markers have diagnostic and prognostic importance in patients with HF. As noted, some of these biomarkers, such as pro-inflammatory cytokines and chemokines, may be involved in the pathogenesis and progression of HF, whereas others such as CRP or the ESR may simply reflect the degree of systemic inflammation. Table 15–2 provides a summary of the inflammatory biomarkers that have been implicated in HF thus far, as well as whether they: (1) are involved in the pathogenesis of HF, (2) correlate with disease severity or prognosis in HF, (3) predict the development of HF in asymptomatic patients, (4) change with HF therapy, or (5) represent potential targets for future therapies.

References

1. Levine B, Kalman J, Mayer L, Fillit HM, Packer M. Elevated circulating levels of tumor necrosis factor in severe chronic heart failure. *N Engl J Med.* 1990;323(4):236–241.
2. Bozkurt B, Kribbs SB, Clubb FJ Jr, et al. Pathophysiologically relevant concentrations of tumor necrosis factor-alpha promote progressive left ventricular dysfunction and remodeling in rats. *Circulation.* 1998;97(14):1382–1391.

3. Aukrust P, Ueland T, Muller F, et al. Elevated circulating levels of C-C chemokines in patients with congestive heart failure. *Circulation.* 1998;97(12):1136–1143.
4. Mann DL. Inflammatory mediators and the failing heart: past, present, and the foreseeable future. *Circ Res.* 2002;91(11):988–998.
5. Torre-Amione G, Kapadia S, Benedict C, Oral H, Young JB, Mann DL. Proinflammatory cytokine levels in patients with depressed left ventricular ejection fraction: a report from the Studies of Left Ventricular Dysfunction (SOLVD). *J Am Coll Cardiol.* 1996;27(5): 1201–1206.
6. Torre-Amione G, Kapadia S, Lee J, et al. Tumor necrosis factor-alpha and tumor necrosis factor receptors in the failing human heart. *Circulation.* 1996;93(4):704–711.
7. Kapadia SR, Yakoob K, Nader S, Thomas JD, Mann DL, Griffin BP. Elevated circulating levels of serum tumor necrosis factor-alpha in patients with hemodynamically significant pressure and volume overload. *J Am Coll Cardiol.* 2000;36(1):208–212.
8. Nathan C, Sporn M. Cytokines in context. *J Cell Biol.* 1991;113(5): 981–986.
9. Torre-Amione G, Kapadia S, Lee J, Bies RD, Lebovitz R, Mann DL. Expression and functional significance of tumor necrosis factor receptors in human myocardium. *Circulation.* 1995;92(6):1487–1493.
10. Matsumori A, Yamada T, Suzuki H, Matoba Y, Sasayama S. Increased circulating cytokines in patients with myocarditis and cardiomyopathy. *Br Heart J.* 1994;72(6):561–566.
11. Dutka DP, Elborn JS, Delamere F, Shale DJ, Morris GK. Tumour necrosis factor alpha in severe congestive cardiac failure. *Br Heart J.* 1993;70(2):141–143.
12. Katz SD, Rao R, Berman JW, et al. Pathophysiological correlates of increased serum tumor necrosis factor in patients with congestive heart failure. Relation to nitric oxide-dependent vasodilation in the forearm circulation. *Circulation.* 1994;90(1):12–16.
13. Aukrust P, Ueland T, Lien E, et al. Cytokine network in congestive heart failure secondary to ischemic or idiopathic dilated cardiomyopathy. *Am J Cardiol.* 1999;83(3):376–382.
14. Weinberg EO, Shimpo M, Hurwitz S, Tominaga S, Rouleau JL, Lee RT. Identification of serum soluble ST2 receptor as a novel heart failure biomarker. *Circulation.* 2003;107(5):721–726.

15. Braunwald E. Biomarkers in heart failure. *N Engl J Med.* 2008; 358(20):2148–2159.

16. Januzzi JL Jr, Peacock WF, Maisel AS, et al. Measurement of the interleukin family member ST2 in patients with acute dyspnea: results from the PRIDE (Pro-Brain Natriuretic Peptide Investigation of Dyspnea in the Emergency Department) Study. *J Am Coll Cardiol.* 2007;50(7):607–613.

17. Anker SD, Egerer KR, Volk HD, Kox WJ, Poole-Wilson PA, Coats AJ. Elevated soluble CD14 receptors and altered cytokines in chronic heart failure. *Am J Cardiol.* 1997;79(10):1426–1430.

18. Wiedermann CJ, Beimpold H, Herold M, Knapp E, Braunsteiner H. Increased levels of serum neopterin and decreased production of neutrophil superoxide anions in chronic heart failure with elevated levels of tumor necrosis factor-alpha. *J Am Coll Cardiol.* 1993;22(7): 1897–1901.

19. Ferrari R, Bachetti T, Confortini R, et al. Tumor necrosis factor soluble receptors in patients with various degrees of congestive heart failure. *Circulation.* 1995;92(6):1479–1486.

20. Munger MA, Johnson B, Amber IJ, Callahan KS, Gilbert EM. Circulating concentrations of proinflammatory cytokines in mild or moderate heart failure secondary to ischemic or idiopathic dilated cardiomyopathy. *Am J Cardiol.* 1996;77(9):723–727.

21. MacGowan GA, Mann DL, Kormos RL, Feldman AM, Murali S. Circulating interleukin-6 in severe heart failure. *Am J Cardiol.* 1997;79(8): 1128–1131.

22. Loppnow H, Werdan K, Werner C. The enhanced plasma levels of soluble tumor necrosis factor receptors (sTNF-R1; sTNF-R2) and interleukin-10 (IL-10) in patients suffering from chronic heart failure are reversed in patients treated with beta-adrenoceptor antagonist. *Auton Autacoid Pharmacol.* 2002;22(2):83–92.

23. Seta Y, Kanda T, Tanaka T, et al. Interleukin-18 in patients with congestive heart failure: induction of atrial natriuretic peptide gene expression. *Res Commun Mol Pathol Pharmacol.* 2000;108(1–2): 87–95.

24. Tsutamoto T, Hisanaga T, Wada A, et al. Interleukin-6 spillover in the peripheral circulation increases with the severity of heart failure, and the high plasma level of interleukin-6 is an important prognostic

predictor in patients with congestive heart failure. *J Am Coll Cardiol.* 1998;31(2):391–398.

25. Dibbs Z, Thornby J, White BG, Mann DL. Natural variability of circulating levels of cytokines and cytokine receptors in patients with heart failure: implications for clinical trials. *J Am Coll Cardiol.* 1999;33(7):1935–1942.
26. Rauchhaus M, Doehner W, Francis DP, et al. Plasma cytokine parameters and mortality in patients with chronic heart failure. *Circulation.* 2000;102(25):3060–3067.
27. Vasan RS, Sullivan LM, Roubenoff R, et al. Inflammatory markers and risk of heart failure in elderly subjects without prior myocardial infarction: the Framingham Heart Study. *Circulation.* 2003;107(11): 1486–1491.
28. Deswal A, Petersen NJ, Feldman AM, White BG, Mann DL. Effects of vesnarinone on peripheral circulating levels of cytokines and cytokine receptors in patients with heart failure: a report from the Vesnarinone Trial. *Chest.* 2001;120(2):453–459.
29. Saraste A, Voipio-Pulkki LM, Heikkila P, Laine P, Nieminen MS, Pulkki K. Soluble tumor necrosis factor receptor levels identify a subgroup of heart failure patients with increased cardiomyocyte apoptosis. *Clin Chim Acta.* 2002;320(1–2):65–67.
30. Testa M, Yeh M, Lee P, et al. Circulating levels of cytokines and their endogenous modulators in patients with mild to severe congestive heart failure due to coronary artery disease or hypertension. *J Am Coll Cardiol.* 1996;28(4):964–971.
31. Anker SD, Ponikowski PP, Clark AL, et al. Cytokines and neurohormones relating to body composition alterations in the wasting syndrome of chronic heart failure. *Eur Heart J.* 1999;20(9):683–693.
32. McMurray J, Abdullah I, Dargie HJ, Shapiro D. Increased concentrations of tumour necrosis factor in "cachectic" patients with severe chronic heart failure. *Br Heart J.* 1991;66(5):356–358.
33. Niebauer J, Volk HD, Kemp M, et al. Endotoxin and immune activation in chronic heart failure: a prospective cohort study. *Lancet.* 1999;353(9167):1838–1842.
34. Deswal A, Petersen NJ, Feldman AM, Young JB, White BG, Mann DL. Cytokines and cytokine receptors in advanced heart failure: an analysis of the cytokine database from the Vesnarinone trial (VEST). *Circulation.* 2001;103(16):2055–2059.

35. Dunlay SM, Weston SA, Redfield MM, Killian JM, Roger VL. Tumor necrosis factor-alpha and mortality in heart failure: a community study. *Circulation.* 2008;118(6):625–631.

36. Seta Y, Shan K, Bozkurt B, Oral H, Mann DL. Basic mechanisms in heart failure: the cytokine hypothesis. *J Card Fail.* 1996;2(3): 243–249.

37. Hansen MS, Stanton EB, Gawad Y, et al. Relation of circulating cardiac myosin light chain 1 isoform in stable severe congestive heart failure to survival and treatment with flosequinan. *Am J Cardiol.* 2002;90(9):969–973.

38. Nowak J, Rozentryt P, Szewczyk M, et al. Tumor necrosis factor receptors sTNF-RI and sTNF-RII in advanced chronic heart failure. *Pol Arch Med Wewn.* 2002;107(3):223–229.

39. Nozaki N, Yamaguchi S, Shirakabe M, Nakamura H, Tomoike H. Soluble tumor necrosis factor receptors are elevated in relation to severity of congestive heart failure. *Jpn Circ J.* 1997;61(8):657–664.

40. Chin BS, Blann AD, Gibbs CR, Chung NA, Conway DG, Lip GY. Prognostic value of interleukin-6, plasma viscosity, fibrinogen, von Willebrand factor, tissue factor and vascular endothelial growth factor levels in congestive heart failure. *Eur J Clin Invest.* 2003;33(11): 941–948.

41. Mohler ER III, Sorensen LC, Ghali JK, et al. Role of cytokines in the mechanism of action of amlodipine: the PRAISE Heart Failure Trial. Prospective Randomized Amlodipine Survival Evaluation. *J Am Coll Cardiol.* 1997;30(1):35–41.

42. Maeda K, Tsutamoto T, Wada A, et al. High levels of plasma brain natriuretic peptide and interleukin-6 after optimized treatment for heart failure are independent risk factors for morbidity and mortality in patients with congestive heart failure. *J Am Coll Cardiol.* 2000;36(5):1587–1593.

43. Kell R, Haunstetter A, Dengler TJ, Zugck C, Kubler W, Haass M. Do cytokines enable risk stratification to be improved in NYHA functional class III patients? Comparison with other potential predictors of prognosis. *Eur Heart J.* 2002;23(1):70–78.

44. Ferrari R. Interleukin-6: a neurohumoral predictor of prognosis in patients with heart failure: light and shadow. *Eur Heart J.* 2002;23(1): 9–10.

45. Wilson Tang WH, Francis GS, Morrow DA, et al. National Academy of Clinical Biochemistry Laboratory Medicine Practice Guidelines: Clinical Utilization of Cardiac Biomarker Testing in Heart Failure. *Circulation.* 2007;116(5):e99–e109.

46. Hernandez-Presa M, Bustos C, Ortego M, et al. Angiotensin-converting enzyme inhibition prevents arterial nuclear factor-kappa B activation, monocyte chemoattractant protein-1 expression, and macrophage infiltration in a rabbit model of early accelerated atherosclerosis. *Circulation.* 1997;95(6):1532–1541.

47. Wei GC, Sirois MG, Qu R, Liu P, Rouleau JL. Subacute and chronic effects of quinapril on cardiac cytokine expression, remodeling, and function after myocardial infarction in the rat. *J Cardiovasc Pharmacol.* 2002;39(6):842–850.

48. Gurlek A, Kilickap M, Dincer I, Dandachi R, Tutkak H, Oral D. Effect of losartan on circulating TNFalpha levels and left ventricular systolic performance in patients with heart failure. *J Cardiovasc Risk.* 2001; 8(5):279–282.

49. Prabhu SD, Chandrasekar B, Murray DR, Freeman GL. beta-adrenergic blockade in developing heart failure: effects on myocardial inflammatory cytokines, nitric oxide, and remodeling. *Circulation.* 2000;101(17):2103–2109.

50. Aronson D, Burger AJ. Effect of beta-blockade on autonomic modulation of heart rate and neurohormonal profile in decompensated heart failure. *Ann Noninvasive Electrocardiol.* 2001;6(2):98–106.

51. de Werra I, Jaccard C, Corradin SB, et al. Cytokines, nitrite/nitrate, soluble tumor necrosis factor receptors, and procalcitonin concentrations: comparisons in patients with septic shock, cardiogenic shock, and bacterial pneumonia. *Crit Care Med.* 1997;25(4):607–613.

52. Gage JR, Fonarow G, Hamilton M, Widawski M, Martinez-Maza O, Vredevoe DL. Beta blocker and angiotensin-converting enzyme inhibitor therapy is associated with decreased Th1/Th2 cytokine ratios and inflammatory cytokine production in patients with chronic heart failure. *Neuroimmunomodulation.* 2004;11(3):173–180.

53. Matsumura T, Tsushima K, Ohtaki E, et al. Effects of carvedilol on plasma levels of interleukin-6 and tumor necrosis factor-alpha in nine patients with dilated cardiomyopathy. *J Cardiol.* 2002;39(5): 253–257.

54. Ohtsuka T, Hamada M, Hiasa G, et al. Effect of beta-blockers on circulating levels of inflammatory and anti-inflammatory cytokines in patients with dilated cardiomyopathy. *J Am Coll Cardiol.* 2001;37(2): 412–417.

55. Tsutamoto T, Wada A, Matsumoto T, et al. Relationship between tumor necrosis factor-alpha production and oxidative stress in the failing hearts of patients with dilated cardiomyopathy. *J Am Coll Cardiol.* 2001;37(8):2086–2092.

56. Gullestad L, Aukrust P, Ueland T, et al. Effect of high- versus low-dose angiotensin converting enzyme inhibition on cytokine levels in chronic heart failure. *J Am Coll Cardiol.* 1999;34(7):2061–2067.

57. Lemaitre JP, Harris S, Fox KA, Denvir M. Change in circulating cytokines after 2 forms of exercise training in chronic stable heart failure. *Am Heart J.* 2004;147(1):100–105.

58. Adamopoulos S, Parissis J, Karatzas D, et al. Physical training modulates proinflammatory cytokines and the soluble Fas/soluble Fas ligand system in patients with chronic heart failure. *J Am Coll Cardiol.* 2002;39(4):653–663.

59. Torre-Amione G, Stetson SJ, Youker KA, et al. Decreased expression of tumor necrosis factor-alpha in failing human myocardium after mechanical circulatory support: a potential mechanism for cardiac recovery. *Circulation.* 1999;100(11):1189–1193.

60. Clark AL, Loebe M, Potapov EV, et al. Ventricular assist device in severe heart failure: effects on cytokines, complement and body weight. *Eur Heart J.* 2001;22(24):2275–2283.

61. Raymond RJ, Dehmer GJ, Theoharides TC, Deliargyris EN. Elevated interleukin-6 levels in patients with asymptomatic left ventricular systolic dysfunction. *Am Heart J.* 2001;141(3):435–438.

62. Ridker PM, Rifai N, Pfeffer M, Sacks F, Lepage S, Braunwald E. Elevation of tumor necrosis factor-alpha and increased risk of recurrent coronary events after myocardial infarction. *Circulation.* 2000;101(18): 2149–2153.

63. Ridker PM, Rifai N, Stampfer MJ, Hennekens CH. Plasma concentration of interleukin-6 and the risk of future myocardial infarction among apparently healthy men. *Circulation.* 2000;101(15): 1767–1772.

64. Joynt KE, Gattis WA, Hasselblad V, et al. Effect of angiotensin-converting enzyme inhibitors, beta blockers, statins, and aspirin on

C-reactive protein levels in outpatients with heart failure. *Am J Cardiol.* 2004;93(6):783–785.

65. Rollins BJ, Yoshimura T, Leonard EJ, Pober JS. Cytokine-activated human endothelial cells synthesize and secrete a monocyte chemoattractant, MCP-1/JE. *Am J Pathol.* 1990;136(6):1229–1233.
66. Shioi T, Matsumori A, Kihara Y, et al. Increased expression of interleukin-1 beta and monocyte chemotactic and activating factor/monocyte chemoattractant protein-1 in the hypertrophied and failing heart with pressure overload. *Circ Res.* 1997;81(5):664–671.
67. Behr TM, Wang X, Aiyar N, et al. Monocyte chemoattractant protein-1 is upregulated in rats with volume-overload congestive heart failure. *Circulation.* 2000;102(11):1315–1322.
68. Kolattukudy PE, Quach T, Bergese S, et al. Myocarditis induced by targeted expression of the MCP-1 gene in murine cardiac muscle. *Am J Pathol.* 1998;152(1):101–111.
69. Damas JK, Eiken HG, Oie E, et al. Myocardial expression of CC- and CXC-chemokines and their receptors in human end-stage heart failure. *Cardiovasc Res.* 2000;47(4):778–787.
70. Black S, Kushner I, Samols D. C-reactive protein. *J Biol Chem.* 2004;279(47):48487–48490.
71. Pye M, Rae AP, Cobbe SM. Study of serum C-reactive protein concentration in cardiac failure. *Br Heart J.* 1990;63(4):228–230.
72. Kaneko K, Kanda T, Yamauchi Y, et al. C-reactive protein in dilated cardiomyopathy. *Cardiology.* 1999;91(4):215–219.
73. Milo O, Cotter G, Kaluski E, et al. Comparison of inflammatory and neurohormonal activation in cardiogenic pulmonary edema secondary to ischemic versus nonischemic causes. *Am J Cardiol.* 2003;92(2):222–226.
74. Alonso-Martinez JL, Llorente-Diez B, Echegaray-Agara M, Olaz-Preciado F, Urbieta-Echezarreta M, Gonzalez-Arencibia C. C-reactive protein as a predictor of improvement and readmission in heart failure. *Eur J Heart Fail.* 2002;4(3):331–336.
75. Cesari M, Penninx BW, Newman AB, et al. Inflammatory markers and onset of cardiovascular events: results from the Health ABC study. *Circulation.* 2003;108(19):2317–2322.
76. Haber HL, Leavy JA, Kessler PD, Kukin ML, Gottlieb SS, Packer M. The erythrocyte sedimentation rate in congestive heart failure. *N Engl J Med.* 1991;324(6):353–358.

77. Parry EH. The erythrocyte sedimentation rate in heart failure. *Acta Med Scand.* 1961;169:79–85.

78. McGinnis AE, Lansche WE, Glaser RJ, Loeb LH. Observations on the erythrocyte sedimentation rate in congestive heart failure. *Am J Med Sci.* 1953;225(6):599–604.

79. Sharma R, Rauchhaus M, Ponikowski PP, et al. The relationship of the erythrocyte sedimentation rate to inflammatory cytokines and survival in patients with chronic heart failure treated with angiotensin-converting enzyme inhibitors. *J Am Coll Cardiol.* 2000;36(2): 523–528.

80. Furman MI, Gore JM, Anderson FA, et al. Elevated leukocyte count and adverse hospital events in patients with acute coronary syndromes: findings from the Global Registry of Acute Coronary Events (GRACE). *Am Heart J.* 2004;147(1):42–48.

81. Menon V, Lessard D, Yarzebski J, Furman MI, Gore JM, Goldberg RJ. Leukocytosis and adverse hospital outcomes after acute myocardial infarction. *Am J Cardiol.* 2003;92(4):368–372.

82. Kyne L, Hausdorff JM, Knight E, Dukas L, Azhar G, Wei JY. Neutrophilia and congestive heart failure after acute myocardial infarction. *Am Heart J.* 2000;139(1 Pt 1):94–100.

83. Maekawa Y, Anzai T, Yoshikawa T, et al. Prognostic significance of peripheral monocytosis after reperfused acute myocardial infarction: a possible role for left ventricular remodeling. *J Am Coll Cardiol.* 2002;39(2):241–246.

84. Ommen SR, Hodge DO, Rodeheffer RJ, McGregor CG, Thomson SP, Gibbons RJ. Predictive power of the relative lymphocyte concentration in patients with advanced heart failure. *Circulation.* 1998;97(1): 19–22.

85. Acanfora D, Gheorghiade M, Trojano L, et al. Relative lymphocyte count: a prognostic indicator of mortality in elderly patients with congestive heart failure. *Am Heart J.* 2001;142(1):167–173.

86. Tang WH, Tong W, Troughton RW, et al. Prognostic value and echocardiographic determinants of plasma myeloperoxidase levels in chronic heart failure. *J Am Coll Cardiol.* 2007;49(24):2364–2370.

87. van Kimmenade RR, Januzzi JL Jr, Ellinor PT, et al. Utility of amino-terminal pro-brain natriuretic peptide, galectin-3, and apelin for the evaluation of patients with acute heart failure. *J Am Coll Cardiol.* 2006;48(6):1217–1224.

88. Sharma UC, Pokharel S, van Brakel TJ, et al. Galectin-3 marks activated macrophages in failure-prone hypertrophied hearts and contributes to cardiac dysfunction. *Circulation.* 2004;110(19): 3121–3128.

89. Tang WH, Brennan ML, Philip K, et al. Plasma myeloperoxidase levels in patients with chronic heart failure. *Am J Cardiol.* 2006; 98(6):796–799.

90. Bozkurt B, Mann DL. Use of biomarkers in the management of heart failure: are we there yet? *Circulation.* 2003;107(9):1231–1233.

91. Anand IS, Fisher LD, Chiang YT, et al. Changes in brain natriuretic peptide and norepinephrine over time and mortality and morbidity in the Valsartan Heart Failure Trial (Val-HeFT). *Circulation.* 2003; 107(9):1278–1283.

92. Milani RV, Mehra MR, Endres S, et al. The clinical relevance of circulating tumor necrosis factor-alpha in acute decompensated chronic heart failure without cachexia. *Chest.* 1996;110(4):992–995.

93. Anker SD, Chua TP, Ponikowski P, et al. Hormonal changes and catabolic/anabolic imbalance in chronic heart failure and their importance for cardiac cachexia. *Circulation.* 1997;96(2):526–534.

94. Nishigaki K, Minatoguchi S, Seishima M, et al. Plasma Fas ligand, an inducer of apoptosis, and plasma soluble Fas, an inhibitor of apoptosis, in patients with chronic congestive heart failure. *J Am Coll Cardiol.* 1997;29(6):1214–1220.

95. Mueller T, Dieplinger B, Gegenhuber A, Poelz W, Pacher R, Haltmayer M. Increased plasma concentrations of soluble ST2 are predictive for 1-year mortality in patients with acute destabilized heart failure. *Clin Chem.* 2008;54(4):752–756.

96. Stenvinkel P, Andersson P, Wang T, et al. Do ACE-inhibitors suppress tumour necrosis factor-alpha production in advanced chronic renal failure? *J Intern Med.* 1999;246(5):503–507.

Section III

Natriuretic Peptides

16 ▪ Biology of the Natriuretic Peptides

TOMOKO ICHIKI, MD, PHD
CANDACE Y.W. LEE, MD, PHD
JOHN C. BURNETT, JR., MD

ACKNOWLEDGMENTS: Supported by the National Institutes of Health (R01 HL36634; P01 HL76611 and R01 HL83231) and the Mayo Foundation (grants to JCB). CYWL was a recipient of a Canadian Institutes of Health Research Clinical Research Initiative Fellowship Award (2006), a 2007 Research Fellowship Award from the Heart Failure Society of America, and the American Society for Clinical Pharmacology and Therapeutics 2007 Young Investigator Award.

DISCLOSURES: Mayo Clinic and Foundation has licensed CD-NP to Nile Therapeutics. Dr. Burnett serves as Chair of the Scientific Advisory Board of Nile Therapeutics.

Introduction

In 1964, Braunwald advanced the concept that the heart is an endocrine organ.[1] Following the discovery that norepinephrine is synthesized in the heart, he speculated that a primary function of the myocardium was to act as an endocrine gland. Now over four decades later, we have come to understand the existence of the natriuretic peptide system (NPS), a peptide hormonal system of cardiac origin, which is represented by structurally similar—but genetically distinct—peptides, which include atrial natriuretic peptide (ANP), B-type natriuretic peptide (BNP), C-type natriuretic peptide (CNP), and urodilatin (URO).[2–4] Studies have established that ANP, BNP, and URO are ligands for a well-characterized particulate guanylylyclase (pGC) receptor known as the natriuretic peptide receptor-A (NPR-A).[5] CNP serves as the endogenous ligand for the NPR-B receptor.[5] All four peptides are cleared by a noncyclic GMP-linked receptor that is termed the NPR-C receptor.[4] It should be noted that all four peptides are degraded by the ectoenzyme neutral endopeptidase (NEP).[6] Recent attention has also been focused on a fourth nonmammalian member of the NP family—Dendroaspis natriuretic peptide (DNP). This peptide is structurally similar to the other NPs, but was isolated from the venom of the green mamba snake.[7] Studies support its existence as a potent NPR-A activator.[8] Great attention has been placed on the NPS because of its diverse biology which—via its second messenger cyclic guanosine monophosphate (cGMP)—has cardiorenal protective actions, as well as its diagnostic and therapeutic potential for cardiovascular disease syndromes.

Cardiac Production and Secretion

Current knowledge is that ANP, BNP, and CNP are genetically distinct, but share structural similarities (Figure 16–1). They are produced as preprohormones, which are subsequently processed into prohormones by cleavage of an N-terminal signal peptide.

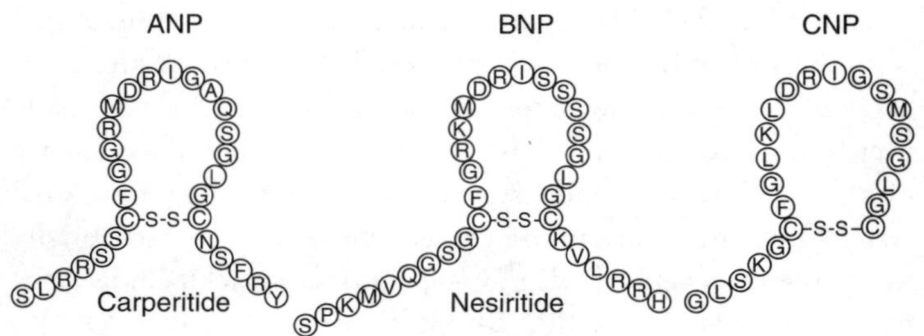

■ **Figure 16–1** Structures and amino acid sequences of atrial natriuretic peptide (ANP), B-type natriuretic peptide (BNP), C-type natriuretic peptide (CNP), Dendroaspis natriuretic peptide (DNP), and urodilatin (URO).

Human preproANP is a 151-amino acid (AA) peptide which is cleaved to the 126-AA proANP, whereas human preproBNP is a 134-AA peptide which is cleaved to the 108-AA proBNP.[9,10] ProANP and proBNP are both stored in secretory granules in atrial cardiomyocytes and are cleaved to form ANP and BNP upon secretion. An emerging concept is that ANP is more the stored peptide released upon immediate stretch and released BNP reflects more active production rather than storage.[11] Processing of proANP to ANP is mediated by corin, while a role for furin has been implicated for BNP as well.[12,13] Alternative processing of proANP in the kidney generates URO, which shares the same AA sequence as ANP, but also has an additional 4 AAs in the N-terminus.[4,14] Both human ANP, a 28-AA peptide, and human BNP, a 32-AA peptide, are released from the myocardium in response to various physiologic and pathophysiologic stimuli, such as myocardial wall stretch. An intriguing emerging concept from our group is that both proANP and proBNP may also be released into the circulation intact and be processed to mature forms in the plasma and within other organ systems. Further research is needed to clarify this possibility.

Studies have established that proCNP consists of 103-AA residues and is processed by furin (an intracellular endoprotease that is enriched in the Golgi apparatus) to the mature 53-AA CNP.[15]CNP-53, which is found primarily in the brain, the heart, and endothelial cells, may be further cleaved to CNP-22.[4] CNP-22 consists of a 17-AA ring structure, including a disulfide bond joining the two cysteine residues, and a single 5-AA extension in the N-terminal position, in contrast to the presence of two terminal extensions (both the N- and the C-termini) in other NPs (see Figure 16–1).

Receptor-Mediated Biological Actions

It is now well established that the NPR-A is the target for ANP, BNP, URO, and DNP (Figure 16–2). The following rank order of potency has been reported for NPR-A: DNP > BNP ~ ANP >>

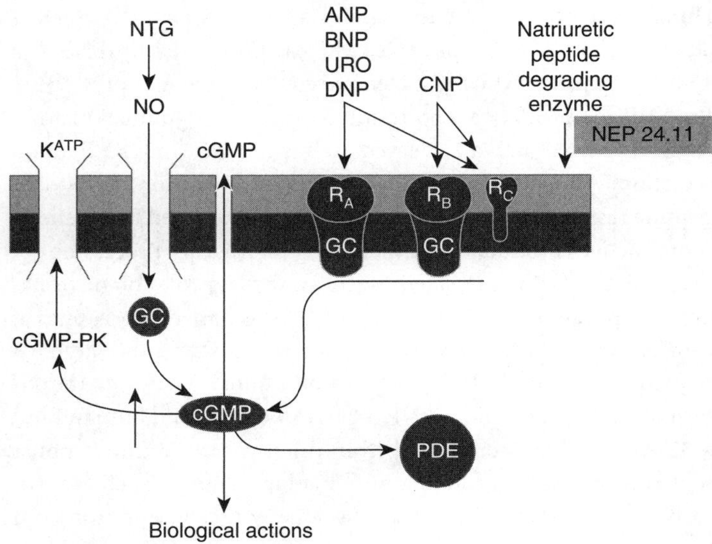

■ **Figure 16–2** Signal transduction pathways of the particulate guanylyl cyclase and the soluble guanylyl cyclase systems. GC = guanylyl cyclase, NTG = nitroglycerin, NO = nitric oxide, cGMP = 3′,5′ cyclic guanosine monophosphate, PDE = phosphodiesterase type V.

CNP in a study that used a radioiodinated analog of DNP to evaluate the selectivity of DNP for NPR-A in the human myocardium.[8] The ligand-receptor interaction activates cGMP, resulting in natriuresis, vasorelaxation, natriuresis, inhibition of renin and aldosterone, enhanced myocardial relaxation, inhibition of fibrosis and hypertrophy, promotion of cell survival, and inhibition of inflammation (see Figure 16–2).[3,4] These pleotropic properties of the NPs are underscored by recent studies observing that the NPs may also be involved in the control of lipolysis in human adipose tissue.[16]

In the kidney, both glomeruli and the inner medullary collecting duct (IMCD) cells are abundant in NP receptors, especially NPR-A and NPR-C. Renal targets for ANP, BNP, URO, and DNP include the glomeruli and the IMCD, as well as the vascular system.[17] Sites of action also include the proximal convoluted tubules, medullary thick ascending limb, and cortical collecting ducts. The biological result of activation of renal NPR-A includes increased natriuresis, diuresis, glomerular filtration rate (GFR), and filtration fraction (FF). The mechanism for NP-induced increases in GFR include relaxation of mesangial cells and an increase in ultrafiltration coefficient, augmentation of glomerular hydrostatic pressure (from afferent arteriolar dilatation and efferent arteriolar constriction), and direct tubular effects. It has been demonstrated that ANP inhibits angiotensin-mediated sodium and fluid reabsorption,[18] as well as the Na^+/H^+ antiporter at the level of the proximal tubule.[19] At the level of the loop of Henle, ANP decreases reabsorption of chloride and inhibits Na^+/K^+-ATPase. Also, it has been reported that in the IMCD, ANP mediates a dose-dependent inhibitory effect on oxygen consumption[20] and blocks the entry of Na.[+21] In addition, ANP also antagonizes the actions of vasopressin and of aldosterone. Moreover, Na^+ delivery to the macula densa is enhanced by ANP, leading to indirect inhibition of renin secretion and subsequent angiotensin II and aldosterone secretion. ANP also suppresses aldosterone production by the adrenal gland, which is underscored by the high density of NPR-A in zona glomerulosa cells.[22] It is important to note too that BNP has been reported to also suppress aldosterone even when stimulated by potent diuretics, such as furosemide.[23]

Studies also have reported that URO is synthesized in the renal distal tubules where it is secreted into the lumen.[24] URO binds to NPR-A on IMCD cells and plays an important role as a paracrine regulator of Na^+ excretion in the kidney.[25] Its cGMP-stimulating action has also been detected in IMCD cells, glomeruli, proximal convoluted tubules, and medullary thick ascending limbs; and its cGMP response is similar to that of ANP. Importantly, URO enhances natriuresis and diuresis in healthy subjects,[26,27] and mediates favorable hemodynamic effects in patients with decompensated heart failure (HF), such as significant reductions in pulmonary capillary wedge pressure (PCWP).[28,29] In experimental studies, attenuation of myocardial ischemia-reperfusion injury (IRI)[30] and possible anticancer effects have also been reported.[31]

Unlike the NPR-A agonists (ANP, BNP, DNP, and URO), CNP is the endogenous ligand for NPR-B, which shares topology with NPR-A and binds NPs in the following rank order: CNP >> ANP ≥ BNP.[4] NPR-B has been reported in epithelial and mesangial cells of human glomeruli,[32] in addition to its wide distribution in the brain, chondrocytes, vascular smooth muscle cells, fibroblasts, myocardium, lung, kidney, adrenal, uterus, and ovary cells.[4] Importantly, the 17-AA core ring structure and the disulfide bond have been shown to be critical for NPR-B selectivity and for its cGMP-stimulating actions in vascular smooth muscle cells.[4] Natural or engineered mutations of the ring may enhance or reduce CNP binding to NPR-B.[33,34]

Importantly, CNP is the most conserved NP across species and is thought to mediate its actions through a paracrine or autocrine mechanism.[4] Both renal production of CNP and NPR-B activation by CNP in the kidney have been demonstrated.[35,36] Moreover, CNP possesses diverse biological actions and is involved in various regulatory processes, such as bone growth and cartilage homeostasis,[37] and control of vascular tone.[38] CNP exerts antiproliferative and anti-inflammatory actions and has been shown to reduce cardiac preload (based upon the greater abundance of NPR-B in veins as compared to arteries), inhibit vascular smooth muscle proliferation, reduce leukocyte recruitment and leukocyte-platelet interactions, protect against cardiac IRI, prevent ventricular remodeling following myocardial infarction, and attenuate cardiac dysfunction and inflammation in experimental acute myocarditis.[39–48] It exhibits greater antifibrotic properties than ANP or BNP,[49] however, it exerts only limited natriuretic and diuretic actions.[50,51]

Clearance and Metabolism

The clearance and degradation of the NPs occurs via two mechanisms. One is a receptor-mediated mechanism and the other is an enzymatic pathway for metabolism. Both are important and will be discussed below.

Others have reported that the extracellular domain of NPR-C shares about 30% homology with NPR-A and NPR-B, but it lacks particulate guanylyl cyclase activity.[4,5] NPR-C is the most abundant receptor subtype, with expression in most tissues, especially in the kidney, the vascular endothelium, smooth muscle cells, and the heart.[4] The rank order for NPR-C binding affinity for NPs (human and rats) is ANP ≥ CNP > BNP.[4] Even though it was initially believed that NPR-C functions as a clearance receptor, accumulating evidence suggests that NPR-C may be involved in the regulation of cell function[52] and may play a role in mediating the antifibrotic effect of BNP in cardiac fibroblasts.[53]

Neutral endopeptidase (NEP) 24.11—which is a membrane-bound metallopeptidase with zinc at its active site that cleaves endogenous peptide at the amino side of hydrophilic residues—is involved in the degradation of NPs and is distributed in the kidney, lung, and vascular wall.[54] In the kidney, NEP is highly expressed in the brush borders of the proximal tubules and this results in rapid degradation of ANP. NEP is often found to colocalize with angiotensin-converting enzyme. The rank order of potency for hydrolysis by NEP in vitro has been reported to be CNP > ANP > BNP.[54] Studies by Chen et al. suggest that DNP is the most resistant of the NPs to NEP degradation.[55]

Natriuretic Peptides in Cardiorenal Regulation in Heart Failure

A hallmark of HF is activation of NPs which serves as a compensatory mechanism to maintain sodium homeostasis and to suppress the renin-angiotensin-aldosterone system (RAAS). In 1986, Burnett et al.[56] identified that plasma ANP was elevated in human HF. Subsequently, elevation of BNP in human HF was reported by Mukoyama and colleagues.[11] In order to preserve and/or enhance renal function in HF, an understanding of intrarenal biology of NPs may provide direction on optimal use of current therapies and also lead to newer therapeutic strategies especially as they relate to the NPs.

Heart failure is a cardiac volume or pressure overload state with release of ANP and BNP, which activates NPR-A/cGMP signaling, including activation of the effector protein kinase G (PKG).[3] NPR-A is the binding site for ANP and BNP, as well as the intrarenal natriuretic peptide URO. Administration of these three NPs in animals and humans with HF results in natriuresis and diuresis and, at certain doses, an increase in GFR.[57] They possess other actions including: suppression of the RAAS, inhibition of fibrosis and cardiomyocyte hypertrophy, and positive lusitropism. In severe experimental or human HF, a renal hyporesponsiveness or renal resistance may occur to the NPs due in part to excessive hypotension, as well as up-regulation of phosphodiesterase type V (PDEV) activity, which degrades NP generated cGMP.[58,59] The importance of the NPs and the NPR-A in renal regulation is underscored by studies of genetic and pharmacologic receptor disruption characterized by impaired renal sodium handling and often hypertension.[60–62]

It is important to note that while cardiac volume overload as in acute HF may result in the release of ANP and BNP, the associated reduction of arterial pressure which may occur activates the intrarenal nitric oxide (NO) pathway in which NO stimulates soluble guanylyl cyclase (sGC) localized to the cell cytosol.

When considering the clinical perspective of acute HF, both sodium nitroprusside (SNP) and nitroglycerin (NTG) are widely used for the treatment and both are sGC activators and potent vasodilators. This is in contrast to ANP and BNP, which also are used for acute HF therapy, but target pGC. To further explore cGMP mechanisms in HF, we recently employed a novel direct activator of sGC (BAY 58–2667) in a model of HF and observed potent renal vasodilatation without natriuresis and diuresis or changes in GFR, although both (i.e., BAY and NTG) produced a significant reduction in arterial pressure together with cardiac unloading.[63] This is in contrast to pGC activation in the kidney by

ANP or BNP that, as discussed above, may be hypotensive, but may augment GFR, natriuresis, and diuresis.

Based upon such studies, what is emerging in cGMP regulation of cardiorenal function is the concept of compartmentalization. Specifically, compartmentalization of cGMP signaling in cells has been advanced especially in the heart in which pGC and sGC have been demonstrated to have distinct roles in cardiomyocyte function.[64,65] Further, Airhart and colleagues have reported that the pGC agonist ANP—but not the sGC agonist S-nitroso-L-acetyl penicillamine—stimulates the translocation of PKG to the plasma membrane of renal cells augmenting the NPR-A receptor to which ANP, BNP, and URO bind.[66] We, therefore, advance the concept that these observations support distinct functional roles for pGC and sGC in the kidney, meaning an NP like ANP or BNP could have different renal actions than NTG or SNP, despite the fact they both activate the second messenger cGMP.

We should state that understanding the intrarenal roles of the NP/pGC/cGMP and NO/sGC/cGMP pathways in vivo in HF in the control of renal function should advance our knowledge of renal adaptations in this syndrome and guide our therapeutic strategies. Therefore, we investigated in vivo, in a large animal model of HF, the physiological properties of the endogenous NP/pGC/cGMP and NO/sGC/cGMP pathways in the control of renal hemodynamic and excretory function.[67] We hypothesized that each pathway would play specific roles in the maintenance of renal function in HF consistent with distinct GC enzymes for each system.

These studies revealed differential and complementary roles for these two endogenous cGMP activating systems in HF whereby the endogenous NPs appear to play a greater role in the preservation of GFR and sodium excretion, while the endogenous NO system was more important in the control of renal blood flow. Thus, the preservation of renal function in experimental acute decompensated HF is mediated by dual cGMP systems which activate both pGC and sGC enzymes.

There exists, however, a paradox in HF: there is elevation of ANP and BNP, yet the kidney is vasoconstricted and sodium avid. The biological significance of this elevation in ANP and BNP is now emerging. We have reported that despite an elevation in BNP1–32 (the active form of BNP as measured by point-of-care testing in subjects with HF and New York Heart Association Class IV symptoms), an absence of BNP1–32 was demonstrated by quantitative mass spectral analysis.[68] This key observation suggests that other molecular forms of BNP might have contributed to the results of point-of-care testing. Indeed, recent investigations have demonstrated reduced biological activities in other molecular forms of BNP, which contributed to the increased BNP immunoreactivity.[69,70] Most importantly, it appears that two processes are functioning in advanced HF to reduce biologically-active BNP1–32. One is excessive accumulation of BNP's precursor—proBNP—possibly due to impaired processing by corin. Secondly, the dipeptidyl peptidase IV (DPPIV) enzyme rapidly degrades BNP1–32 to a form that has reduced renal natriuretic and renovasodilating actions (BNP3–32) and may also partially explain the absence of BNP1–32 in advanced HF.[71]

What we have come to understand from clinical investigations of BNP in HF is the following: Commercially available assays for BNP are not specific and detect other nonactive forms. As discussed above, assays are detecting forms of BNP which include abundant nonactive forms, such as proBNP. Of note, some investigators reported that the propeptide convertase enzymes, furin and corin, may have important roles in disease state because they can convert proBNP. Because of the importance of this issue, we will briefly summarize some key points related to corin and furin.

Corin is a transmembrane cardiac serine protease which exists in the heart and can convert proANP or proBNP into active ANP or BNP.[12] Tran et al. reported that both corin and ANP mRNA were increased in phenylephrine-stimulated rat neonatal cardiomyocytes and corin mRNA and ANP protein were also increased in a rat model of HF.[72] In contrast, Lagenickel et al. reported that corin mRNA expression was decreased in both atria in the infrarenal aortocaval shunt model.[73] Importantly, Chan at al. reported findings in corin-deficient mice ($Cor^{-/-}$).[74] They showed that $Cor^{-/-}$ mice had elevated levels of pro-ANP, but no detectable levels of mature ANP, had spontaneous hypertension as compared with wild-type mice, and exhibited cardiac hypertrophy resulting in a mild decline in cardiac function later in life. Interestingly, some investigators reported human corin single nucleotide polymorphisms (SNPs) (Q568P and T555I).[75] Further, Wang et al. reported that the corin variant T555I/Q568P reduced pro-ANP and pro-BNP processing activity compared to that of wild-type in HEK293 cells.[76] In humans, corin SNPs were common in African Americans and was associated with higher blood pressure and an increased risk for prevalent hypertension and left ventricular hypertrophy in the presence of untreated hypertension.[77] These corin SNPs data suggest that corin could affect cardiac function by modulating natriuretic peptide activation.

Furin, an intracellular endoprotease enriched in the Golgi apparatus, functions to cleave proproteins into their mature and active forms. Wu et al. reported that furin converts proCNP into CNP but not in furin-deficient cells.[15] Sawada et al. reported that both furin and BNP mRNA were increased in the atria and ventricles in a model of myocardial infarction (MI) and showed furin could process the BNP precursor to BNP-45 by using furin-specific inhibitors in cardiocytes.[13,78] In addition, Semenov et al. reported that proBNP that was not glycosylated in the region of the cleavage site could effectively be processed into BNP by furin.[79] Taken together, these studies suggest that both corin and furin convert proNPs into active NPs—corin for ANP and BNP, furin for BNP and CNP—and that they may have important roles in mediating the conversion of the proNP hormones into mature biologically-active peptides.

References

1. Braunwald E, Harrison DC, Chidsey CA. The heart as an endocrine organ. *Am J Med.* 1964;36:1–4.
2. Lee CY, Burnett JC Jr. Natriuretic peptides and therapeutic applications. *Heart Fail Rev.* 2007;12:131–142.
3. Garbers DL, Chrisman TD, Wiegn P, et al. Membrane guanylyl cyclase receptors: an update. *Trends Endocrinol Metab.* 2006;17:251–258.
4. Potter LR, Abbey-Hosch S, Dickey DM. Natriuretic peptides, their receptors, and cyclic guanosine monophosphate-dependent signaling functions. *Endocr Rev.* 2006;27:47–72.
5. van den Akker F. Structural insights into the ligand binding domains of membrane bound guanylyl cyclases and natriuretic peptide receptors. *J Mol Biol.* 2001;311:923–937.
6. Chen HH, Cataliotti A, Burnett JC Jr. Role of the natriuretic peptides in the cardiorenal and humoral actions of omapatrilat: insights from experimental heart failure. *Curr Hypertens Rep.* 2001;3 Suppl 2:S15–S21.
7. Schweitz H, Vigne P, Moinier D, Frelin C, Lazdunski M. A new member of the natriuretic peptide family is present in the venom of the green mamba (Dendroaspis angusticeps). *J Biol Chem.* 1992;267:13928–13932.
8. Singh G, Kuc RE, Maguire JJ, Fidock M, Davenport AP. Novel snake venom ligand Dendroaspis natriuretic peptide is selective for natriuretic peptide receptor-A in human heart: Downregulation of natriuretic peptide receptor-A in heart failure. *Circ Res.* 2006;99:183–190.
9. de Bold AJ, Borenstein HB, Veress AT, Sonnenberg H. A rapid and potent natriuretic response to intravenous injection of atrial myocardial extract in rats. *Life Sci.* 1981;28:89–94.
10. Sudoh T, Kangawa K, Minamino N, Matsuo H. A new natriuretic peptide in porcine brain. *Nature.* 1988;332:78–81.
11. Mukoyama M, Nakao K, Hosoda K, et al. Brain natriuretic peptide as a novel cardiac hormone in humans. Evidence for an exquisite dual natriuretic peptide system, atrial natriuretic peptide and brain natriuretic peptide. *J Clin Invest.* 1991;87:1402–1412.

12. Yan W, Wu F, Morser J, Wu Q. Corin, a transmembrane cardiac serine protease, acts as a pro-atrial natriuretic peptide-converting enzyme. *Proc Natl Acad Sci U S A.* 2000;97:8525–8529.

13. Sawada Y, Inoure M, Kanda T, et al. Co-elevation of BNP and pro-protein-processing endoprotease furin after MI in rats. *FEBS Lett.* 1997;400:177–182.

14. Schulz-Knappe P, Forssmann K, Herbst F, Hock D, Pipkorn R, Forssmann WG. Isolation and structural analysis of "urodilatin," a new peptide of the cardiodilatin-(ANP)-family, extracted from human urine. *Klin Wochenschr.* 1988;66:752–759.

15. Wu C, Wu F, Pan J, Morser J, Wu Q. Furin-mediated processing of pro-C-type natriuretic peptide. *J Biol Chem.* 2003;278:25847–25852.

16. Sengenes C, Berlan M, De Glisezinski I, Lafontan M, Galitzky J. Natriuretic peptides: a new lipolytic pathway in human adipocytes. *FASEB J.* 2000;14:1345–1351.

17. Candido R, Burrell LM, Jandeleit-Dahm KAM, Cooper ME. Vasoactive peptides and the kidney. In: Brenner BM, ed. *Brenner & Rector's The Kidney*, 8th ed. Philadelphia, PA: Saunders;2008:333–362.

18. Harris PJ, Thomas D, Morgan TO. Atrial natriuretic peptide inhibits angiotensin-stimulated proximal tubular sodium and water reabsorption. *Nature.* 1987;326:697–698.

19. Winaver J, Burnett JC, Tyce GM, Dousa TP. ANP inhibits Na^+-H^+ antiport in proximal tubular brush border membrane: role of dopamine. *Kidney Int.* 1990;38:1133–1140.

20. Zeidel ML, Seifter JL, Lear S, Brenner BM, Silva P. Atrial peptides inhibit oxygen consumption in kidney medullary collecting duct cells. *Am J Physiol.* 1986;251:F379–F383.

21. Gunning M, Silva P, Brenner BM, Zeidel ML. Characteristics of ANP-sensitive guanylate cyclase in inner medullary collecting duct cells. *Am J Physiol.* 1989;256:F766–F775.

22. Kudo T, Baird A. Inhibition of aldosterone production in the adrenal glomerulosa by atrial natriuretic factor. *Nature.* 1984;312:756–757.

23. Cataliotti A, Boerrigter G, Costello-Boerrigter LC, et al. Brain natriuretic peptide enhances renal actions of furosemide and suppresses furosemide-induced aldosterone activation in experimental heart failure. *Circulation.* 2004;109:1680–1685.

24. Hirsch JR, Meyer M, Forssmann WG. ANP and urodilatin: Who is who in the kidney. *Eur J Med Res.* 2006;11:447–454.

25. Goetz K, Drummer C, Zhu JL, Leadley R, Fiedler F, Gerzer R. Evidence that urodilatin, rather than ANP, regulates renal sodium excretion. *J Am Soc Nephrol.* 1990;1:867–874.

26. Carstens J, Jensen KT, Pedersen EB. Metabolism and action of urodilatin infusion in healthy volunteers. *Clin Pharmacol Ther.* 1998;64: 73–86.

27. Dorner GT, Selenko N, Kral T, Schmetterer L, Eichler HG, Wolzt M. Hemodynamic effects of continuous urodilatin infusion: a dose-finding study. *Clin Pharmacol Ther.* 1998;64:322–330.

28. Mitrovic V, Luss H, Nitsche K, et al. Effects of the renal natriuretic peptide urodilatin (ularitide) in patients with decompensated chronic heart failure: a double-blind, placebo-controlled, ascending-dose trial. *Am Heart J.* 2005;150:1239:e1–e8.

29. Mitrovic V, Seferovic PM, Simeunovic D, et al. Haemodynamic and clinical effects of ularitide in decompensated heart failure. *Eur Heart J.* 2006;27:2823–2832.

30. Padilla F, Garcia-Dorado D, Agullo L, et al. Intravenous administration of the natriuretic peptide urodilatin at low doses during coronary reperfusion limits infarct size in anesthetized pigs. *Cardiovasc Res.* 2001;51:592–600.

31. Vesely BA, Eichelbaum EJ, Alli AA, Sun Y, Gower WR Jr, Vesely DL. Urodilatin and four cardiac hormones decrease human renal carcinoma cell numbers. *Eur J Clin Invest.* 2006;36:810–819.

32. Nir A, Beers KW, Clavell AL, et al. CNP is present in canine renal tubular cells and secreted by cultured opossum kidney cells. *Am J Physiol.* 1994;267:R1653–R1657.

33. Furuya M, Tawaragi Y, Minamitake Y, et al. Structural requirements of C-type natriuretic peptide for elevation of cyclic GMP in cultured vascular smooth muscle cells. *Biochem Biophys Res Commun.* 1992; 183:964–969.

34. Dickey D, Burnett JC Jr, Potter L. Novel bifunctional natriuretic peptides as potential therapeutics. *J Bio Chem.* 2008;283:35003–35009.

35. Zhao J, Ardaillou N, Lu CY, et al. Characterization of C-type natriuretic peptide receptors in human mesangial cells. *Kidney Int.* 1994;46:717–725.

36. Canaan-Kuhl S, Jamison RL, Myers BD, Pratt RE. Identification of "B" receptor for natriuretic peptide in human kidney. *Endocrinology.* 1992;130:550–552.

37. Espiner EA, Prickett TC, Yandle TG, et al. ABCs of natriuretic peptides: growth. *Horm Res.* 2007;67:81–90.

38. Ahluwalia A, Hobbs AJ. Endothelium-derived C-type natriuretic peptide: more than just a hyperpolarizing factor. *Trends Pharmacol Sci.* 2005;26:162–167.

39. Pagel-Langenickel I, Buttgereit J, Bader M, Langenickel TH. Natriuretic peptide receptor B signaling in the cardiovascular system: Protection from cardiac hypertrophy. *J Mol Med.* 2007;85:797–810.

40. Kelsall CJ, Chester AH, Sarathchandra P, Singer DRJ. Expression and localization of C-type natriuretic peptide in human vascular smooth muscle cells. *Vascul Pharmacol.* 2006;45:368–373.

41. Xia W, Mruk DD, Cheng CY. C-type natriuretic peptide regulates blood-testis barrier dynamics in adult rat testes. *Proc Natl Acad Sci.* 2007;104:3841–3846.

42. Soeki T, Kishimoto I, Okumura H, et al. C-type natriuretic peptide, a novel antifibrotic and antihypertrophic agent, prevents cardiac remodeling after myocardial infarction. *J Am Coll Cardiol.* 2005;45: 608–616.

43. Wei CM, Aarhus LL, Miller VM, Burnett JC Jr. Action of C-type natriuretic peptide in isolated canine arteries and veins. *Am J Physiol.* 1993;264:H71–H73.

44. Scotland RS, Cohen M, Foster P, et al. C-type natriuretic peptide inhibits leukocyte recruitment and platelet-leukocyte interactions via suppression of P-selectin expression. *Proc Natl Acad Sci U S A.* 2005;102:14452–14457.

45. Hobbs A, Foster P, Prescott C, Scotland R, Ahluwalia A. Natriuretic peptide receptor-C regulates coronary blood flow and prevents myocardial ischemia/reperfusion injury: novel cardioprotective role for endothelium-derived C-type natriuretic peptide. *Circulation.* 2004; 110:1231–1235.

46. Tokudome T, Horio T, Soeki T, et al. Inhibitory effect of C-type natriuretic peptide (CNP) on cultured cardiac myocyte hypertrophy: interference between CNP and endothelin-1 signaling pathways. *Endocrinology.* 2004;145:2131–2140.

47. Obata H, Yanagawa B, Tanaka K, et al. CNP infusion attenuates cardiac dysfunction and inflammation in myocarditis. *Biochem Biophys Res Commun.* 2007;356:60–66.

48. Wang Y, de Waard MC, Sterner-Kock A, et al. Cardiomyocyte-restricted over-expression of C-type natriuretic peptide prevents cardiac hypertrophy induced by myocardial infarction in mice. *Eur J Heart Fail.* 2007;9:548–557.

49. Horio T, Tokudome T, Maki T, et al. Gene expression, secretion, and autocrine action of C-type natriuretic peptide in cultured adult rat cardiac fibroblasts. *Endocrinology.* 2003;144:2279–2284.

50. Stingo AJ, Clavell AL, Aarhus LL, Burnett JC Jr. Cardiovascular and renal actions of C-type natriuretic peptide. *Am J Physiol.* 1992;262: H308–H312.

51. Hunt PJ, Richards AM, Espiner EA, Nicholls MG, Yandle TG. Bioactivity and metabolism of C-type natriuretic peptide in normal man. *J Clin Endocrinol Metab.* 1994;78:1428–1435.

52. Anand-Srivastava MB. Natriuretic peptide receptor-C signaling and regulation. *Peptides.* 2005;26:1044–1059.

53. Huntley BK, Sandberg SM, Noser JA, et al. BNP-induced activation of cGMP in human cardiac fibroblasts: interactions with fibronectin and natriuretic peptide receptors. *J Cell Physiol.* 2006;209:943–949.

54. Kenny AJ, Bourne A, Ingram J. Hydrolysis of human and pig brain natriuretic peptides, urodilatin, C-type natriuretic peptide and some C-receptor ligands by endopeptidase-24.11. *Biochem J.* 1993;291(Pt 1):83–88.

55. Chen HH, Lainchbury JG, Burnett JC Jr. Natriuretic peptide receptors and neutral endopeptidase in mediating the renal actions of a new therapeutic synthetic natriuretic peptide dendroaspis natriuretic peptide. *J Am Coll Cardiol.* 2002;40:1186–1191.

56. Burnett JC Jr, Kao PC, Hu DC, et al. Atrial natriuretic peptide elevation in congestive heart failure in the human. *Science.* 1986;231: 1145–1147.

57. Chen HH, Cataliotti A, Schirger JA, Martin FL, Burnett JC Jr. Equimolar doses of atrial and brain natriuretic peptides and urodilatin have differential renal actions in overt experimental heart failure. *Am J Physiol Regul Integr Comp Physiol.* 2005;288:R1093–R1097.

58. Margulies KB, Heublein DM, Perrella MA, Burnett JC Jr. ANF-mediated renal cGMP generation in congestive heart failure. *Am J Physiol.* 1991;260:F562–F568.

59. Supaporn T, Sandberg SM, Borgeson DD, et al. Blunted cGMP response to agonists and enhanced glomerular cyclic 3′,5′-nucleotide phosphodiesterase activities in experimental congestive heart failure. *Kidney Int.* 1996;50:1718–1725.

60. Patel JB, Valencik ML, Pritchett AM, Burnett JC Jr, McDonald JA, Redfield MM. Cardiac-specific attenuation of natriuretic peptide A receptor activity accentuates adverse cardiac remodeling and mortality in response to pressure overload. *Am J Physiol Heart Circ Physiol.* 2005;289:H777–H784.

61. John SW, Veress AT, Honrath U, et al. Blood pressure and fluid-electrolyte balance in mice with reduced or absent ANP. *Am J Physiol.* 1996;271:R109–R114.

62. Borgeson DD, Stevens TL, Heublein DM, Matsuda Y, Burnett JC. Activation of myocardial and renal natriuretic peptides during acute intravascular volume overload in dogs: functional cardiorenal responses to receptor antagonism. *Clin Sci (Lond).* 1998;95:195–202.

63. Boerrigter G, Costello-Boerrigter LC, Cataliotti A, Lapp H, Stasch J-P, Burnett JC Jr. Targeting heme-oxidized soluble guanylate cyclase in experimental heart failure. *Hypertension.* 2007;49:1128–1133.

64. Fischmeister R, Castro LR, Abi-Gerges A, et al. Compartmentation of cyclic nucleotide signaling in the heart: the role of cyclic nucleotide phosphodiesterases. *Circ Res.* 2006;99:816–828.

65. Castro LR, Verde I, Cooper DM, Fischmeister R. Cyclic guanosine monophosphate compartmentation in rat cardiac myocytes. *Circulation.* 2006;113:2221–2228.

66. Airhart N, Yang YF, Roberts CT Jr, Silberbach M. Atrial natriuretic peptide induces natriuretic peptide receptor-cGMP-dependent protein kinase interaction. *J Biol Chem.* 2003;278:38693–386938.

67. Martin FL, Supaporn T, Chen HH, et al. Distinct roles for renal particulate and soluble guanylyl cyclases in preserving renal function in experimental acute heart failure. *Am J Physiol Regul Integr Comp Physiol.* 2007;293:R1580–R1585.

68. Hawkridge AM, Heublein DM, Bergen HR III, Cataliotti A, Burnett JC Jr, Muddiman DC. Quantitative mass spectral evidence for the absence of circulating brain natriuretic peptide (BNP-32) in severe human heart failure. *Proc Natl Acad Sci U S A.* 2005;102: 17442–17447.

69. Liang F, O'Rear J, Schellenberger U, et al. Evidence for functional heterogeneity of circulating B-type natriuretic peptide. *J Am Coll Cardiol.* 2007;49:1071–1078.

70. Heublein DM, Huntley BK, Boerrigter G, et al. Immunoreactivity and guanosine 3′,5′-cyclic monophosphate activating actions of various molecular forms of human B-type natriuretic peptide. *Hypertension.* 2007;49:1114–1119.

71. Boerrigter G, Costello-Boerrigter LC, Harty GJ, Lapp H, Burnett JC. Des-serine-proline B-type natriuretic peptide (BNP 3-32) in cardiorenal regulation. *Am. J. Physiol. Renal Fluid Electrolyte Physiol.* 2007;292:R897–R901.

72. Tran KL, Lu X, Lei M, Feng Q, Wu Q. Upregulation of corin gene expression in hypertrophic cardiomyocytes and failing myocardium. *Am J Physiol Heart Circ Physiol.* 2004;287:H1625–H1631.

73. Lagenickel TH, Pagel I, Buttgereit J, et al. Rat corin gene: molecular cloning and reduced expression in experimental heart failure. *Am J Physiol Heart Circ Physiol.* 2004;287:H1516–H1521.

74. Chan JCY, Knudson O, Wu F, Morser J, Dole WP, Wu Q. Hypertension in mice lacking the proatrial natriuretic peptide convertase corin. *Proc Natl Acad Sci U S A.* 2005;102:785–790.

75. Wang W, Liao X, Fukuda K, et al. Corin gene minor allele defined by 2 missense mutations in common in blacks and associated with high blood pressure and hypertension. *Circulation.* 2005;112:2403–2410.

76. Dries DL, Victor RG, Rame E, et al. Corin variant associated with hypertension and cardiac hypertrophy exhibits impaired zymogen activation and NP processing activity. *Circ Res.* 2008;103:502–508.

77. Rame JE, Drazner MH, Post W, et al. Corin I555(P568) allele is associated with enhanced cardiac hypertrophic response to increased systemic afterload. *Hypertension.* 2007;49:857–864.

78. Sawada Y, Suda M, Yokoyama H, et al. Stretch-induced hypertrophic growth of cardiocytes and processing of BNP are controlled by furin. *J Biol Chem.* 1997;272:20545–20554.

79. Semenov AG, Postnikov AB, Tamm NN, Seferian KR, Karpova NS, Bloshchitsyna MN, Koshkina EV, Krasnoselsky MI, Serebryanaya DV, and Katrukha AG. *Clin Chem.* 2009;55(2):489–498.

17 ■ Natriuretic Peptides: Laboratory Considerations

Jordi Ordóñez-Llanos MD PhD
Javier Mercé-Muntañola MD

Introduction

The first immunologic assay for B-type natriuretic peptides (NPs) measurement in human plasma was described two decades ago.[1] Since then, numerous reports have demonstrated the utility of BNP (B-type natriuretic peptide) and NT-proBNP (N-terminal pro-B-type natriuretic peptide) in different clinical settings in which myocyte overload or damage exists. To satisfy the requirement of measuring NPs with sufficient accuracy and imprecision and, particularly, in large series of samples, a number of immunoassays have been developed and adapted to a wide range of instruments ranging from the largest, fully-automated immunoassay platforms to the smallest point-of-care devices. Such proliferation of methods, using different sets of antibodies and standards and producing different results for the same NP measurement, have generated some degree of confusion in the laboratory and clinical communities.

Furthermore, NPs are relatively small peptide molecules, whose concentration in clinical samples may be influenced by a number of preanalytical variables, such as the blood specimen they are measured in, the anticoagulant used when blood is drawn up, the time and temperature of sample storage, etc. The lack of accurate control of all these factors can lead to a false increase or decrease in NP concentrations, hampering their clinical utility.

Bearing in mind all these issues, international organizations, such as the National Academy of Clinical Biochemistry (NACB) and the International Federation of Clinical Chemistry (IFCC, Committee of Standardization of Cardiac Markers Damage), have released guidelines highlighting the most important preanalytical, analytical, and postanalytical issues that the laboratory and clinical community should know for the correct interpretation of NP measurements. The purpose of this chapter is to summarize current knowledge of these subjects.

Nomenclature

There are different circulating peptides released in the context of BNP gene activation, whose nomenclature should be clarified to avoid confusion. $ProBNP_{1-108}$—produced by cleavage of pre-proBNP—contains 108 amino acids and has been found in both myocardium and plasma.[2] BNP_{1-32}—one of the physiologically-active forms of BNP—is produced from the carboxy-terminal portion (amino acids 77–108) of $proBNP_{1-108}$ and is present in both myocardium and plasma. Finally, NT-$proBNP_{1-76}$ is the entire N-terminal fragment of $proBNP_{1-108}$. It lacks physiological activity and is also found in both myocardium and plasma.

Degradation products of BNP_{1-32} (BNP_{3-32}, as well as BNP_{6-32}) are more abundant than the progenitor compound and may possess reduced biological activity. Similarly, glycosylated molecules of NPs (notably NT-proBNP) also exist and their immunoreactions with NP assays are relevant for the correct interpretation of NP concentrations. Oligomeric products of NPs have also been described,[3] although recent evidence questions their existence.[4]

It is now well established that all the commercially-available assays for BNP and NT-proBNP actually detect a mixture of peptides (discussed in more detail below). Practically speaking, this is of less importance to the clinician as the assays are valuable for their clinical applications, but it is worthy to note and acknowledge. Given the heterogeneity of NP forms in the circulation and the NP recognition by the different assays, it is recommended, however, that NP concentrations be expressed in ng/L or pg/mL, not in pmol/L.

Preanalytical Issues

The preanalytical phase of testing is responsible for more than two-thirds of all laboratory errors;[5] however, when measuring biological compounds, preanalytical variability is assumed to be zero (or close to zero). Thus, the control of the preanalytical phase is a matter of major importance. There are many preanalytical factors that could influence NP measurements; their effects on such measurements are described below.

Sample Type

Circulating NT-proBNP can be measured in different specimens. Serum and heparin plasma produce similar results; both specimen types are considered to be interchangeable and recommendable for NT-proBNP measurement. Although testing of NT-proBNP in ethylenediaminetetraacetic acid (EDTA) plasma produces lower values than those of serum or heparin plasma (10 to 13% depending on the method), this sample has been used with the Ortho Vitros NT-proBNP assay[6] and the results were similar to those of serum. NT-proBNP fragmentation appears to be more intense in serum than in EDTA plasma;[7] in this regard, the use of EDTA (or antiprotease agents, such as aprotinin to avoid proteolysis) may be advisable. However, until the existence and the relevance of such fragments to NT-proBNP measurement and its clinical utility are unequivocally demonstrated, serum or heparin plasma remain the specimens of choice for NT-proBNP measurement. Citrate and oxalate plasma are not recommended for NT-proBNP analysis. Heparinized[8,9] or EDTA-whole blood[10] has been used as a sample for the point-of-care systems whose evaluation has been reported.

The recommended specimen for BNP measurement is EDTA plasma because in heparin plasma serum BNP concentrations show values between 25 and 40% lower than those obtained in EDTA.[11] However, heparin plasma produces results and clinical classification of patients similar to that of EDTA plasma in the Beckman Access BNP assay.[12]

Ideal Tube Types

Blood for NT-proBNP analysis can be drawn into either glass or plastic tubes—siliconized or not—without affecting the stability of the molecule. Moreover, BNP analysis mandatorily requires blood to be drawn into plastic tubes because proteases implicated in BNP proteolysis become activated on contact with glass.[13]

Effect of Storage Time and Temperature

NT-proBNP concentrations are stable in serum, plasma, and whole blood under a variety of storage conditions. The immunoreactivity of the molecule is not significantly increased or decreased after seven days at room temperature, one to three days in the refrigerator at 4°C, or several months at −20°C or lower temperatures;[14,15] freeze-thaw cycles do not significantly modify NT-proBNP concentrations.[14,16] When whole blood is used in point-of-care devices, NT-proBNP is also stable at room temperature for a prolonged period. Stability at room temperature facilitates the handling of specimens for NT-proBNP measurement in often-busy clinical laboratories. In this regard, NT-proBNP is a more convenient molecule to work with than BNP, which is largely unstable under any storage conditions.

BNP is largely unstable at room temperature and even after freezing (Figure 17–1),[17,18] and its stability is dependent on the specific assay being used.[17] This instability is likely because the BNP proteolysis occurring during storage affects the molecular regions recognized by some assays, but not involved in the antigenic reaction in other assays. Moreover, BNP degradation during storage is more pronounced in samples with high BNP values than in samples with low values that show no decrease during three months at −20°C or one year −80°C.[19] To avoid BNP instability during storage, it is recommended to add protease inhibitors to specimens. Belenky has shown increased stability of BNP during storage for ten days in the refrigerator when such inhibitors are added to clinical samples.[20] The IFCC Committee on Standardization of Cardiac Markers Damage recommended in its guideline for

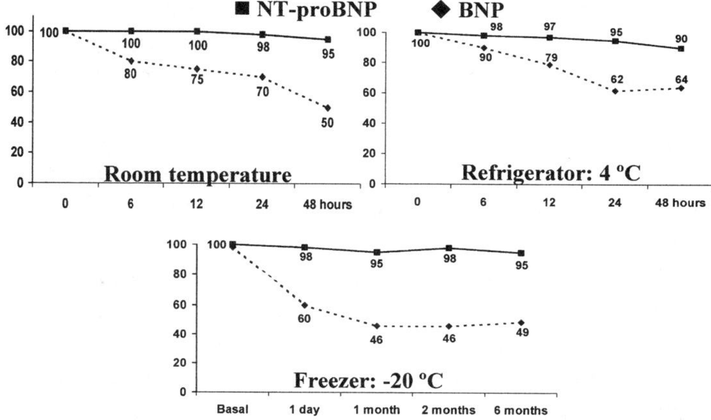

■ **Figure 17–1** Stability (as % decrease of original concentration) of BNP and NT-proBNP during different storage conditions.

BNP measurement that BNP should be measured within 4 h of collection if the sample is stored at room temperature. If the testing cannot be performed within 4 h, the sample should be processed, a protease inhibitor should be added, and the plasma should be stored and refrigerated at 4°C for up to 72 h or frozen (ideally at −70°C) if stored for longer periods.[21]

Conditions of the Subject

For NP measurements, the conditions required prior to and during blood sampling to decrease preanalytical variation are not fully known; the most studied condition is the effect of physical exercise on NP measurements.

Effects of exercise testing on NP measurements in patients with heart failure (HF) or coronary disease have been thoroughly described; however, it is important to know the effect of practicing regular physical exercise because it could be a preanalytical source of variation in NP measurements.

In patients with HF, previous physical exercise at 50% of the maximal heart rate increased BNP by 30% over pre-exercise levels, but such an increase was not observed in reference individuals. Although not analyzed, NT-proBNP is expected to follow the same pattern.[22] Therefore, as a general rule, patients should be sampled after resting, preferably in an upright position for at least 10–15 minutes. As with many other biochemical variables, the use of a tourniquet should be as short as possible.

Finally, after strenuous exercise (like a marathon or ultramarathon), BNP and NT-proBNP concentrations are increased over pre-race values and return to baseline values in one to three days.[23,24] The increase of NPs was associated with echocardiographic signs and cardiac troponin T or I elevations, which demonstrate cardiac dysfunction; NPs are also markers of such dysfunction.[23]

Analytical Issues

Earlier methods used to measure NPs required cumbersome radioimmunoassay, typically requiring an extractive step for the sample.[25] A methodological improvement was achieved when competitive enzyme immunoassays were developed;[26] however, automated methods have greatly facilitated BNP and NT-proBNP measurement and are widely accepted and used in the clinical setting.[27,28]

NT-proBNP: Available Assays and Their Characteristics

Currently, assays based on the same design used by the Roche Diagnostics (Elecsys, Modular, Cardiac reader) assay are available from bioMérieux (in the Vidas systems), while Siemens markets the Dade Behring (Dimension, Stratus CS) and DPC (Immulite 1000, 2000, and 2500) methods. In addition, Mitsubishi (Pathfast), Nanogen (LifeSign EXpress), Ortho Clinical Diagnostics (Vitros ECI), and Response Biomedical (RAMP) methods are available; a second generation, monoclonal NT-proBNP assay is under evaluation by several companies (Table 17–1).

Table 17–1: Currently-available methods for NT-proBNP measurement.[1]

Manufacturer	Instruments
Roche Diagnostics	Elecsys, Modular, Cardiac Reader (POC)
Dade-Behring	Dimension, Stratus CS (POC)
Diagnostics Products Co.	Immulite (different versions)
Ortho Clinical Diagnostics	Vitros
bioMérieux	Vidas, Mini Vidas (POC)
Mitsubishi Kagaku Iatron	Pathfast (POC)
Nanogen	LifeSign EXpress Reader (POC)
Response Biomedical	RAMP (POC)

[1]The original manufacturer of each method is reported.

The first generation NT-proBNP method developed by Roche Diagnostics is based in a noncompetitive chemoimmunoanalysis using a pair of polyclonal antibodies: one biotinylated directed at amino acids 1–21 (capture antibody) and the other labeled with a ruthenium complex (detection antibody) and directed at amino acids 39–50. The original, first generation NT-proBNP assay from Roche Diagnostics is calibrated with a preparation of synthetic human NT-proBNP$_{1-76}$-amide in which methionine on position 67 has been replaced by norleucine. The material is traceable to pure synthetic human NT-proBNP and it is used by the remaining NT-proBNP Roche-licensed assays.

Use of the same calibration material and antibodies by most of the NT-proBNP assays explains the lower than 20% difference detected in the NT-proBNP values by the different assays; this fact is shown in Figure 17–2 where the percent difference—obtained from regression equations—between the first generation Roche assay and the remaining marketed methods at the concentrations

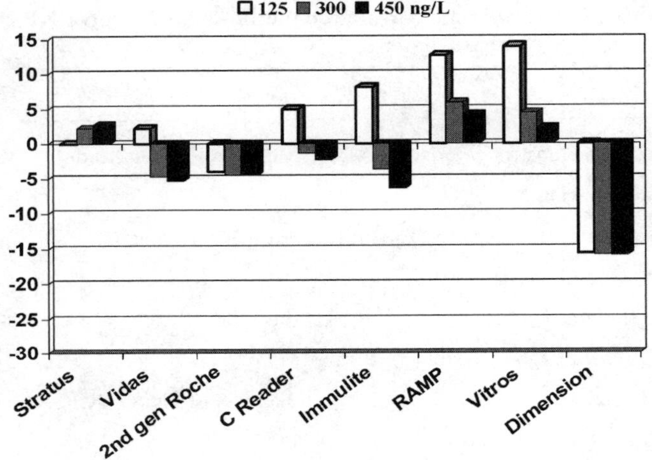

■ **Figure 17–2** Difference (in %) between the Roche Diagnostics 1st generation assay and the remaining methods at the recommended cutpoint values.

recommended as cutoff points are shown. The main characteristics of the assays in terms of imprecision, in accordance with the IFCC recommendation of total imprecision, is less than 15% for evaluating values in the reference range and less than 10% for evaluating serial changes,[21] accuracy, detection limit, and others are shown in Table 17–2.

Antibody Characteristics of NT-proBNP Assays

It is notable that the antibodies used by the first generation of the Roche Diagnostics assay are shared by the remaining assays, except for the point-of-care (POC) system from Roche (Cardiac Reader), which claims to use a monoclonal and a polyclonal antibody.[9] The second generation of the Roche Diagnostics assay using a pair of monoclonal antibodies (which recognized the epitopes shown in Figure 17–3) has been recently evaluated. Although the "in vitro" crossreactivity experiments show an immunoreactivity around

Table 17–2: Main analytical features† of the available NT-proBNP assays.

Linearity (range)	10–39,000 ng/L
Imprecision (%):	
Within-run	1.5–3.9%
Total	1.8–4.5%
Range assayed	67–27,449 ng/L
Accuracy (as % recovery)	92–100%
Limit of detection	3.8–<20 ng/L
Concentration at 20% of coefficient variation	9.4–21 ng/L
Hook effect (absent up to a concentration of)	285,000–500,000 ng/L

†Values are expressed as the minimum and maximum values of different evaluations.

half that of the first generation assay, clinical samples measured by both systems give the same NT-proBNP concentrations owing to the calibration characteristics of both assays.[29]

Biology of NT-proBNP and Antibody Binding

The amino-terminal ends of the pre-pro molecule of B-type natriuretic peptides, $proBNP_{1-108}$, and $NT\text{-}proBNP_{1-76}$, contain seven glycosylation sites.[30] Glycosylation is known to affect the reactivity of both molecules with the antibodies used in the NT-proBNP assays. When clinical samples are deglycosylated, the amount of NT-proBNP detected with the Roche assay (and with all the remaining NT-proBNP assays licensed by Roche) increases.[4] This occurs because there are two glycosylation sites in the aminoacid sequence 39–50 to which the detection antibody is directed (Figure 17–3); thus, glycosylation interferes with the antigenic reaction. Recently, a second generation of the Roche NT-proBNP assay has

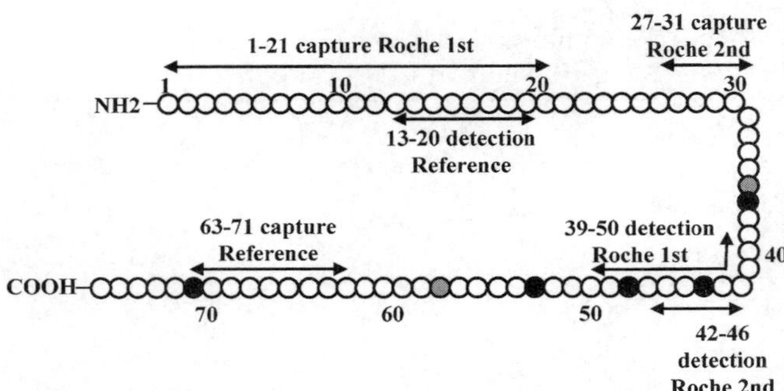

■ **Figure 17–3** NT-proBNP immunoassays. Epitopes recognized by the antibodies used in available methods.

Table 17–3: Reactivity of different NP molecules with NT-proBNP assays.

Molecular form	Reactivity
BNP_{1-32}	No reaction
Glycosylated $proBNP_{1-108}$	No reaction
Nonglycosylated $proBNP_{1-108}$	Low to very high
Glycosylated $NT\text{-}proBNP_{1-76}$	No reaction to low
Nonglycosylated $NT\text{-}proBNP_{1-76}$	Low to very high

been developed using antibodies directed against different sequences, however its reactivity with glycosylated NT-proBNP has yet to be thoroughly tested. Furthermore, the nonglycosylated NT-proBNP form is highly recognized (Table 17–3) by all existing NT-proBNP assays.

Fragments of NT-proBNP have been described in the circulation;[7] proteolysis can exist at both carboxyl- and amino-terminal ends of the molecule. As in the case of glycosylation, fragmentation could expose or hide epitopes recognized by the antibodies used in the NT-proBNP immunoassays. By using the pair of antibodies of the Roche first generation assay (against amino acids 1–21 and 39–50), the assays should recognize part of fragmented NT-proBNP forms because most of them are detected by any antibody recognizing the amino acid sequence 10–29.[7]

ProBNP_{1-108} has been found in plasma of patients and reference subjects in a truncated form, lacking the amino acids 1 and 2 of the original molecule; its reactivity in the NT-proBNP assays is dependent on the glycosylation status. As in the case of NT-proBNP, the glycosylated form is less detected by NT-proBNP assays, whereas the nonglycosylated form exhibits variable degrees of cross reaction, from low to high.[31] Therefore, proBNP_{1-108} is also a potential source of analytical variability for NT-proBNP measurements.

BNP: Available Assays and Characteristics

The first BNP assay from Biosite, Inc. was approved in the year 2000 by the Food and Drug Administration (FDA) of the United States. The assay is based on an immunofluorimetric detection of BNP in a point-of-care device (Triage) using whole blood as the sample. The method is easily applicable to clinical routine. After the Biosite assay was introduced, it was licensed to Beckman Coulter; later, Bayer and Abbott assays were launched. The Bayer assay is currently marketed by Siemens Medical Solutions, whereas the Biosite assay is currently property of Inverness Medical. The Abbott, Bayer, and Beckman assays are designed to be run in different immunoassay platforms (Table 17–4). Unlike the case of NT-proBNP, BNP-available assays are characterized by the use of different calibrator materials and antibodies, except in the case of the Beckman assay which uses the same calibrator and antibodies as the Biosite assay. Recombinant BNP is used as calibrator of

Table 17–4: Currently-available methods for BNP measurement.†

Manufacturer	Instruments
Abbott Laboratories	AxSym, Architect, i-STAT
Bayer	ADVIA Centaur
Beckman Coulter	Access 2, Synchron LXi, UniCel DeI
Biosite Diagnostics	Triage

†The original manufacturer of each method is reported.

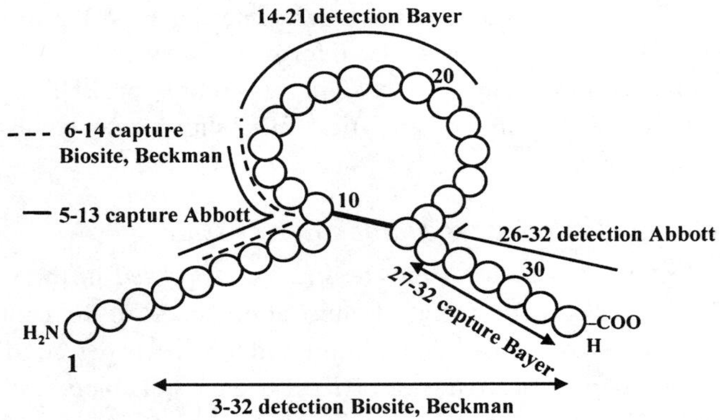

■ **Figure 17–4** BNP immunoassays. Epitopes recognized by the antibodies used in currently available methods.

the Biosite and Beckman BNP assays, whereas synthetic BNP is used by the Bayer and Abbott assays. As mentioned, the antibodies used by the different BNP assays are directed to quite different regions of the BNP molecule (Figure 17–4). This would imply a significant difference between the BNP results obtained with the different methods.

Table 17–5: Main analytical features† of the available BNP assays.

	Biosite assay	Remaining BNP assays
Linearity (range)	Up to 5000 ng/L	Up to 5000 ng/L
Imprecision (%):		
Within-run	9.4–15%	1.8–6%
Total	11–16%	0–10%
Range assayed	40–800 ng/L	44–2080 ng/L
Limit of detection	6 ng/L	5 ng/L
Hook effect (absent up to)	100,000 ng/L	285,000–500,000 ng/L

†Values are expressed as the minimum and maximum values of different evaluations.

The currently-automated BNP assay has overcome the main drawback of the Biosite assay; i.e., its high total imprecision owing to its manual steps; this and other features of BNP assays are shown in Table 17–5. The total imprecision of the automated assays is in accordance with the previously-cited values recommended by the IFCC.[21]

The harmonization of BNP assays will not be as easy as it may be in the case of NT-proBNP assays; the diversity of the calibration material and epitopes recognized by the BNP assays produce inter-method differences ranging from −30 to +10%.

Antibody Characteristics of BNP Assays

As shown in Figure 17–4, the assays currently available use three pairs of antibodies directed against different parts of the BNP molecule. Recognition of the ring sequence of the BNP molecule by the antibodies is required for identification of the BNP; all the assays use antibodies directed against different zones of this ring structure. Biosite and Beckman assays use a capture antibody recognizing the 6–14 amino acid sequence, whereas the capture antibody of the Abbott assay is directed against the 5–13 sequence. The Bayer assay recognizes the ring sequence by the detection antibody which is directed against the 14–21 sequence. The other antibodies not directed to the ring structure recognize the COOH-terminal sequence (Abbott detection antibody against 26–32, Bayer capture antibody against 27–32) or the 3–32 sequence (Biosite and Beckman detection antibodies). The dissimilarity of the BNP regions recognized by the antibodies greatly contributes to the high intermethod variability existing among BNP results by different methods. The percent difference (obtained from regression equations) between the Biosite assay (considered as the reference) and the remaining methods at the BNP concentrations recommended as cutoff points are shown in Figure 17–5.

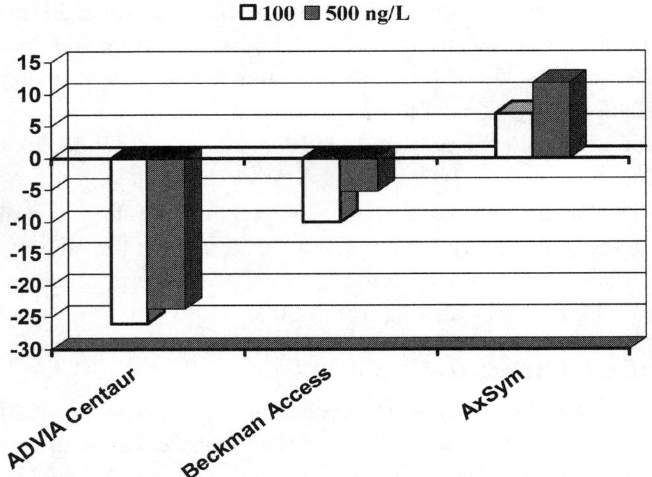

■ **Figure 17–5** Difference (in %) between the Biosite assay and the remaining methods at the recommended cutpoint values.

Biology of BNP and Antibody Binding

The reaction of the NP molecules to the different BNP assays is less complex than that of the reactions to the NT-proBNP assays. All of the BNP assays react strongly with nonglycosylated BNP_{1-32} (Table 17–6), a form known to be rapidly cleared from the circulation; there is a much weaker reaction with nonglycosylated BNP_{3-32},[32] the form considered to represent the "true" circulating BNP.[33] No data are available on the reactivity of the BNP_{6-32} form described by Pankow.[34] No reactivity exists with NT-$proBNP_{1-76}$, whether glycosylated or nonglycosylated. Finally, $proBNP_{1-108}$ is detected in BNP assays in a variable manner: glycosylated proBNP reacted one to ten times more often than nonglycosylated proBNP.

Shared Features of BNP and NT-proBNP Assays

Crossreactivity with Related Molecules

Natriuretic peptides are a family of molecules with shared chemical characteristics. Thus, the potential crossreactivity of BNP and

Table 17–6: Reactivity of different NP molecules with BNP assays.

Molecular form	Reactivity with BNP assays	Observations
BNP_{1-32}	High to very high	Rapidly cleared from circulation
BNP_{3-32}	Low	The major form detected in HF patients
Glycosylated $proBNP_{1-108}$	Medium	
Nonglycosylated $proBNP_{1-108}$	Low	
Glycosylated NT-$proBNP_{1-76}$	No reaction	
Nonglycosylated NT-$proBNP_{1-76}$	No reaction	

NT-proBNP assays with these (or other related) peptides must be checked. The assays have been tested for a number of such potential cross-reactants, e.g., atrial natriuretic peptide (ANP), amino-terminal proANP, and C-type natriuretic peptide (urodilatin), with no significant (<0.1%) cross reaction. Other tested molecules that also do not show cross reaction are: adrenomedullin; aldosterone; angiotensins I, II, and III; arginine vasopressin; endothelin; and renin. Therefore, NP assays are not affected by these molecules whose concentrations can be greatly altered under the same conditions that alter BNP and NT-proBNP.

Interferences from Biological Interferents or Drugs

No significant interferences (<10%) have been shown from classical biological variables, such as hemolysis (up to a free hemoglobin concentration of 400–500 mg/L), except for the NT-proBNP Ortho Vitros assay where an interference of 13% due to chylomicronemia (up to a triglyceride concentration of 30 g/L) and hyperbilirubinemia (at concentrations up to 200 mg/L) was observed. Some of the assays have also been tested for possible interference of drugs used in heart diseases (antiarrhythmics, anticoagulants, antiplatelets, beta blockers, diuretics, fibrinolytics, and statins) or most commonly-used drugs (analgesics, antibiotics, antipyretics). No interference was found.

Postanalytical Issues

Reference Limits and Ethnicity

Galasko and colleagues[35] reported data for the expected normal NT-proBNP values. Of 734 subjects aged greater than or equal to 45 years in the general population, only those without a history of ischemic heart disease, peripheral arterial disease, hypertension, diabetes, heart failure, or loop diuretic use were included. Moreover, they required blood pressure to be less than 160/90 mm Hg, an estimated glomerular filtration rate (eGFR) greater than or equal to 60 mL/min, and that no significant abnormalities be present on the echocardiogram. The normal range data (n = 397

Table 17–7: Reference NT-proBNP values (ng/L) in healthy subjects aged 40 to 82 years by the Roche Diagnostics assay.

Age (years)	Male			Female		
	Median	97.5th	95% CI	Median	97.5th	95% CI
40–65[1]	54	184	162–206	79	268	228–314
5–59[1]	20	100	78–173	49	164	150–281
>60[1]	40	172	144–173	78	225	180–254
66–76[1]	79	269	223–306	115	391	339–446
65–75[2]	25	NA	NA	36	NA	NA
70–75[2]	85	NA	NA	93	NA	NA
>75[2] to 82	127	NA	NA	161	NA	NA

Note: Median and 97.5th percentile and corresponding 95% confidence interval (CI) are shown.
*NA = Results not available
[1]From References 35 and 39
[2]From Reference 36

subjects) are shown in Table 17–7, which also includes results from another well-controlled population aged up to 82 years.[36] The BNP reference values were obtained in a population of 767 healthy subjects participating in the Olmsted County Study with no evidence of any disease influencing NP values and normal systolic, diastolic, and valvular function by echocardiography (Table 17–8).[37] Both studies on reference NP values have shown that a gender- and age-related difference exists for both BNP and NT-proBNP, whereas ethnicity has little, if any, effect on NP values.

In apparently healthy subjects, women presented higher NT-proBNP concentrations than men.[38] However, when subjects with mild impairment in renal function or glycemic control or with

Table 17–8: Reference BNP values (in ng/L) in healthy subjects aged 45 to 83 years by the Biosite assay.†

	Male			Female		
Age (years)	Median	5th	95th	Median	5th	95th
45–54	7	4	40	18	8	73
55–64	11	5	52	27	10	93
65–74	40	7	67	56	13	120
75–83	21	9	86	67	16	155

†From Reference 37
Note: Median and 5th and 95th percentiles are shown.

modest increases in blood pressure were excluded, these differences tended to decrease.[39] The same gender-related differences have been described for BNP.[37] This difference does not seem to interfere with the NP discriminant capacity to detect HF; a large study of 600 dyspneic patients with suspected HF reported no influence of gender on the capacity of NT-proBNP to rule in or rule out HF as the origin of dyspnea.[40]

Both BNP and NT-proBNP show a trend towards increased concentrations with advanced age. According to this fact, age should be taken into account when evaluating NP values both in reference subjects and in patients. The International Collaborative of NT-proBNP (ICON) study[41] showed the increase in diagnostic accuracy of NT-proBNP values when age-dependent cut points were used in the evaluation of subjects with acute dyspnea. However, for BNP values, a single age-independent cut point is still used,[42] despite reduced diagnostic value of this approach in older subjects.

The effect of ethnicity on the diagnostic capacity of NT-proBNP has been analyzed. In a Caucasian population with suspected acute coronary syndromes, NT-proBNP values were higher than those of African Americans;[40] however, these differences seem to be related to demographic or physiological variables, such as age or renal function when analyzed by multivariate analysis. The same results were observed for BNP with increased values in white compared to African American subjects.[42] Again, and as it was for the NT-proBNP values, the effect of ethnicity on the diagnostic accuracy of BNP was very small. Therefore, the ethnicity of the evaluated subjects could be ruled out as a relevant cause of interindividual variation of NP values.

Biological Variation

Serial measurements of biological variables are used to monitor changes due to physiological or pathophysiological causes. However, whether a difference between serial measurements is significant should be interpreted on the basis of the total variability of the variable, i.e., the sum of its analytical and individual variability. Individual variability is the highest contributor to biological variation; it can be calculated from the serial evaluation of a variable not only in reference subjects, but also in diseased individuals in their most stable condition. Preanalytical variation is also a component of the biological variability, although given the difficulty in controlling the numerous causes contributing to this variability, it is usually assumed to be zero or near zero. However, as already mentioned, this assumption is not always entirely true for NP measurements and the main causes of preanalytical variation must be known and their impact on NP measurements minimized.

Once the biological variation is known, critical differences (also called reference change values [RCVs]) considered as significant changes between consecutive measurements can be calculated. There are reports in the literature on the RCVs for both NT-proBNP and BNP. NT-proBNP variations of at least 92% in reference subjects[43] and 98% in stable HF patients were initially described as significant;[44] the same figures for BNP were 132% and

113%, respectively. These data suggest that NT-proBNP may be more sensitive than BNP for detecting significant changes in serial measurements.[43] However, the main interest in serial NP changes is its ability to detect significant changes in diseased patients. In the case of HF patients, to obtain the most accurate estimate of the minimum RCV indicating significant variation in patient status, biological variation must be estimated in very stable HF patients when their volume overload is minimal, i.e., the so-called "dry status." In a group of such well-controlled HF patients, much lower values than those previously reported for a 1-week RCV (23% for NT-proBNP and 43% for BNP) have been described;[45] again, NT-proBNP emerged with lower individual variation than BNP.

Calculations used for RCV estimation assume that measurements from which it is derived are normally distributed; this would not be the case for NPs. Fokkema[46] showed that after normalization of NT-proBNP values obtained in HF patients by log transformation, RCVs became asymmetric; thus, higher RCVs are needed for a week-to-week increase (157%) than for a decrease (−61%) to be considered significant. A later refinement came from Araujo,[47] who reported lower differences among consecutive NT-proBNP values in HF patients while NT-proBNP increased, e.g., the lowest differences (−30 to 40%) were observed for NT-proBNP values higher than 1300 ng/L.

Conclusion

In summary, although the biology of NT-proBNP and BNP are complex, the assays for their clinical measurement are robust and provide useful information to the clinician.

References

1. Togashi K, Hirata Y, Ando K, Takei Y, Kawakami M, Marumo F. Brain natriuretic peptide-like immunoreactivity is present in human plasma. *FEBS Lett.* 1989;250:235–237.
2. Hunt PJ, Espiner EA, Nicholls MG, Richards AM, Yandle TG. The role of circulation in processing pro-brain natriuretic peptide

(proBNP) to amino-terminal BNP and BNP-32. *Peptides.* 1997;18: 1475–1481.

3. Seidler T, Pemberton C, Yandle T, Espiner E, Nicholls G, Richards M. The amino terminal regions of proBNP and proANP oligomerise through leucine zipper-like coiled-coil motifs. *Biochem Biophys Res Commun.* 1999;255:495–501.
4. Seferian KR, Tamm NN, Semenov AG, Tolstaya AA, Koshkina EV, Krasnoselsky MI, et al. Immunodetection of glycosylated NT-proBNP circulating in human blood. *Clin Chem.* 2008;54:866–873.
5. Lippi G, Guidi GC, Mattiuzzi C, Plebani M. Preanalytical variability: the dark side of the moon in laboratory testing. *Clin Chem Lab Med.* 2006;44:358–365.
6. Januzzi JL, Lewandrowski KB, Bashirians G, Jackson S, Freyler D, Smith K, et al. Analytical and clinical performance of the Ortho-Clinical Diagnostics VITROS® amino-terminal pro-B type natriuretic peptide assay. *Clin Chim Acta.* 2008;387:48–54.
7. Ala-Kopsala M, Magga J, Peuhkurinen K, Leipala J, Ruskoaho H, Leppaluoto J, et al. Molecular heterogeneity has a major impact on the measurement of circulating N-terminal fragments of A- and B-type natriuretic peptides. *Clin Chem.* 2004;50:1576–1588.
8. Chenevier-Gobeaux C, Guillot D, Ursulet J, Paul JL, Ekindjian OG, Desmoulins D, et al. The N-terminal pro-brain natriuretic peptide (NT-proBNP) assay with the Stratus CS analyzer. *Ann Biol Clin (Paris).* 2007;65:77–82.
9. Zugck C, Nelles M, Katus HA, Collinson PO, Gaze DC, Dikkeschei B, et al. Multicentre evaluation of a new point-of-care test for the determination of NT-proBNP in whole blood. *Clin Chem Lab Med.* 2006;44:1269–1277.
10. Lee-Lewandrowski E, Januzzi JL, Green SM, Tannous B, Wu AHB, Smith A, et al. Multi-center validation of the Response Biomedical Corporation RAMP NT-proBNP assay with comparison to the Roche Diagnostics GmbH Elecsys proBNP assay. *Clin Chim Acta.* 2007; 386:20–24.
11. Lippi G, Fortunato A, Salvagno GL, Montagnana M, Sofiatti G, Guidi GC. Influence of sample matrix and storage on BNP measurement on the Bayer Advia Centaur. *J Clin Lab Anal.* 2007;21:293–297.
12. Dupuy AM, Terrier N, Dubois M, Boularan AM, Cristol JP. Heparin plasma sampling as an alternative to EDTA for BNP determination

on the Access-Beckman Coulter—effect of storage at −20 degrees C. *Clin Lab.* 2006;52:393–397.

13. Shimizu H, Aono K, Masuta K, Asada H, Misaki A, Teraoka H. Degradation of human brain natriuretic peptide (BNP) by contact activation of blood coagulation system. *Clin Chim Acta.* 2001;305: 181–186.
14. Sokoll LJ, Baum H, Collinson PO, et al. Multicenter analytical performance evaluation of the Elecsys proBNP assay. *Clin Chem Lab Med.* 2004;42:965–972.
15. Yeo KT, Wu AH, Apple FS, Kroll MH, Christenson RH, Lewandrowski KB, et al. Multicenter evaluation of the Roche NT-proBNP assay and comparison to the Biosite Triage BNP assay. *Clin Chim Acta.* 2003;338:107–115.
16. Barnes SC, Collinson PO, Galasko G, Lahiri A, Senior R. Evaluation of N-terminal pro-B type natriuretic peptide analysis on the Elecsys 1010 and 2010 analysers. *Ann Clin Biochem.* 2004;41:459–463.
17. Christenson RH, Azzazy HM, Duh SH. Stability of B-type natriuretic peptide (BNP) in whole blood and plasma stored under different conditions when measured with the Biosite Triage or Beckman-Coulter Access systems. *Clin Chim Acta.* 2007;384:176–178.
18. Mueller T, Gegenhuber A, Dieplinger B, Poelz W, Haltmayer M. Long-term stability of endogenous B-type natriuretic peptide (BNP) and amino terminal proBNP (NT-proBNP) in frozen plasma samples. *Clin Chem Lab Med.* 2004;42:942–944.
19. Pereira M, Azevedo A, Severo M, Barros H. Long-term stability of endogenous B-type natriuretic peptide after storage at −20 °C or −80 °C. *Clin Chem Lab Med.* 2008;46:1171–1174.
20. Belenky A, Smith A, Zhang B, Lin S, Despres N, Wu AH, Bluestein BI. The effect of class-specific protease inhibitors on the stabilization of B-type natriuretic peptide in human plasma. *Clin Chim Acta.* 2004;340:163–172.
21. Apple FS, Panteghini M, Ravkilde J, Mair J, Wu AHB, Tate J, et al. on behalf of the Committee on Standardization of Markers of Cardiac Damage of the IFCC. Quality specifications for B-type natriuretic peptide assays. *Clin Chem.* 2005;51:486–493.
22. Kjaer A, Appel J, Hildebrandt P, Petersen CL. Basal and exercise-induced neuroendocrine activation in patients with heart failure and in normal subjects. *Eur J Heart Fail.* 2004;6:29–39.

23. Neilan TG, Januzzi JL, Lee-Lewandrowski E, Ton-Nu TT, Yoerger DM, Jassal DS, et al. Myocardial injury and ventricular dysfunction related to training levels among nonelite participants in the Boston Marathon. *Circulation.* 2006;114:2325–2333.

24. Ohba H, Takada H, Musha H, Nagashima J, Mori N, Awaya T, et al. Effects of prolonged strenuous exercise on plasma levels of atrial natriuretic peptide and brain natriuretic peptide in healthy men. *Am Heart J.* 2001;141:751–758.

25. Hunt PJ, Yandle TG, Nicholls MG, Richards AM, Espiner EA. The amino-terminal portion of pro-brain natriuretic peptide (pro-BNP) circulates in human plasma. *Biochem Biophys Res Comm.* 1995; 214:1175–1183.

26. Missbichler A, Hawa G, Woloszczuk W, Schmal N, Hartter E. Enzymimmunoassays für proBNP fragmente (8–29) und (32–57). *J Lab Med.* 1999;23:241–244.

27. Vogeser M, Jacob K. B-type natriuretic peptide (BNP)—validation of an immediate response assay. *Clin Lab.* 2001;47:29–33.

28. Karl J, Borgya A, Gallusser A, Huber E, Krueger K, Rollinger W, Schenk J. Development of a novel, N-terminal-proBNP (NT-proBNP) assay with a low detection limit. *Scand J Clin Lab Invest.* 1999;59 (Suppl. 230):177–181.

29. Garcia-Beltran L, Gremmler B, Hensel-Wiegel K, Luthe H, Meisel S, Merce J, et al. Multicentre evaluation of the second generation Elecsys® NT-ProBNP assay. *Clin Chem.* 2008;54:A93–A93 [Abstract B-137].

30. Schellenberger U, O'Rear J, Guzzetta A, Jue RA, Protter AA, Pollitt NS. The precursor to B-type natriuretic peptide is an O-linked glycoprotein. *Arch Biochem Biophys.* 2006;451:160–166.

31. Luckenbill KN, Christenson RH, Jaffe AS, Mair J, Ordonez-Llanos J, Pagani F, et al. Cross-reactivity of BNP, NT-proBNP, and proBNP in commercial BNP and NT-proBNP assays: preliminary observations from the IFCC Committee for Standardization of Markers of Cardiac Damage. *Clin Chem.* 2008;54:619–621 [Letter].

32. Apple FS, Luckenbill KN, Jaffe AS, Mair J, Ordonez-Llanos J, Wu AH, et al. Cross-reactivity studies of BNP, proBNP, and NT-proBNP in commercial NT-proBNP assays. *Clin Chem.* 2008;54:A84–A84 [Abstract B-109].

33. Hawkridge AM, Heublein DM, Bergen R, Cataliotti A, Burnett JC Jr, Muddiman DC. Quantitative mass spectral evidence for the absence

of circulating brain natriuretic peptide (BNP-32) in severe human heart failure. *Proc Natl Acad Sci U S A*. 2005;102:17442–17447.

34. Pankow K, Wang Y, Gembardt F, Krause E, Sun X, Krause G, et al. Successive action of meprin A and neprilysin catabolizes B-type natriuretic peptide. *Circ Res*. 2007;101:875–882.

35. Galasko GI, Lahiri A, Barnes SC, Collinson P, Senior R. What is the normal range for N-terminal pro-brain natriuretic peptide? How well does this normal range screen for cardiovascular disease? *Eur Heart J*. 2005;26:2269–2276.

36. Alehagen U, Goetze JP, Dahlström U. Reference intervals and decision limits for B-type natriuretic peptide (BNP) and its precursor (NT-proBNP) in the elderly. *Clin Chim Acta*. 2007;382:8–14.

37. Redfield MM, Rodeheffer RJ, Jacobsen SJ, Mahoney DW, Bailey KR, Burnett JC. Plasma brain natriuretic peptide concentration: impact of age and gender. *J Am Coll Cardiol*. 2002;40:976–982.

38. Raymond I, Groenning BA, Hildebrandt PR, Nilsson JC, Baumann M, Trawinski J, et al. The influence of age, sex and other variables on the plasma level of N-terminal pro brain natriuretic peptide in a large sample of the general population. *Heart*. 2003;89:745–751.

39. Johnston N, Jernberg T, Lindahl B, et al. Biochemical indicators of cardiac and renal function in a healthy elderly population. *Clin Biochem*. 2004;37:210–216.

40. Krauser DG, Chen AA, Tung R, Anwaruddin S, Baggish AL, Januzzi JL Jr. Neither race nor gender influences the usefulness of amino-terminal pro-brain natriuretic peptide testing in dyspneic subjects: a ProBNP Investigation of Dyspnea in the Emergency Department (PRIDE) substudy. *J Card Fail*. 2006;12:452–457.

41. Januzzi JL, van Kimmenade R, Lainchbury J, et al. NT-proBNP testing for diagnosis and short-term prognosis in acute destabilized heart failure: an international pooled analysis of 1256 patients: the International Collaborative of NT-proBNP Study. *Eur Heart J*. 2006;27: 330–337.

42. Maisel AS, Clopton P, Krishnaswamy P, Nowak RM, McCord J, Hollander JE, et al. Impact of age, race, and sex on the ability of B-type natriuretic peptide to aid in the emergency diagnosis of heart failure: results from the Breathing Not Properly (BNP) multinational study. *Am Heart J*. 2004;147:1078–1084.

43. Wu AH. Serial testing of B-type natriuretic peptide and NT-proBNP for monitoring therapy of heart failure: the role of biologic variation in the interpretation of results. *Am Heart J.* 2006;152:828–834.

44. Bruins S, Fokkema MR, Romer JW, Dejongste MJ, van der Dijs FP, van den Ouweland JM, et al. High intraindividual variation of B-type natriuretic peptide (BNP) and amino-terminal proBNP in patients with stable chronic heart failure. *Clin Chem.* 2004;50:2052–2058.

45. Schou M, Gustafsson F, Kjaer A, Hildebrandt PR. Long-term clinical variation of NT-proBNP in stable chronic heart failure patients. *Eur Heart J.* 2007;28:177–182.

46. Fokkema MR, Herrmann Z, Muskiet FA, Moecks J. Reference change values for brain natriuretic peptides revisited. *Clin Chem.* 2006;52: 1602–1603 [Letter].

47. Araujo JP, Azevedo A, Lourenco P, Rocha-Goncalves F, Ferreira A, Bettencourt P. Intraindividual variation of amino-terminal pro-B-type natriuretic peptide levels in patients with stable heart failure. *Am J Cardiol.* 2006;98:1248–1250.

18 ■ Natriuretic Peptides and Structural Heart Disease: Cardiac Correlates of Natriuretic Peptide Elevation

SABE DE, MD
W. H. WILSON TANG, MD

Introduction

Cardiac structural alterations are important determinants of natriuretic peptide expression in the setting of heart failure. Much of the understanding of atrial natriuretic peptide (ANP) and B-type natriuretic peptide (BNP) production and secretion has come from animal models, demonstrating that increased mechanical stretch on the atria and ventricles results in increased ANP and BNP levels.[1,2] Natriuretic peptides may also play a role in preventing progressive collagen accumulation and remodeling associated with worsening heart failure, as mice with targeted disruption of BNP had increased fibrosis in response to left ventricular (LV) pressure overload.[3] This chapter summarizes our current understanding of the production of natriuretic peptides as it relates to alterations in cardiac structure and function. We will focus our discussion primarily on BNP and its by-product, amino-terminal pro-B-type natriuretic peptide (NT-proBNP), because they are commonly measured in the clinical setting.

Impact of Left Ventricular Systolic Dysfunction and Wall Stress

The release of BNP is clearly triggered in response to increased ventricular pressures leading to increased wall stretch,[4–6] thereby increasing BNP gene expression and protein production and release.[7–10] LV wall stress, as defined by Laplace (wall stress = pressure radius/wall thickness), is perhaps the most important

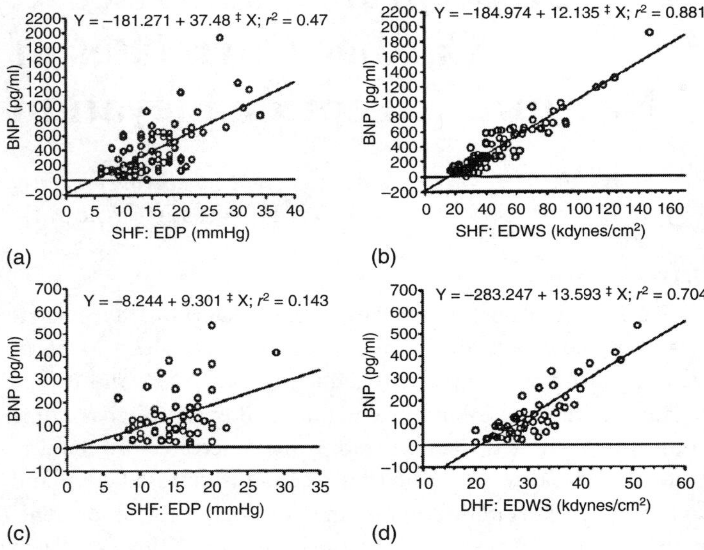

■ **Figure 18–1** Correlation between B-type natriuretic peptide and left ventricular functional parameters (including left ventricular end-diastolic pressure [EDP] and end-diastolic wall-stress [EDWS]) in patients with systolic heart failure (SHF) and diastolic heart failure (DHF).

Reproduced from Iwanaga, et al. B-Type Natriuretic Peptide Strongly Reflects Diastolic Wall Stress in Patients With Chronic Heart Failure: Comparison Between Systolic and Diastolic Heart Failure. *J Am Coll Cardiol.* 2006;47(2): 742–8.

determinant of BNP expression and production (Figure 18–1).[8,11,12] Other common cardiac and noncardiac causes of elevated natriuretic peptide levels are shown in Table 18–1.

When considering the contribution of mass, 70% of cardiac BNP arises from the ventricles. BNP is far more up-regulated in failing ventricular myocardium than ANP. However, the relationship among BNP and NT-proBNP and LV systolic dysfunction is far more complex. In studies evaluating their diagnostic utilities,

Table 18–1: Common cardiac and noncardiac causes of elevated natriuretic peptide levels.

Cardiac Causes
Heart Muscle Disease
—Hypertrophic heart muscle disease
—Infiltrative cardiomyopathies, including amyloidosis
—Acute cardiomyopathies, including apical balloon syndrome
—Inflammatory, including myocarditis and chemotherapy
Valvular Heart Disease
—Aortic stenosis and regurgitation
—Mitral stenosis and regurgitation
Arrhythmia
—Atrial fibrillation and flutter
Congenital Heart Disease
Pulmonary heart disease
—Sleep apnea
—Pulmonary embolism
—Pulmonary hypertension
Noncardiac Causes
Renal insufficiency
Anemia
Critical illness
—Bacterial sepsis
—Burns
—Acute respiratory distress syndrome (ARDS)
Metabolic disorders
Thyroid diseases

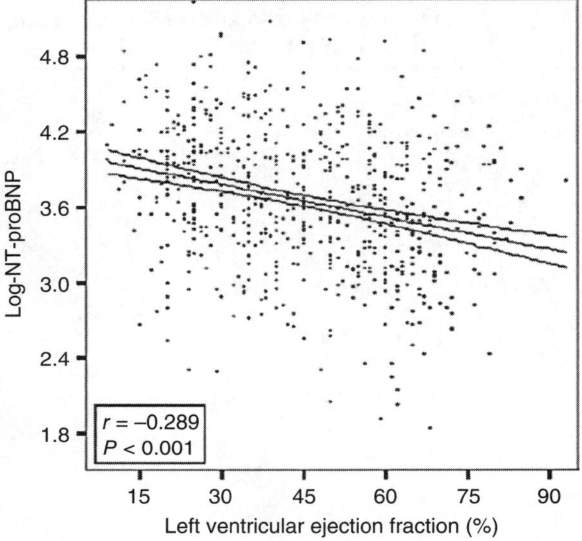

■ **Figure 18–2** BNP relates to left ventricular ejection fraction (LVEF) in a population of patients with Acute Decompensated Heart Failure.

Reproduced from Januzzi J.L., et al. NT-proBNP testing for diagnosis and short-term prognosis in acute destabilized heart failure: an international pooled analysis of 1256 patients: the International Collaborative of NT-proBNP Study. *Eur Heart J.* 2006;27(3): 330–7.

natriuretic peptide levels are weakly inversely correlated with LV ejection fraction (r = −0.289 for NT-proBNP, p < 0.001, Figure 18–2).[13] This is likely due to the variability of compensation observed across the spectrum of LV end-diastolic volumes—leading to differential wall stress. Different loading conditions, presence of LV hypertrophy without significant cardiac remodeling, or ventricular interdependency between the left and right ventricles may also affect BNP or NT-proBNP levels. Clearly, such variations may indirectly affect the clinical utility for natriuretic peptide testing to distinguish those with versus those without LV systolic dysfunction in population screening for cardiac dysfunction, which will be discussed in Chapter 19.

Impact of Left Ventricular Diastolic Dysfunction

Heart failure severity is often characterized by progressive elevation of LV filling pressures and echocardiographic evidence of progressive restrictive filling, with or without ventricular dilatation and dysfunction. Most modern echocardiography protocols currently report diastolic dysfunction based on pulsed wave Doppler transmitral inflow. Elevations of mitral E wave to tissue Doppler early diastolic lateral annulus velocity ratio (E/Ea) have been proposed as noninvasive surrogate indicators of elevated LV filling pressures.[14,15] A study of 50 patients in the intensive care unit with pulmonary artery catheters examined the predictive power of elevated BNP levels and the E/Ea ratio based on elevated pulmonary capillary wedge pressure (PCWP). Both BNP elevations at a cutoff of greater than 300 pg/ml and a mitral E/Ea cutoff of greater than 15 had a high sensitivity for predicting a PCWP greater than 15 mm Hg.[16] In this study, E/Ea was found to correlate better with PCWP ($r = 0.69$; $P < 0.001$) than with BNP ($r = 0.32$; $P = 0.02$ for log-transformed BNP). The correlation between the E/Ea ratio and natriuretic peptide levels has also been confirmed in other studies.[17,18] Interestingly, the area under the receiver operating characteristic (ROC) curve can be higher for the diagnosis of systolic and diastolic function combined (0.95), compared to systolic dysfunction alone in the absence of diastolic function assessment (0.82).[19]

A very powerful and often disregarded interplay among left- and right-sided chambers and echocardiographically-derived diastolic filling indices exists when attempting to interpret elevations of natriuretic peptide levels in symptomatic patients with chronic heart failure with underlying LV systolic dysfunction. Plasma BNP levels not only correlated with the patient's symptomatic status, as defined by NYHA functional class, but also with diastolic dysfunction stages, mitral regurgitation severity, and impairment of right ventricular (RV) systolic function—all independent echocardiographic predictors of BNP levels (Figure 18–3).[18] Similar observations were made with NT-BNP levels in the acute setting, whereby one-year mortality was independently predicted by NT-proBNP level, LVEF, right ventricular dilation, and systolic blood pressure.[20]

Impact of Left Ventricular Mass and Stiffness

Myocardial diseases that result in abnormal LV wall thickening consist of a spectrum of entities including hypertensive heart disease, hypertrophic cardiomyopathy, and infiltrative diseases (such as cardiac amyloidosis). Hypertension may directly increase LV cavity pressure, and thus increases wall stress. However, in the presence of LV hypertrophy, the increased wall thickness can normalize wall stress in the absence of intrinsic myocardial stiffness. If there is chamber enlargement from possible confounding variables like systolic dysfunction or mitral regurgitation, the wall stress will further increase, unless there is a hypertrophic response. BNP has been shown to be elevated in patients with hypertension and to correlate with LV mass index and relative wall thickness.[21] In population studies, a modest correlation between LVH and BNP levels has been observed.[22] Interestingly, in multivariate analysis, increased LV mass index displaced diastolic dysfunction and was a significantly greater predictor of BNP elevation.

Hypertrophic cardiomyopathy (HCM) is an inherited myocardial disorder characterized by myofibril disarray commonly expressed as asymmetric septal hypertrophy in a nondilated left ventricle. HCM is characterized by increased BNP expression in ventricular myocytes.[23] Higher BNP expression can also be found in the presence of LV outflow tract obstruction causing increasing intracardiac filling pressures.[24] Furthermore, a rise in natriuretic peptide levels has been shown to be predictive of a subgroup of patients who may eventually develop LV dilatation with immunohistochemistry, demonstrating an increase in BNP-positive myocytes that highly correlate with raised LV end-diastolic pressures.[25]

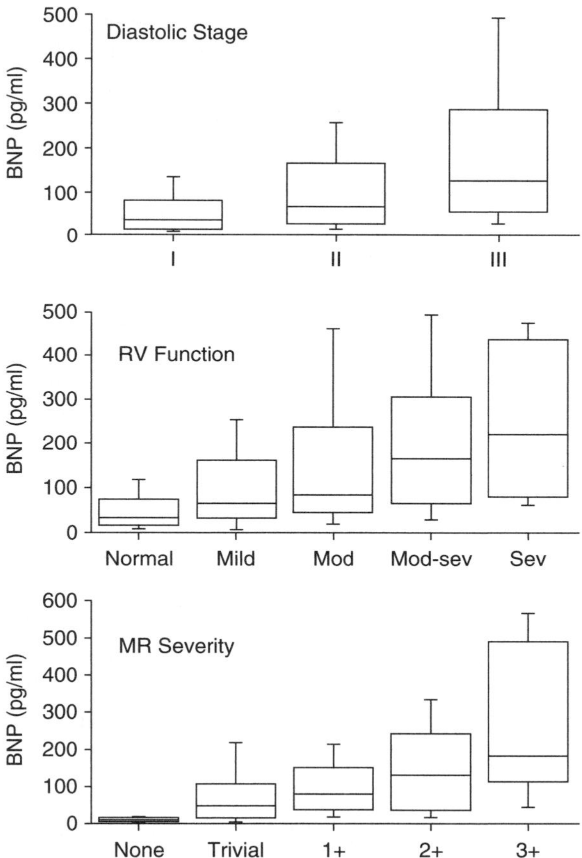

■ **Figure 18–3** Relationships of BNP with diastolic dysfunction Stage, right ventricular (RV) systolic function, and mitral regurgitation (MR) severity based on echocardiography in patients with chronic systolic heart failure.

Reproduced from Troughton R.W., et al. Plasma B-type natriuretic peptide levels in systolic heart failure: importance of left ventricular diastolic function and right ventricular systolic function. *J Am Coll Cardiol.* 2004;43(3): 416–22.

In addition to wall stretch, cytotoxic or metabolic heart muscle injury, such as that seen with exposure to chemotherapeutic agents, bacterial sepsis, critical illness, or thyroid disease, has been shown to elevate both BNP and NT-proBNP, often in the presence of low filling pressures and normal cardiac hemodynamics. Indeed, in this context, studies have suggested a higher prevalence of septic-mediated LV dysfunction among those with sepsis and elevated BNP concentrations.

Intrinsic myocardial stiffness is another major determinant of BNP expression and production in a wide range of heart failure conditions.[26] Clearly, an inability for the myocardium to compensate for increasing load (pressure or volume) due to a stiff ventricle may result in raised intracardiac pressures and myocyte stretch, leading to elevated BNP levels. Patients with cardiac amyloidosis, for example, have increased ANP and BNP levels in addition to increased gene expression in their ventricular myocytes.[27] NT-proBNP is a sensitive marker of cardiac involvement and restrictive physiology in patients with AL amyloidosis and elevated levels are associated with a worsening clinical prognosis, with one study suggesting that the sensitivity of NT-proBNP for predicting disease progression is greater than that of conventional echocardiographic parameters.[28] Other studies of amyloidosis, however, have found BNP levels to be similar for patients with and without overt heart failure.[29]

In contrast to restrictive heart disease, lower BNP levels have generally been observed in constrictive pericarditis.[30] While patients with secondary constrictive pericarditis did not have a significant difference in BNP versus those with restrictive physiology, the absolute level was relatively lower (278 ng/L versus 499 ng/L), and the difference between idiopathic constrictive and restrictive cardiomyopathy was significantly apparent (80 ng/L versus 499 ng/L, respectively; $P < 0.05$).[31] It has been postulated that the thickened pericardium constraints may act to oppose the myocardial stretch. This diminished stretch results in lessened wall tension and a lower stimulus for BNP release and subsequent natriuretic peptide levels. Larger studies are required, but BNP may play an additive role beyond hemodynamic assessment in distinguishing restriction from constriction.[8]

Impact of Pulmonary Hypertension and the Right Ventricular Dysfunction

The right ventricle plays an important pathophysiologic role in explaining BNP elevation in patients with systolic and/or diastolic dysfunction. Natriuretic peptide levels are often elevated in animal models and in patients with pulmonary hypertension.[32,33] Nagaya et al. attempted to delineate the relationship between BNP, right ventricular volume overload (RVVO), and right ventricular pressure overload (RVPO) by comparing BNP levels in patients with atrial septal defect versus patients with thromboembolic pulmonary hypertension.[34] The study incorporated echocardiographic data and invasive hemodynamic data, together with electron beam CT-derived data of RV volume and mass. Plasma BNP showed a positive correlation with mean right atrial and pulmonary artery pressures, as well as with pulmonary vascular resistance and RV myocardial mass. As expected, BNP negatively correlated with cardiac output and RV ejection fraction. Plasma BNP was significantly higher in patients with RVPO compared to those with RVVO (294 versus 48 pg/mL; $P < 0.05$). Both BNP and ANP were elevated in RVVO, yet BNP was predominantly elevated in RVPO. These findings were mirrored by a more recent study showing that BNP correlates with indices of pulmonary pressure and inversely correlates with RV function.[35] Clearly, RV dysfunction is an important source of BNP and NT-proBNP elevation, as secretion mediated by pressure overload and increased wall stretch can affect the RV in a manner similar to the LV. Furthermore, these findings are also of prognostic and clinical significance in the setting of pulmonary hypertension, as vasodilator therapy and the subsequent drop in pulmonary vascular resistance result in seemingly lower concentrations of natriuretic peptides.

The relationship between RV dysfunction and natriuretic peptide levels can also been found in other predominantly RV disorders. In patients presenting with pulmonary embolism, echocardiographic evidence of RV dysfunction is associated both with raised natriuretic peptide levels and a poorer prognosis.[36–38]

In patients with arrhythmogenic right ventricular dysplasia, natriuretic peptide levels have correlated with the degree of RV dysfunction and the electrophysiology study-derived amount of arrhythmogenic substrate. More interestingly, myocytes with fibro-fatty infiltrate demonstrate strong BNP immunoreactivity.[39]

Impact of Valvular Dysfunction

Rarely mentioned, but a potentially important determinant of ventricular wall stress and dysfunction, as well as an important contributor for heart failure, is the presence of underlying valvular dysfunction. For example, patients with mitral stenosis (MS) have higher natriuretic peptide levels than do healthy subjects,[40] but this was evident primarily in those patients with increased left atrium diameter or raised pulmonary artery pressures. Since MS is generally characterized by normal LV function and a relatively low LV end-diastolic pressure (LVEDP) due to underfilling, the correlation between BNP or NT-proBNP levels and PCWP may be modest, and potentially less tight than of that between ANP and PCWP.[41] Only ANP levels have been shown to consistently decline after balloon valvuloplasty for MS,[42–49] whereas BNP levels do not seem to change significantly despite correlating with LVEDP.[48] Furthermore, patients with MS who develop atrial fibrillation (AF) may also have higher NT-proBNP levels than those without the condition.[44] However, plasma natriuretic peptide levels may not decrease following valvuloplasty in patients with MS and AF.[49,50]

There have been discrepancies in the literature regarding the relationship between the severity of mitral regurgitation (MR) and natriuretic peptide levels.[18,51] This is likely due to the fact that BNP and NT-proBNP levels can vary based on the etiology and the pace of progression of MR. Functional or secondary MR typically denotes structurally normal valve leaflets, with regurgitation on the basis of altered geometry from ventricular dilatation, and annular enlargement or papillary muscle displacement from tethering or tenting of the leaflet. Compared to organic or primary MR, natriuretic peptide levels are higher in those with functional MR. Regardless, for patients with chronic severe MR, elevated natriuretic peptide levels carry important prognostic implications of symptom status. Asymptomatic patients with elevated natriuretic peptide levels are at increased likelihood of requiring surgery within one year.[52] Those with elevated natriuretic peptide levels may also face an increased risk of post-operative LV dysfunction.[53]

Aortic stenosis (AS) represents a state of pressure overload on the left ventricle. Since this pathophysiology is the basis for BNP gene expression and plasma secretion, BNP and NT-proBNP levels are more elevated in AS versus other valve conditions, largely in response to increases in end-systolic wall stress.[54] To support this concept, natriuretic peptide levels have been shown to correlate with LVH, aortic valve pressure gradient, and symptom status.[55,56] Elevations of BNP and NT-proBNP can also be highly sensitive and specific for the identification of patients with symptomatic AS and provide independent risk prediction for both symptomatic and asymptomatic AS patients.[57–59] Interestingly, there was a steep increase in plasma peptide levels with the onset of LV dysfunction related to AS.[60] In a subsequent follow-up paper, the average increase in BNP per year was most predictive of developing symptoms in an asymptomatic AS population.[61]

The increased regurgitant volume in chronic aortic regurgitation (AR) results in a slow, but steady, increase in LV end-diastolic volume. Compensatory hypertrophy and dilatation attempt to reduce this wall stress and maintain stroke volume, hence natriuretic peptide levels tend to be relatively low in this setting. Nevertheless, natriuretic peptide levels tend to be higher in symptomatic patients than those who are asymptomatic.[62,63] However, correlations between ANP, BNP, and NT-proBNP with LV volumes, diameters, LV mass, and LV wall stress, are weaker in AR compared to AS. A small study of only 12 patients suggested elevated BNP levels correlated mostly with LV mass index.[64]

Impact of Atrial Fibrillation and Myocardial Ischemia

Beyond structural alterations, AF and myocardial ischemia are the two major confounders of natriuretic peptide levels in patients with cardiac diseases. AF may occur as a result of previously mentioned pathologies, including LV hypertrophy, systolic or diastolic dysfunction, or valvular heart disease. Natriuretic peptide levels may be elevated as a result of these comorbidities alone, or from the influence of AF. While BNP is mostly produced in the ventricle, patients with AF show increased atrial secretion of BNP when measured from the coronary sinus.[65] AF has shown to be associated with increased mRNA gene expression of NT-proBNP at the atrial level.[66] Atrial production of BNP is subsequently reduced with cardioversion to sinus rhythm.[67]

Clinically, the associations between BNP and NT-proBNP with AF may be important because this arrhythmia is a common cause of dyspnea, even in the absence of heart failure.[68] In a study of 599 patients presenting to the emergency room with dyspnea, 13% were found to have AF. For those patients not in overt heart failure, the presence of AF was associated with higher NT-proBNP concentrations. For such patients, AF was the strongest predictor of having an NT-proBNP concentration at a level suggestive of acute heart failure. Similarly, the presence of AF is an important confounding factor in the interpretation of BNP levels in patients with heart failure, as AF has been shown to reduce the diagnostic specificity of BNP in this setting. This was best demonstrated in the Breathing Not Properly study, in which the specificity of a BNP of 100 pg/ml was 40% for patients with AF versus 79% for those without.[69]

With respect to coronary ischemia, increased ventricular wall stress can be caused by localized ventricular ischemia resulting in

LV systolic or diastolic dysfunction. Furthermore, animal studies have suggested that ischemia alone may stimulate BNP secretion independent of increases in wall stress.[70] In pigs, in particular, acute myocardial hypoxia has been shown to result in an increase of BNP mRNA production, with a rapid release noted of newly synthesized NT-proBNP.[71] Human studies have also shown that BNP mRNA and plasma natriuretic peptide levels are increased in patients with coronary artery disease in the absence of LV dysfunction.[72] In large-scale clinical trials, BNP and NT-proBNP levels have been found to be consistently elevated in patients presenting with non-ST elevation acute coronary syndromes.[73–74] These elevations are also independently predictive of poor outcomes beyond other biomarkers (as discussed in Chapter 22). In a study of 112 patients undergoing nuclear perfusion imaging, there were notable increases with exercise in BNP, NT-proBNP, as well as NT-proANP levels.[75] Inducible ischemia by dobutamine stress echocardiography (DSE) was associated with higher NT-proBNP levels,[76] but that was not confirmed in another smaller study.[77] In addition to ischemia related to coronary artery disease, other forms of tissue ischemia—including hypoxia and anemia—have also been reported to be associated with elevations in BNP and NT-proBNP.

Conclusion

This chapter discussed many cardiac determinants of natriuretic peptide elevation, and because all these factors can directly or indirectly lead to worsening symptom status, natriuretic peptide expression or production should be better characterized as an integrated marker of altered cardiac structure and function leading to signs and symptoms of heart failure and cardiac dysfunction. This is likely to explain the fact that BNP and NT-proBNP are both powerfully prognostic across a wide array of cardiac pathological states. As cardiac imaging continues to evolve and provides more insight into cardiomyopathies and valvular lesions, BNP assessment will yield incremental information for diagnostic and prognostic purposes as an indicator of heightened wall stress and pressure overload. Future studies are necessary to understand the biological processing and mechanisms of production and release of BNP and other cardiac peptides to refine our understanding of their potential clinical utilities.

References

1. Ogawa T, Linz W, Stevenson M, et al. Evidence for load-dependent and load-independent determinants of cardiac natriuretic peptide production. *Circulation.* 1996;93:2059–2067.
2. Luchner A, Stevens TL, Borgeson DD, et al. Differential atrial and ventricular expression of myocardial BNP during evolution of heart failure. *Am J Physiol.* 1998;274:H1684–H1689.
3. Tamura N, Ogawa Y, Chusho H, et al. Cardiac fibrosis in mice lacking brain natriuretic peptide. *Proc Natl Acad Sci U S A.* 2000;97:4239–4244.
4. Nakamura M, Niinuma H, Chiba M, et al. Effect of the maze procedure for atrial fibrillation on atrial and brain natriuretic peptide. *Am J Cardiol.* 1997;79:966–970.
5. Richards AM, Crozier IG, Yandle TG, Espiner EA, Ikram H, Nicholls MG. Brain natriuretic factor: regional plasma concentrations and correlations with haemodynamic state in cardiac disease. *Br Heart J.* 1993;69:414–417.
6. Yasue H, Yoshimura M, Sumida H, et al. Localization and mechanism of secretion of B-type natriuretic peptide in comparison with those of A-type natriuretic peptide in normal subjects and patients with heart failure. *Circulation.* 1994;90:195–203.
7. Nakagawa O, Ogawa Y, Itoh H, et al. Rapid transcriptional activation and early mRNA turnover of brain natriuretic peptide in cardiocyte hypertrophy. Evidence for brain natriuretic peptide as an "emergency" cardiac hormone against ventricular overload. *J Clin Invest.* 1995;96:1280–1287.
8. Alter P, Rupp H, Rominger MB, et al. B-type natriuretic peptide and wall stress in dilated human heart. *Mol Cell Biochem.* 2008;314:179–191.
9. Vanderheyden M, Goethals M, Verstreken S, et al. Wall stress modulates brain natriuretic peptide production in pressure overload cardiomyopathy. *J Am Coll Cardiol.* 2004;44:2349–2354.

10. Wiese S, Breyer T, Dragu A, et al. Gene expression of brain natriuretic peptide in isolated atrial and ventricular human myocardium: influence of angiotensin II and diastolic fiber length. *Circulation.* 2000;102:3074–3079.

11. Krittayaphong R, Boonyasirinant T, Saiviroonporn P, Thanapiboonpol P, Nakyen S, and Udompunturak S. Correlation between NT-pro BNP levels and left ventricular wall stress, sphericity index and extent of myocardial damage: a magnetic resonance imaging study. *J Card Fail.* 2008;14:687–694.

12. Iwanaga Y, Nishi I, Furuichi S, et al. B-type natriuretic peptide strongly reflects diastolic wall stress in patients with chronic heart failure: comparison between systolic and diastolic heart failure. *J Am Coll Cardiol.* 2006;47:742–748.

13. Januzzi JL, van Kimmenade R, Lainchbury J, et al. NT-proBNP testing for diagnosis and short-term prognosis in acute destabilized heart failure: an international pooled analysis of 1256 patients: the International Collaborative of NT-proBNP Study. *Eur Heart J.* 2006;27:330–337.

14. Nagueh SF, Middleton KJ, Kopelen HA, Zoghbi WA, Quinones MA. Doppler tissue imaging: a noninvasive technique for evaluation of left ventricular relaxation and estimation of filling pressures. *J Am Coll Cardiol.* 1997;30:1527–1533.

15. Ommen SR, Nishimura RA, Appleton CP, et al. Clinical utility of Doppler echocardiography and tissue Doppler imaging in the estimation of left ventricular filling pressures: a comparative simultaneous Doppler-catheterization study. *Circulation.* 2000;102:1788–1794.

16. Dokainish H, Zoghbi WA, Lakkis NM, et al. Optimal noninvasive assessment of left ventricular filling pressures: a comparison of tissue Doppler echocardiography and B-type natriuretic peptide in patients with pulmonary artery catheters. *Circulation.* 2004;109(20):2432–2439.

17. Dong SJ, de las Fuentes L, Brown AL, Waggoner AD, Ewald GA, Davila-Roman VG. N-terminal pro B-type natriuretic peptide levels: correlation with echocardiographically determined left ventricular diastolic function in an ambulatory cohort. *J Am Soc Echocardiogr.* 2006;19:1017–1025.

18. Troughton RW, Prior DL, Pereira JJ, et al. Plasma B-type natriuretic peptide levels in systolic heart failure: importance of left ventricular

diastolic function and right ventricular systolic function. *J Am Coll Cardiol.* 2004;43:416–422.

19. Krishnaswamy P, Lubien E, Clopton P, et al. Utility of B-natriuretic peptide levels in identifying patients with left ventricular systolic or diastolic dysfunction. *Am J Med.* 2001;111:274–279.
20. Chen AA, Wood MJ, Krauser DG, et al. NT-proBNP levels, echocardiographic findings, and outcomes in breathless patients: results from the ProBNP Investigation of Dyspnoea in the Emergency Department (PRIDE) echocardiographic substudy. *Eur Heart J.* 2006;27:839–845.
21. Kohno M, Horio T, Yokokawa K, et al. Brain natriuretic peptide as a marker for hypertensive left ventricular hypertrophy: changes during 1-year antihypertensive therapy with angiotensin-converting enzyme inhibitor. *Am J Med.* 1995;98:257–265.
22. Lukowicz TV, Fischer M, Hense HW, et al. BNP as a marker of diastolic dysfunction in the general population: importance of left ventricular hypertrophy. *Eur J Heart Fail.* 2005;7:525–531.
23. Hasegawa K, Fujiwara H, Doyama K, et al. Ventricular expression of brain natriuretic peptide in hypertrophic cardiomyopathy. *Circulation.* 1993;88:372–380.
24. Nishigaki K, Tomita M, Kagawa K, et al. Marked expression of plasma brain natriuretic peptide is a special feature of hypertrophic obstructive cardiomyopathy. *J Am Coll Cardiol.* 1996;28:1234–1242.
25. Pieroni M, Bellocci F, Sanna T, et al. Increased brain natriuretic peptide secretion is a marker of disease progression in nonobstructive hypertrophic cardiomyopathy. *J Card Fail.* 2007;13:380–388.
26. Watanabe S, Shite J, Takaoka H, et al. Myocardial stiffness is an important determinant of the plasma brain natriuretic peptide concentration in patients with both diastolic and systolic heart failure. *Eur Heart J.* 2006;27:832–838.
27. Takemura G, Takatsu Y, Doyama K, et al. Expression of atrial and brain natriuretic peptides and their genes in hearts of patients with cardiac amyloidosis. *J Am Coll Cardiol.* 1998;31:754–765.
28. Palladini G, Campana C, Klersy C, et al. Serum N-terminal pro-brain natriuretic peptide is a sensitive marker of myocardial dysfunction in AL amyloidosis. *Circulation.* 2003;107:2440–2445.

29. Nordlinger M, Magnani B, Skinner M, Falk RH. Is elevated plasma B-natriuretic peptide in amyloidosis simply a function of the presence of heart failure? *Am J Cardiol.* 2005;96:982–984.

30. Leya FS, Arab D, Joyal D, et al. The efficacy of brain natriuretic peptide levels in differentiating constrictive pericarditis from restrictive cardiomyopathy. *J Am Coll Cardiol.* 2005;45:1900–1902.

31. Babuin L, Alegria JR, Oh JK, Nishimura RA, Jaffe AS. Brain natriuretic peptide levels in constrictive pericarditis and restrictive cardiomyopathy. *J Am Coll Cardiol.* 2006;47:1489–1491.

32. Hill NS, Klinger JR, Warburton RR, Pietras L, Wrenn DS. Brain natriuretic peptide: possible role in the modulation of hypoxic pulmonary hypertension. *Am J Physiol.* 1994;266:L308–L315.

33. Nootens M, Kaufmann E, Rector T, et al. Neurohormonal activation in patients with right ventricular failure from pulmonary hypertension: relation to hemodynamic variables and endothelin levels. *J Am Coll Cardiol.* 1995;26:1581–1585.

34. Nagaya N, Nishikimi T, Okano Y, et al. Plasma brain natriuretic peptide levels increase in proportion to the extent of right ventricular dysfunction in pulmonary hypertension. *J Am Coll Cardiol.* 1998;31: 202–208.

35. Leuchte HH, Holzapfel M, Baumgartner RA, et al. Clinical significance of brain natriuretic peptide in primary pulmonary hypertension. *J Am Coll Cardiol.* 2004;43:764–770.

36. Kruger S, Graf J, Merx MW, et al. Brain natriuretic peptide predicts right heart failure in patients with acute pulmonary embolism. *Am Heart J.* 2004;147:60–65.

37. Kline JA, Zeitouni R, Marchick MR, Hernandez-Nino J, Rose GA. Comparison of 8 biomarkers for prediction of right ventricular hypokinesis 6 months after submassive pulmonary embolism. *Am Heart J.* 2008;156:308–314.

38. Coutance G, Le Page O, Lo T, Hamon M. Prognostic value of brain natriuretic peptide in acute pulmonary embolism. *Crit Care.* 2008;12:R109.

39. Matsuo K, Nishikimi T, Yutani C, et al. Diagnostic value of plasma levels of brain natriuretic peptide in arrhythmogenic right ventricular dysplasia. *Circulation.* 1998;98:2433–2440.

40. Golbasy Z, Ucar O, Yuksel AG, Gulel O, Aydogdu S, Ulusoy V. Plasma brain natriuretic peptide levels in patients with rheumatic heart disease. *Eur J Heart Fail.* 2004;6:757–760.

41. Yoshimura M, Yasue H, Okumura K, et al. Different secretion patterns of atrial natriuretic peptide and brain natriuretic peptide in patients with congestive heart failure. *Circulation.* 1993;87:464–469.

42. Ledoux S, Dussaule JC, Michel PL, et al. Acute and delayed hormonal changes in mitral stenosis treated by balloon valvulotomy. *Am J Cardiol.* 1993;72:932–938.

43. Davutoglu V, Celik A, Aksoy M, Sezen Y, Soydinc S, Gunay N. Plasma NT-proBNP is a potential marker of disease severity and correlates with symptoms in patients with chronic rheumatic valve disease. *Eur J Heart Fail.* 2005;7:532–536.

44. Arat-Ozkan A, Kaya A, Yigit Z, et al. Serum N-terminal pro-BNP levels correlate with symptoms and echocardiographic findings in patients with mitral stenosis. *Echocardiography.* 2005;22:473–478.

45. Iltumur K, Karabulut A, Yokus B, Yavuzkir M, Taskesen T, Toprak N. N-terminal proBNP plasma levels correlate with severity of mitral stenosis. *J Heart Valve Dis.* 2005;14:735–741.

46. Hung JS, Fu M, Cherng WJ, et al. Rapid fall in elevated plasma atrial natriuretic peptide levels after successful catheter balloon valvuloplasty of mitral stenosis. *Am Heart J.* 1989;117:381–385.

47. Waldman HM, Palacios IF, Block PC, et al. Responsiveness of plasma atrial natriuretic factor to short-term changes in left atrial hemodynamics after percutaneous balloon mitral valvuloplasty. *J Am Coll Cardiol.* 1988;12:649–655.

48. Nakamura M, Kawata Y, Yoshida H, et al. Relationship between plasma atrial and brain natriuretic peptide concentration and hemodynamic parameters during percutaneous transvenous mitral valvulotomy in patients with mitral stenosis. *Am Heart J.* 1992;124:1283–1288.

49. Shang YP, Lai L, Chen J, Zhang F, Wang X. Effects of percutaneous balloon mitral valvuloplasty on plasma B-type natriuretic peptide in rheumatic mitral stenosis with and without atrial fibrillation. *J Heart Valve Dis.* 2005;14:453–459.

50. Razzolini R, Leoni L, Cafiero F, et al. Neurohormones in mitral stenosis before and after percutaneous balloon mitral valvotomy. *J Heart Valve Dis.* 2002;11:185–190.

51. Detaint D, Messika-Zeitoun D, Avierinos JF, et al. B-type natriuretic peptide in organic mitral regurgitation: determinants and impact on outcome. *Circulation.* 2005;111:2391–2397.

52. Brookes CI, Kemp MW, Hooper J, Oldershaw PJ, Moat NE. Plasma brain natriuretic peptide concentrations in patients with chronic mitral regurgitation. *J Heart Valve Dis.* 1997;6:608–612.

53. Sutton TM, Stewart RA, Gerber IL, et al. Plasma natriuretic peptide levels increase with symptoms and severity of mitral regurgitation. *J Am Coll Cardiol.* 2003;41:2280–2287.

54. Ikeda T, Matsuda K, Itoh H, et al. Plasma levels of brain and atrial natriuretic peptides elevate in proportion to left ventricular end-systolic wall stress in patients with aortic stenosis. *Am Heart J.* 1997;133:307–314.

55. Qi W, Mathisen P, Kjekshus J, et al. Natriuretic peptides in patients with aortic stenosis. *Am Heart J.* 2001;142:725–732.

56. Talwar S, Downie PF, Squire IB, Davies JE, Barnett DB, Ng LL. Plasma N-terminal pro BNP and cardiotrophin-1 are elevated in aortic stenosis. *Eur J Heart Fail.* 2001;3:15–19.

57. Lim P, Monin JL, Monchi M, et al. Predictors of outcome in patients with severe aortic stenosis and normal left ventricular function: role of B-type natriuretic peptide. *Eur Heart J.* 2004;25:2048–2053.

58. Nessmith MG, Fukuta H, Brucks S, Little WC. Usefulness of an elevated B-type natriuretic peptide in predicting survival in patients with aortic stenosis treated without surgery. *Am J Cardiol.* 2005;96:1445–1448.

59. Bergler-Klein J, Mundigler G, Pibarot P, et al. B-type natriuretic peptide in low-flow, low-gradient aortic stenosis: relationship to hemodynamics and clinical outcome: results from the Multicenter Truly or Pseudo-Severe Aortic Stenosis (TOPAS) study. *Circulation.* 2007;115:2848–2855.

60. Gerber IL, Stewart RA, Legget ME, et al. Increased plasma natriuretic peptide levels reflect symptom onset in aortic stenosis. *Circulation.* 2003;107:1884–1890.

61. Gerber IL, Legget ME, West TM, Richards AM, Stewart RA. Usefulness of serial measurement of N-terminal pro-brain natriuretic peptide plasma levels in asymptomatic patients with aortic stenosis to predict symptomatic deterioration. *Am J Cardiol.* 2005;95:898–901.

62. Gerber IL, Stewart RA, French JK, et al. Associations between plasma natriuretic peptide levels, symptoms, and left ventricular function in patients with chronic aortic regurgitation. *Am J Cardiol.* 2003; 92:755–758.
63. Ozkan M, Baysan O, Erinc K, et al. Brain natriuretic peptide and the severity of aortic regurgitation: is there any correlation? *J Int Med Res.* 2005;33:454–459.
64. Eimer MJ, Ekery DL, Rigolin VH, Bonow RO, Carnethon MR, Cotts WG. Elevated B-type natriuretic peptide in asymptomatic men with chronic aortic regurgitation and preserved left ventricular systolic function. *Am J Cardiol.* 2004;94:676–678.
65. Inoue S, Murakami Y, Sano K, Katoh H, Shimada T. Atrium as a source of brain natriuretic polypeptide in patients with atrial fibrillation. *J Card Fail.* 2000;6:92–96.
66. Tuinenburg AE, Brundel BJ, Van Gelder IC, et al. Gene expression of the natriuretic peptide system in atrial tissue of patients with paroxysmal and persistent atrial fibrillation. *J Cardiovasc Electrophysiol.* 1999;10:827–835.
67. Shin DI, Jaekel K, Schley P, et al. Plasma levels of NT-pro-BNP in patients with atrial fibrillation before and after electrical cardioversion. *Z Kardiol.* 2005;94:795–800.
68. Morello A, Lloyd-Jones DM, Chae CU, et al. Association of atrial fibrillation and amino-terminal pro-brain natriuretic peptide concentrations in dyspneic subjects with and without acute heart failure: results from the ProBNP Investigation of Dyspnea in the Emergency Department (PRIDE) study. *Am Heart J.* 2007;153:90–97.
69. Knudsen CW, Omland T, Clopton P, et al. Impact of atrial fibrillation on the diagnostic performance of B-type natriuretic peptide concentration in dyspneic patients: an analysis from the breathing not properly multinational study. *J Am Coll Cardiol.* 2005;46:838–844.
70. Tóth M, Vuorinen KH, Vuolteenaho O, et al. Hypoxia stimulates release of ANP and BNP from perfused rat ventricular myocardium. *Am J Physiol.* 1994;266:H1572–H1580.
71. Goetze JP, Gore A, Moller CH, Steinbruchel DA, Rehfeld JF, Nielsen LB. Acute myocardial hypoxia increases BNP gene expression. *FASEB J.* 2004;18:1928–1930.
72. Goetze JP, Christoffersen C, Perko M, et al. Increased cardiac BNP expression associated with myocardial ischemia. *FASEB J.* 2003;17: 1105–1117.

73. Jernberg T, Stridsberg M, Venge P, Lindahl B. N-terminal pro brain natriuretic peptide on admission for early risk stratification of patients with chest pain and no ST-segment elevation. *J Am Coll Cardiol.* 2002;40:437–445.

74. Heeschen C, Hamm CW, Mitrovic V, Lantelme NH, White HD. N-terminal pro-B-type natriuretic peptide levels for dynamic risk stratification of patients with acute coronary syndromes. *Circulation.* 2004;110:3206–3212.

75. Sabatine MS, Morrow DA, de Lemos JA, et al. Acute changes in circulating natriuretic peptide levels in relation to myocardial ischemia. *J Am Coll Cardiol.* 2004;44:1988–1995.

76. Karabinos I, Karvouni E, Chiotinis N, et al. Acute changes in N-terminal pro-brain natriuretic peptide induced by dobutamine stress echocardiography. *Eur J Echocardiogr.* 2007;8:265–274.

77. Salinas G, Daher IN, Okorodudu AO, Ahmad M. B-type natriuretic peptide is not a marker of ischemia during dobutamine stress echocardiography. *J Am Soc Echocardiogr.* 2007;20:23–26.

19 ■ Population Testing with Natriuretic Peptides: Potential Promises and Pitfalls

Estelle Docteur, MD
Thomas J. Wang, MD

Introduction

The utility of natriuretic peptide measurements in acutely-ill patients with suspected heart failure is well established. Much less is known about the value of assessing natriuretic peptides in the preclinical setting, although recent studies have generated interest in this area. The idea of population testing originated with the observation that natriuretic peptide levels are raised in individuals with asymptomatic left ventricular dysfunction, suggesting a potentially useful screening strategy for the early detection of individuals at risk for heart failure (HF). The rationale for screening to prevent heart failure is reviewed in the first section of this chapter. The next section reviews the evidence that natriuretic peptide levels are a marker of global cardiovascular risk, and describes ongoing work to sort out the potential implications of natriuretic peptides in populations. The final part of the chapter summarizes what is known about the influence of extracardiac factors on circulating natriuretic peptide levels.

Screening with Natriuretic Peptides to Reduce Heart Failure

Heart failure is a major public health problem in the United States,[1,2] with approximately 5.3 million patients affected, and over 660,000 new cases diagnosed each year.[3] It was the primary cause of death for 57,120 patients in 2004, and was responsible for over 1 million hospital discharges in 2005. The direct and indirect cost of heart failure is estimated to be $38.4 billion nationally in 2008.[3]

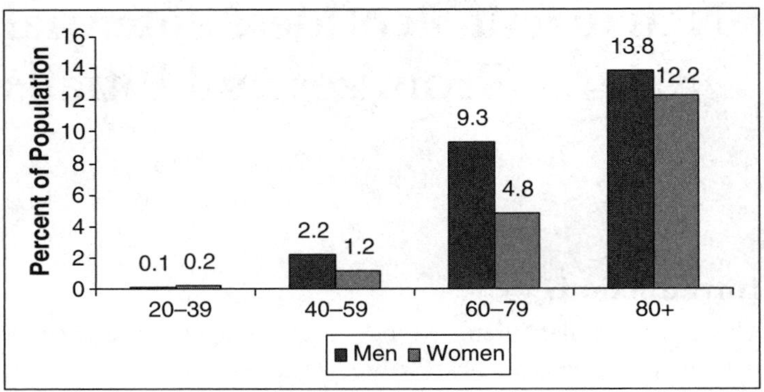

Sources: NCHS and NHLBI.
*NHANES is the National Health and Nutrition Examination Survey.

■ **Figure 19–1** Prevalence of Heart Failure by sex and age (NHANES: 1999-2004). Percentages are age adjusted for Americans ≥20 years of age. These data are based on self-reports. *NHANES is the National Health and Nutrition Examination Survey.

Adapted from Rosamond W, et al. Heart disease and stroke statistics–2008 update: a report from the American Heart Association Statistics Committee and Stroke Statistics Subcommittee. *Circulation*. 2008;117(4):e25–e146.

From an epidemiological standpoint, heart failure is primarily a disease of the elderly (Figure 19–1), with an incidence of 10 per 1000 population in individuals over the age of 65 years.[2] Accordingly, the burden of disease will continue to increase as the elderly population continues to grow and as survival rates after myocardial infarction continue to improve.[2,4]

Heart failure continues to have a high mortality rate in spite of advances made in treatment of this disorder.[1] This has led to considerable effort directed toward identifying and treating individuals prior to the onset of clinical disease.

When it progresses in at-risk patients (or those with so-called Stage A heart failure according to the current American College of Cardiology/American Heart Association [ACC/AHA] practice guidelines),[1] heart failure typically begins with a latent phase, referred to as asymptomatic left ventricular systolic dysfunction

(LVSD),[4] or Stage B in the guidelines. Data from randomized controlled trials indicate that treatment of LVSD with angiotensin-converting enzyme (ACE) inhibitors and beta blockers may significantly improve health outcomes in patients with asymptomatic LVSD.[5,6] For instance, in the Studies of Left Ventricular Dysfunction (SOLVD) Prevention trial, there was a 29% risk reduction in the incidence of death and heart failure, and a 20% risk reduction in the rate of heart failure requiring hospitalizations in the group treated with enalapril compared to placebo.[5] The Survival and Ventricular Enlargement (SAVE) trial showed that patients with asymptomatic LVSD who received long-term captopril after myocardial infarction had a 19% reduction in all-cause mortality, and a 22% reduction in the incidence of heart failure requiring hospitalization.[6] Retrospective analysis of the SAVE data further suggested that treatment with beta blockers resulted in a significant reduction in the risk of heart failure (21%).[7] Hence, the current ACC/AHA guidelines advocate treatment with ACE inhibitors in patients at high risk for developing heart failure, and treatment with beta blockers in patients with reduced ejection fraction (EF).[1]

The results from SOLVD and SAVE have led many to consider widespread screening for asymptomatic LVSD,[8] particularly among patients at high risk for developing LVSD, such as those with diabetes mellitus.[9,10] Asymptomatic LVSD is as prevalent as heart failure in the general population, with estimates of prevalence ranging from 0.9% to 12.9% in various studies (Table 19–1).[11] The time course to progression to heart failure in individuals with mild LVSD (EF 40–50%) is approximately ten years, suggesting a window of opportunity in which high-risk patients could be identified and possibly treated.[4]

For diagnosing LVSD, echocardiography is considered the gold standard. However, widespread screening with echocardiography is not possible given issues of cost and limited access.[12,13] Another potential screening tool is the electrocardiogram because a normal electrocardiogram is associated with a low risk of LVSD.[14] However, the electrocardiogram has low specificity for the detection of asymptomatic LSVD.[11] In a study by Galasko et al., the

Table 19–1 Prevalence of LVSD by ejection fraction threshold.

Study (reference)	Country	N	Age	Male	LVSD Criteria	Prevalence of LVSD	Prevalence of LVSD without CHF
EF above 40% or equivalent							
Strong Heart Study (American Indians)[104]	U.S.	3184	58	37%	EF ≤ 54%	14.0%	12.5%
HyperGEN Study[105]	U.S.	2086	55	38%	EF ≤ 54%	14.0%	12.9%
Redfield et al.[106]	U.S.	2042	62	48%	EF ≤ 50%	6.0%	4.7%
Davies et al.[107]	England	3960	61	50%	EF ≤ 50%	5.3%	3.3%
MONICA project (Augsburg)[108]	Germany	1566	50	48%	EF < 48%	2.7%	1.1%*
Hedberg et al.[109]	Sweden	412	75	50%	WMI < 1.7	6.8%	3.2%
Nielsen et al.[110]	Denmark	126	70	55%	WMI ≤ 1.5 or FS < 0.26	2.9%	1.0%
Rotterdam Study[111]	Netherlands	2267	66	45%	FS ≤ 25%	3.7%	2.9%†
Helsinki Aging Study[112]	Finland	501	–‡	27%	FS < 25%	10.8%	8.6%

EF 40% or below							
Strong Heart Study[104]	U.S.	3184	58	37%	EF < 40%	2.9%	2.1%
HyperGEN Study[105]	U.S.	2086	55	38%	EF < 40%	4.0%	3.4%
Redfield et al.[106]	U.S.	2042	62	48%	EF ≤ 40%	2.0%	1.0%
Davies et al.[107]	England	3960	61	50%	EF < 40%	1.8%	0.9%
MONICA project (Glasgow)[113]	Scotland	1467	50	48%	EF ≤ 35%	7.7%	5.9%
MONICA project (Glasgow)[113]	Scotland	1467	50	48%	EF ≤ 30%	2.9%	1.4%
Qualitatively "reduced" EF							
Cardiovascular Health Study[114]	U.S.	5532	73	42%	Qualitative§	3.5%	2.5%
Morgan et al.[115]	England	817	76	46%	Qualitative	7.5%	3.9%

*Without symptoms or known cardiovascular disease.

†Based on 1698 subjects.

‡Range 75–86 years.

§Categorized as "impaired" systolic dysfunction.

Notes: CHF: congestive heart failure; EF: ejection fraction; FS: fractional shortening; HyperGEN: Hypertension Genetic Epidemiology Network study; LVSD: left ventricular systolic dysfunction; MONICA: Monitoring Trends and Determinants in Cardiovascular Disease study; WMI: wall motion index.

Source: Modified and adapted with permission from Wang TJ, Levy D, Benjamin EJ, Vasan RS. The epidemiology of "asymptomatic" left ventricular systolic dysfunction: implications for screening. *Ann Intern Med.* 2003;138(11):907–916.

electrocardiogram had a sensitivity of 90% to 92% for LVSD in the general population, but a specificity of only 64–78% and a positive predictive value of only 14–19%.[12]

The natriuretic peptides have emerged as a potential screening tool because of their availability, low cost for serial testing, and elevation in LVSD.[15] McDonagh and colleagues found that BNP levels were significantly higher in participants with LVSD (mean 24.0 pg/mL) than in those with normal LV function (mean 7.7 pg/mL), levels that are well below the conventional cutoff values used for the diagnosis of heart failure in acutely dyspneic patients (BNP < 100 pg/mL,[16] NT-proBNP < 300 pg/mL[17]). For detecting LVSD in the McDonagh study, plasma BNP levels of 17.9 pg/mL or greater had a sensitivity of 77% and specificity of 87%. Sensitivity and specificity rose to 92% and 72% in participants aged 55 years or older.[15]

Other studies examining the performance of natriuretic peptides as screening tests for LVSD in the general population are shown in Table 19–2. Performance of these assays is influenced by the prevalence of LVSD and the ejection fraction threshold values used to define LV dysfunction.[18] In population-based studies using different BNP and amino-terminal pro atrial natriuretic peptide (NT-proANP) partition values, the sensitivities and specificities for detecting LSVD ranged from 26% to 92%, and 34% to 89%, respectively. The area under the receiver-operating-characteristic curve (AUC) estimates ranged from 0.56 to 0.88.[11] In addition, the threshold values for detecting LVSD have varied up to fourfold in different studies.[19]

The Framingham Heart Study group evaluated the diagnostic performance of BNP for detecting elevated left ventricular (LV) mass and LVSD in healthy participants, and found that the AUC estimates for detecting any LVSD (EF ≤ 50% and/or fractional shortening <29%), and moderate to severe LVSD (EF ≤ 40%, and/or fractional shortening <22%) were 0.72 and 0.79 in men, and 0.56 and 0.85 in women, respectively. The diagnostic performance in women improved when the natriuretic peptides were evaluated

Table 19–2: Use of natriuretic peptides for identifying left ventricular systolic dysfunction.

Study/setting	N	Definition of LVSD	Discrimination Limit	Sensitivity	Specificity	AUC
Community-based studies						
Framingham Heart Study[19]	1470 (men)	FS < 29%*	BNP level > 21 pg/ml	53%	84%	0.72
Framingham Heart Study[19]	1707 (women)	FS < 29%*	BNP level > 21 pg/ml	26%	89%	0.56
Olmsted County[106]	2042	EF < 40%	BNP level > 25.9 pg/ml	62%	63%	0.79
MONICA project (Augsburg)[116]	479	FS < 28%	BNP level > 34 pg/ml	28%	86%	0.61
Uppsala, Sweden[117]	205 (men)	EF ≤ 40%	NT-ANP level > 398 pmol/l	86%	75%	0.83
MONICA project (Glasgow)[15]	1252	EF < 35%	BNP level > 17.9 pg/ml	43%	88%	–
MONICA project (Glasgow)[15]	1252	EF < 30%	BNP level > 17.9 pg/ml	77%	87%	0.88

Table 19–2: (Continued)

Study/setting	N	Definition of LVSD	Discrimination Limit	Sensitivity	Specificity	AUC
Referral series						
Echocardiography laboratory[118]	466	EF < 45%	BNP level > 37 pg/ml	79%	64%	0.79
Echocardiography laboratory[119]	400	EF < 50%†	BNP level > 87 pg/ml	90%	67%	0.82
Nuclear laboratory[120]	75	EF ≤ 0.55	BNP level > 30 pg/ml	58%	76%	0.70
Nuclear laboratory[121]	180	EF < 45%‡	NT-ANP level > 54 pmol/l	90%	92%	–
Nuclear laboratory[122]	87	EF ≤ 35%	BNP level > 13.8 pg/ml	100%	58%	0.88
Catheterization laboratory[13]	94	EF < 45%	BNP level > 61.2 pg/ml	83%	81%	0.85
Catheterization laboratory[123]	254	EF < 45%	–	–	–	0.74

*or mild or greater reduction in EF on visual estimation.
†or wall motion abnormalities.
‡at rest, or <55% with exercise.
Notes: AUC: area under the receiver-operating characteristic curve; BNP: brain natriuretic peptide; EF: ejection fraction; FS: fractional shortening; MONICA: Monitoring Trends and Determinants in Cardiovascular Disease study; NT-ANP: N-terminal pro-atrial natriuretic peptide.
Source: Modified and adapted with permission from Wang TJ, Levy D, Benjamin EJ, Vasan RS. The epidemiology of "asymptomatic" left ventricular systolic dysfunction: implications for screening. *Ann Intern Med.* 2003;138(11):907–916.

in the high-risk group, with an AUC of 0.86. The plasma BNP levels used to yield 95% specificity for detection of LVSD were 45 pg/mL in men and 50 pg/mL in women. These investigators concluded that insufficient evidence existed to recommend use of natriuretic peptides for widespread community screening for LVSD.[19] Similarly, data from Olmsted County showed that BNP had a suboptimal screening performance for asymptomatic LVSD in that population. The AUC estimates for the detection of an EF less than 50% or diastolic dysfunction were both less than 0.70. In the high-risk subgroup, the AUC estimates for the detection of an EF less than or equal to 40% were 0.85 in men and 0.74 in women. These investigators reported that 10% to 40% of patients screened with plasma BNP would require confirmatory testing with an echocardiogram as a result of a high BNP level. However, most of these echocardiograms would be negative. Furthermore, up to 60% of those affected with LVSD would be missed with this strategy.[20]

Plasma NT-proBNP levels appear to be at least equivalent to plasma BNP levels for detecting LVSD,[21,22] and may be superior in detecting LVSD in men and in elderly patients.[23] The Copenhagen City Heart Study examined the use of plasma NT-proBNP for detecting LVSD or increased LV mass.[24] Normal plasma NT-proBNP levels had a high negative predictive value (≥ 99%) in excluding LVSD compared to echocardiography, but the positive predictive values for detecting any cardiovascular disease in the general population and high-risk population were only 56% and 62%, respectively.[25]

Based on the above data, the current National Academy of Clinical Biochemistry Laboratory Medicine Practice Guidelines do not recommend routine screening with plasma BNP or NT-proBNP for the detection of left ventricular dysfunction in the asymptomatic patient population.[26] In addition to performance characteristics for detecting subclinical LVSD, however, considerations such as cost may influence the usefulness of a screening strategy. Hendrich and colleagues evaluated a strategy of screening asymptomatic individuals with BNP by only referring those with elevated BNP levels (BNP > 24 pg/mL in men and > 34 pg/mL in women) for echocardiography. The gender-specific sensitivity and specificity of BNP testing for detecting LVSD were based on data from the Framingham and Olmsted County cohorts, and the assumption regarding treatment benefit with ACE inhibitors was based on the data from the SOLVD prevention study. The investigators concluded that a screening strategy using echocardiography to confirm an abnormal BNP tests was cost-effective in men at age 60 years, and perhaps in women at age 60 years. This screening strategy was estimated to provide a health benefit at a cost of < \$50,000 per quality-adjusted life year (QALY), provided that the prevalence of LVSD (EF < 40%) was at least 1%. A cost-effectiveness ratio of < \$20,000 per QALY was attainable if the prevalence of LVSD exceeded 3% for women and 4% for men.[27]

Nielsen and colleagues performed a retrospective analysis of the cost-effectiveness of BNP in screening for LVSD, and reported that screening may be of greater utility in higher risk groups.[28] The investigators stratified the subjects into three groups: those with symptomatic ischemic heart disease; those with blood pressure > 160/95 mmHg and/or abnormal electrocardiogram (high risk); and healthy subjects with no risk factors (low risk). Screening in high-risk patients with BNP could potentially reduce the cost per detected case of LVSD by 21% to 26% compared with echocardiography alone.[28]

Ultimately, the cost-effectiveness of BNP or NT-proBNP testing for screening will depend in part on cost issues, such as the pricing of the echocardiogram and the natriuretic peptide assay,[28] in addition to the specificity of the assay used to screen for LVSD, which will determine how many echocardiograms are ordered.[29] On the other hand, it is worthwhile to emphasize that the benefits of screening also need to be established more precisely. Existing trials with ACE inhibitors have focused on patients with an EF less than or equal to 35%.[5,6] The majority of the individuals in the general population with asymptomatic LVSD would have been excluded from the SOLVD and SAVE trials because most have milder systolic dysfunction (EF 40–50%). Furthermore, the prevalence of underlying coronary disease was higher in the SOLVD and SAVE populations compared with those with LVSD in the community. Thus, it remains an open question whether unselected individuals would benefit to the same extent as those enrolled in the trials.

Natriuretic Peptides as Markers of Global Cardiovascular Risk: Potential Promises

Emerging literature suggests that the information provided by natriuretic peptide levels is not limited to LVSD or risk of future heart failure. Studies such as those summarized below indicate that mild elevations in natriuretic peptide levels in ambulatory individuals predict a higher risk of a variety of cardiovascular events. Interest in identifying new global markers of cardiovascular risk factors stems in part from the recognition that many cases of cardiovascular disease occur in individuals without traditional risk factors, such as hypertension, hyperlipidemia, smoking, or diabetes.[30,31]

The Framingham Heart Study investigators examined natriuretic peptide levels in ambulatory individuals without evidence of heart failure or renal failure and found that plasma BNP and NT-proANP levels predicted the risk of death and cardiovascular events after adjustment for traditional risk factors (Figure 19–2). A graded relationship existed between levels of BNP within the normal range and the risk for cardiovascular events. Thus, each increment of one standard deviation (SD) in log BNP values was associated with increased risk for all-cause mortality (by 27%), a first major cardiovascular event (28%), heart failure (77%), atrial fibrillation (66%), and stroke or transient ischemic attack (53%). BNP values above the 80th percentile (20 pg/mL for men and 23.3 pg/mL for women) were associated with a 62% increased risk of death and 76% increased risk for a first major cardiovascular event. The strongest associations were seen with heart failure and

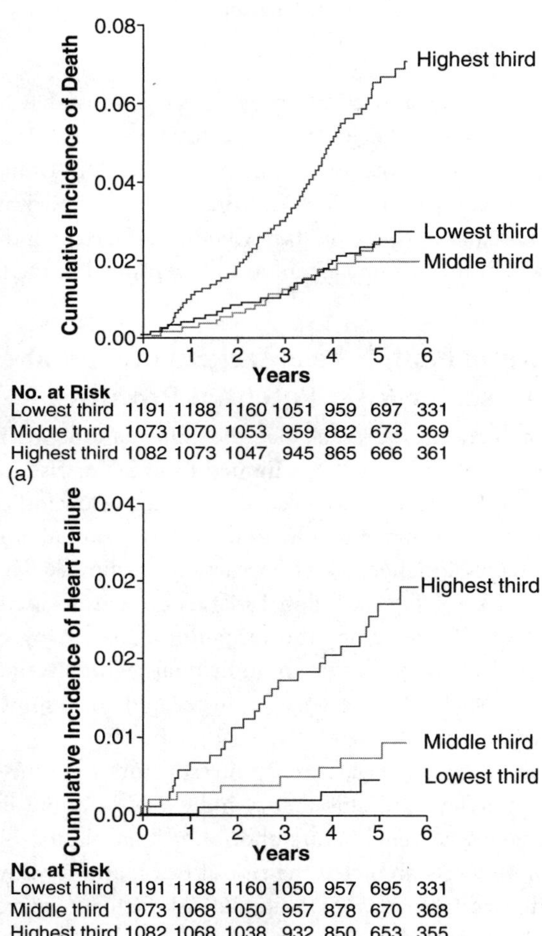

■ **Figure 19–2** Cumulative Incidence of Death (Panel A) and Heart Failure (Panel B), According to the Plasma B-Type Natriuretic Peptide Level at Base Line. The lowest third, middle third, and highest third of plasma B-type natriuretic peptide levels were 4.0 pg per milliliter or less, 4.1 to 12.7 pg per milliliter, and 12.8 pg per milliliter or more, respectively, for men and 5.9 pg per illiliter or less, 6.0 to 15.7 pg per milliliter, and 15.8 pg per milliliter or more, respectively, for women. Follow-up results are truncated after six years.

Adapted from Wang TJ, Larson MG, Levy D, et al. Plasma natriuretic peptide levels and the risk of cardiovascular events and death. *N Eng J Med.* 2004;350(7): 655–663.

atrial fibrillation, with multivariable-adjusted hazard ratios of 3.07 and 1.91, respectively.[30]

The prognostic value of natriuretic peptides for future cardiovascular events in the general population was also demonstrated in the Olmsted County cohort. The investigators compared NT-proBNP and BNP using three different assays and found that BNP and NT-proBNP levels predicted mortality above and beyond traditional and echocardiographic risk factors. Compared to BNP levels, NT-proBNP had a higher predictive value for mortality—after adjusting for clinical and echocardiographic variables[32]—suggesting possible superiority of NT-proBNP for the prognostication of apparently normal individuals.

The natriuretic peptides have also been shown to predict future cardiovascular risk and mortality in other large population studies outside of the United States.[33–36] In the Glasgow MONICA (Monitoring Trends and Determinants in Cardiovascular Disease) project, BNP was an independent predictor of death in the general population aged 25–74 years. The median plasma BNP levels in the participants who died was 16.9 pg/mL compared to 7.8 pg/mL in those who survived, using four years of follow-up data. Patients with an EF greater than 40% had a mortality rate of 8.5% if the plasma BNP level was greater than 17.9 pg/mL, compared to 2% in those with plasma BNP levels less than 17.9 pg/mL.[37] Another population-based study of individuals aged 50 to 89 years (mean age 67.9 years) in the ambulatory setting in Copenhagen, Denmark, showed that the prognostic information from NT-proBNP was independent of traditional risk factors, pre-existing cardiac disease, LVSD, and renal function.[38] Further, NT-proBNP was a better predictor of mortality and first major cardiovascular events than C-reactive protein (CRP) or urinary microalbumin. Each SD increase in log NT-proBNP was associated with a 92% increased risk for first major cardiovascular event and a 76% increased risk for ischemic stroke.[38] BNP has also been shown to be a strong and independent predictor of all-cause mortality in older populations (aged 80 years or higher).[34,36]

A strategy incorporating both traditional risk factors and cardiac biomarkers can potentially enhance the efforts of both primary and secondary preventive therapies. However, there has been much debate over the utility and validity of biomarkers for primary prevention.[39] The area under the receiver-operating-characteristic curve (c-statistic) is currently used in most of the models for risk prediction in cardiovascular research, but some argue that the c-statistic may not be the best method for assessing models that predict future risk or stratify individuals into risk categories.[40] To assess the predictive accuracy of biomarkers for cardiovascular events, the investigators from the Framingham Heart Study group examined ten biomarkers (including BNP, NT-proANP, CRP, homocysteine, and urinary albumin-to-creatine ratio) from different biological pathways. As evidenced by small changes in the c-statistic, these ten biomarkers did not clearly contribute substantially to conventional risk factors. That said, BNP was a better predictor of death and first major cardiovascular events when compared to the other nine biomarkers[41] and the approach to using c-statistic change as the gold standard for validating importance of biomarkers has been questioned.

Recent data from participants in the Uppsala Longitudinal Study of Adult Men (USLAM) project suggest that the risk stratification for death from cardiovascular disease in elderly men (mean age 71 years) improved with the addition of several biomarkers, including NT-proBNP. In those without cardiovascular disease, the c-statistic increased from 0.688 to 0.748 when four biomarkers (NT-proBNP, troponin I, cystatin C, and CRP) were added into a risk model with traditional risk factors.[42] Differences with the Framingham data have been attributed to the contrasting study populations, with the Swedish study focusing on a sample that was not only older, but also at higher risk, and in which conventional risk factors fared relatively poorly (c-statistic less than 0.70).

The concept that natriuretic peptides may be useful in relatively high-risk, though ambulatory, populations is supported by several secondary prevention studies. In the Heart and Soul Study cohort, composed of individuals with known coronary disease, each SD increase in log NT-proBNP level was associated with a 1.7-fold adjusted hazard ratio for cardiovascular events. The c-statistic improved from 0.76 to 0.80 with the addition of NT-proBNP to traditional risk factors and echocardiographic parameters.[43] In the Heart Outcomes Prevention Evaluation (HOPE) Study, the addition of NT-proBNP to conventional risk factors provided the best prediction of recurrent cardiovascular events, compared with nine other inflammatory biomarkers, and raised the c-statistic significantly. Nearly all patients in this study had some form of established cardiovascular disease.[44] Similarly, in the Heart Protection Study, baseline NT-proBNP levels were predictive of future heart failure and major cardiovascular events, after adjustment for other clinical characteristics.[45]

In summary, the natriuretic peptides are independent predictors of cardiovascular events, heart failure, and death in asymptomatic individuals,[37] and provide important prognostic information beyond the traditional cardiovascular risk factors;[30] BNP and NT-proBNP appear to be better predictors of cardiovascular disease[13,46,47] and mortality[29] when compared with ANP. Some data suggest that NT-proBNP may have a higher predictive value for mortality compared with BNP, but few studies have compared the peptides head-to-head.[32] Importantly, for the clinician, plasma natriuretic peptide values associated with increased risk of death and cardiovascular outcomes in apparently well subjects are well below the standard cutoff values used for the diagnosis of heart failure in acutely dyspneic patients (BNP $<$ 100 pg/mL ([16]), NT-proBNP $<$ 300pg/mL ([17])). Thus, natriuretic peptide values below the heart failure cutoffs cannot necessarily be regarded as "normal" or indicative of low cardiovascular risk.[30]

The recent interest in biomarker testing for prediction of global cardiovascular risk has also revealed limitations of current tests, and engendered an ongoing debate over the appropriate ways to assess the usefulness of a biomarker test and the appropriate subgroups to consider for testing. These questions are only likely to be answered with data from additional large studies. Overall, the role for natriuretic peptides, as well as other biomarkers, in population screening for cardiovascular disease remains an active area of investigation.

Effect of Various Noncardiac Influences on Natriuretic Peptides: Potential Pitfalls

Natriuretic peptide levels are elevated in a variety of settings other than acute[16] and chronic heart failure.[48,49] Accordingly, these confounding factors must be taken into account when interpreting BNP and NT-proBNP values, particularly in the ambulatory setting. Several physiological and pathological conditions,[50] including advanced age and female gender,[51,52] obesity,[53] metabolic traits,[54,55] renal disease,[56] acute coronary syndromes,[57,58] pulmonary disease,[59] pulmonary embolism,[60] atrial fibrillation,[61] and drugs[62] have been shown to affect plasma natriuretic peptide levels. We will focus our discussion on the effects of age, sex, obesity, and metabolic traits.

Advanced Age

Both plasma BNP[52] and NT-proBNP[63] levels increase with age. Initial clinical studies argued that the higher BNP levels were the result of renal dysfunction, systolic or diastolic dysfunction, and increased myocardial mass.[64] However, recent studies suggest that plasma BNP levels are elevated in healthy elderly patients without any evidence of cardiovascular disease or valvular heart disease.[51,53] The Framingham Heart Study investigators examined plasma BNP levels in healthy subjects, and found that a ten-year increase in age was associated with a 1.4-fold increase in plasma BNP levels. The use of age-pooled reference limits compared with age-specific limits classified a higher percentage of healthy elderly subjects (17% versus 2.5%) as "abnormal," but a lower percentage of healthy young subjects without cardiovascular disease as "abnormal" (1% versus 2.5%).[52] Data from the Mayo Clinic showed that the age relation persisted even after excluding patients with abnormal systolic and diastolic on a research echocardiogram.[51]

The exact physiological basis for the age-related increase in natriuretic peptide levels is unclear. The higher prevalence of subclinical cardiac disease in the elderly population does not seem to fully explain the several-fold differences observed across age groups.[64,65] Potential mechanisms for the increased natriuretic peptide levels with advancing age include chamber-specific increases in natriuretic peptide gene expression,[66] and a reduction in expression of the clearance receptor.[48,67–69]

Sex

In the absence of severe heart failure, concentrations of BNP and NT-proBNP are higher in women compared to men across all ages.[51,52,63] Data from the Framingham Heart Study showed that compared with healthy men, healthy women had 1.6-fold higher BNP levels.[52] The mechanisms whereby gender influences BNP levels are unclear, but may in part be related to the effect of sex hormones. In animal studies, female sex hormones have a stimulatory effect on natriuretic peptide gene expression.[70] One study in postmenopausal women showed an increase in plasma BNP levels after three months of hormone replacement therapy (HRT) with transdermal estradiol.[71] Redfield and colleagues showed that older women on HRT had higher BNP levels compared with women not on HRT.[51] Circulating plasma BNP levels were 99% higher in women on HRT compared with men, and were 21% higher in women on HRT compared with women not on HRT. The use of estrogen also influenced NT-proBNP levels in the same community cohort, but to a lesser extent after adjusting for age and gender.[23] Data from healthy, premenopausal women (aged 35 to 49 years) in the Reynolds Women's Study, which is a substudy of the Dallas Heart study, suggest that circulating free testosterone—and not estradiol—is associated with differences in BNP and NT-proBNP levels.[72] In the context of acute heart failure, sex-related differences in BNP or NT-proBNP concentrations are no longer seen.

Obesity

Concentrations of natriuretic peptide levels are significantly lower in overweight and obese patients compared with nonobese patients.[53,73] The inverse relationship between natriuretic peptides and body mass index (BMI) has been observed in patients with acute[74,75] and chronic heart failure as well.[76]

The Framingham Heart Study investigators examined the relationship of BMI to plasma BNP and NT-proANP in healthy participants without evidence of heart failure and found a strong inverse correlation. The mean plasma BNP levels in lean (BMI < 25 kg/m^2), overweight (BMI 25–29.9 kg/m^2), and obese (BMI > 30 kg/m^2) men were 21.4, 15.5, and 12.7 pg/mL, respectively. Corresponding plasma BNP values in women were 21.1, 16.3, and 13.1 pg/mL, and all differences were statistically significant (Figure 19–3). This inverse relationship was independent of age, clinical, and echocardiographic variables.[53]

It has been postulated that obese individuals have an impaired natriuretic peptide response, called a natriuretic handicap, and that this phenomenon contributes to the increased susceptibility of obese patients to fluid retention, hypertension, and heart failure.[77] Nonetheless, in spite of the lower natriuretic peptide levels in obese patients, higher BNP values within any BMI category portend a worse prognosis.[78]

The exact mechanism for the lower natriuretic peptide levels in obese patients is unknown, but presumably involves either reduced secretion,[79] impaired synthesis,[80] increased clearance (least likely), or some combination of the above. Natriuretic peptide clearance receptors (NPR-Cs) are expressed on adipocytes cells[81,82] and neutral endopeptidases are secreted by fat tissue; both would be expected to lead to lower BNP values. However, the N-terminal pro-peptides (NT-proANP and NT-proBNP) neither bind to NPR-Cs, nor are they degraded by neutral endopeptidases; both are reduced in parallel to BNP in obesity, suggesting that reduced secretion or synthesis is a more important mechanism than

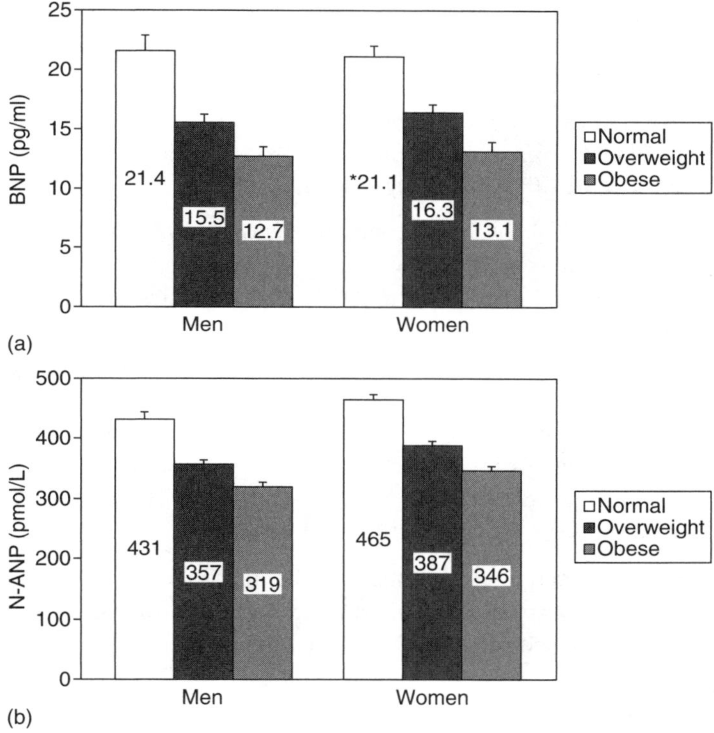

■ **Figure 19–3** Adjusted means for plasma BNP (A) and N-ANP (B) by BMI category. Bars indicate SE.

Adapted from Wang TJ, Larson MG, Levy D, et al. Impact of obesity on plasma natriuretic peptide levels. *Circulation*. 2004;109(5):594–600.

increased clearance.[73,83] Investigators from the Dallas Heart Study showed that the negative association between BMI and BNP and NT-proBNP was more closely linked with lean mass than fat mass, leading them to postulate that sex steroid hormones played a mediating role because they are produced in the lean mass.[73] The association between higher BMI and lean mass with natriuretic peptides was not present after adjustment for free testosterone levels.[72]

Metabolic Risk Factors

The National Cholesterol Education Program (NCEP) Adult Treatment Panel (ATP III) definition of the metabolic syndrome,[84] with modifications recommended by the American Heart Association and National Heart, Lung, and Blood Institute,[85] includes three or more of the following five criteria:

1. abdominal obesity (waist circumference ≥ 102 cm in men, ≥ 88 cm in women);
2. fasting triglycerides ≥ 150 mg/dL or use of fibrates or nicotinic acid;
3. reduced high-density lipoprotein (HDL) (< 40 mg/dL in men, < 50 mg/dL in women);
4. systolic blood pressure ≥ 130 mmHg, diastolic blood pressure ≥ 85mmHg), or use of antihypertensive medications; and
5. fasting glucose ≥ 100 mg/dL or use of hypoglycemic medications.

The main underlying risk factors for the metabolic syndrome are abdominal obesity and insulin resistance and these two risk factors are associated with increased risk for cardiovascular disease and diabetes.[86]

Early data on the association between metabolic risk factors and natriuretic peptides were conflicting.[63,87–90] However, two recent, large, population-based studies have demonstrated consistent negative correlations between metabolic traits and natriuretic peptide levels, even after adjusting for BMI.[54,55] Olsen et al. showed in a Danish cohort that serum NT-proBNP was inversely associated with serum insulin, cholesterol, and triglycerides. The prevalence of metabolic syndrome was relatively low in that sample. The Framingham Heart Study group evaluated the association of plasma BNP levels with metabolic risk factors, the metabolic syndrome, and insulin resistance in healthy participants without evidence of heart failure. With the exception of blood pressure, all of the metabolic risk factors were inversely associated with plasma natriuretic peptides, even after adjusting for BMI (Figure 19–4).[55] Plasma BNP levels were 24% lower in men and 29% lower in

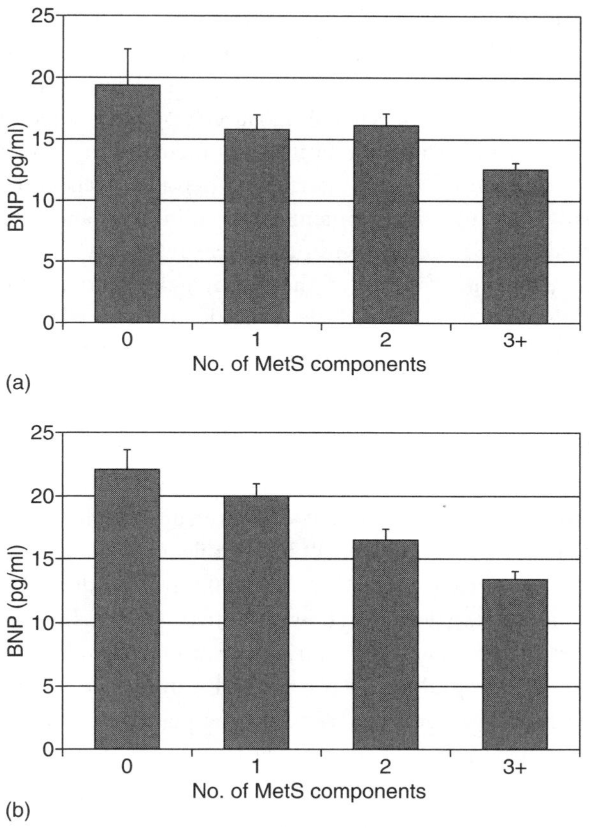

■ **Figure 19–4** Multivariable-adjusted mean plasma BNP levels in men (A) and women (B) according to number of metabolic syndrome criteria. Bars indicate SE.

Adapted from Wang TJ, Larson MG, Keyes MJ, Levy D, Benjamin EJ, Vasan RS. Association of plasma natriuretic peptide levels with metabolic risk factors in ambulatory individuals. *Circulation.* 2007;115(11):1345–1353.

women with the metabolic syndrome. Hypertension is associated with elevated plasma natriuretic peptide levels, likely attributable to the effect of systemic blood pressure on ventricular wall stress.[91,92]

Given the association between natriuretic peptide levels and metabolic risk factors, it is conceivable that natriuretic peptides could influence lipid and glucose metabolism.[55] Prior experimental studies have suggested that the natriuretic peptides affect lipolysis,[93,94] modulate insulin secretion and/or metabolism,[95] and inhibit glucagon secretion.[96] Low natriuretic peptide levels could also predispose to the development of insulin resistance through increased activation of the renin-angiotensin system.[97] The mechanisms by which activation of the renin-angiotensin system promotes insulin resistance[55] include: inhibition of intracellular insulin signaling,[97] enhanced oxidative stress,[98,99] inflammation,[100] and reduced adipocyte differentiation.[101,102]

Conclusion

The natriuretic peptides are released from cardiomyocytes in response to ventricular stretch and pressure overload, and the actions of these molecules result in vasodilatation, natriuresis, and diuresis.[103] A variety of factors, including age, gender, BMI, and metabolic traits, have been shown to affect the baseline levels of natriuretic peptide, and these variables must be taken into account when interpreting BNP and NT-proBNP values.

There has been great interest in using plasma natriuretic peptides as a widespread screening tool for the detection of asymptomatic LVSD.[15] The available evidence does not yet support routine screening in the general population, but it remains possible that testing could be beneficial in selected subgroups.[19,20] Two proposed screening strategies would be to screen all high-risk individuals with plasma BNP,[28] or to screen men over the age of 60 years with plasma BNP, provided that the prevalence of LVSD is at least 1% in the population.[27] An important caveat to screening is that effective treatment with ACE inhibitors has only been shown to improve outcome in patients with an EF less than or equal to 35%, which is uncommon in the community.[5,6] Further studies are needed to establish whether individuals who would be picked up by community screening would benefit similarly from this treatment strategy.[11] In addition, there is less information about the projected costs and benefits of identifying individuals with asymptomatic LVSD, although this ailment is also an important precursor of heart failure.

For global risk prediction, plasma natriuretic peptide levels provide prognostic information that is incremental to traditional risk factors. Indeed, levels within the range currently regarded as "normal" (BNP < 100 pg/mL, NT-proBNP < 300 pg/mL) are still associated with an increased risk of death and cardiovascular events.[30] The cardiovascular risk associated with elevated natriuretic peptide levels may be continuous rather than restricted to values above a threshold. Ultimately, a better understanding of the normal biological and physiological variability in natriuretic peptide levels in healthy individuals is needed so that results in the preclinical setting can be interpreted more reliably.

References

1. Hunt SA, et al. ACC/AHA 2005 Guideline Update for the Diagnosis and Management of Chronic Heart Failure in the Adult: a report of the American College of Cardiology/American Heart Association Task Force on Practice Guidelines (Writing Committee to Update the 2001 Guidelines for the Evaluation and Management of Heart Failure): developed in collaboration with the American College of Chest Physicians and the International Society for Heart and Lung Transplantation: endorsed by the Heart Rhythm Society. *Circulation.* 2005;112(12):e154–e235.
2. Lloyd-Jones DM, et al. Lifetime risk for developing congestive heart failure: the Framingham Heart Study. *Circulation.* 2002;106(24): 3068–3072.
3. Rosamond W, et al. Heart disease and stroke statistics–2008 update: a report from the American Heart Association Statistics Committee and Stroke Statistics Subcommittee. *Circulation.* 2008;117(4):e25–e146.
4. Wang TJ, et al. Natural history of asymptomatic left ventricular systolic dysfunction in the community. *Circulation.* 2003;108(8): 977–982.

5. Effect of enalapril on mortality and the development of heart failure in asymptomatic patients with reduced left ventricular ejection fractions. The SOLVD Investigators. *N Engl J Med.* 1992;327(10): 685–691.
6. Pfeffer MA, et al. Effect of captopril on mortality and morbidity in patients with left ventricular dysfunction after myocardial infarction. Results of the survival and ventricular enlargement trial. The SAVE Investigators. *N Engl J Med.* 1992;327(10): 669–677.
7. Vantrimpont P, et al. Additive beneficial effects of beta-blockers to angiotensin-converting enzyme inhibitors in the Survival and Ventricular Enlargement (SAVE) Study. SAVE Investigators. *J Am Coll Cardiol.* 1997;29(2):229–236.
8. McMurray JV, et al. Should we screen for asymptomatic left ventricular dysfunction to prevent heart failure? *Eur Heart J.* 1998; 19(6):842–846.
9. Struthers AD, Morris AD. Screening for and treating left-ventricular abnormalities in diabetes mellitus: a new way of reducing cardiac deaths. *Lancet.* 2002;359(9315):1430–1432.
10. Epshteyn V, et al. Utility of B-type natriuretic peptide (BNP) as a screen for left ventricular dysfunction in patients with diabetes. *Diabetes Care.* 2003;26(7):2081–2087.
11. Wang TJ, et al. The epidemiology of "asymptomatic" left ventricular systolic dysfunction: implications for screening. *Ann Intern Med.* 2003;138(11):907–916.
12. Galasko GI, et al. What is the most cost-effective strategy to screen for left ventricular systolic dysfunction: natriuretic peptides, the electrocardiogram, hand-held echocardiography, traditional echocardiography, or their combination? *Eur Heart J.* 2006;27(2):193–200.
13. Yamamoto K, et al. Superiority of brain natriuretic peptide as a hormonal marker of ventricular systolic and diastolic dysfunction and ventricular hypertrophy. *Hypertension.* 1996;28(6):988–994.
14. Nielsen OW, et al. Risk assessment of left ventricular systolic dysfunction in primary care: cross sectional study evaluating a range of diagnostic tests. *BMJ.* 2000;320(7229):220–224.
15. McDonagh TA, et al. Biochemical detection of left-ventricular systolic dysfunction. *Lancet.* 1998;351(9095):9–13.

16. Maisel AS, et al. Rapid measurement of B-type natriuretic peptide in the emergency diagnosis of heart failure. *N Engl J Med.* 2002; 347(3):161–167.

17. Januzzi JL, Jr, et al. The N-terminal Pro-BNP investigation of dyspnea in the emergency department (PRIDE) study. *Am J Cardiol.* 2005;95(8):948–954.

18. Nakamura M, et al. B-type natriuretic peptide testing for structural heart disease screening: a general population-based study. *J Card Fail.* 2005;11(9):705–712.

19. Vasan RS, et al. Plasma natriuretic peptides for community screening for left ventricular hypertrophy and systolic dysfunction: the Framingham heart study. *JAMA.* 2002;288(10):1252–1259.

20. Redfield MM, et al. Plasma brain natriuretic peptide to detect preclinical ventricular systolic or diastolic dysfunction: a community-based study. *Circulation.* 2004;109(25):3176–3181.

21. Hobbs FD, et al. Reliability of N-terminal proBNP assay in diagnosis of left ventricular systolic dysfunction within representative and high risk populations. *Heart.* 2004;90(8):866–870.

22. Pfister R, et al. Use of NT-proBNP in routine testing and comparison to BNP. *Eur J Heart Fail.* 2004;6(3):289–293.

23. Costello-Boerrigter LC, et al. Amino-terminal pro-B-type natriuretic peptide and B-type natriuretic peptide in the general community: determinants and detection of left ventricular dysfunction. *J Am Coll Cardiol.* 2006;47(2):345–353.

24. Goetze JP, et al. Plasma pro-B-type natriuretic peptide in the general population: screening for left ventricular hypertrophy and systolic dysfunction. *Eur Heart J.* 2006;27(24):3004–3010.

25. Galasko GI, et al. What is the normal range for N-terminal pro-brain natriuretic peptide? How well does this normal range screen for cardiovascular disease? *Eur Heart J.* 2005;26(21):2269–2276.

26. Tang WH, et al. National Academy of Clinical Biochemistry Laboratory Medicine practice guidelines: Clinical utilization of cardiac biomarker testing in heart failure. *Circulation.* 2007;116(5):e99–e109.

27. Heidenreich PA, et al. Cost-effectiveness of screening with B-type natriuretic peptide to identify patients with reduced left ventricular ejection fraction. *J Am Coll Cardiol.* 2004;43(6):1019–1026.

28. Nielsen OW, et al. Retrospective analysis of the cost-effectiveness of using plasma brain natriuretic peptide in screening for left ventricular systolic dysfunction in the general population. *J Am Coll Cardiol.* 2003;41(1):113–120.
29. Omland T, et al. Plasma brain natriuretic peptide as an indicator of left ventricular systolic function and long-term survival after acute myocardial infarction. Comparison with plasma atrial natriuretic peptide and N-terminal proatrial natriuretic peptide. *Circulation.* 1996;93(11):1963–1969.
30. Wang TJ, et al. Plasma natriuretic peptide levels and the risk of cardiovascular events and death. *N Engl J Med.* 2004;350(7): 655–663.
31. Ridker PM, et al. Established and emerging plasma biomarkers in the prediction of first atherothrombotic events. *Circulation.* 2004;109(25 Suppl 1):6–19.
32. McKie PM, et al. Amino-terminal pro-B-type natriuretic peptide and B-type natriuretic peptide: biomarkers for mortality in a large community-based cohort free of heart failure. *Hypertension.* 2006; 47(5):874–880.
33. Wallen T, et al. Atrial natriuretic peptides predict mortality in the elderly. *J Intern Med.* 1997;241(4):269–275.
34. Wallen T, et al. Brain natriuretic peptide predicts mortality in the elderly. *Heart.* 1997;77(3):264–267.
35. Knight EL, et al. Atrial natriuretic peptide level contributes to a model of future mortality in the oldest old. *J Am Geriatr Soc.* 1998; 46(4):453–457.
36. Ueda R, et al. Prognostic value of high plasma brain natriuretic peptide concentrations in very elderly persons. *Am J Med.* 2003; 114(4):266–270.
37. McDonagh TA, et al. Left ventricular dysfunction, natriuretic peptides, and mortality in an urban population. *Heart.* 2001;86(1): 21–26.
38. Kistorp C, et al. N-terminal pro-brain natriuretic peptide, C-reactive protein, and urinary albumin levels as predictors of mortality and cardiovascular events in older adults. *JAMA.* 2005;293(13): 1609–1616.
39. Wang TJ. New cardiovascular risk factors exist, but are they clinically useful? *Eur Heart J.* 2008;29(4):441–444.

40. Cook NR, Use and misuse of the receiver operating characteristic curve in risk prediction. *Circulation.* 2007;115(7):928–935.

41. Wang TJ, et al. Multiple biomarkers for the prediction of first major cardiovascular events and death. *N Engl J Med.* 2006;355(25): 2631–2639.

42. Zethelius B, et al. Use of multiple biomarkers to improve the prediction of death from cardiovascular causes. *N Engl J Med.* 2008; 358(20):2107–2116.

43. Bibbins-Domingo K, et al. N-terminal fragment of the prohormone brain-type natriuretic peptide (NT-proBNP), cardiovascular events, and mortality in patients with stable coronary heart disease. *JAMA.* 2007;297(2):169–176.

44. Blankenberg S, et al. Comparative impact of multiple biomarkers and N-Terminal pro-brain natriuretic peptide in the context of conventional risk factors for the prediction of recurrent cardiovascular events in the Heart Outcomes Prevention Evaluation (HOPE) Study. *Circulation.* 2006;114(3):201–208.

45. Heart Protection Study Collaborative, G, et al. N-terminal Pro-B-type natriuretic peptide, vascular disease risk, and cholesterol reduction among 20,536 patients in the MRC/BHF heart protection study. *J Am Coll Cardiol.* 2007;49(3):311–319.

46. Omland T, Aakvaag A, Vik-Mo H. Plasma cardiac natriuretic peptide determination as a screening test for the detection of patients with mild left ventricular impairment. *Heart.* 1996;76(3):232–237.

47. Davis M, et al. Plasma brain natriuretic peptide in assessment of acute dyspnoea. *Lancet.* 1994;343(8895):440–444.

48. Tsutamoto T, et al. Attenuation of compensation of endogenous cardiac natriuretic peptide system in chronic heart failure: prognostic role of plasma brain natriuretic peptide concentration in patients with chronic symptomatic left ventricular dysfunction. *Circulation.* 1997;96(2):509–516.

49. Maeda K, et al. High levels of plasma brain natriuretic peptide and interleukin-6 after optimized treatment for heart failure are independent risk factors for morbidity and mortality in patients with congestive heart failure. *J Am Coll Cardiol.* 2000;36(5):1587–1593.

50. Daniels LB, Maisel AS. Natriuretic peptides. *J Am Coll Cardiol.* 2007; 50(25):2357–2368.

51. Redfield MM, et al. Plasma brain natriuretic peptide concentration: impact of age and gender. *J Am Coll Cardiol.* 2002;40(5):976–982.

52. Wang TJ, et al. Impact of age and sex on plasma natriuretic peptide levels in healthy adults. *Am J Cardiol.* 2002;90(3):254–258.

53. Wang TJ, et al. Impact of obesity on plasma natriuretic peptide levels. *Circulation.* 2004;109(5):594–600.

54. Olsen MH, et al. N-terminal pro brain natriuretic peptide is inversely related to metabolic cardiovascular risk factors and the metabolic syndrome. *Hypertension.* 2005;46(4):660–666.

55. Wang TJ, et al. Association of plasma natriuretic peptide levels with metabolic risk factors in ambulatory individuals. *Circulation.* 2007;115(11):1345–1353.

56. Tsutamoto T, et al. Relationship between renal function and plasma brain natriuretic peptide in patients with heart failure. *J Am Coll Cardiol.* 2006;47(3):582–586.

57. Morita E, et al. Increased plasma levels of brain natriuretic peptide in patients with acute myocardial infarction. *Circulation.* 1993;88(1):82–91.

58. de Lemos JA, et al. The prognostic value of B-type natriuretic peptide in patients with acute coronary syndromes. *N Engl J Med.* 2001;345(14):1014–1021.

59. Nagaya N, et al. Plasma brain natriuretic peptide levels increase in proportion to the extent of right ventricular dysfunction in pulmonary hypertension. *J Am Coll Cardiol.* 1998;31(1):202–208.

60. Kucher N, Printzen G, Goldhaber SZ. Prognostic role of brain natriuretic peptide in acute pulmonary embolism. *Circulation.* 2003;107(20):2545–2547.

61. Ellinor PT, et al. Discordant atrial natriuretic peptide and brain natriuretic peptide levels in lone atrial fibrillation. *J Am Coll Cardiol.* 2005;45(1):82–86.

62. Balion CM, et al. Physiological, pathological, pharmacological, biochemical and hematological factors affecting BNP and NT-proBNP. *Clin Biochem.* 2008;41(4–5):231–239.

63. Raymond I, et al. The influence of age, sex and other variables on the plasma level of N-terminal pro brain natriuretic peptide in a large sample of the general population. *Heart.* 2003;89(7):745–751.

64. Sayama H, et al. Why is the concentration of plasma brain natriuretic peptide in elderly inpatients greater than normal? *Coron Artery Dis.* 1999;10(7):537–540.

65. Davis KM, et al. Atrial natriuretic peptide levels in the elderly: differentiating normal aging changes from disease. *Journals of Gerontology Series A-Biological Sciences & Medical Sciences.* 1996;51(3): M95–M101.

66. Raizada V, et al. Cardiac chamber-specific alterations of ANP and BNP expression with advancing age and with systemic hypertension. *Mol Cell Biochem.* 2001;216(1–2):137–140.

67. Kawai K, et al. Attenuation of biologic compensatory action of cardiac natriuretic peptide system with aging. *Am J Cardiol.* 2004; 93(6):719–723.

68. Clark BA, et al. Influence of age and dose on the end-organ responses to atrial natriuretic peptide in humans. *Am J Hypertens.* 1991;4(6): 500–507.

69. Giannessi D, et al. Possibility of age regulation of the natriuretic peptide C-receptor in human platelets. *J Endocrinol Invest.* 2001; 24(1):8–16.

70. Hong M, et al. Estradiol, progesterone and testosterone exposures affect the atrial natriuretic peptide gene expression in vivo in rats. *Biol Chem Hoppe-Seyler.* 1992;373(4):213–218.

71. Maffei S, et al. Increase in circulating levels of cardiac natriuretic peptides after hormone replacement therapy in postmenopausal women. *Clin Sci.* 2001;101(5):447–453.

72. Chang AY, et al. Associations among androgens, estrogens, and natriuretic peptides in young women: observations from the Dallas Heart Study. *J Am Coll Cardiol.* 2007;49(1):109–116.

73. Das SR, et al. Impact of body mass and body composition on circulating levels of natriuretic peptides: results from the Dallas Heart Study. *Circulation.* 2005;112(14):2163–2168.

74. Krauser DG, et al. Effect of body mass index on natriuretic peptide levels in patients with acute congestive heart failure: a ProBNP Investigation of Dyspnea in the Emergency Department (PRIDE) substudy. *Am Heart J.* 2005;149(4):744–750.

75. Daniels LB, et al. How obesity affects the cut-points for B-type natriuretic peptide in the diagnosis of acute heart failure. Results

from the Breathing Not Properly Multinational Study. *Am Heart J.* 2006;151(5):999–1005.

76. Mehra MR, et al. Obesity and suppressed B-type natriuretic peptide levels in heart failure. *J Am Coll Cardiol.* 2004;43(9):1590–1595.
77. Dessi-Fulgheri P, et al. Plasma atrial natriuretic peptide and natriuretic peptide receptor gene expression in adipose tissue of normotensive and hypertensive obese patients. *J Hypertens.* 1997;15(12 Pt 2):1695–1699.
78. Horwich TB, Hamilton MA, Fonarow GC. B-type natriuretic peptide levels in obese patients with advanced heart failure. *J Am Coll Cardiol.* 2006;47(1):85–90.
79. Licata G, et al. Salt-regulating hormones in young normotensive obese subjects. Effects of saline load. *Hypertension.* 1994;23(1 Suppl): 20–24.
80. Morabito D, Vallotton MB, Lang U. Obesity is associated with impaired ventricular protein kinase C-MAP kinase signaling and altered ANP mRNA expression in the heart of adult Zucker rats. *J Investig Med.* 2001;49(4):310–318.
81. Sarzani R, et al. Comparative analysis of atrial natriuretic peptide receptor expression in rat tissues. *J Hypertens—Suppl.* 1993;11(5): S214–S215.
82. Sarzani R, et al. Expression of natriuretic peptide receptors in human adipose and other tissues. *J Endocrinol Invest.* 1996;19(9): 581–585.
83. Martinez-Rumayor A, et al. Biology of the natriuretic peptides. *Am J Cardiol.* 2008;101(3A):3–8.
84. Expert Panel on Detection, E.a.T.o.H.B.C.i.A., Executive Summary of The Third Report of The National Cholesterol Education Program (NCEP) Expert Panel on Detection, Evaluation, And Treatment of High Blood Cholesterol In Adults (Adult Treatment Panel III). *JAMA.* 2001;285(19):2486–2497.
85. American Heart Association. National Heart, Lung, and Blood Institute, G.S.C.J.D.S.D.K.E.R.F.B.G.D.K.R.S.P.S.S.J.S.J.C.F., Diagnosis and management of the metabolic syndrome: an American Heart Association/National Heart, Lung, and Blood Institute Scientific Statement. *Circulation.* 2005;112(17):2735–2752.
86. Eckel RH, Grundy SM, Zimmet PZ. The metabolic syndrome. *Lancet.* 2005;365(9468):1415–1428.

87. Chattington PD, et al. Atrial natriuretic peptide in type 2 diabetes mellitus: response to a physiological mixed meal and relationship to renal function. *Diabet Med.* 1998;15(5):375–379.

88. Bell GM, et al. Increased plasma atrial natriuretic factor and reduced plasma renin in patients with poorly controlled diabetes mellitus. *Clin Sci.* 1989;77(2):177–182.

89. Yano Y, et al. Plasma brain natriuretic peptide levels in normotensive noninsulin-dependent diabetic patients with microalbuminuria. *J Clin Endocrinol Metab.* 1999;84(7):2353–2356.

90. Kanda H, et al. What factors are associated with high plasma B-type natriuretic peptide levels in a general Japanese population? *J Hum Hypertens.* 2005;19(2):165–172.

91. Sagnella GA, et al. Raised circulating levels of atrial natriuretic peptides in essential hypertension. *Lancet.* 1986;1(8474):179–181.

92. Buckley MG, et al. Plasma concentrations and comparisons of brain and atrial natriuretic peptide in normal subjects and in patients with essential hypertension. *J Hum Hypertens.* 1993;7(3):245–250.

93. Lafontan M, et al. An unsuspected metabolic role for atrial natriuretic peptides: the control of lipolysis, lipid mobilization, and systemic nonesterified fatty acids levels in humans. *Arterioscler, Thromb Vasc Biol.* 2005;25(10):2032–2042.

94. Sengenes C, et al. Natriuretic peptides: a new lipolytic pathway in human adipocytes. *FASEB J.* 2000;14(10):1345–1351.

95. Uehlinger DE, et al. Increase in circulating insulin induced by atrial natriuretic peptide in normal humans. *J Cardiovasc Pharmacol.* 1986; 8(6):1122–1129.

96. Verspohl EJ, Bernemann IK. Atrial natriuretic peptide (ANP)-induced inhibition of glucagon secretion: mechanism of action in isolated rat pancreatic islets. *Peptides.* 1996;17(6):1023–1029.

97. Velloso LA, et al. Cross-talk between the insulin and angiotensin signaling systems. *Proceedings of the National Academy of Sciences of the United States of America.* 1996;93(22):12490–12495.

98. Prasad A, Prasad A.A. Quyyumi, Renin-angiotensin system and angiotensin receptor blockers in the metabolic syndrome. *Circulation.* 2004;110(11):1507–1512.

99. Rajagopalan S, et al. Angiotensin II-mediated hypertension in the rat increases vascular superoxide production via membrane NADH/

NADPH oxidase activation. Contribution to alterations of vasomotor tone. *J Clin Invest.* 1996;97(8):1916–1923.

100. Fliser D.B.K.H.H.E.T.o.O.a.P.i.I.a.A.I., Antiinflammatory effects of angiotensin II subtype 1 receptor blockade in hypertensive patients with microinflammation. *Circulation.* 2004;110(9):1103–1107.

101. Janke J, et al. Mature adipocytes inhibit in vitro differentiation of human preadipocytes via angiotensin type 1 receptors. *Diabetes.* 2002;51(6):1699–1707.

102. Yvan-Charvet L, et al. Deletion of the angiotensin type 2 receptor (AT2R) reduces adipose cell size and protects from diet-induced obesity and insulin resistance. *Diabetes.* 2005;54(4):991–999.

103. de Lemos, JA, McGuire DK, Drazner MH. B-type natriuretic peptide in cardiovascular disease. *Lancet.* 2003;362(9380):316–322.

104. Devereux RB, et al. A population-based assessment of left ventricular systolic dysfunction in middle-aged and older adults: the Strong Heart Study. *Am Heart J.* 2001;141(3):439–446.

105. Devereux RB, et al. Left ventricular systolic dysfunction in a biracial sample of hypertensive adults: The Hypertension Genetic Epidemiology Network (HyperGEN) Study. *Hypertension.* 2001;38(3):417–423.

106. Redfield MM, et al. Burden of systolic and diastolic ventricular dysfunction in the community: appreciating the scope of the heart failure epidemic. *JAMA.* 2003;289(2):194–202.

107. Davies M, et al. Prevalence of left-ventricular systolic dysfunction and heart failure in the Echocardiographic Heart of England Screening study: a population based study. *Lancet.* 2001;358(9280):439–444.

108. Schunkert H, et al. Left-ventricular dysfunction. *Lancet.* 1998; 351(9099):372.

109. Hedberg P, et al. Left ventricular systolic dysfunction in 75-year-old men and women; a population-based study. *Eur Heart J.* 2001;22(8): 676–683.

110. Nielsen OW, et al. Cross sectional study estimating prevalence of heart failure and left ventricular systolic dysfunction in community patients at risk. *Heart.* 2001;86(2):172–178.

111. Mosterd A, et al. Prevalence of heart failure and left ventricular dysfunction in the general population; The Rotterdam Study. *Eur Heart J.* 1999;20(6):447–455.

112. Kupari M, et al. Congestive heart failure in old age: prevalence, mechanisms and 4-year prognosis in the Helsinki Ageing Study. *J Intern Med.* 1997;241(5):387–394.

113. McDonagh TA, et al. Symptomatic and asymptomatic left-ventricular systolic dysfunction in an urban population. *Lancet.* 1997;350(9081):829–833.

114. Gottdiener JS, et al. Outcome of congestive heart failure in elderly persons: influence of left ventricular systolic function. The Cardiovascular Health Study. *Ann Intern Med.* 2002;137(8):631–639.

115. Morgan S, et al. Prevalence and clinical characteristics of left ventricular dysfunction among elderly patients in general practice setting: cross sectional survey. *BMJ.* 1999;318(7180):368–372.

116. Luchner A, et al. Evaluation of brain natriuretic peptide as marker of left ventricular dysfunction and hypertrophy in the population. *J Hypertens.* 2000;18(8):1121–1128.

117. Arnlov J, et al. N-terminal atrial natriuretic peptide and left ventricular geometry and function in a population sample of elderly males. *J Intern Med.* 2000;247(6):699–708.

118. Yamamoto K, et al. Clinical criteria and biochemical markers for the detection of systolic dysfunction. *J Card Fail.* 2000;6(3):194–200.

119. Krishnaswamy P, et al. Utility of B-natriuretic peptide levels in identifying patients with left ventricular systolic or diastolic dysfunction. *Am J Med.* 2001;111(4):274–279.

120. Friedl W, et al. Natriuretic peptides and cyclic guanosine 3′,5′-monophosphate in asymptomatic and symptomatic left ventricular dysfunction. *Heart.* 1996;76(2):129–136.

121. Lerman A, et al. Circulating N-terminal atrial natriuretic peptide as a marker for symptomless left-ventricular dysfunction. *Lancet.* 1993;341(8853):1105–1109.

122. Davidson NC, et al. Comparison of atrial natriuretic peptide B-type natriuretic peptide, and N-terminal proatrial natriuretic peptide as indicators of left ventricular systolic dysfunction. *Am J Cardiol.* 1996;77(10):828–831.

123. Muders F, et al. Evaluation of plasma natriuretic peptides as markers for left ventricular dysfunction. *Am Heart J.* 1997;134(3):442–449.

20 ▪ Natriuretic Peptide Testing in Symptomatic Primary Care Patients

Per Hildebrandt, MD

Introduction

Although widely used in the hospital setting for the diagnostic evaluation of patients with acute symptoms, natriuretic peptide testing has great promise in the primary care arena. This chapter will address the burden of heart failure (HF) on the primary care community, and how natriuretic peptide testing might be most optimally applied in this setting.

Chronic Stable HF

HF is a large and increasing challenge for the health care system. It is a common disease, with an expected increase in the prevalence due to several reasons. The mortality for the underlying diseases—ischemic heart disease and hypertension—has been reduced substantially, thus leaving an increasing pool of patients with chronic heart disease, including HF. The pharmacological and nonpharmacological treatment of HF has improved, thus reducing the mortality and increasing the number of patients. As HF primarily is a disease of the elderly, the general aging of the population will furthermore increase the prevalence of HF.

Despite this, we have, in general, observed a decrease in admissions for HF during the last ten years due to an impressive effect of the treatment and an improvement in the organization of HF treatment and follow-up, primarily the use of HF clinics.[1,2]

The modern treatment of HF includes a variety of options that impact the mortality and morbidity of the patient. These include: angiotensin-converting enzyme (ACE) inhibitors, angiotensin-receptor blockers (ARB), beta blockers, aldosterone antagonists,

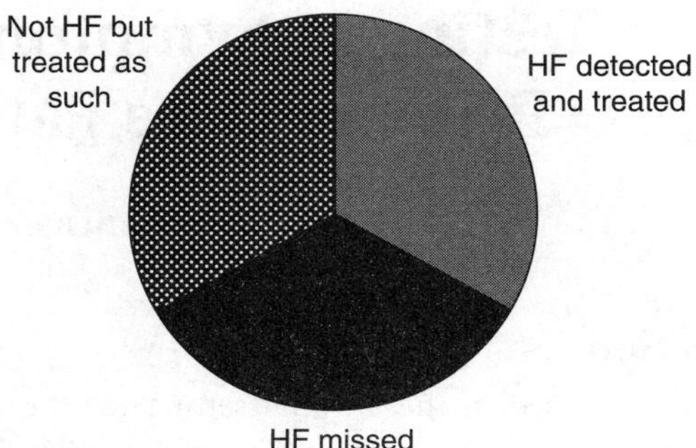

■ **Figure 20–1** The proportion of heart failure (HF) patients known, unknown, and misdiagnosed in a population analysis from Denmark. In this analysis, roughly 40,000 patients were in each group.

implantable cardioverter defibrillators, and cardiac resynchronization therapy.[1,2] Using this arsenal of treatment, the mortality can be reduced by more than two-thirds. But to intervene with this treatment we have to overcome a major problem—finding the right patients! It is generally anticipated that only 50% of the patients with HF have been identified, and of the patients treated for HF, 50% of them have no objective evidence of this disease, but have other explanations for their symptoms (Figure 20–1). A major problem is that the symptoms of HF can be fairly vague and nonspecific, characteristics shared with many other diseases. For example, the major HF symptoms of dyspnea and fatigue may also present with other diseases and can be misinterpreted as HF, when they are actually indications of obstructive airway disease, or simply deconditioning. In a Danish population survey of patients 55 years and older,[3] 25% of the persons complained of dyspnea, but only a minority of these had objective evidence of (systolic) HF (Figure 20–2).

A widespread definition of HF is the one put forward by the European Society of Cardiology.[1] It requires the existence of symptoms of HF and objective evidence of cardiac dysfunction. The diagnosis is supported by an effect of treatment to improve

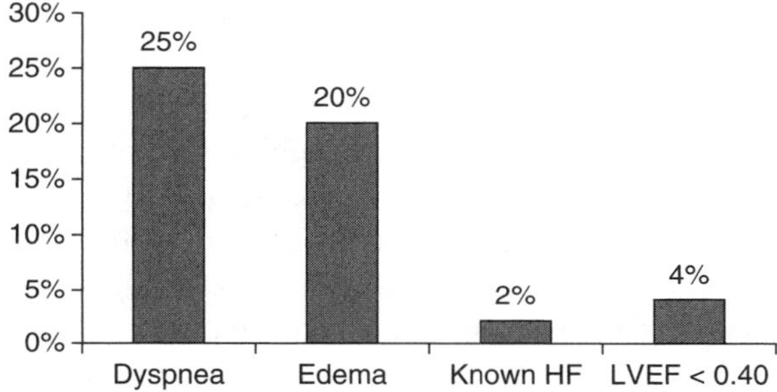

■ **Figure 20–2** The low prevalence of HF among persons older than 55 years relative to symptoms of dyspnea and/or edema and/or a known diagnosis of HF.

symptoms. The objective evidence of HF may, in some patients, be from the electrocardiogram (e.g., atrial fibrillation [AF]), but the vast majority will require diagnostic imaging—most often echocardiography. Because the number of patients with symptoms suggestive of HF is huge and echocardiography demands expensive equipment and skilled investigators, rather often the availability of this type of diagnostic imaging will be limited.

To make up for this shortage of easy screening tools, a screening marker for ruling out HF would be very valuable, reserving more expensive methods, such as echocardiography, for those with elevated values. This approach would be cost-effective and reduce the number of echocardiograms. B-type natriuretic peptide (BNP) and its inactive split-product N-terminal proBNP (NT-proBNP) have shown great promise for this purpose and are increasingly being used for primary care evaluation of the HF symptomatic patient.

Evidence for the Use of Natriuretic Peptides in Patients with Symptoms Suggestive of Chronic HF

Reduced cardiac function will have different causes and pathophysiology. The major distinction will be between HF due to left ventricular systolic dysfunction (LVSD) with reduced left ventricular ejection fraction (LVEF), and nonsystolic HF. HF with LVSD is the better characterized entity between the two. This is a condition easily diagnosed using diagnostic imaging, most often echocardiography, and with solid evidence-based treatment.

As for the use of natriuretic peptides (NPs) in HF, it is important to stress that the NPs correlate only vaguely with the structure and function of the left ventricle,[4] even using MRI. Thus, results from BNP or NT-proBNP testing will not resemble echocardiography, but by excluding patients with a very low likelihood for HF, the number of echocardiograms done can be reduced, or reserved for patients with elevated NP levels.

HF with Reduced Left Ventricular Systolic Dysfunction

The majority of studies on the use of NPs for screening and diagnostics concern systolic HF. Evidence supports the role of BNP or NT-proBNP screenings for symptomatic HF in general practice.

Several studies have investigated the value of NT-proBNP testing for the evaluation of patients with symptoms suggestive of HF. Notably, Wright et al. showed that the use of NT-proBNP in the General Practice Study significantly improved diagnostic accuracy compared to clinical findings alone, and improved the ability to rule out HF.[5] Along these lines, in all of the studies performed, the value of NT-proBNP for ruling out HF in primary care was clearly superior to that for diagnosing HF. Accordingly, the focus for use of NT-proBNP in the symptomatic outpatient is based on its very high negative predictive value (NPV), as it is essential that the risk for overlooking a patient with HF is minimized. Thus, the optimal cut point for ruling out HF must be that with an NPV as close to 100% as possible. Furthermore, in order to minimize the number of false-positive results—which might lead to unnecessary cardiologic evaluation—an acceptable specificity/positive predictive value should be retained.[6]

In each of the studies examining the value of NT-proBNP for outpatients,[7–11] the optimal "rule-out" value has been suggested to

Table 20–1: Diagnostic value as a function of NT-proBNP cut points for excluding heart failure in primary care setting.

Study	N	Optimal cutoff	NPV	PPV
Zaphiriou[9]	306	125 pg/mL	97%	44%
Nielsen[10]	345	93 pg/mL (male)	97%	57%
		144 pg/mL (female)	97%	48%
Gustafsson[11]	367	125 pg/mL	99%	15%
Fuat[7]	279	150 pg/mL	92%	48%
Al-Barjas[8]	220	125 pg/mL	97%	76%
Lim[14]	137	160 pg/mL	100%	27%

Notes: NPV: negative predictive value; PPV: positive predictive value

be between 100 and 160 pg/mL, yielding an NPV of 92–100%, while retaining positive predictive values of 15–76%, depending on the prevalence of HF in the populations (Table 20–1). One study took a confirmatory approach, by using a predefined value of 125 pg/mL, derived from a previous study.[11] In this study, a very high sensitivity (97%) was demonstrated, retaining a specificity of approximately 50%. The very high sensitivity implies a very low risk to overlook a patient with HF, a fact essential for a good screening method. There is now a general agreement of a "rule-out" value of 125 pg/mL in patients with symptoms suggestive of HF.

For BNP, the cut point for stable outpatients with symptoms suggestive of HF is more inconsistent and not adequately tested. In a study examining BNP cut points, a value of 20 pg/mL was suggested,[12] while a recent review suggests 50–100 pg/mL as the range to consider for this application.[13] For both of the peptides, one of the major problems with their use is increasing values with increasing age. As a result, age-dependent rule-out values have been suggested as resolutions. This topic will be dealt with more thoroughly in the section on age.

The value of combining NPs with other tests, especially electrocardiography, has been examined. The results are not consistent, but in general, electrocardiography adds little to NP testing in the evaluation of patients with dyspnea in the outpatient setting[14] (although this has been disputed in regards to the elderly). Nevertheless, in clinical practice most often both tests will be carried out in tandem.

HF with Preserved Systolic Function: Diastolic Dysfunction

A substantial proportion of HF patients have nonsystolic HF caused by many different etiologies of the condition. According to the European Society of Cardiology definition for HF, the definition of diastolic HF includes objective evidence for reduced diastolic function, the major problem being the lack of diagnostic "gold standards." Partly due to this, the value of the natriuretic peptides in evaluation for diastolic HF is less thoroughly investigated. In a study on BNP, very fine diagnostic accuracy for significant diastolic abnormalities were demonstrated, and the presence of even minor diastolic abnormalities were in general identified.[15] In another study, NT-proBNP was demonstrated to be useful for evaluation of patients with diastolic HF,[16] although generally lower values for the NPs are expected in this case. The use of the natriuretic peptides in systolic, as well as diastolic, dysfunction determination has very strong prognostic value even in diastolic dysfunction.[17–19]

HF with Preserved Systolic Dysfunction: Other Forms

Most other forms of nonsystolic HF will often induce a substantial rise in NPs.

Valvular Heart Disease

Valvular heart disease is an important cause of HF with preserved systolic function. Testing for BNP and NT-proBNP may be of value for evaluating those with valvular heart disease.

Aortic Valve Stenosis and Regurgitation

Several studies have shown a strong correlation between the degree of aortic stenosis and NPs.[20] Thus, screening with an NP will catch the patients with even mild to moderate aortic stenosis before any intervention is warranted. It could even be speculated that NT-proBNP could replace echocardiography for the follow-up of aortic stenosis, at least in milder cases. A similar, although weaker, relation between NPs and aortic valve regurgitation has been demonstrated.[21] It is reasonable to expect that both BNP and NT-proBNP will be elevated by the time when either aortic stenosis or regurgitation is clinically relevant.

Mitral Valve Disease

Natriuretic peptides are related to the severity of the regurgitation,[22] as well as to death and incidence of HF.[23] Even in mitral stenosis, the NP levels are correlated to severity of the disease.[24]

Arrhythmia

Atrial fibrillation (AF) is a common arrhythmia, which can cause symptoms of HF due to the hemodynamic consequences of the high heart rate. Furthermore, AF can cause tachycardia-induced LVSD, most often reversible with treatment of the tachycardia. It is important for the clinician to know that levels of natriuretic peptides are increased in atrial fibrillation, even without HF or structural heart disease.[25] Such levels are said to also predict recurrence of AF after cardioversion.

Noncardiac Factors Influencing the Levels of Natriuretic Peptides

When using NPs for ruling out HF, a number of potential pitfalls must be taken into account (Table 20–2), the most important being age.

Table 20–2: Important variables to consider in primary care interpretation of BNP or NT-proBNP.

Major:
Age: increasing values with age
Renal function: increasing values with worse renal function
Minor:
Gender: slightly higher values in women
Obesity: slightly lower values with rising body mass index
Nonsystolic HF: values typically elevated, but less so than systolic HF
Valve disease: increased values in the absence of HF possible
Atrial fibrillation: increased values in the absence of HF possible
Left ventricular hypertrophy: increased values in the absence of HF possible
Medication treatment: decreased values with most vasoactive drugs (β-blockers may transiently increase concentrations of BNP or NT-proBNP)

Age and Optimal Cut Points

A major problem of using NPs as a screening tool for further cardiac evaluation of patients with suspected HF is that increasing concentrations of natriuretic peptides are observed with increasing age—even in those patients without any clinically-overt cardiac disease.[3,26] The reason for this could be age-related changes in the heart, renal function, and in the metabolism of natriuretic peptides.

An NT-proBNP value of 125 pg/mL has been explored as a common cut point for all patients with symptoms suggestive of HF, giving an excellent NPV. However, this value will tend to give excellent sensitivity, but inadequate specificity in younger patients. At the same time, it will provide low sensitivity (and thus creating a risk for overlooking HF), while retaining specificity in elderly patients.

Table 20–3: Proposed age-related values for the use of NT-proBNP to rule out heart failure.

Age category	Proposed cut point
<50 years	50 pg/mL
50–75 years	75 pg/mL
>75 years	250 pg/mL

Preliminary analysis of available studies suggests that age-specific cut points (Table 20–3) will optimize the sensitivity, retaining an acceptable specificity of approximately 50%. For younger patients (those less than 50 years of age), the optimal cutoff value is 50 pg/mL, while for middle-aged patients (ages 50–75 years), 75 pg/mL is superior to 125 pg/mL. Because the mean value of NT-proBNP in 80-year-old persons is approximately 150 pg/mL and as symptoms suggestive of HF are common in older persons, the uncritical use of a rule-out value of 125 pg/mL could potentially induce further cardiologic evaluation in a larger percentage of older persons.[3] To avoid this, the Food and Drug Administration has approved a value of 450 pg/mL for those greater than or equal to 75 years of age. However, this may be too high, resulting in inadequate sensitivity;[27] thus a value of 250 pg/mL is proposed for those over 75 years to be more useful. These age-related cut point values have yet to be validated.

Unfortunately, while age exerts the same effects on BNP, age-dependent cut points for outpatient use of BNP are not known. Thus, it is reasonable for the clinician to expect that an unadjusted BNP cut point of 20 pg/mL will deliver unacceptable specificity for HF in older subjects.

Renal Impairment

Natriuretic peptides increase with decreasing renal function,[28] but mild renal dysfunction with an estimated glomerular filtration rate (eGFR) > 60 mL/min per 1,73 m2, and presumably even a little lower, probably does not impact screening. In moderate-to-severe renal dysfunction, the levels of NPs are frequently elevated. This should be kept in mind when such testing is performed on those with chronic kidney disease.

In contrast to age and renal failure, the magnitude of the impact of most other factors affecting NPs is fairly small and of no real importance in outpatient testing. Thus, the same cutoff value can be used regardless of these factors.

Gender

The values of BNP or NT-proBNP is higher in females than males,[3,26] but the magnitude of these differences is fairly small and of only minor importance in the clinical use of screening. Thus, the same cutoff value can be used in both females and males.

Obesity

Obese patients have lower NP values, but presumably this difference is small and without any clinical importance for the use in screening.[29]

Thyroid Function

NT-proBNP levels increase in hyperthyroidism and decrease in hypothyroidism even in the subclinical states.[30] Stabilization of thyroid function normalizes the NT-proBNP level. In general, the impact of thyroid dysfunction will have no impact on the screening utility of the marker.

Left Ventricular Hypertrophy

Natriuretic peptide values are increased in **left ventricular hypertrophy**,[31] but as cardiologic evaluation is warranted in this setting, an elevated NP level, prompting echocardiography, is a screening advantage rather than a disadvantage.

Chronic Obstructive Pulmonary Disease

Chronic obstructive pulmonary disease (COPD) is a major differential diagnosis to HF, but fortunately, NP levels are unaffected by this ailment,[10] and NP determination has been shown to be of large value for demonstrating a putative concomitant HF in these patients.[32] Only in states with significantly elevated pulmonary artery pressure, as in primary pulmonary hypertension, does the level increase.[33]

Medications

Both BNP and NT-proBNP levels are influenced by medication treatment. ACE inhibitors,[34] ARBs,[35] aldosterone antagonists,[36] and diuretics[37] all reduce NP concentrations, while nonvasodilating beta blockers may induce a small increase or decrease.[38,39] The decrease caused by these drugs can be fairly large—sometimes driving the NP value below the cutoff level—thus creating a distortion when using NP as a screening tool. Practically speaking, however, this is not likely to be an issue, as BNP or NT-proBNP elevations in those with significant HF are typically quite significant.

Cost-Benefit Analysis

A discussion on diagnostic evaluation requires some cost-benefit considerations for the strategy associated with the diagnostic tool applied. For outpatient evaluation, NP testing to exclude diagnosis of HF is used to direct the focus away from unnecessary and costly diagnostic efforts. Accordingly, when an NP value is below the reference limit, alternative diagnoses should be considered, while an elevated NP value would direct diagnostic focus to the cardiovascular system. The very high sensitivity implies a very low risk of failing to diagnose a patient with HF—a fact essential for a good screening method. Prospective evaluation of NT-proBNP as a gatekeeper screening test in the primary care setting has been conclusively demonstrated to be cost-effective[40] when used in the logical manner detailed above and in Figure 20–3.

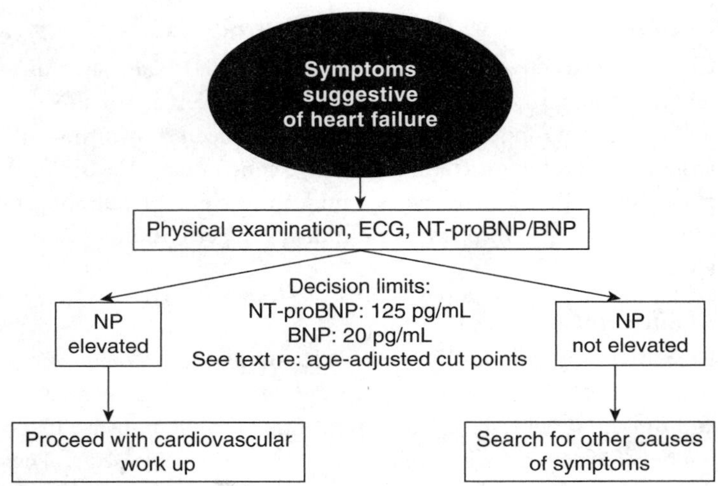

■ **Figure 20–3** Recommended approach for use of NT-proBNP or BNP in primary care setting.

Conclusion

The aforementioned hard evidence now supports the use of natriuretic peptide measurements for evaluation of outpatients with suspected HF, when using the appropriate decision levels. A strategy for use of the markers is proposed in Figure 20–3. If NP levels are below the rule-out value, HF is exceedingly unlikely; performing further diagnostic cardiovascular tests, such as echocardiography, is neither likely to be cost-effective, nor yield positive results. Thus, given the sensitivity at selected cut points, if elevated levels are detected, proceeding with a cardiovascular evaluation, including echocardiography, would be supported.

References

1. The Task Force for the Diagnosis and Treatment of Acute and Chronic Heart Failure 2008 of the European Society of Cardiology. ESC Guidelines for the diagnosis and treatment of acute and chronic heart failure 2008. *Eur Heart J.* 2008;29:2388–2442.

2. American College of Cardiology/American Heart Association Task Force on Practice Guidelines. ACC/AHA 2005 Guideline Update for the Diagnosis and Management of Chronic Heart Failure in the Adult. *Circulation.* 2005;112:1825–1852.

3. Raymond I, Groenning BA, Hildebrandt PR, et al. The influence of age, sex and other variables on the plasma level of N-terminal pro brain natriuretic peptide in a large sample of the general population. *Heart.* 2003;89:745–751.

4. Groenning BA, Nilsson JC, Sondergaard L, et al. Detection of left ventricular enlargement and impaired systolic function with plasma N-terminal pro brain natriuretic peptide concentrations. *Am Heart J.* 2002;143(5):923–929.

5. Wright SP, Doughty RN, Pearl A, et al. Plasma amino-terminal pro-brain natriuretic peptide and accuracy of heart-failure diagnosis in primary care: a randomized, controlled trial. *J Am Coll Cardiol.* 2003;42:1793–1800.

6. Hildebrandt P, Collinson PO. Amino-terminal pro-B-type natriuretic peptide testing to assist the diagnostic evaluation of heart failure in symptomatic primary care patients. *Am J Cardiol.* 2008;101(3A): 25–28.

7. Fuat A, Murphy JJ, Hungin AP, et al. The diagnostic accuracy and utility of a B-type natriuretic peptide test in a community population of patients with suspected heart failure. *Br J Gen Pract.* 2006;56: 327–333.

8. Al-Barjas M, Nair D, Ayrton P, Morris R, Davar J. How can the role of N terminal pro B natriuretic peptide (NT-proBNP) be optimised in heart failure screening? A prospective observational comparative study. *Eur J Heart Fail Suppl.* 2004;3:51 [abstract].

9. Zaphiriou A, Robb S, Murray-Thomas T, et al. The diagnostic accuracy of plasma BNP and NTproBNP in patients referred from primary care with suspected heart failure: results of the UK natriuretic peptide study. *Eur J Heart Fail.* 2005;7:537–541.

10. Nielsen LS, Svanegaard J, Klitgaard NA, Egeblad H. N-terminal pro-brain natriuretic peptide for discriminating between cardiac and non-cardiac dyspnoea. *Eur J Heart Fail.* 2004;6:63–70.

11. Gustafsson F, Steensgaard-Hansen F, Badskjaer J, Poulsen AH, Corell P, Hildebrant P. Diagnostic and prognostic performance of

N-terminal ProBNP in primary care patients with suspected heart failure. *J Card Fail.* 2005;11:S15–S20.

12. Atisha D, Bhalla MA, Morrison LK, et al. A prospective study in search of an optimal B-natriuretic peptide level to screen patients for cardiac dysfunction. *Am Heart J.* 2004;148(3):518–523.
13. McDonald K, Dahlström U, Aspromonte N, et al. B-type natriuretic peptide: application in the community. *Congest Heart Fail.* 2008; 14(4):12–16.
14. Lim TK, Collinson PO, Celik E, Gaze D, Senior R. Value of primary care electrocardiography for the prediction of left ventricular systolic dysfunction in patients with suspected heart failure. *Int J Cardiol.* 2007;115:73–74.
15. Atisha, D, Bhalla, MA, Morrison LK, et al. A prospective study in search of an optimal B-natriuretic peptide level to screen patients for cardiac dysfunction. *Am Heart J.* 2004;148(3):518–523.
16. Tschope C, Kasner M, Westermann D, et al. The role of NT-proBNP in the diagnostics of isolated diastolic dysfunction: correlation with echocardiographic and invasive measurements. *Eur Heart J.* 2005; 26:2277–2784.
17. Hartmann F, Packer M, Coats AJ, et al. Prognostic impact of plasma N-terminal pro-brain natriuretic peptide in severe chronic congestive heart failure: a substudy of the Carvedilol Prospective Randomized Cumulative Survival (COPERNICUS) trial. *Circulation.* 2004;110:178.
18. Anand IS, Fisher LD, Chiang YT, et al. Val-HeFT Investigators. Changes in brain natriuretic peptide and norepinephrine over time and mortality and morbidity in the Valsartan Heart Failure Trial (Val-HeFT). *Circulation.* 2003;107(9):1278–1283.
19. Cleland JG, Tendera M, Adamus J, Freemantle N, Polonski L, Taylor J. PEP-CHF Investigators. The perindopril in elderly people with chronic heart failure (PEP-CHF) study. *Eur Heart J.* 2006;27(19): 2338–2345.
20. Weber M, Arnold R, Rau M, et al. Relation of N-terminal pro B-type natriuretic peptide to progression of aortic valve disease. *Eur Heart J.* 2005;26:1023–1030.
21. Gerber IL, Stewart RA, French JK, et al. Associations between plasma natriuretic peptide levels, symptoms, and left ventricular function in patients with chronic aortic regurgitation. *Am J Cardiol.* 2003;92: 755–758.

22. Sutton TM, Stewart RAH, Gerber IL, et al. Plasma natriuretic peptide levels increase with symptoms and severity of mitral regurgitation. *J Am Coll Cardiol.* 2003;41:2280–2287.

23. Detaint D, Messika-Zeitoun D, Avierinos JF, et al. B-type natriuretic peptide in organic mitral regurgitation: determinants and impact on outcome. *Circulation.* 2005;111:2391–2397.

24. Arat-Ozkan A, Kaya A, Yigit Z, et al. Serum N-terminal pro-BNP levels correlate with symptoms and echocardiographic findings in patients with mitral stenosis. *Echocardiography.* 2005;22:473–478.

25. Shelton RJ, Clark AL, Goode K, Rigby AS, Cleland JG. The diagnostic utility of N-terminal pro-B-type natriuretic peptide for the detection of major structural heart disease in patients with atrial fibrillation. *Eur Heart J.* 2006;27:2353–2361.

26. Costello-Boerrigter, LC, Boerrigter G, Redfield MM, et al. Amino-terminal pro-B-type natriuretic peptide and B-type natriuretic peptide in the general community: determinants and detection of left ventricular dysfunction. *J Am Coll Cardiol.* 2006;47:345–353.

27. Gustafsson F, Badskjaer J, Steensgaard-Hansen F, Poulsen AH, Hildebrandt P. Value of N-proBNP in the diagnosis of left ventricular systolic dysfunction in primary care patients referred for echocardiography. *Heartdrug.* 2003;3:141–146.

28. deFilippi C, Seliger SL, Maynard S, Christenson RH. Impact of renal disease on natriuretic peptide testing for diagnosing decompensated heart failure and predicting mortality. *Clin Chem.* 2007;53(8): 1511–1519.

29. Das SR, Drazner MH, Dries DL, et al. Impact of body mass and body composition on circulating levels of natriuretic peptides: results from the Dallas Heart Study. *Circulation.* 2005;112:2163–2168.

30. Schultz M, Faber J, Kistorp C, et al. N-terminal-pro-B-type natriuretic peptide (NT-pro-BNP) in different thyroid function states. *Clin Endocrinol (Oxf).* 2004;60(1):54–59.

31. Hildebrandt P, Boesen M, Wachtell K, et al. N-terminal pro brain natriuretic peptide in arterial hypertension—a marker for left ventricular dimensions and prognosis. *Eur J Heart Fail.* 2004;6: 313–317.

32. Rutten FH, Moons KGM, Cramer MJM, et al. Recognising heart failure in elderly patients with stable chronic obstructive pulmonary

disease in primary care: cross sectional diagnostic study. *Br Med J.* 2005;331(7529):1379.

33. Gøtze JP, Videbaek R, Boesgaard S, et al. Pro-brain natriuretic peptide as marker of cardiovascular or pulmonary causes of dyspnea in patients with terminal parenchymal lung disease. *J Heart Lung Transplant.* 2004;23:80–87.

34. Murdoch DR, McDonagh TA, Byrne J, et al. Titration of vasodilator therapy in chronic heart failure according to plasma brain natriuretic peptide concentration: randomized comparison of the hemodynamic and neuroendocrine effects of tailored versus empirical therapy. *Am Heart J.* 1999;138:1126–1132.

35. Latini R, Masson S, Anand I, et al. Valsartan Heart Failure Trial Investigators. Effects of valsartan on circulating brain natriuretic peptide and norepinephrine in symptomatic chronic heart failure: the Valsartan Heart Failure Trial (Val-HeFT). *Circulation.* 2002;106: 2454–2458.

36. Tsutamoto T, Wada A, Maeda K, et al. Effect of spironolactone on plasma brain natriuretic peptide and left ventricular remodelling in patients with congestive heart failure. *J Am Coll Cardiol.* 2001;37:1228–1233.

37. van Kraaij DJ, Jansen RW, Sweep FC, et al. Neurohormonal effects of furosemide withdrawal in elderly heart failure patients with normal systolic function. *Eur J Heart Fail.* 2003;5:47–53.

38. Davis ME, Richards AM, Nicholls MG, et al. Introduction of metoprolol increases plasma B-type cardiac natriuretic peptides in mild, stable heart failure. *Circulation.* 2006;113:977–985.

39. Yoshizawa A, Yoshikawa T, Nakamura I, et al. Brain natriuretic peptide response is heterogeneous during betablocker therapy for congestive heart failure. *J Card Fail.* 2004;10:310–315.

40. Collinson PO. The cost effectiveness of B-Type natriuretic peptide measurement in the primary care setting—a UK perspective. *Congest Heart Fail.* 2006;12:103–107.

21 ▪ Natriuretic Peptide Testing for Diagnostic Evaluation of Patients with Suspected Acute Heart Failure

Asim A. Mohammed, MD
James L. Januzzi, Jr., MD

Introduction

The discovery of atrial natriuretic factor highlighted the endocrine function of the heart.[1] Since then, there has been tremendous progress in our understanding of the natriuretic peptides. The natriuretic peptide assays used clinically are for measurement of B-type natriuretic peptide (BNP) and its amino-terminal cleavage equivalent (NT-proBNP); both are being used worldwide in clinical medicine for numerous indications, such as diagnosis and exclusion of heart failure (HF).[2]

Natriuretic Peptide Biology

Biology and Physiology

The BNP gene is located on the chromosome 1. The nuclear transcription factor, GATA 4, plays a dominant role in regulating the process of BNP gene transcription.[3,4] Although originally viewed as a 'ventricular' marker, it turns out that the BNP gene is expressed in both the atria and the ventricles,[5] and the synthesis and release of BNP and NT-proBNP may be triggered by changes in the cardiomyocyte wall tension of either chamber, including those on the right side of the heart. Although wall tension is known to be a primary trigger for BNP and NT-proBNP release, other less recognized factors, such as norepinephrine,[6] proinflammatory cytokines, glucocorticoids, and myocardial ischemia,[7] may lead to considerable release of natriuretic peptides.

Once BNP gene transcription and translation occurs, a 108 amino acid intracellular precursor molecule, $proBNP_{108}$, is generated within the myocyte; this precursor is subsequently cleaved in various amounts by corin to yield the 76 amino acid NT-proBNP, and the biologically-active C-terminal fragment, BNP. However, the biology of NT-proBNP and BNP is considerably more complex. In the circulation, NT-proBNP may be glycosylated to a varying degree;[8] as well, while liberated as a 32 amino acid protein, BNP_{1-32} is rapidly degraded to BNP_{3-32} by neutral endopeptidases, as well as BNP_{6-32} by meprin-A.[9] Lastly, a considerable amount of biologically-inactive $proBNP_{108}$ is released, which is cross-identified by commercial assays for detection of BNP and NT-proBNP.[10]

In the context of HF, natriuretic peptides may be loosely viewed as the body's response to the volume overload, neurohormonal derangement, and activation of the renin-angiotensin system. The principle actions of BNP are: natriuresis, reduction in peripheral vascular resistance, hypotension, and diuresis. These effects are mediated by binding to natriuretic peptide receptors (NPRs), which are expressed in the cardiovascular system, lungs, kidneys, skin, platelets, and central nervous system.[11] There are three types of NPRs: NPR-A, NPR-B and NPR-C. The NPR-A and -B receptors are widely distributed in the myocardium and blood vessels and the NPR-C is a clearance receptor. The activation of NPR-A receptor triggers production of guanylyl cyclase leading to a rise in cyclic guanylyl monophosphate, which subsequently leads to the mentioned actions of BNP.[12]

Half-Life and Clearance

The half-life of BNP is estimated to be 21 minutes[13] and that of NT-proBNP is estimated to be 70 minutes.[14] There are at least three mechanisms of clearance of BNP: receptor binding to NPR-C,[15] degradation by neutral endopeptidases, as well as passive clearance by the kidneys.[16,17] In contrast, NT-proBNP is passively cleared by organs with high blood flows and, hence, has a longer half-life.[17]

Role of BNP and NT-proBNP in HF Diagnosis and Exclusion

Diagnosis of HF has traditionally been made on clinical grounds. However, HF may present with nonspecific symptoms, such as fatigue and dizziness, making it a challenging diagnosis to secure; delays in HF diagnosis are not uncommon. Complicating matters, other conditions—such as acute coronary syndrome, sepsis, and pulmonary embolism—may present with dyspnea and mimic HF. Thoughtful application of natriuretic peptide testing has been shown to be a potential solution to this conundrum,[18,19] and as such, natriuretic peptide testing is incorporated in contemporary clinical guidelines for the diagnostic evaluation of heart failure.[20–23]

Role of Natriuretic Peptides in Acute Dyspnea

Following several smaller pilot studies suggesting value from BNP for the diagnostic evaluation of the dyspneic patient, the Breathing Not Properly Multinational Study,[18] a landmark study of natriuretic peptide testing, solidified the value of BNP measurement in acute dyspnea. In this large, multicenter trial involving 1586 dyspneic patients, BNP values partitioned with heart failure symptom severity (Figure 21–1) and a BNP concentration over 100 ng/L had 83% accuracy for the clinical diagnosis of HF, which was superior to the NHANES and Framingham criteria (which had 67% and 73% accuracy, respectively). In addition, results of BNP testing were superior to clinical judgment alone, but the additive value of BNP plus clinical judgment was superior to either alone.[24]

While a BNP of 100 ng/L had a reasonable negative predictive value (NPV) of 88%, it is necessary to point out that a value of BNP to "exclude" acute HF with confidence (i.e., with an NPV of 95% or more) was considerably lower—in the range of 30 ng/L (Figure 21–2a). While the positive predictive value (PPV) of BNP for HF was a robust 79%, it is obvious that several other diagnoses are necessary to consider when confronted with a BNP in this

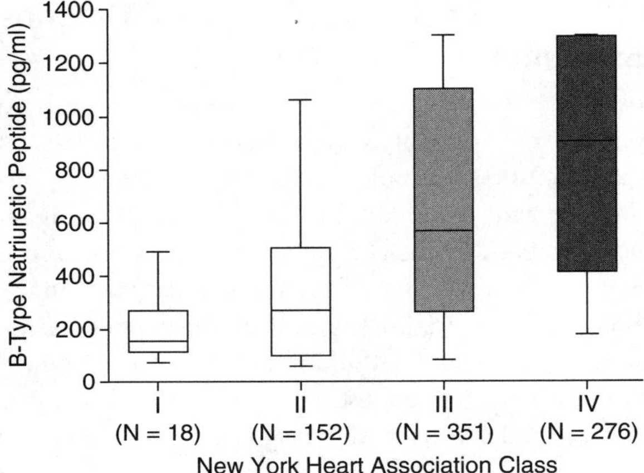

■ **Figure 21–1** Box Plots Showing Median Levels of B-Type Natriuretic Peptide among Patients in Each of the Four New York Heart Association Classifications.

Source: Maisel A.S., et al. Rapid measurement of B-type natriuretic peptide in the emergency diagnosis of heart failure. *N Engl J Med.* 2002;347(3):161–167 © Massachusetts Medical Society.

range, as many situations are associated with a high BNP in the absence of HF, including advancing age (Table 21–1).[25] Nonetheless, BNP testing in the Breathing Not Properly study was valuable across a wide range of patient types, including those with prior HF,[18] and those with chronic kidney disease.[26] In fact, BNP was more valuable than chest radiography for diagnosis of HF.[18]

With respect to NT-proBNP studies, early data from Barcelona[27] suggested that NT-proBNP was of value for the diagnosis of acute HF, and further suggested a dual-modality application of NT-proBNP by identifying cutoffs to “rule in” and “rule out” the diagnosis of acute heart failure. Subsequent data from Christchurch, New Zealand,[28] demonstrated that the NT-proBNP concentrations were significantly higher in acute HF and of comparable value to BNP for this indication. Similarly, Mueller et al.[29] compared NT-proBNP and BNP in 251 dyspneic patients and found

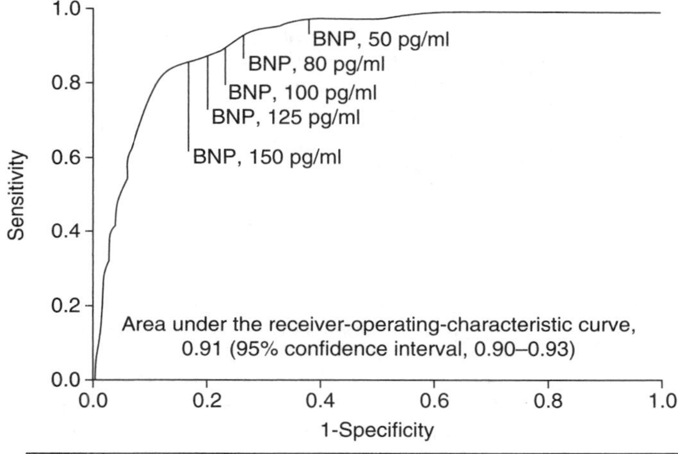

BNP pg/ml	Sensitivity	Specificity	Positive Predictive Value	Negative Predictive Value	Accuracy
50	97%	62%	71%	96%	79%
80	93%	74%	77%	92%	83%
100	90%	76%	79%	89%	83%
125	87%	79%	80%	87%	83%
150	85%	83%	83%	85%	84%

(a)

■ **Figure 21–2** Receiver-Operating-Characteristic Curve for Various Cutoff Levels of A) BNP and B) NT-proBNP. Both peptides were highly sensitive and specific for the diagnosis of acute HF, both with a highly significant area under the curve.

Source(s): (A) Maisel A.S., et al. Rapid measurement of B-type natriuretic peptide in the emergency diagnosis of heart failure. *N Engl J Med.* 2002;347(3):161–167 © Massachusetts Medical Society; (B) Januzzi J.L., Jr., et al. The N-terminal Pro-BNP Investigation of Dyspnea in the Emergency department (PRIDE) study. *Am J Cardiol.* 2005;95(8):948–954. © Elsevier.

no difference between the two. More definitive data supporting NT-proBNP testing came from the ProBNP Investigation of Dyspnea in the Emergency Department (PRIDE) study,[19] a large prospective analysis of 599 acutely dyspneic patients, of whom 209

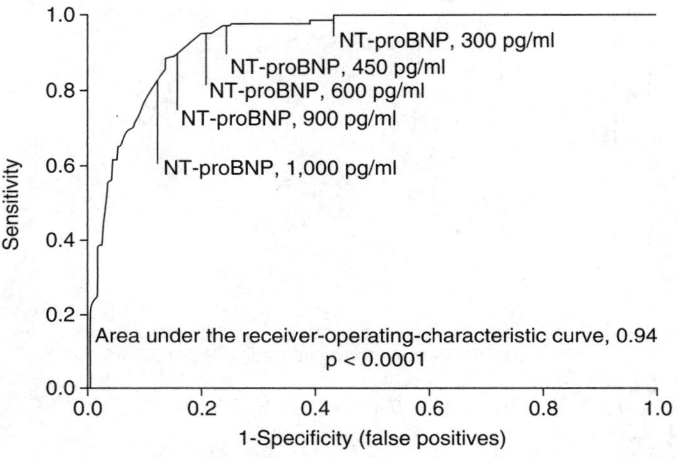

Cut Point pg/ml	Sensitivity	Specificity	Positive Predictive Value	Negative Predictive Value	Accuracy
300	99%	68%	62%	99%	79%
450	98%	76%	68%	99%	83%
600	96%	81%	73%	97%	86%
900	90%	85%	86%	94%	87%
1000	87%	86%	78%	91%	87%

(b)

Figure 21–2 (Continued)

Table 21–1: Differential diagnosis for increased and decreased natriuretic peptides levels.

Increased natriuretic peptides

Physiologic

Age

Female gender

Cardiovascular disease

Heart failure

Table 21–1: (Continued)

Ischemia
Arrhythmia
Valvular heart disease
Hypertension with LVH
Asymptomatic LV dysfunction
Noncardiac causes
Pulmonary embolism
Cor pulmonale
Sepsis
Pulmonary hypertension
Hyperthyroidism
Kidney failure
Tumors
Intracerebral hemorrhage
Advanced liver disease
Excessive cortisol levels
Decreased natriuretic peptides
Obesity
Cardiac medicine ACE inhibitors
ARB
Diuretics
Spironolactone
Beta blocker*
Nonpharmacological factors
Exercise
Cardiac resynchronization therapy
Left ventricular assist devices

*Beta blockers may initially raise natriuretic peptide levels.

had HF. The PRIDE study demonstrated that an NT-proBNP value of 900 ng/L had a PPV of 76% for diagnosis of acute HF, similar to those findings for a BNP of 100 ng/L in the Breathing Not Properly study (Figure 21–2b); significant elevations in NT-proBNP were seen among those with acute HF compared to those without (4435 ng/L versus 131 ng/L) (Figure 21–3). In the PRIDE study, NT-proBNP concentrations correlated with symptom severity in HF, and multivariable analysis showed that an elevation of NT-proBNP was the strongest predictor of HF in acutely dyspneic patients. Also, and importantly, NT-proBNP was superior (and additive) to clinical judgment for correctly securing (or excluding) the diagnosis of HF in this setting (Figure 21–4), findings reflected in the Rapid Emergency Department Heart Failure Outpatient Trial (REDHOT)[30] study.

Subsequent randomized, prospective decision-making trials performed in Switzerland and Canada lent further support to the use of BNP and NT-proBNP, respectively. As demonstrated by Mueller and colleagues,[31] use of BNP to evaluate dyspnea was associated with less resource utilization, while a prospective Canadian multicenter study further validated this point for NT-proBNP;[32] in both studies, acutely dyspneic patients were randomized to unblinded versus blinded NP testing. In addition to shorter lengths of stay in both studies, a significant reduction of 35% in rehospitalization in two months follow-up was seen in the latter trial. In both studies, NP testing was cost-effective and results were reminiscent of decision-analytic framework analysis data from PRIDE.[33]

The explanation for these findings likely reflects reductions in clinician indecision, a common phenomenon when evaluating dyspnea,[24,34] and one that is associated with more resource utilization, longer lengths of stay, and worse outcomes.[34] As earlier and more routine measurement of NP are associated with better outcomes,[35] reductions in clinician indecision about the correct diagnosis—with more secure and early treatment—is most likely linked to these differences in outcome.

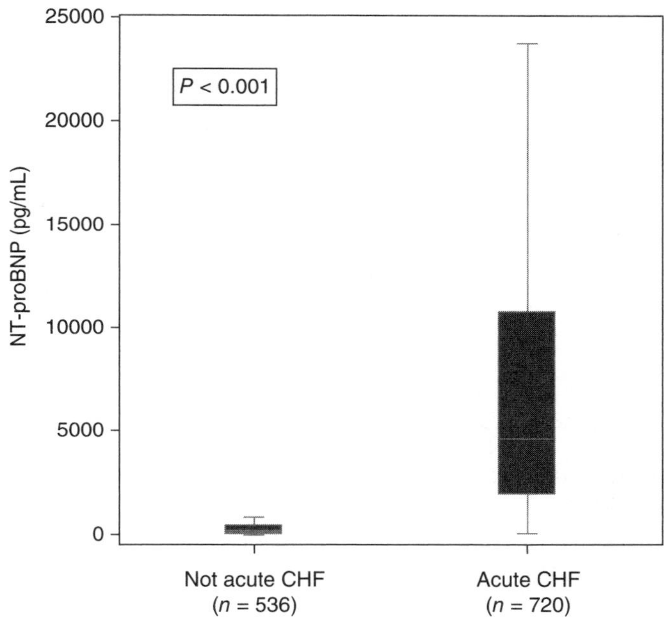

Diagnostic category	Median NT-proBNP	IQR
Not acute CHF	108 pg/mL	37–381 pg/mL
Acute CHF	4639 pg/mL	1882–10818 pg/mL

■ **Figure 21–3** NT-proBNP values as function of final diagnosis in acutely dyspneic patients.

Source: Januzzi J.L., Jr., et al. The N-terminal Pro-BNP Investigation of Dyspnea in the Emergency department (PRIDE) study. *Am J Cardiol.* 2005;95(8):948–954. © Elsevier.

Natriuretic Peptide Cut Points: Rational Application

Natriuretic peptides are continuously distributed variables with a degree of overlap between those with and without HF. In addition, the degree of overlap between health and disease is not static, with significant influence by several variables in the absence of HF,

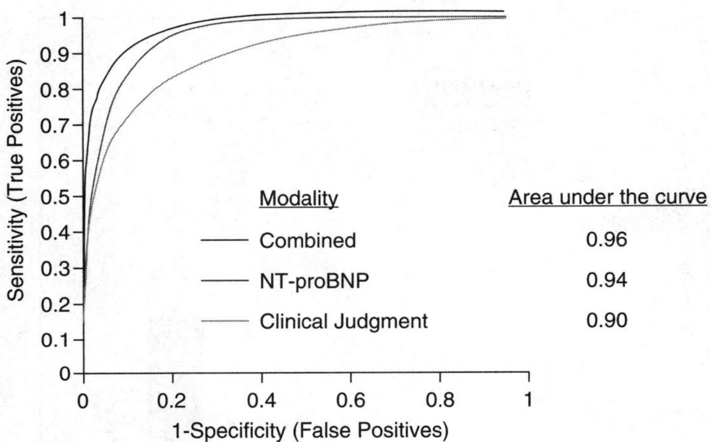

■ **Figure 21–4** Receiver-operating characteristic curve comparison of results from NT-proBNP testing relative to clinical judgment.

Source: Januzzi J.L., Jr., et al. The N-terminal Pro-BNP Investigation of Dyspnea in the Emergency department (PRIDE) study. *Am J Cardiol.* 2005;95(8):948–954. © Elsevier.

including normative processes, such as age, as well as relevant structural heart disease, including abnormalities in heart rhythm, ischemic heart disease, valvular disease, and pulmonary hypertension. Accordingly, it is not at all surprising that a single cut point for either peptide is less useful than considering the markers as continuous variables, whereas higher concentrations are more likely to be associated with HF. This, notwithstanding the need for discrete cut points, is important for simplicity of application.

With respect to BNP and NT-proBNP for excluding acute HF in symptomatic patients, it has been shown that very low values are necessary to exclude the diagnosis. For NT-proBNP, a cut point that equates with an NPV of 98–99% is 300 ng/L.[19,27,36] For BNP, the value is approximately 20–30 ng/L. Values above these concentrations, whether or not they are below the "rule in" cut point, may be associated with HF.

To identify acute HF, it has been argued that an "advantage" of BNP is the mandate to use a single cut point of 100 ng/L across all patient types. This overly-simplistic approach ignores the point that this cut point is unable to "rule out" HF; furthermore, several diagnoses may lead to a BNP above 100 ng/L in the absence of HF,[37] most notably due to age. Indeed, there is no manifest advantage of BNP over NT-proBNP when using a single cut point: the PRIDE investigators found that an NT-proBNP concentration of 900 ng/L provides an equally beneficial diagnostic value as a BNP level of 100 ng/L,[19] yet superior diagnostic accuracy could be had by simply adjusting for age, a significant confounder when interpreting natriuretic peptide (NP) values. Accordingly, an age-stratified approach of 450/900/1800 ng/L for ages <50/50–75/>75 years was found to be superior to a single cut point approach.[38] Age-appropriate cut points for BNP are not known.

The Gray Zone

When partitioning values of NP between lower and higher likelihood for the diagnosis of HF, an intermediate zone of indecision, or "gray zone," is created. For BNP, these values are between 100 ng/L and 500 ng/L, while for NT-proBNP, the zone is between 300 ng/dl and the age-adjusted cut point (450 ng/L, 900 ng/L and 1800 ng/L).[39,40] It is worthwhile to consider that a BNP value greater than 30 ng/L could indicate HF, and thus, there is a risk for underdiagnosis for values just below 100 ng/L in particular.

Causes of "gray zone" values include: mild HF, nonsystolic HF or effects from other cardiac diseases, such as coronary ischemia and atrial fibrillation, as well as pulmonary embolism, and severe infections. According to a subanalysis of the International Collaborative of NT-proBNP (ICON) study, clinical parameters—including absence of cough, prior history of HF, presence of paroxysmal nocturnal dyspnea, jugular venous distention, and use of loop diuretics on presentation—predict a diagnosis of HF.[40] Hence, clinical judgment assumes extra importance when NP levels are in "gray zone."

Special Topics: Elevated NP Values in the Absence of HF

NPs in Chronic Renal Failure Patients

Chronic kidney disease (CKD) is prevalent in heart failure patients. It is noted that 33–56% of heart failure patients have CKD,[41,42] while, conversely, CKD patients have relevant structural heart disease that is in parallel to the loss of renal function. As noted above, both NPs are partially cleared by the kidneys.[43,44] Hence, patients with CKD are expected to have elevated concentrations of BNP or NT-proBNP. Although this finding was originally considered a "false positive," it is now known that elevated NPs in CKD patients predict structural heart disease and particularly poor outcome,[45] which makes it much less likely that the values of BNP and NT-proBNP observed in those with CKD are spurious.

When used for diagnosis of HF in patients with CKD, BNP and NT-proBNP appear to be equally affected by loss of renal function and have worse diagnostic accuracy than those without CKD. That being said, both markers retain utility for diagnosis of HF if adjusted for renal function. Subanalysis from PRIDE and the Breathing Not Properly multicenter study demonstrated that the accuracy of both the NPs is only modestly worse when compared to patients with normal renal function with slightly elevated cut points (200 ng/L for BNP and 1200 ng/L for NT-proBNP).[18,19,26] Using the age-adjusted cut points recommended by the ICON study, there was no need for change in the cut points for CKD patients to diagnose HF.[36]

NPs in Chronic HF Patients

Among patients with prior HF, elevations of BNP and NT-proBNP are expected, as they are sensitive measures of HF presence and severity, and are directly associated with outcomes. However, when a dyspneic patient with prior HF is evaluated using BNP and NT-proBNP measurements, it may be challenging to differentiate acute-on-chronic HF from other causes of dyspnea. In this situation, it is important to compare current NP levels with previously available NP values, or ideally with the "dry NP value." As above, with the knowledge that the biological variation in a stable chronic HF is 25%,[46,47] a change in NP values of greater than 25% is supportive of acute destabilization.

NPs and Non-HF Structural Heart Disease

Ischemic Coronary Artery Disease

As noted, expression of the cardiac BNP gene is increased in myocardial ischemia, resulting in elevation of both BNP and NT-proBNP.[48,49] It is unclear how ischemia triggers BNP release, but it may be related in part to ischemia-mediated wall stress or tissue-level hypoxia. Indeed, based on basic[49] and clinical observations, hypoxia has been noted as an independent trigger for BNP release.[50,51] NPs may not be diagnostic of acute coronary syndrome (ACS), but are excellent predictors of mortality and morbidity in this context.[52–57]

Atrial Fibrillation

Both BNP and NT-proBNP levels are elevated in patients with acute and chronic atrial fibrillation (AF).[58–60] NT-proBNP levels are higher in HF patients with AF than in HF patients with sinus rhythm and have an independent prognostic value despite the presence of AF.[61] Moreover, the NP levels decrease after restoration of sinus rhythm by cardioversion.[62] Furthermore, the NP levels have also been shown to predict the recurrence of AF following direct current cardioversion,[63,64] and to predict development of AF following pacemaker placement for sick sinus rhythm[65] and postcardiac surgery.[66]

Valvular Heart Disease

Diseases of cardiac valves may lead to chronic pressure and volume overload, which leads to increases in myocardial wall stress; hence, increased secretion of BNP and NT-proBNP may be seen in this context, even in the absence of HF.

Among patients with aortic stenosis, NP levels correlate well, not only with the mean pressure gradient, valve area, and left ventricular wall stress,[67–70] but also with the symptom status (determined by the NYHA classification).[71–73] Furthermore, NP levels were predictive of development symptoms in asymptomatic patients and outcomes after valve replacement surgery.[74] Similar data exist for aortic regurgitation.[75,76]

With respect to the mitral valve, it is known that both BNP and NT-proBNP rise in parallel with the severity of regurgitation—even in the absence of symptoms—and predict outcomes in this setting.[77–79] Similarly, among patients with mitral stenosis, it has been reported that BNP and NT-proBNP rise in proportion to the severity of the valve lesion, which runs counter to the concept that they are 'ventricular' markers. Lastly, right-sided valvular heart disease may lead to lower elevations of BNP and NT-proBNP than left-sided lesions, but nonetheless is important to keep in mind when interpreting concentrations of these markers.[80]

Pulmonary Diseases

Both BNP and NT-proBNP have been shown to be of value for sorting out the diagnosis causing dyspnea among those patients with both chronic obstructive airway disease and concomitant HF, and may be able to identify a significant percentage of patients with chronic lung disease who had unexpected—or "masked"—HF.[27,81] Having said this, NPs have been shown to be elevated in non-HF disorders that cause chronic right ventricular (RV) dysfunction, such as primary pulmonary hypertension, chronic obstructive pulmonary disease, thromboembolic pulmonary hypertension, and left-to-right cardiac shunts.[82–87]

With respect to pulmonary thromboembolism, a low NP level has a high negative predictive value in ruling out adverse outcome[88] and a high NP level with acute pulmonary embolism suggests right ventricular dysfunction and warrants further evaluation.[88–94] A persistent elevation of NT-proBNP levels within 24 hours after an acute pulmonary embolism suggests severe right ventricular dysfunction and hence a poor prognosis warranting aggressive management.[90] Based on this correlation, investigators have incorporated NT-proBNP in a risk stratification algorithm for patients with acute pulmonary embolism.[88]

In chronic pulmonary hypertension, an increase in NPs not only correlates with the degree of RV dysfunction and functional status,[82,86,87] but also with the risk for mortality.[86]

Critical Illness

Sepsis, major trauma, complicated major surgery, or other critical illness can directly insult the cardiovascular system leading to poor outcomes.[95] Elevations of both BNP and NT-proBNP levels occur in these settings and are directly predictive of adverse outcomes like death[96,97]—independent of HF[98]—left ventricular mass, or intracardiac filling pressures—reflecting a possible myocardial depression from direct toxic effect of inflammatory mediators.[99–101] Both BNP and NT-proBNP are independent predictors of outcomes in unselected critically-ill patients.[81,102–104]

Special Topics: Low NP Values in the Presence of HF

NPs and Nonsystolic HF

Affecting up to 50% of patients afflicted with HF in modern medicine, HF with preserved systolic function is an important consideration when applying NP testing. As was shown by Maisel[39] and O'Donoghue,[105] the presence of nonsystolic HF is associated with BNP and NT-proBNP values that are typically lower than those of patients with systolic HF. This may mean a higher likelihood for an NP value below the "rule-in" threshold, but rarely does it lead to a result below the "rule-out" cut point of 30 ng/L and 300 ng/L for BNP and NT-proBNP, respectively.

NPs and Body Mass Index

Concentrations of both NPs are significantly lower in overweight and obese patients in a manner parallel to body mass index

(BMI),[106,107] and independent of the elevated filling pressures in these patients.[108] The effects of BMI-mediated NP suppression include a change in optimal cut points for BNP. The authors of the Breathing Not Properly Multinational Study substudy proposed a lower cut point of BNP (54 ng/L) in obese patients to improve sensitivity in this population. Although the level of NT-proBNP is also lower in obese patients, a subanalysis of the ICON study demonstrated no need for cut point adjustment for BMI,[38,109] and NT-proBNP retained its prognostic ramification across all weight categories.

Conclusion

The use of BNP and NT-proBNP have revolutionized the evaluation and management of patients with acute symptoms suggestive of HF. The optimal method of use for both BNP and NT-proBNP is to integrate the results from testing for either with clinical judgment. Knowledge of the wide range of physiologic and pathophysiologic factors that affect concentrations of BNP or NT-proBNP helps to better understand the results gained from their testing. When used in this manner, cost effective care may be expected.

References

1. de Bold AJ, Borenstein HB, Veress AT, Sonnenberg H. A rapid and potent natriuretic response to intravenous injection of atrial myocardial extracts in rats. *Life Sci.* 1981;28:89–94.
2. Braunwald E. Biomarkers in heart failure. *N Engl J Med.* 2008; 358(20):2148–2159.
3. Grepin C, Dagnino L, Robitaille L, et al. A hormone-encoding gene identifies a pathway for cardiac but not skeletal muscle gene transcription. *Mol Cell Biol.* 1994;14(5):3115–3129.
4. Thuerauf DJ, Hanford DS, Glembotski CC. Regulation of rat brain natriuretic peptide transcription. A potential role for GATA-related transcription factors in myocardial cell gene expression. *J Biol Chem.* 1994;269(27):17772–17775.
5. Yasue H, Yoshimura M, Sumida H, et al. Localization and mechanism of secretion of B-type natriuretic peptide in comparison with

those of A-type natriuretic peptide in normal subjects and patients with heart failure. *Circulation*. 1994;90(1):195–203.

6. Magga J, Marttila M, Mantymaa P, Vuolteenaho O, Ruskoaho H. Brain natriuretic peptide in plasma, atria, and ventricles of vasopressin- and phenylephrine-infused conscious rats. *Endocrinology*. 1994; 134(6):2505–2515.
7. Cameron VA, Rademaker MT, Ellmers LJ, et al. Atrial (ANP) and brain natriuretic peptide (BNP) expression after myocardial infarction in sheep: ANP is synthesized by fibroblasts infiltrating the infarct. *Endocrinology*. 2000;141(12):4690–4697.
8. Schellenberger U, O'Rear J, Guzzetta A, et al. The precursor to B-type natriuretic peptide is an O-linked glycoprotein. *Arch Biochem Biophys*. 2006;451(2):160–166.
9. Brandt I, Lambeir AM, Ketelslegers JM, et al. Dipeptidyl-peptidase IV converts intact B-type natriuretic peptide into its des-SerPro form. *Clin Chem*. 2006;52(1):82–87.
10. Luckenbill KN, Christenson RH, Jaffe AS, et al. Cross-reactivity of BNP, NT-proBNP, and proBNP in commercial BNP and NT-proBNP assays: preliminary observations from the IFCC Committee for Standardization of Markers of Cardiac Damage. *Clin Chem*. 2008;54(3):619–621.
11. Koller KJ, Goeddel DV. Molecular biology of the natriuretic peptides and their receptors. *Circulation*. 1992;86(4):1081–1088.
12. Tremblay J, Desjardins R, Hum D, Gutkowska J, Hamet P. Biochemistry and physiology of the natriuretic peptide receptor guanylyl cyclases. *Mol Cell Biochem*. 2002;230(1–2):31–47.
13. Richards AM, Crozier IG, Holmes SJ, et al. Brain natriuretic peptide: natriuretic and endocrine effects in essential hypertension. *J Hypertens*. 1993;11(2):163–170.
14. Pemberton CJ, Johnson ML, Yandle TG, Espiner EA. Deconvolution analysis of cardiac natriuretic peptides during acute volume overload. *Hypertension*. 2000;36(3):355–359.
15. Suga S, Nakao K, Hosoda K, et al. Receptor selectivity of natriuretic peptide family, atrial natriuretic peptide, brain natriuretic peptide, and C-type natriuretic peptide. *Endocrinology*. 1992;130(1):229–239.
16. Schou M, Dalsgaard MK, Clemmesen O, et al. Kidneys extract BNP and NT-proBNP in healthy young men. *J Appl Physiol*. 2005;99(5): 1676–1680.

17. Martinez-Rumayor A, Richards AM, Burnett JC, Januzzi JL, Jr. Biology of the natriuretic peptides. *Am J Cardiol.* 2008;101(3A): 3–8.

18. Maisel AS, Krishnaswamy P, Nowak RM, et al. Rapid measurement of B-type natriuretic peptide in the emergency diagnosis of heart failure. *N Engl J Med.* 2002;347(3):161–167.

19. Januzzi JL, Jr, Camargo CA, Anwaruddin S, et al. The N-terminal Pro-BNP Investigation of Dyspnea in the Emergency department (PRIDE) study. *Am J Cardiol.* 2005;95(8):948–954.

20. Arnold JM, Liu P, Demers C, et al. Canadian Cardiovascular Society consensus conference recommendations on heart failure 2006: diagnosis and management. *Can J Cardiol.* 2006;22(1):23–45.

21. Hunt SA, Abraham WT, Chin MH, et al. ACC/AHA 2005 Guideline Update for the Diagnosis and Management of Chronic Heart Failure in the Adult: a report of the American College of Cardiology/American Heart Association Task Force on Practice Guidelines (Writing Committee to Update the 2001 Guidelines for the Evaluation and Management of Heart Failure): developed in collaboration with the American College of Chest Physicians and the International Society for Heart and Lung Transplantation: endorsed by the Heart Rhythm Society. *Circulation.* 2005;112(12):e154–e235.

22. Swedberg K, Cleland J, Dargie H, et al. Guidelines for the diagnosis and treatment of chronic heart failure: executive summary (update 2005): The Task Force for the Diagnosis and Treatment of Chronic Heart Failure of the European Society of Cardiology. *Eur Heart J.* 2005;26(11):1115–1140.

23. Tang WH, Francis GS, Morrow DA, et al. National Academy of Clinical Biochemistry Laboratory Medicine practice guidelines: Clinical utilization of cardiac biomarker testing in heart failure. *Circulation.* 2007;116(5):e99–e109.

24. McCullough PA, Nowak RM, McCord J, et al. B-type natriuretic peptide and clinical judgment in emergency diagnosis of heart failure: analysis from Breathing Not Properly (BNP) Multinational Study. *Circulation.* 2002;106(4):416–422.

25. Knudsen CW, Riis JS, Finsen AV, et al. Diagnostic value of a rapid test for B-type natriuretic peptide in patients presenting with acute dyspnoe: effect of age and gender. *Eur J Heart Fail.* 2004;6(1): 55–62.

26. McCullough PA, Duc P, Omland T, et al. B-type natriuretic peptide and renal function in the diagnosis of heart failure: an analysis from the Breathing Not Properly Multinational Study. *Am J Kidney Dis.* 2003;41(3):571–579.
27. Bayes-Genis A, Santalo-Bel M, Zapico-Muniz E, et al. N-terminal probrain natriuretic peptide (NT-proBNP) in the emergency diagnosis and in-hospital monitoring of patients with dyspnoea and ventricular dysfunction. *Eur J Heart Fail.* 2004;6(3):301–308.
28. Lainchbury JG, Campbell E, Frampton CM, et al. Brain natriuretic peptide and n-terminal brain natriuretic peptide in the diagnosis of heart failure in patients with acute shortness of breath. *J Am Coll Cardiol.* 2003;42(4):728–735.
29. Mueller T, Gegenhuber A, Poelz W, Haltmayer M. Head-to-head comparison of the diagnostic utility of BNP and NT-proBNP in symptomatic and asymptomatic structural heart disease. *Clin Chim Acta.* 2004;341(1–2):41–48.
30. Maisel A, Hollander JE, Guss D, et al. Primary results of the Rapid Emergency Department Heart Failure Outpatient Trial (REDHOT). A multicenter study of B-type natriuretic peptide levels, emergency department decision making, and outcomes in patients presenting with shortness of breath. *J Am Coll Cardiol.* 2004;44(6):1328–1333.
31. Mueller C, Laule-Kilian K, Schindler C, et al. Cost-effectiveness of B-type natriuretic peptide testing in patients with acute dyspnea. *Arch Intern Med.* 2006;166(10):1081–1087.
32. Moe GW, Howlett J, Januzzi JL, Zowall H. N-terminal pro-B-type natriuretic peptide testing improves the management of patients with suspected acute heart failure: primary results of the Canadian prospective randomized multicenter IMPROVE-CHF study. *Circulation.* 2007;115(24):3103–3110.
33. Siebert U, Januzzi JL, Jr, Beinfeld MT, Cameron R, Gazelle GS. Cost-effectiveness of using N-terminal pro-brain natriuretic peptide to guide the diagnostic assessment and management of dyspneic patients in the emergency department. *Am J Cardiol.* 2006;98(6): 800–805.
34. Green SM, Martinez-Rumayor A, Gregory SA, et al. Clinical uncertainty, diagnostic accuracy, and outcomes in emergency department patients presenting with dyspnea. *Arch Intern Med.* 2008;168(7): 741–748.

35. Maisel AS, Peacock WF, McMullin N, et al. Timing of immunoreactive B-type natriuretic peptide levels and treatment delay in acute decompensated heart failure: an ADHERE (Acute Decompensated Heart Failure National Registry) analysis. *J Am Coll Cardiol.* 2008;52(7):534–540.

36. Januzzi JL, Jr, van Kimmenade RRJ, Lainchbury JG, et al. NT-proBNP Testing for Diagnosis and Short-Term Prognosis in Acute Congestive Heart Failure: An International Pooled Analysis of 1256 Patients. The International Collaborative of NT-proBNP (ICON) Study. *Eur Heart J.* 2006;27(3):330–337.

37. Knudsen CW, Clopton P, Westheim A, et al. Predictors of elevated B-type natriuretic peptide concentrations in dyspneic patients without heart failure: an analysis from the breathing not properly multinational study. *Ann Emerg Med.* 2005;45(6):573–580.

38. Januzzi JL, van Kimmenade R, Lainchbury J, et al. NT-proBNP testing for diagnosis and short-term prognosis in acute destabilized heart failure: an international pooled analysis of 1256 patients: the International Collaborative of NT-proBNP Study. *Eur Heart J.* 2006; 27(3):330–337.

39. Maisel AS, McCord J, Nowak RM, et al. Bedside B-Type natriuretic peptide in the emergency diagnosis of heart failure with reduced or preserved ejection fraction. Results from the Breathing Not Properly Multinational Study. *J Am Coll Cardiol.* 2003;41(11):2010–2017.

40. van Kimmenade RRJ, Pinto YM, Bayes-Genis A, et al. Usefulness of Intermediate Amino-Terminal Pro-Brain Natriuretic Peptide Concentrations for Diagnosis and Prognosis of Acute Heart Failure. *Am J Cardiol.* 2006;98(3):386–390.

41. Mahon NG, Blackstone EH, Francis GS, et al. The prognostic value of estimated creatinine clearance alongside functional capacity in ambulatory patients with chronic congestive heart failure. *J Am Coll Cardiol.* 2002;40(6):1106–1113.

42. McAlister FA, Ezekowitz J, Tonelli M, Armstrong PW. Renal Insufficiency and Heart Failure: Prognostic and Therapeutic Implications From a Prospective Cohort Study. *Circulation.* 2004;109(8):1004–1009.

43. Cameron SJ, Green GB. Cardiac Biomarkers in Renal Disease: The Fog Is Slowly Lifting. *Clin Chem.* 2004;50(12):2233–2235.

44. Apple FS, Murakami MM, Pearce LA, Herzog CA. Multi-Biomarker Risk Stratification of N-Terminal Pro-B-Type Natriuretic Peptide, High-Sensitivity C-Reactive Protein, and Cardiac Troponin T and I in End-Stage Renal Disease for All-Cause Death. *Clin Chem.* 2004; 50(12):2279–2285.

45. van Kimmenade R, Januzzi JL, Jr, Baggish AL, et al. Amino-terminal Pro-Brain Natriuretic Peptide, Renal Function and Outcomes in Acute Heart Failure; Re-defining the Cardio-Renal Interaction? *J Am Coll Cardiol.* 2006;48(8):1621–1627.

46. Wu AH. Serial testing of B-type natriuretic peptide and NTpro-BNP for monitoring therapy of heart failure: the role of biologic variation in the interpretation of results. *Am Heart J.* 2006;152(5): 828–834.

47. Schou M, Gustafsson F, Kjaer A, Hildebrandt PR. Long-term clinical variation of NT-proBNP in stable chronic heart failure patients. *Eur Heart J.* 2007;28(2):177–182.

48. Goetze JP, Christoffersen C, Perko M, et al. Increased cardiac BNP expression associated with myocardial ischemia. *Faseb J.* 2003; 17(9):1105–1107.

49. Toth M, Vuorinen KH, Vuolteenaho O, et al. Hypoxia stimulates release of ANP and BNP from perfused rat ventricular myocardium. *Am J Physiol.* 1994;266(4 Pt 2):H1572–H1580.

50. Marumoto K, Hamada M, Hiwada K. Increased secretion of atrial and brain natriuretic peptides during acute myocardial ischaemia induced by dynamic exercise in patients with angina pectoris. *Clin Sci (Lond).* 1995;88(5):551–556.

51. Kyriakides ZS, Markianos M, Michalis L, et al. Brain natriuretic peptide increases acutely and much more prominently than atrial natriuretic peptide during coronary angioplasty. *Clin Cardiol.* 2000; 23(4):285–288.

52. Mega JL, Morrow DA, De Lemos JA, et al. B-type natriuretic peptide at presentation and prognosis in patients with ST-segment elevation myocardial infarction: an ENTIRE-TIMI-23 substudy. *J Am Coll Cardiol.* 2004;44(2):335–339.

53. Khan SQ, Dhillon O, Kelly D, et al. Plasma N-terminal B-Type natriuretic peptide as an indicator of long-term survival after acute myocardial infarction: comparison with plasma midregional pro-atrial natriuretic peptide: the LAMP (Leicester Acute Myocardial

Infarction Peptide) study. *J Am Coll Cardiol.* 2008;51(19):1857–1864.

54. de Lemos, JA, Morrow DA, Bentley JH, et al. The prognostic value of B-type natriuretic peptide in patients with acute coronary syndromes. *N Engl J Med.* 2001;345(14):1014–1021.

55. Omland T, Aakvaag A, Bonarjee VV, et al. Plasma brain natriuretic peptide as an indicator of left ventricular systolic function and long-term survival after acute myocardial infarction. Comparison with plasma atrial natriuretic peptide and N-terminal proatrial natriuretic peptide. *Circulation.* 1996;93(11):1963–1969.

56. Drewniak W, Snopek G, Zarukiewicz M, Borys M, Dabrowski M. Prognostic value of the N-terminal pro-B-type natriuretic peptide in the elderly with acute myocardial infarction. *Kardiol Pol.* 2008; 66(7):750–755.

57. Ashley KE, Galla JM, Nicholls SJ. Brain natriuretic peptides as biomarkers for atherosclerosis. *Prev Cardiol.* 2008;11(3):172–176.

58. Rossi A, Enriquez-Sarano M, Burnett JC, Jr, et al. Natriuretic peptide levels in atrial fibrillation: a prospective hormonal and Doppler-echocardiographic study. *J Am Coll Cardiol.* 2000;35(5):1256–1262.

59. Morello A, Lloyd-Jones DM, Chae CU, et al. Association of atrial fibrillation and amino-terminal pro-brain natriuretic peptide concentrations in dyspneic subjects with and without acute heart failure: results from the ProBNP Investigation of Dyspnea in the Emergency Department (PRIDE) study. *Am Heart J.* 2007;153(1):90–97.

60. Silvet H, Young-Xu Y, Walleigh D, Ravid S. Brain natriuretic peptide is elevated in outpatients with atrial fibrillation. *Am J Cardiol.* 2003; 92(9):1124–1127.

61. Corell P, Gustafsson F, Kistorp C, et al. Effect of atrial fibrillation on plasma NT-proBNP in chronic heart failure. *Int J Cardiol.* 2007; 117(3):395–402.

62. Jourdain P, Bellorini M, Funck F, et al. Short-term effects of sinus rhythm restoration in patients with lone atrial fibrillation: a hormonal study. *Eur J Heart Fail.* 2002;4(3):263–267.

63. Mabuchi N, Tsutamoto T, Maeda K, Kinoshita M. Plasma cardiac natriuretic peptides as biochemical markers of recurrence of atrial

fibrillation in patients with mild congestive heart failure. *Jpn Circ J.* 2000;64(10):765–771.

64. Mabuchi N, Tsutamoto T, Maeda K, Masahiko K. [Plasma cardiac natriuretic peptide as a biological marker of recurrence of atrial fibrillation in elderly people]. *Nippon Ronen Igakkai Zasshi.* 2000; 37(7):535–540.

65. Horie H, Tsutamoto T, Minai K, et al. Brain natriuretic peptide predicts chronic atrial fibrillation after ventricular pacing in patients with sick sinus syndrome. *Jpn Circ J.* 2000;64(12):965–970.

66. Wazni OM, Martin DO, Marrouche NF, et al. Plasma B-type natriuretic peptide levels predict postoperative atrial fibrillation in patients undergoing cardiac surgery. *Circulation.* 2004;110(2): 124–127.

67. Ikeda T, Matsuda K, Itoh H, et al. Plasma levels of brain and atrial natriuretic peptides elevate in proportion to left ventricular end-systolic wall stress in patients with aortic stenosis. *Am Heart J.* 1997;133(3):307–314.

68. Kupari M, Turto H, Lommi J, Makijarvi M, Parikka H. Transcardiac gradients of N-terminal B-type natriuretic peptide in aortic valve stenosis. *Eur J Heart Fail.* 2005;7(5):809–814.

69. Qi W, Mathisen P, Kjekshus J, et al. Natriuretic peptides in patients with aortic stenosis. *Am Heart J.* 2001;142(4):725–732.

70. Talwar S, Downie PF, Squire IB, et al. Plasma N-terminal pro BNP and cardiotrophin-1 are elevated in aortic stenosis. *Eur J Heart Fail.* 2001;3(1):15–19.

71. Gerber IL, Stewart RA, Legget ME, et al. Increased plasma natriuretic peptide levels reflect symptom onset in aortic stenosis. *Circulation.* 2003;107(14):1884–1890.

72. Gerber IL, Legget ME, West TM, Richards AM, Stewart RA. Usefulness of serial measurement of N-terminal pro-brain natriuretic peptide plasma levels in asymptomatic patients with aortic stenosis to predict symptomatic deterioration. *Am J Cardiol.* 2005;95(7): 898–901.

73. Bergler-Klein J, Klaar U, Heger M, et al. Natriuretic peptides predict symptom-free survival and postoperative outcome in severe aortic stenosis. *Circulation.* 2004;109(19):2302–2308.

74. Weber M, Arnold R, Rau M, et al. Relation of N-terminal pro B-type natriuretic peptide to progression of aortic valve disease. *Eur Heart J.* 2005;26(10):1023–1030.

75. Eimer MJ, Ekery DL, Rigolin VH, et al. Elevated B-type natriuretic peptide in asymptomatic men with chronic aortic regurgitation and preserved left ventricular systolic function. *Am J Cardiol.* 2004; 94(5):676–678.

76. Ozkan M, Baysan O, Erinc K, et al. Brain natriuretic peptide and the severity of aortic regurgitation: is there any correlation? *J Int Med Res.* 2005;33(4):454–459.

77. Sutton TM, Stewart RAH, Gerber IL, et al. Plasma natriuretic peptide levels increase with symptoms and severity of mitral regurgitation. *Journal of the American College of Cardiology.* 2003;41(12):2280–2287.

78. Yusoff R, Clayton N, Keevil B, Morris J, Ray S. Utility of plasma N-terminal brain natriuretic peptide as a marker of functional capacity in patients with chronic severe mitral regurgitation. *Am J Cardiol.* 2006;97(10):1498–1501.

79. Brookes CI, Kemp MW, Hooper J, Oldershaw PJ, Moat NE. Plasma brain natriuretic peptide concentrations in patients with chronic mitral regurgitation. *J Heart Valve Dis.* 1997;6(6):608–612.

80. Chen AA, Wood MJ, Krauser DG, et al. NT-proBNP levels, echocardiographic findings, and outcomes in breathless patients: results from the ProBNP Investigation of Dyspnoea in the Emergency Department (PRIDE) echocardiographic substudy. *Eur Heart J.* 2006;27(7):839–845.

81. Tung RH, Camargo CA, Jr, Krauser D, et al. Amino-terminal pro-brain natriuretic peptide for the diagnosis of acute heart failure in patients with previous obstructive airway disease. *Ann Emerg Med.* 2006;48(1):66–74.

82. Nagaya N, Nishikimi T, Uematsu M, et al. Plasma brain natriuretic peptide as a prognostic indicator in patients with primary pulmonary hypertension. *Circulation.* 2000;102(8):865–870.

83. Nagaya N, Nishikimi T, Okano Y, et al. Plasma brain natriuretic peptide levels increase in proportion to the extent of right ventricular dysfunction in pulmonary hypertension. *J Am Coll Cardiol.* 1998; 31(1):202–208.

84. Bando M, Ishii Y, Sugiyama Y, Kitamura S. Elevated plasma brain natriuretic peptide levels in chronic respiratory failure with cor pulmonale. *Respir Med.* 1999;93(7):507–514.

85. Ishii J, Nomura M, Ito M, et al. Plasma concentration of brain natriuretic peptide as a biochemical marker for the evaluation of right ventricular overload and mortality in chronic respiratory disease. *Clin Chim Acta.* 2000;301(1–2):19–30.

86. Leuchte HH, El Nounou M, Tuerpe JC, et al. N-terminal pro-brain natriuretic peptide and renal insufficiency as predictors of mortality in pulmonary hypertension. *Chest.* 2007;131(2):402–409.

87. Leuchte HH, Holzapfel M, Baumgartner RA, et al. Clinical significance of brain natriuretic peptide in primary pulmonary hypertension. *J Am Coll Cardiol.* 2004;43(5):764–770.

88. Binder L, Pieske B, Olschewski M, et al. N-terminal pro-brain natriuretic peptide or troponin testing followed by echocardiography for risk stratification of acute pulmonary embolism. *Circulation.* 2005;112(11):1573–1579.

89. Kurose M, Yoshimura M, Yasue H. Raised plasma BNP in a patient with acute pulmonary thromboembolism. *Heart.* 1997;78(3):320–321.

90. Kostrubiec M, Pruszczyk P, Kaczynska A, Kucher N. Persistent NT-proBNP elevation in acute pulmonary embolism predicts early death. *Clin Chim Acta.* 2007;382(1–2):124–128.

91. Logeart D, Lecuyer L, Thabut G, et al. Biomarker-based strategy for screening right ventricular dysfunction in patients with non-massive pulmonary embolism. *Intensive Care Med.* 2007;33(2):286–292.

92. Pieralli F, Olivotto I, Vanni S, et al. Usefulness of bedside testing for brain natriuretic peptide to identify right ventricular dysfunction and outcome in normotensive patients with acute pulmonary embolism. *Am J Cardiol.* 2006;97(9):1386–1390.

93. Kruger S, Graf J, Merx MW, et al. Brain natriuretic peptide predicts right heart failure in patients with acute pulmonary embolism. *Am Heart J.* 2004;147(1):60–65.

94. Tulevski II, Hirsch A, Sanson BJ, et al. Increased brain natriuretic peptide as a marker for right ventricular dysfunction in acute pulmonary embolism. *Thromb Haemost.* 2001;86(5):1193–1196.

95. Parrillo JE. Pathogenetic mechanisms of septic shock. *N Engl J Med.* 1993;328(20):1471–1477.
96. Hoffmann U, Brueckmann M, Bertsch T, et al. Increased plasma levels of NT-proANP and NT-proBNP as markers of cardiac dysfunction in septic patients. *Clin Lab.* 2005;51(7–8):373–379.
97. Charpentier J, Luyt CE, Fulla Y, et al. Brain natriuretic peptide: A marker of myocardial dysfunction and prognosis during severe sepsis. *Crit Care Med.* 2004;32(3):660–665.
98. Stewart D, Waxman K, Brown CA, et al. B-type natriuretic peptide levels may be elevated in the critically injured trauma patient without congestive heart failure. *J Trauma.* 2007;63(4):747–750.
99. Price S, Anning PB, Mitchell JA, Evans TW. Myocardial dysfunction in sepsis: mechanisms and therapeutic implications. *Eur Heart J.* 1999;20(10):715–724.
100. He Q, LaPointe MC. Interleukin-1beta regulation of the human brain natriuretic peptide promoter involves Ras-, Rac-, and p38 kinase-dependent pathways in cardiac myocytes. *Hypertension.* 1999;33(1 Pt 2):283–289.
101. Groeneveld AB, Hartemink KJ, de Groot MC, Visser J, Thijs LG. Circulating endothelin and nitrate-nitrite relate to hemodynamic and metabolic variables in human septic shock. *Shock.* 1999;11(3):160–166.
102. Januzzi JL, Jr, Sakhuja R, O'Donoghue M, et al. Utility of amino-terminal pro-brain natriuretic peptide testing for prediction of 1-year mortality in patients with dyspnea treated in the emergency department. *Arch Intern Med.* 2006;166(3):315–320.
103. Meyer B, Huelsmann M, Wexberg P, et al. N-terminal pro-B-type natriuretic peptide is an independent predictor of outcome in an unselected cohort of critically ill patients. *Crit Care Med.* 2007;35(10):2268–2273.
104. Almog Y, Novack V, Megralishvili R, et al. Plasma level of N terminal pro-brain natriuretic peptide as a prognostic marker in critically ill patients. *Anesth Analg.* 2006;102(6):1809–1815.
105. O'Donoghue M, Chen A, Baggish AL, et al. The effects of ejection fraction on N-terminal ProBNP and BNP levels in patients with acute CHF: analysis from the ProBNP Investigation of Dyspnea in the Emergency Department (PRIDE) study. *J Card Fail.* 2005;11(5 Suppl):S9–S14.

106. Horwich TB, Hamilton MA, Fonarow GC. B-type natriuretic peptide levels in obese patients with advanced heart failure. *J Am Coll Cardiol.* 2006;47(1):85–90.

107. Krauser DG, Lloyd-Jones DM, Chae CU, et al. Effect of body mass index on natriuretic peptide levels in patients with acute congestive heart failure: a ProBNP Investigation of Dyspnea in the Emergency Department (PRIDE) substudy. *Am Heart J.* 2005;149(4):744–750.

108. Taylor JA, Christenson RH, Rao K, Jorge M, Gottlieb SS. B-type natriuretic peptide and N-terminal pro B-type natriuretic peptide are depressed in obesity despite higher left ventricular end diastolic pressures. *Am Heart J.* 2006;152(6):1071–1076.

109. Bayes-Genis A, Lloyd-Jones DM, van Kimmenade RR, et al. Effect of body mass index on diagnostic and prognostic usefulness of amino-terminal pro-brain natriuretic peptide in patients with acute dyspnea. *Arch Intern Med.* 2007;167(4):400–407.

22 ■ Natriuretic Peptide Testing for Patients with Acute and Chronic Coronary Disease

Torbjørn Omland, MD, PhD, MPH, FESC

Introduction

B-type natriuretic peptide (BNP) and the N-terminal fragment (NT-proBNP) of its prohormone (proBNP) are associated with indices of cardiac function and are established markers for diagnosis and risk assessment in heart failure. Recent data demonstrate that both BNP and NT-proBNP are strong and independent prognostic markers in acute and chronic coronary disease. Whereas associations with recurrent ischemic events are relatively weak or nonexistent after adjustment for confounding factors, associations with incident death and heart failure are strong and consistent. Prospective data demonstrating that BNP or NT-proBNP are clinically useful guides to therapy in patients with unstable or stable coronary artery disease are still lacking.

Ischemic heart disease is the most prevalent chronic, life-threatening disease in the Western world.[1] In North America, an estimated 20 million people have significant, symptomatic or asymptomatic, coronary artery disease. Stable coronary disease may progress to an acute coronary syndrome, a condition associated with significant risk of ventricular dysfunction, serious cardiac arrhythmias, and death. In the United States, approximately eight million patients present annually to emergency departments with nontraumatic chest pain and a suspected acute coronary syndrome.[2] Additionally, each year an estimated 300,000 North Americans die suddenly of undiagnosed coronary artery disease. Accordingly, new and better diagnostic methods for detection of coronary artery disease and prognostic tools for identifying patients who may require intensified therapy are desirable.

Acute Coronary Syndrome

The measurement of natriuretic peptides is of value in those with acute coronary syndromes. This is based on the observation that coronary ischemia may lead to elevation in both BNP and NT-proBNP, and when this occurs, it is a prognostically meaningful situation.

BNP Synthesis and Release in Myocardial Ischemia

The cardiac BNP system is activated following acute ischemic injury.[3–5] In a rat coronary ligation model, BNP tissue levels doubled by 12 hours and increased by a factor of five 24 hours after the ischemic injury.[3] Increased BNP levels were detected in both the infarcted and noninfarcted regions of the ventricle, showing that increased circulating BNP concentrations are not only secondary to tissue necrosis, but reflect synthesis and release from viable cardiomyocytes.

In the clinical setting, the plasma concentration of BNP and NT-proBNP increases rapidly after the onset of acute myocardial infarction;[4,6] the magnitude and duration of the rise is proportional to infarct size, as assessed by cardiac enzyme levels in the circulation[7] by single photon-computed tomography[8] or contrast-enhanced magnetic resonance imaging.[9,10] Accordingly, circulating levels of BNP and NT-proBNP are predictive of the subsequent degree of left ventricular dysfunction.[6,10] Anterior wall infarctions are associated with higher levels of circulating BNP and NT-proBNP than inferior wall infarcts, and a biphasic pattern with a second peak on days 2–5 may be more commonly associated with an anterior than an inferior infarct location.[4] Circulating concentrations of BNP and NT-proBNP decline gradually during the course of weeks after an acute coronary syndrome.[11]

Systolic dysfunction and pump failure of the left ventricle have long been considered major stimuli for BNP and NT-proBNP synthesis and release.[12,13] Ventricular relaxation abnormalities, an early sign of ischemia preceding electrocardiographic changes and anginal pain,[14] may also increase the synthesis and release of BNP and NT-proBNP. Accordingly, during the processes of infarct expansion and ventricular remodeling that occur early after myocardial infarction, both elevated intracavitary pressure and volume increase may result in higher levels of BNP and NT-proBNP in the circulation.

Brief periods of ischemia may cause release of BNP without concomitant change in left ventricular end-diastolic pressure, suggesting that ischemia *per se* is a stimulus for BNP release.[15,16] Indeed, in rats trained in hypobaric hypoxic conditions, BNP gene expression is induced,[17] while in human atrial myocytes, incubation in a hypoxic buffer results in increased natriuretic peptide release.[18] The theory that ischemia/hypoxia itself may act as a stimulus for BNP and NT-proBNP release is also favored by the fact that unstable angina is associated with increased BNP and NT-proBNP levels,[19,20] which return to normal following successful percutaneous coronary intervention.[19] Similarly, in stress testing, BNP and NT-proBNP concentrations at rest reflect the size of subsequently ischemic territories,[21–25] and increase in proportion to the severity of ischemia.[22,26–28] Moreover, circulating BNP concentrations are elevated and are associated with BNP mRNA expression in patients with normal left ventricular systolic function during coronary bypass surgery,[29] and euvolemic patients with cyanotic heart disease have higher NT-proBNP levels than noncyanotic patients with repaired congenital heart defects.[18] Also suggesting a role for BNP and NT-proBNP in coronary artery disease is the demonstration of BNP and NT-proBNP immunoreactivity in human coronary arteries,[30] perhaps indicating an autocrine or paracrine role in modulating the process of atherosclerosis. In aggregate, the data are compelling to support the contention that ischemia and ischemic heart disease may trigger release of BNP or NT-proBNP.

Diagnostic Value of BNP and NT-proBNP in Acute Coronary Syndromes

BNP and NT-proBNP production and release are both stimulated by myocardial ischemia. That notwithstanding, natriuretic peptides are poor diagnostic markers in the setting of suspected acute coronary syndromes. Whereas cardiac-specific troponins measured with conventional assays are commonly considered highly specific and sometimes almost considered a qualitative test by many clinicians ("troponin positive versus troponin negative"), BNP and NT-proBNP tend to be less specific because concentrations in the circulation are associated with numerous cardiac and noncardiac factors (e.g., age, gender, body mass index). In comparison with cardiac-specific troponins which display a narrow normal range with conventional assays, BNP and NT-proBNP normal levels are relatively wide. Important for diagnostic purposes, the signal-noise ratio is not particularly favorable for diagnosing myocardial infarction or unstable angina: the magnitude of the increase in circulating BNP and NT-proBNP is usually considerably lower than what is typically seen in patients with acutely destabilized cardiac failure. In particular, if the patient's own "normal" value is unknown because of lack of prior measurements, it may be difficult to correctly interpret a single, mildly-elevated BNP or NT-proBNP test result.

Risk Assessment in Acute Coronary Syndrome

The term "acute coronary syndrome" describes a pathophysiological process of varying degrees of impairment of coronary artery blood flow and subsequent reduction of myocardial oxygen supply, combined with a constellation of clinical symptoms secondary to myocardial ischemia. Based on findings of the electrocardiogram at presentation, acute coronary syndromes are subdivided according to the presence or absence of ST segment elevation. Patients without ST segment elevation are further subdivided into unstable angina with no biochemical evidence of myocardial necrosis and myocardial infarction without electrocardiographic ST segment elevation. Traditionally, clinical signs of heart failure, systolic ventricular dysfunction, and larger left ventricular dimensions have been linked to poor outcomes after acute myocardial infarction.[31,32] Following advances in therapies for acute coronary syndromes during the past two decades, fewer patients will develop large transmural infarctions complicated with acute heart failure. Moreover, redefinition of the diagnosis of acute myocardial infarction and introduction of more sensitive biomarkers of myocardial necrosis have resulted in a relative increase in the incidence of non-ST segment myocardial infarctions.

To mirror the evolving change in the panorama of acute coronary syndromes and to reflect more contemporary therapeutic practices, multiple models for risk prediction have been generated for various subsets of the acute coronary syndrome.[33,34] These models have to a large extent been derived from large-scale clinical trials and the generalizability to the patients encountered by the practicing clinicians has been questioned. Even more recently, attempts have been made to develop risk scores based on more unbiased and representative populations. One such example is the Global Registry of Acute Coronary Events (GRACE), which is based on a multinational cooperative effort of 94 hospitals in 14 countries and encompasses all types of ACS and is applicable to both short-term and long-term mortality.[35] The variables identified to predict mortality at six months in GRACE are presented in Table 22–1. The overall prognostic accuracy of the GRACE prediction model, expressed as areas under the receiver-operating characteristic curve (ROC), or C statistic, are 0.81 in the derivation and 0.75 in the validation cohort. Accordingly, one important criterion for demonstrating improvement in overall risk stratification by a candidate biomarker is to increase the C statistic

Table 22–1: Predictors of mortality at six months in the Global Registry of Acute Coronary Events (GRACE).[35]
Older age
History of myocardial infarction
History of heart failure
Increased pulse rate at presentation
Lower systolic blood pressure at presentation
Elevated initial serum creatinine concentration
Elevated initial cardiac biomarker (troponin) level
ST segment depression on presenting electrocardiogram
Not having a percutaneous coronary intervention in hospital

significantly above and beyond that of the conventional risk factor model.[36]

Prognostic Value of BNP and NT-proBNP in Acute Coronary Syndromes

The first studies showing that BNP obtained in the acute or subacute phase of myocardial infarction are predictive of subsequent mortality were published in 1996.[5,37] Despite a relatively modest number of patients (<150) in each study, these investigations demonstrated that BNP provides prognostic information complementary to conventional risk markers, including left ventricular systolic function. Similar results for NT-proBNP were published in 1998.[38] Starting in 2001, several large-scale studies have confirmed and extended these results to show that BNP and NT-proBNP concentrations are strong, independent predictors of both short-term and long-term cardiovascular mortality as well as total mortality across the spectrum of acute coronary syndromes, from unstable angina

Table 22–2: Key points regarding BNP and NT-proBNP in acute and chronic coronary disease.

Acute coronary disease

- BNP and NT-proBNP are both independently associated with death and heart failure development in patients with acute coronary disease.
- The association with recurrent ischemic events is weaker and attenuated after adjustment for other risk markers.
- The risk associated with BNP and NT-proBNP elevation is directly proportional to circulating levels, with highest risk in those with most marked elevation of the marker.
- Although retrospective analyses in different studies yield different theoretically optimal cutoffs, the aggregate of existing data suggests that persistently elevated levels of BNP (>80 pg/mL) and NT-pro-BNP (>250 pg/mL) are associated with adverse outcome.
- In patients with a suspected acute coronary syndrome, it is recommended to measure BNP or NT-proBNP at (or near) the time of admission.
- Prospective studies demonstrating usefulness of BNP or NT-proBNP determination as a guide to therapy in acute coronary disease—including the use of early revascularization or use of glycoprotein IIb/IIIa inhibitors—are lacking.
- Based on retrospective data, early cardiac catheterization and coronary intervention should be considered in patients presenting with an elevated BNP or NT-proBNP measurements, particularly if troponin levels are also elevated.
- As BNP and NT-proBNP measurements performed in the subacute or early convalescent phase provide more accurate information concerning long-term outcome than measurements at presentation, repeat BNP or NT-proBNP measurement may be performed after 24–72 hours and again at 3–6 months.

Chronic coronary disease

- BNP and NT-proBNP are both independently associated with the incidence of death, heart failure development, and stroke in patients with chronic coronary disease.
- The association with the incidence of myocardial infarction is weaker and attenuated after adjustment for other risk markers.

Table 22–2: (Continued)

- Persistently elevated levels of BNP (>80 pg/mL) and NT-pro-BNP (>250 pg/mL) are associated with adverse outcome.
- Studies demonstrating usefulness of BNP or NT-proBNP determination as a guide to therapy in chronic coronary disease—including the use of angiotensin converting enzyme inhibitors, high-dose statin therapy, or prolonged clopidogrel therapy—are lacking.
- In chronic coronary disease, repeat BNP and NT-proBNP measurements may be considered at 6–18 month intervals. A new sample may also be considered in the case of clinical suspicion of disease progression, and in particular if heart failure development is suspected.

Source: Adapted from Omland and Lemos, 2008.[78]

to non-ST and ST elevation myocardial infarction. The risk of death increases proportionally with circulating levels of BNP and NT-proBNP. For instance, in a substudy of the Orbofiban in Patients with Unstable Coronary Syndromes—Thrombolysis in Myocardial Infarction 16 trial (OPUS-TIMI 16), BNP was measured in 2525 patients with unstable angina, non-ST elevation myocardial infarction, or ST elevation myocardial infarction. After subdividing the patients according to quartiles of BNP and using the first quartile as the reference, the adjusted odds ratio estimates for death at ten months were 3.8, 4.0, and 5.8 for the second, third, or fourth quartiles (Figure 22–1).[39] Similar results have been observed for NT-proBNP,[40–42] even after adjustment for left ventricular ejection fraction.[41] Recently, the prognostic value of NT-proBNP has also been examined in a large cohort of acute coronary syndrome patients with normal troponin values on admission. Even in this patient group, commonly considered to be at low risk, NT-proBNP discriminated well between subjects at high and low risk for death.[43]

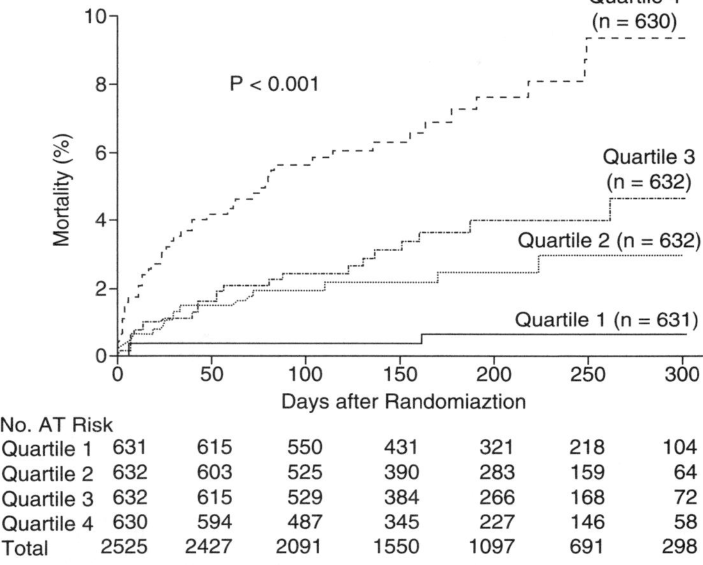

No. AT Risk							
Quartile 1	631	615	550	431	321	218	104
Quartile 2	632	603	525	390	283	159	64
Quartile 3	632	615	529	384	266	168	72
Quartile 4	630	594	487	345	227	146	58
Total	2525	2427	2091	1550	1097	691	298

■ **Figure 22–1** Association between NT-proBNP levels by quartiles and all cause mortality at 10 months in patients with acute coronary syndromes. First quartile, <43.6 ng/L; second quartile, 43.7–81.2 ng/L; third quartile, 81.3–137.8 ng/L; and fourth quartile, more than 137.9 ng/L.

de Lemos JA, Morrow DA, Bentley JH, et al. The prognostic value of B-type natriuretic peptide in patients with acute coronary syndromes. *N Engl J Med.* 2001; 345(14):1014–1021.

Prediction of death following acute coronary syndromes by BNP and NT-proBNP suggests that these peptides are associated with the risk of recurrent ischemic events, arrhythmic events, heart failure, or a combination of these. Several studies have convincingly demonstrated that BNP and NT-proBNP are predictive of the incidence of heart failure after an episode of unstable coronary disease.[39,44,45] In contrast, the association between BNP and NT-proBNP and the incidence of recurrent myocardial infarction is weak or nonexistent after adjusting for potential confounders.[39,40] Given the associations between BNP and NT-proBNP with the severity of coronary artery disease and the extent of myocardial ischemia, this observation may seem surprising. However, it is possible that elevation of BNP or NT-proBNP on admission reflects a large ischemic territory and that a recurrent infarction in such patients is more likely to be fatal. Whether BNP and NT-proBNP are specifically predictive of malignant arrhythmias in patients with acute coronary syndromes remains to be determined. Taken together, the prevailing view is that the ability of BNP and NT-proBNP to predict death in acute coronary syndromes is largely explained by its ability to predict heart failure, rather than a recurrent ischemic event.

The incremental prognostic value of adding BNP and NT-proBNP to existing acute coronary syndrome risk score models for death and heart failure has also been evaluated.[46,47] Data from the OPUS-TIMI 16 and the TACTICS-TIMI 18 suggest that the addition of BNP > 80 pg/mL improved the performance of a risk score to predict the incidence of congestive heart failure.[46] Adding NT-proBNP to the TIMI risk score and to the 2002 ACC/AHA risk classification also resulted in improved prediction of death.[47]

Timing of Measurement

The optimal timing of biomarker measurements in patients with acute coronary syndromes depends on the intended use of the test result. If the biomarker is measured for diagnostic purposes, e.g., to distinguish between an acute coronary syndrome and noncardiac chest pain, or for the assessment of in-hospital outcomes, measurement on admission is clearly desirable. On the other hand, if the intended use is long-term risk stratification, measurement in the subacute phase or at the time discharge may be optimal. The second important point to consider is the plasma profile of the biomarker. As mentioned above, circulating concentrations of BNP and NT-proBNP increase rapidly following acute ischemic injury and are highest on admission, fall markedly during the first

24 hours in uncomplicated cases, and decrease gradually over the following six months.[4,6,11] In contrast, a complicated course is associated with persistent elevation. Accordingly for long-term prognostic purposes, samples obtained in the subacute phase appear to be preferable to those obtained very early, suggesting a favorable signal-noise ratio in the subacute phase. Based on the complementary information derived from early and late samples, it seems logical to perform serial sampling. The clinical utility of such a strategy has been tested, and a second NT-proBNP measurement performed 72 hours following admission improved short-term risk prediction. Regardless of the NT-proBNP value on admission, an NT-proBNP concentration of greater than 250 ng/L at 72 hours was associated with increased risk.[48] In addition, BNP levels obtained four months after the acute events seem to provide additional prognostic information to that obtained from early measurements. Accordingly, BNP levels greater than 80 pg/mL four months after the index hospitalization were associated with the risk of future deaths and heart failure hospitalizations.[45] Conversely, BNP levels less than 80 pg/mL were associated with reduced risk regardless of baseline concentrations.[45]

Prediction of Therapeutic Effects

Cardiac troponin measurements are performed routinely in patients with suspected acute coronary syndromes, not only because it is a *sine qua non* criterion for myocardial infarction, but also because it permits the clinician to identify patients who are likely to benefit from more aggressive therapy (e.g., with glycoprotein IIb/IIIa receptor inhibitors or an early invasive strategy).[49] Documenting that BNP or NT-proBNP can be used to tailor therapy in acute coronary syndromes would be considered by most clinicians more immediately useful than demonstration of an association with risk alone and would imply a clear clinical application for the use of BNP or NT-proBNP. Unfortunately, robust evidence for such an association is currently relatively limited. One contributing factor is that in contrast to troponins, which are powerful predictors of recurrent ischemic events, BNP and NT-proBNP are primarily predictors of mortality and heart failure, and few therapeutic strategies in acute coronary syndrome are associated with a reduction in mortality. The following evidence suggests that BNP or NT-proBNP can be used to identify subjects with non-ST elevation acute coronary syndromes who benefit from revascularization: In the Fragmin and Fast Revascularization During Instability in Coronary Artery Disease (FRISC)-II trial, a trend towards greater mortality reduction in the early invasive arm was observed in the highest NT-proBNP tertile, whereas no beneficial effect of the early invasive strategy was observed in those in the lower two NT-proBNP tertiles.[50] In a retrospective propensity score analysis from the Global Use of Strategies to Open Coronary Arteries (GUSTO)-IV trial, patients with higher NT-proBNP levels appeared to have a survival benefit from coronary revascularization, particularly if they had a concomitant increase in troponin, whereas those with normal value of both biomarkers had a significant increase in mortality at one year if they underwent revascularization.[51] However, the TACTICS-TIMI 18 trial and the Invasive Versus Conservative Treatment in Unstable Coronary Syndromes (ICTUS) trial both failed to find an association between BNP or NT-proBNP levels and the effect of an early invasive strategy.[44,52] Potential reasons for the discrepant results include differences in endpoint definitions and the frequency of crossover to an invasive strategy from the conservative arms of the respective trials.

Chronic Coronary Disease

Many of the same considerations that apply to natriuretic peptide testing in those with acute coronary syndromes apply to those with chronic coronary disease.

Diagnostic Value of BNP and NT-proBNP in Chronic Coronary Disease

A potential application of BNP and NT-proBNP measurement in chronic coronary disease is for the detection of significant coronary artery stenoses, with the measurement either used as a screening test prior to coronary angiography or as an adjunct to improve the diagnostic accuracy of stress testing.

Multiple studies have demonstrated a relation between circulating BNP and NT-proBNP concentrations and the extent and severity of angiographic coronary artery disease.[23,53–56] Although attenuated, the association remains significant after controlling for confounding factors. Still, the strength of the association appears not to be sufficiently strong for BNP and NT-proBNP to be of real clinical utility.[52–54]

Numerous clinical studies have also assessed potential associations between BNP and NT-proBNP levels at rest and the magnitude of the ischemic territory, as assessed by nuclear imaging methods or stress echocardiography. However, the results are not uniform, probably due to differences in methodology and patient selection. An association between resting BNP and NT-proBNP levels and the extent of myocardial ischemia have been reported by some investigators,[23–25] but not others.[22,57,58] An association between the exercise-induced increments in BNP and NT-proBNP levels and the degree of myocardial ischemia has also been assessed. For instance, in a study including 260 patients with suspected coronary artery disease referred to as SPECT, patients with the greatest increase in NT-proBNP levels during exercise had increased risk of inducible ischemia. Diagnostic accuracy was comparable with that of the exercise electrocardiogram, and combining the two resulted in only slight improvement in diagnostic performance.[26] In another study of 112 patients referred for exercise testing with nuclear perfusion imaging, baseline levels of BNP—but not NT-proBNP—were associated with the subsequent degree of provoked ischemia (Figure 22–2).[22] Exercise-induced increments in BNP were greater in patients with myocardial ischemia than in patients without inducible ischemia. A similar pattern was evident for NT-proBNP, but the change in concentrations were less pronounced than for BNP, which is not surprising given the different kinetics of the two peptides. In a selected group of 74

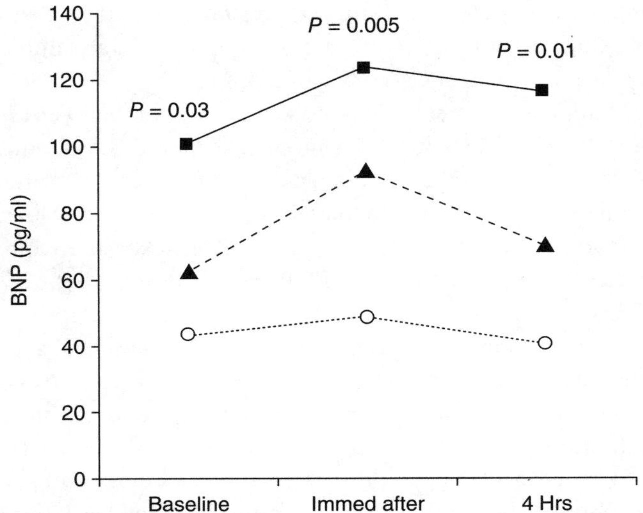

Ischemia	n	Median BNP (IQR) pg/ml		
Severe	14	101 (67–151)	123 (64–263)	115 (54–183)
Mild/Mod	42	62 (43–104)	92 (54–141)	70 (35–97)
No	40	43 (29–114)	49 (22–125)	40 (21–90)

■ **Figure 22–2** Association between circulating BNP and the extent of myocardial ischemia during stress testing. Median BNP levels in patients with no (open circles), mild to moderate (black triangles), and severe (black squares) ischemia at three timepoints (baseline, immediately after and 4 hrs after stress testing). The p-values are for trends across ischemic categories.

Sabatine MS, Morrow DA, de Lemos JA, et al. Acute changes in circulating natriuretic peptide levels in relation to myocardial ischemia. *J Am Coll Cardiol.* 2004; 44(10):1988–1995. © American College of Cardiology Foundation Published by Elsevier Inc.

patients with established coronary artery disease, normal ventricular function, and normal NT-proBNP levels, increments were greater for patients with signs of inducible ischemia than for those without such signs.[27] Compared to exercise electrocardiography,

NT-proBNP measurement performed better, with higher sensitivity at the same levels of specificity.[27] In conclusion, although results from some studies are encouraging, the practical value of adding BNP or NT-proBNP to enhance the diagnostic accuracy of stress testing remains to be determined. Clearly, prior to a general recommendation to include BNP or NT-proBNP measurements routinely during stress testing, new prediction algorithms including these peptides must be developed and validated.

Another potential application of BNP and NT-proBNP in patients with chronic coronary artery disease is detection of left ventricular systolic or diastolic dysfunction. In a study comprising 815 patients with chronic coronary artery disease and no history of heart failure, the usefulness of NT-proBNP for identifying patients with echocardiographic evidence of systolic or diastolic left ventricular dysfunction was assessed.[59] Overall diagnostic accuracy for detecting systolic or diastolic dysfunction, expressed as the area under the ROC, was moderately strong (0.78).

Prognostic Value of BNP and NT-proBNP in Chronic Coronary Disease

Patients with chronic, stable coronary artery disease are commonly believed to carry a favorable prognosis. However, several lines of evidence suggest that BNP and NT-proBNP are predictive of outcome in this patient group, as well:

- BNP and NT-proBNP are known to be associated with left ventricular systolic and diastolic function in patients with established coronary artery disease;
- myocardial ischemia is a strong stimulus for myocardial release of BNP and NT-proBNP;
- levels of BNP and NT-proBNP are associated with the severity and extent of atherosclerosis; and
- the strong association between BNP and NT-proBNP and outcome in unstable coronary disease suggests that the two peptides might be predictive of adverse events in patients with stable coronary artery disease.

This hypothesis has recently been confirmed by a series of studies investigating the association between BNP and NT-proBNP levels and prognosis.[60–67]

Kragelund et al. examined the association between NT-proBNP and mortality in 1034 patients referred for coronary angiography because of symptoms or signs of coronary heart disease.[61] During almost ten years of follow-up, 288 patients died. NT-proBNP levels were significantly lower in survivors than nonsurvivors. NT-proBNP levels correlated with increasing patient age, decreasing left ventricular ejection fraction, increasing left ventricular filling pressure, decreasing estimated glomerular filtration rate, and a history of diabetes mellitus and myocardial infarction. After adjustment for these and other risk factors, a graded, independent association between NT-proBNP concentrations and all-cause mortality was observed (Figure 22–3). These associations were also observed in subgroups of patients with preserved left ventricular systolic function, defined as a ventricular ejection fraction greater than 60%, as well as in diabetic patients.[68]

Richards et al. prospectively assessed the prognostic value of BNP and NT-proBNP in 1049 patients with chronic coronary artery disease.[69] The peptide levels were measured by in-house, closely correlated, noncommercial assays, and they displayed similar associations with traditional markers of risk. BNP and NT-proBNP appeared to be equally predictive of mortality from all causes and the combined endpoint mortality or heart failure. As 292 patients were recruited from a chronic heart failure trial, the study population included a substantial number of patients at relatively high risk.

Even more recently, the association between levels of BNP and/or NT-proBNP and the incidence of specific cardiovascular endpoints—cardiovascular death, myocardial infarction, stroke, and heart failure—recently has been assessed in three large-scale studies. These results may illuminate potential pathophysiological connections between BNP and NT-proBNP and adverse events in chronic coronary artery disease.

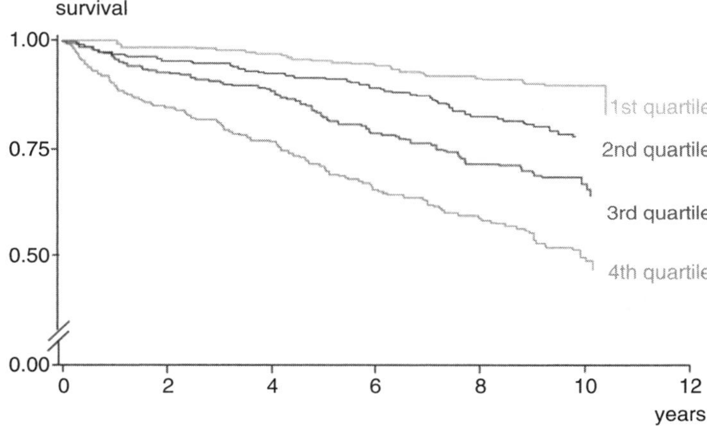

■ **Figure 22–3** Association between NT-proBNP levels by quartiles and all cause mortality in patients with stable coronary artery disease. First quartile, <64 ng/L; second quartile, 64–169 ng/L; third quartile, 170–455 ng/L; and fourth quartile, more than 455 ng/L.

Kragelund C, Gronning B, Kober L, Hildebrandt P, Steffensen R. N-terminal pro-B-type natriuretic peptide and long-term mortality in stable coronary heart disease. *N Engl J Med.* 2005;352(7):666–675.

The California-based Heart and Soul study included 987 stable coronary artery disease patients, and a comprehensive set of examinations of cardiovascular function, including transthoracic echocardiography and exercise testing followed by echocardiographic assessment of wall motion abnormalities. During follow-up, a total of 256 participants experienced a cardiovascular event or died. NT-proBNP levels at baseline were closely and independently associated with the incidence of cardiovascular events and death.[70] Importantly, NT-proBNP provided incremental prognostic information to clinical assessment and echocardiographic indices of cardiac function and exercise-induced ischemia. Considering individual cardiovascular endpoints, NT-proBNP was independently associated with the incidence of cardiovascular death and heart failure, but not with the incidence of myocardial infarction or stroke.

The relationship between NT-proBNP concentrations and the incidence of myocardial infarction, stroke, or cardiovascular death was examined in 3199 patients participating in the Heart Outcomes Prevention Evaluation (HOPE) Study.[71] Approximately 86% of patients had established coronary artery disease. During 4.5 years, 501 patients experienced one or more of the components of the primary outcome. NT-proBNP was independently associated with the primary outcome after adjusting for traditional markers of risk factors and other circulating biomarkers. Considering individual endpoints, NT-proBNP levels were associated with the incidence of myocardial infarction, but not stroke. In contrast to other biomarkers, NT-proBNP significantly increased the area under the ROC when included in a traditional risk factor model (Figure 22–4).

The Prevention of Events with Angiotensin-Converting Enzyme Inhibition Trial (PEACE), compared the effect of trandolapril and placebo in patients with stable coronary artery disease and preserved left ventricular function, defined as a documented left ventricular ejection fraction greater than 40%. In the biomarker substudy of the PEACE trial, plasma BNP and NT-proBNP concentrations at baseline were measured in 3761 patients.[72] The objective of the PEACE substudy was to address some of the still unresolved questions concerning BNP, NT-proBNP and prognosis. These unresolved questions included:

- whether BNP and NT-proBNP are associated with increased risk of specific cardiovascular events in a low-risk population with chronic coronary disease in the absence of impaired left ventricular function and symptoms and signs of heart failure;
- whether the association between BNP and NT-proBNP and the incidence of cardiovascular death can be attributed to prediction of heart failure or not;
- whether BNP and NT-proBNP measurements provide prognostic information above and beyond conventional risk factors as assessed by C-statistic calculations; and

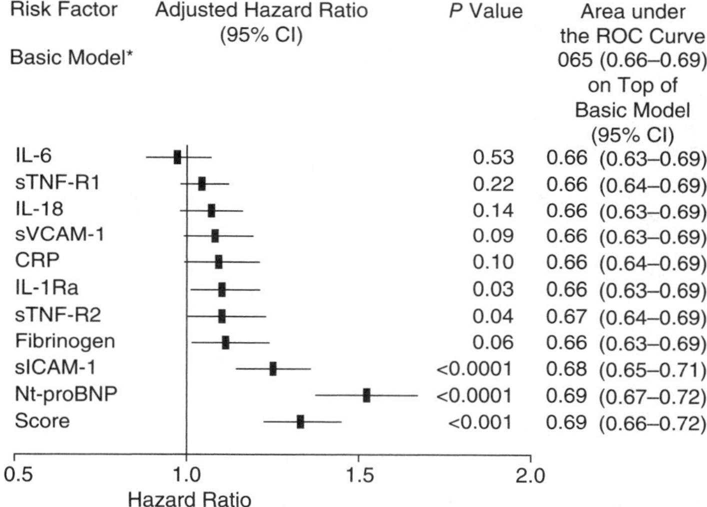

Risk Factor
Adjusted Hazard Ratio (95% CI)
P Value
Area under the ROC Curve
Basic Model*
065 (0.66–0.69)
on Top of Basic Model (95% CI)
IL-6
0.53
0.66 (0.63–0.69)
sTNF-R1
0.22
0.66 (0.64–0.69)
IL-18
0.14
0.66 (0.63–0.69)
sVCAM-1
0.09
0.66 (0.63–0.69)
CRP
0.10
0.66 (0.64–0.69)
IL-1Ra
0.03
0.66 (0.63–0.69)
sTNF-R2
0.04
0.67 (0.64–0.69)
Fibrinogen
0.06
0.66 (0.63–0.69)
sICAM-1
<0.0001
0.68 (0.65–0.71)
Nt-proBNP
<0.0001
0.69 (0.67–0.72)
Score
<0.001
0.69 (0.66–0.72)
0.5
1.0
1.5
2.0
Hazard Ratio

■ **Figure 22–4** Assosciation between the incidence of myocardial infarction, stroke, or cardiovascular death and the concentration of various inflammatory biomarkers, microalbuminuria and NT-proBNP.

Blankenberg S, McQueen MJ, Smieja M, et al. Comparative impact of multiple biomarkers and N-Terminal pro-brain natriuretic peptide in the context of conventional risk factors for the prediction of recurrent cardiovascular events in the Heart Outcomes Prevention Evaluation (HOPE) Study. *Circulation.* 2006; 114(3):201–208.

- whether BNP and NT-proBNP measurements are useful for identifying patients who benefit from angiotensin-converting-enzyme (ACE) inhibitors.

The following observations were made: BNP and NT-proBNP were predictive of cardiovascular death, congestive heart failure, and stroke (Figures 22–5, 22–6, 22–7), but neither one was associated with the incidence of myocardial infarction; both peptides were predictive of the incidence of congestive heart failure after adjustment for conventional risk markers, but only NT-proBNP

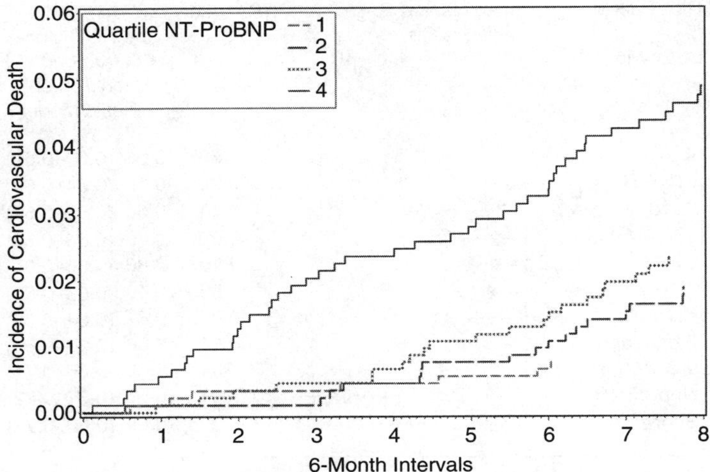

■ **Figure 22–5** Cumulative incidence of death due to a cardiovascular cause in patients with stable coronary artery disease and preserved ventricular function according to quartiles of plasma NT-proBNP concentrations.

Omland T, Sabatine MS, Jablonski KA, et al. Prognostic value of B-Type natriuretic peptides in patients with stable coronary artery disease: the PEACE Trial. *J Am Coll Cardiol.* 2007;50(3):205–214. © American College of Cardiology Foundation Published by Elsevier Inc.

provided independent prognostic information concerning the endpoints of cardiovascular death and stroke; adjustment or censoring for incident heart failure only marginally affected the risk estimates for cardiovascular death—the association between NT-proBNP and cardiovascular death must be explained by other pathophysiological mechanisms; adding BNP or NT-proBNP to a conventional risk marker model significantly increased the C-statistic, an index of overall prognostic accuracy, for the prediction of heart failure, but only NT-proBNP improved overall accuracy for prediction of cardiovascular death; and finally, neither BNP nor NT-proBNP was able to identify patients who experience a greater degree of benefit with ACE-inhibition.

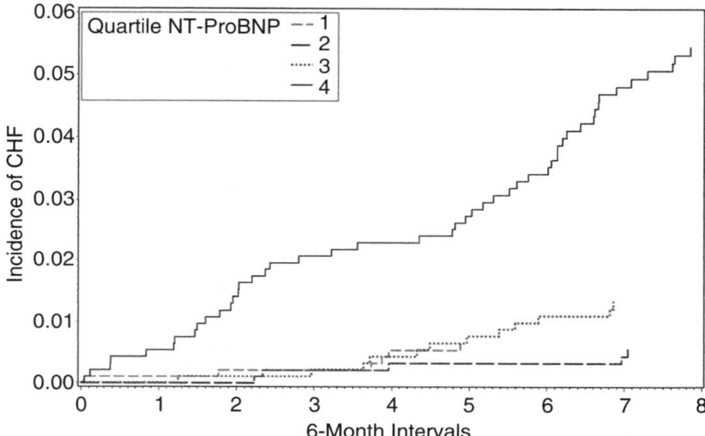

■ **Figure 22–6** Cumulative incidence of new fatal or nonfatal congestive heart failure (CHF) in patients with stable coronary artery disease and preserved ventricular function according to quartiles of plasma NT-proBNP concentrations.

Omland T, Sabatine MS, Jablonski KA, et al. Prognostic value of B-Type natriuretic peptides in patients with stable coronary artery disease: the PEACE Trial. *J Am Coll Cardiol.* 2007;50(3):205–214. © American College of Cardiology Foundation Published by Elsevier Inc.

Although BNP and NT-proBNP are relatively weak predictors of recurrent ischemic events in stable coronary artery disease, they seem to provide important prognostic information during nonurgent percutaneous coronary intervention. For instance, in the Clopidogrel for the Reduction of Events During Observation (CREDO) Study, NT-proBNP was independently associated with the incidence of death and myocardial infarction, but not stroke.[66] In a study from Taiwan encompassing 345 patients recruited after successful nonurgent percutaneous coronary intervention, NT-proBNP and the angiographic severity were significant, independent predictors of clinical restenosis.[73]

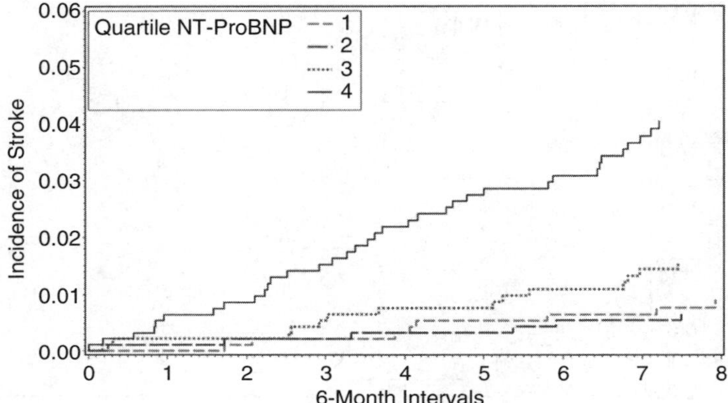

■ **Figure 22–7** Cumulative incidence of fatal or nonfatal stroke in patients with stable coronary artery disease and preserved ventricular function according to quartiles of plasma NT-proBNP concentrations.

Omland T, Sabatine MS, Jablonski KA, et al. Prognostic value of B-Type natriuretic peptides in patients with stable coronary artery disease: the PEACE Trial. *J Am Coll Cardiol.* 2007;50(3):205–214. © American College of Cardiology Foundation Published by Elsevier Inc.

Prediction of Therapeutic Effects

The clinical applications of BNP and NT-proBNP in chronic coronary artery disease would be more obvious if such measurements permitted identification of patients who experience greater benefit from therapeutic intervention. Unfortunately, only limited data exist to support use of BNP and NT-proBNP for this purpose. In a retrospective analysis, the benefit of carvedilol in patients with chronic heart failure secondary to ischemic heart disease was predicted by baseline levels of both BNP and NT-proBNP.[74,75] In contrast, in patients with stable coronary artery disease without heart failure, the effect of ACE inhibition was not predicted by baseline levels of BNP or NT-proBNP, i.e., the ACE inhibitor treatment was ineffective regardless of the baseline BNP or NT-proBNP concentrations.[72] One could argue that this finding could be due to the failure of the PEACE trial to demonstrate any beneficial effect of ACE inhibition on the primary outcome. However, NT-proBNP also failed to identify patients who experienced particular benefit from ACE-inhibitor therapy in the HOPE study, in which ACE inhibition was associated with improved outcome.[76] The failure of BNP and NT-proBNP to identify coronary artery disease patients who might benefit from ACE inhibition may partly be related to their relative inability to predict myocardial infarction.

Finally, the Heart Protection Study assessed the effect of simvastatin in a cohort of 20,536 individuals at high risk for vascular disease. Patients with higher NT-proBNP levels at baseline tended to have a less, but still significant, benefit from simvastatin in preventing major cardiovascular events. Still, because baseline risk was associated with NT-proBNP levels, the absolute benefit from therapy with simvastatin was similar at all levels of NT-proBNP,[77] suggesting that NT-proBNP should not be used to select patients who would benefit from statin therapy.

Conclusion

During the relatively short period of time since measurements have become readily available to clinicians, a remarkable amount of data has emerged consistently showing that BNP and NT-proBNP are extremely powerful predictors of short- and long-term outcomes across the spectrum of coronary artery disease. The associations are strongest for prediction of death and heart failure, and weaker for prediction of recurrent ischemic events. The strong associations with adverse outcome have resulted in Food and Drug Administration approval for the use of BNP and NT-proBNP for risk assessment in coronary artery disease. Moreover, the National Academy of Clinical Biochemistry Laboratory Medicine Guidelines have recently given BNP and NT-proBNP a firm class IIa recommendation for risk assessment in patients with a clinical syndrome consistent with acute coronary syndrome.[49] However, the guidelines also point out the main reason why clinicians have been slow to adopt the use of natriuretic peptides for risk stratification, is that benefits of therapy based on natriuretic peptide measurement remain uncertain. Future work should, therefore, be directed at clarifying the potential therapeutic implications of BNP and NT-proBNP test results in patients with acute and chronic coronary artery disease.

References

1. Hemingway H, McCallum A, Shipley M, Manderbacka K, Martikainen P, Keskimaki I. Incidence and prognostic implications of stable angina pectoris among women and men. *JAMA*. 2006;295(12): 1404–1411.
2. Storrow AB, Gibler WB. Chest pain centers: diagnosis of acute coronary syndromes. *Ann Emerg Med*. 2000;35(5):449–461.
3. Hama N, Itoh H, Shirakami G, et al. Rapid ventricular induction of brain natriuretic peptide gene expression in experimental acute myocardial infarction. *Circulation*. 1995;92(6):1558–1564.
4. Morita E, Yasue H, Yoshimura M, et al. Increased plasma levels of brain natriuretic peptide in patients with acute myocardial infarction. *Circulation*. 1993;88(1):82–91.
5. Omland T, Aakvaag A, Bonarjee VV, et al. Plasma brain natriuretic peptide as an indicator of left ventricular systolic function and long-term survival after acute myocardial infarction. Comparison with plasma atrial natriuretic peptide and N-terminal proatrial natriuretic peptide. *Circulation*. 1996;93(11):1963–1969.
6. Talwar S, Squire IB, Downie PF, et al. Profile of plasma N-terminal proBNP following acute myocardial infarction; correlation with left ventricular systolic dysfunction. *Eur Heart J*. 2000;21(18): 1514–1521.
7. Arakawa N, Nakamura M, Aoki H, Hiramori K. Relationship between plasma level of brain natriuretic peptide and myocardial infarct size. *Cardiology*. 1994;85(5):334–340.
8. Nakagawa K, Umetani K, Fujioka D, et al. Correlation of plasma concentrations of B-type natriuretic peptide with infarct size quantified by tomographic thallium-201 myocardial scintigraphy in asymptomatic patients with previous myocardial infarction. *Circ J*. 2004; 68(10):923–927.

9. Cochet A, Zeller M, Cottin Y, et al. The extent of myocardial damage assessed by contrast-enhanced MRI is a major determinant of N-BNP concentration after myocardial infarction. *Eur J Heart Fail.* 2004;6(5): 555–560.

10. Steen H, Futterer S, Merten C, Junger C, Katus HA, Giannitsis E. Relative role of NT-pro BNP and cardiac troponin T at 96 hours for estimation of infarct size and left ventricular function after acute myocardial infarction. *J Cardiovasc Magn Reson.* 2007;9(5):749–758.

11. Lindahl B, Lindback J, Jernberg T, et al. Serial analyses of N-terminal pro-B-type natriuretic peptide in patients with non-ST-segment elevation acute coronary syndromes: a Fragmin and fast Revascularisation during InStability in coronary artery disease (FRISC)-II substudy. *J Am Coll Cardiol.* 2005;45(4):533–541.

12. Mukoyama M, Nakao K, Hosoda K, et al. Brain natriuretic peptide as a novel cardiac hormone in humans. Evidence for an exquisite dual natriuretic peptide system, atrial natriuretic peptide and brain natriuretic peptide. *J Clin Invest.* 1991;87(4):1402–1412.

13. Ruskoaho H. Cardiac hormones as diagnostic tools in heart failure. *Endocr Rev.* 2003;24(3):341–356.

14. Cohn PF, Fox KM, Daly C. Silent myocardial ischemia. *Circulation.* 2003;108(10):1263–1277.

15. D'Souza SP, Yellon DM, Martin C, et al. B-type natriuretic peptide limits infarct size in rat isolated hearts via KATP channel opening. *Am J Physiol Heart Circ Physiol.* 2003;284(5):H1592–H1600.

16. D'Souza SP, Baxter GF. B Type natriuretic peptide: a good omen in myocardial ischaemia? *Heart.* 2003;89(7):707–709.

17. Perhonen M, Takala TE, Vuolteenaho O, Mantymaa P, Leppaluoto J, Ruskoaho H. Induction of cardiac natriuretic peptide gene expression in rats trained in hypobaric hypoxic conditions. *Am J Physiol.* 1997;273(1 Pt 2):R344–R352.

18. Hopkins WE, Chen Z, Fukagawa NK, Hall C, Knot HJ, LeWinter MM. Increased atrial and brain natriuretic peptides in adults with cyanotic congenital heart disease: enhanced understanding of the relationship between hypoxia and natriuretic peptide secretion. *Circulation.* 2004;109(23):2872–2877.

19. Kikuta K, Yasue H, Yoshimura M, et al. Increased plasma levels of B-type natriuretic peptide in patients with unstable angina. *Am Heart J.* 1996;132(1 Pt 1):101–107.

20. Talwar S, Squire IB, Downie PF, Davies JE, Ng LL. Plasma N terminal pro-brain natriuretic peptide and cardiotrophin 1 are raised in unstable angina. *Heart.* 2000;84(4):421–424.

21. Bibbins-Domingo K, Ansari M, Schiller NB, Massie B, Whooley MA. B-type natriuretic peptide and ischemia in patients with stable coronary disease: data from the Heart and Soul study. *Circulation.* 2003;108(24):2987–2992.

22. Sabatine MS, Morrow DA, de Lemos JA, et al. Acute changes in circulating natriuretic peptide levels in relation to myocardial ischemia. *J Am Coll Cardiol.* 2004;44(10):1988–1995.

23. Weber M, Dill T, Arnold R, et al. N-terminal B-type natriuretic peptide predicts extent of coronary artery disease and ischemia in patients with stable angina pectoris. *Am Heart J.* 2004;148(4): 612–620.

24. Feringa HH, Elhendy A, Bax JJ, et al. Baseline plasma N-terminal pro-B-type natriuretic peptide is associated with the extent of stress-induced myocardial ischemia during dobutamine stress echocardiography. *Coron Artery Dis.* 2006;17(3):255–259.

25. Chatha K, Alsoud M, Griffiths MJ, et al. B-type natriuretic peptide in reversible myocardial ischaemia. *J Clin Pathol.* 2006;59(11): 1216–1217.

26. Staub D, Jonas N, Zellweger MJ, et al. Use of N-terminal pro-B-type natriuretic peptide to detect myocardial ischemia. *Am J Med.* 2005; 118(11):1287.

27. Foote RS, Pearlman JD, Siegel AH, Yeo KT. Detection of exercise-induced ischemia by changes in B-type natriuretic peptides. *J Am Coll Cardiol.* 2004;44(10):1980–1987.

28. Asada J, Tsuji H, Iwasaka T, Thomas JD, Lauer MS. Usefulness of plasma brain natriuretic peptide levels in predicting dobutamine-induced myocardial ischemia. *Am J Cardiol.* 2004;93(6):702–704.

29. Goetze JP, Christoffersen C, Perko M, et al. Increased cardiac BNP expression associated with myocardial ischemia. *FASEB J.* 2003; 17(9):1105–1107.

30. Casco VH, Veinot JP, Kuroski de Bold ML, Masters RG, Stevenson MM, De Bold AJ. Natriuretic peptide system gene expression in human coronary arteries. *J Histochem Cytochem.* 2002;50(6): 799–809.

31. Killip T III, Kimball JT. Treatment of myocardial infarction in a coronary care unit. A two year experience with 250 patients. *Am J Cardiol.* 1967;20(4):457–464.

32. White HD, Norris RM, Brown MA, Brandt PW, Whitlock RM, Wild CJ. Left ventricular end-systolic volume as the major determinant of survival after recovery from myocardial infarction. *Circulation.* 1987;76(1):44–51.

33. Antman EM, Cohen M, Bernink PJ, et al. The TIMI risk score for unstable angina/non-ST elevation MI: A method for prognostication and therapeutic decision making. *JAMA.* 2000;284(7):835–842.

34. Boersma E, Pieper KS, Steyerberg EW, et al. Predictors of outcome in patients with acute coronary syndromes without persistent ST-segment elevation. Results from an international trial of 9461 patients. The PURSUIT Investigators. *Circulation.* 2000;101(22): 2557–2567.

35. Eagle KA, Lim MJ, Dabbous OH, et al. A validated prediction model for all forms of acute coronary syndrome: estimating the risk of 6-month postdischarge death in an international registry. *JAMA.* 2004;291(22):2727–2733.

36. Vasan RS. Biomarkers of cardiovascular disease: molecular basis and practical considerations. *Circulation.* 2006;113(19):2335–2362.

37. Arakawa N, Nakamura M, Aoki H, Hiramori K. Plasma brain natriuretic peptide concentrations predict survival after acute myocardial infarction. *J Am Coll Cardiol.* 1996;27(7):1656–1661.

38. Richards AM, Nicholls MG, Yandle TG, et al. Plasma N-terminal pro-brain natriuretic peptide and adrenomedullin: new neurohormonal predictors of left ventricular function and prognosis after myocardial infarction. *Circulation.* 1998;97(19):1921–1929.

39. de Lemos JA, Morrow DA, Bentley JH, et al. The prognostic value of B-type natriuretic peptide in patients with acute coronary syndromes. *N Engl J Med.* 2001;345(14):1014–1021.

40. James SK, Lindahl B, Siegbahn A, et al. N-terminal pro-brain natriuretic peptide and other risk markers for the separate prediction of mortality and subsequent myocardial infarction in patients with unstable coronary artery disease: a Global Utilization of Strategies To Open occluded arteries (GUSTO)-IV substudy. *Circulation.* 2003; 108(3):275–281.

41. Omland T, Persson A, Ng L, et al. N-terminal pro-B-type natriuretic peptide and long-term mortality in acute coronary syndromes. *Circulation*. 2002;106(23):2913–2918.

42. Galvani M, Ottani F, Oltrona L, et al. N-terminal pro-brain natriuretic peptide on admission has prognostic value across the whole spectrum of acute coronary syndromes. *Circulation*. 2004;110: 128–134.

43. Weber M, Bazzino O, Navarro Estrada JL, et al. N-terminal B-type natriuretic peptide assessment provides incremental prognostic information in patients with acute coronary syndromes and normal troponin T values upon admission. *J Am Coll Cardiol*. 2008;51(12): 1188–1195.

44. Morrow DA, de Lemos JA, Sabatine MS, et al. Evaluation of B-type natriuretic peptide for risk assessment in unstable angina/non-ST-elevation myocardial infarction: B-type natriuretic peptide and prognosis in TACTICS-TIMI 18. *J Am Coll Cardiol*. 2003;41(8): 1264–1272.

45. Morrow DA, de Lemos JA, Blazing MA, et al. Prognostic value of serial B-type natriuretic peptide testing during follow-up of patients with unstable coronary artery disease. *JAMA*. 2005;294(22):2866–2871.

46. Wylie JV, Murphy SA, Morrow DA, de Lemos JA, Antman EM, Cannon CP. Validated risk score predicts the development of congestive heart failure after presentation with unstable angina or non-ST-elevation myocardial infarction: results from OPUS-TIMI 16 and TACTICS-TIMI 18. *Am Heart J*. 2004;148(1):173–180.

47. Bazzino O, Fuselli JJ, Botto F, Perez de Arenaza AD, Bahit C, Dadone J; PACS Group of Investigators. Relative value of N-terminal probrain natriuretic peptide, TIMI risk score, ACC/AHA prognostic classification and other risk markers in patients with non-ST-elevation acute coronary syndromes. *Eur Heart J*. 2004;25(10):859–866.

48. Heeschen C, Hamm CW, Mitrovic V, Lantelme NH, White HD. N-terminal pro-B-type natriuretic peptide levels for dynamic risk stratification of patients with acute coronary syndromes. *Circulation*. 2004;110(20):3206–3212.

49. Morrow DA, Cannon CP, Jesse RL, et al. National Academy of Clinical Biochemistry Laboratory Medicine Practice Guidelines: Clinical characteristics and utilization of biochemical markers in acute coronary syndromes. *Circulation*. 2007;115(13):e356–e375.

50. Jernberg T, Lindahl B, Siegbahn A, et al. N-terminal pro-brain natriuretic peptide in relation to inflammation, myocardial necrosis, and the effect of an invasive strategy in unstable coronary artery disease. *J Am Coll Cardiol.* 2003;42(11):1909–1916.

51. James SK, Lindback J, Tilly J, et al. Troponin-T and N-terminal pro-B-type natriuretic peptide predict mortality benefit from coronary revascularization in acute coronary syndromes: a GUSTO-IV substudy. *J Am Coll Cardiol.* 2006;48(6):1146–1154.

52. Windhausen F, Hirsch A, Sanders GT, et al. N-terminal pro-brain natriuretic peptide for additional risk stratification in patients with non-ST-elevation acute coronary syndrome and an elevated troponin T: an Invasive versus Conservative Treatment in Unstable coronary Syndromes (ICTUS) substudy. *Am Heart J.* 2007;153(4):485–492.

53. Kragelund C, Gronning B, Omland T, et al. Is N-terminal pro B-type natriuretic peptide (NT-proBNP) a useful screening test for angiographic findings in patients with stable coronary disease? *Am Heart J.* 2006;151(3):712.

54. Wolber T, Maeder M, Rickli H, et al. N-terminal pro-brain natriuretic peptide used for the prediction of coronary artery stenosis. *Eur J Clin Invest.* 2007;37(1):18–25.

55. Sakai H, Tsutamoto T, Ishikawa C, et al. Direct comparison of brain natriuretic peptide (BNP) and N-terminal pro-BNP secretion and extent of coronary artery stenosis in patients with stable coronary artery disease. *Circ J.* 2007;71(4):499–505.

56. Ndrepepa G, Braun S, Mehilli J, et al. Plasma levels of N-terminal pro-brain natriuretic peptide in patients with coronary artery disease and relation to clinical presentation, angiographic severity, and left ventricular ejection fraction. *Am J Cardiol.* 2005;95(5):553–557.

57. Karabinos I, Karvouni E, Chiotinis N, et al. Acute changes in N-terminal pro-brain natriuretic peptide induced by dobutamine stress echocardiography. *Eur J Echocardiogr.* 2007;8(4):265–274.

58. Conen D, Jander N, Trenk D, Neumann FJ, Mueller C. The use of B-type natriuretic peptides in the detection of myocardial ischemia in settings with rapid access to coronary angiography. *Int J Cardiol.* 2007;119(3):416–418.

59. Corteville DC, Bibbins-Domingo K, Wu AH, Ali S, Schiller NB, Whooley MA. N-terminal pro-B-type natriuretic peptide as a diagnostic test for ventricular dysfunction in patients with coronary

disease: data from the Heart and Soul study. *Arch Intern Med.* 2007;167(5):483–489.

60. de Winter RJ, Stroobants A, Koch KT, et al. Plasma N-terminal pro-B-type natriuretic peptide for prediction of death or nonfatal myocardial infarction following percutaneous coronary intervention. *Am J Cardiol.* 2004;94(12):1481–1485.
61. Kragelund C, Gronning B, Kober L, Hildebrandt P, Steffensen R. N-terminal pro-B-type natriuretic peptide and long-term mortality in stable coronary heart disease. *N Engl J Med.* 2005;352(7):666–675.
62. Ndrepepa G, Braun S, Niemoller K, et al. Prognostic value of N-terminal pro-brain natriuretic peptide in patients with chronic stable angina. *Circulation.* 2005;112(14):2102–2107.
63. Schnabel R, Rupprecht HJ, Lackner KJ, et al. Analysis of N-terminal-pro-brain natriuretic peptide and C-reactive protein for risk stratification in stable and unstable coronary artery disease: results from the AtheroGene study. *Eur Heart J.* 2005;26(3):241–249.
64. Schnabel R, Lubos E, Rupprecht HJ, et al. B-type natriuretic peptide and the risk of cardiovascular events and death in patients with stable angina: results from the AtheroGene study. *J Am Coll Cardiol.* 2006;47(3):552–558.
65. Omland T, Richards AM, Wergeland R, Vik-Mo H. B-type natriuretic peptide and long-term survival in patients with stable coronary artery disease. *Am J Cardiol.* 2005;95(1):24–28.
66. Tang WH, Steinhubl SR, Van LF, et al. Risk stratification for patients undergoing nonurgent percutaneous coronary intervention using N-terminal pro-B-type natriuretic peptide: a Clopidogrel for the Reduction of Events During Observation (CREDO) substudy. *Am Heart J.* 2007;153(1):36–41.
67. West MJ, Nestel PJ, Kirby AC, et al. The value of N-terminal fragment of brain natriuretic peptide and tissue inhibitor of metalloproteinase-1 levels as predictors of cardiovascular outcome in the LIPID study. *Eur Heart J.* 2008;29(7):923–931.
68. Kragelund C, Gustafsson I, Omland T, et al. Prognostic value of NH2-terminal pro B-type natriuretic peptide in patients with diabetes and stable coronary heart disease. *Diabetes Care.* 2006;29(6):1411–1413.
69. Richards M, Nicholls MG, Espiner EA, et al. Comparison of B-type natriuretic peptides for assessment of cardiac function and prognosis

in stable ischemic heart disease. *J Am Coll Cardiol.* 2006;47(1): 52–60.

70. Bibbins-Domingo K, Gupta R, Na B, Wu AH, Schiller NB, Whooley MA. N-terminal fragment of the prohormone brain-type natriuretic peptide (NT-proBNP), cardiovascular events, and mortality in patients with stable coronary heart disease. *JAMA.* 2007;297(2): 169–176.

71. Blankenberg S, McQueen MJ, Smieja M, et al. Comparative impact of multiple biomarkers and N-Terminal pro-brain natriuretic peptide in the context of conventional risk factors for the prediction of recurrent cardiovascular events in the Heart Outcomes Prevention Evaluation (HOPE) Study. *Circulation.* 2006;114(3):201–208.

72. Omland T, Sabatine MS, Jablonski KA, et al. Prognostic value of B-Type natriuretic peptides in patients with stable coronary artery disease: the PEACE Trial. *J Am Coll Cardiol.* 2007;50(3):205–214.

73. Dai DF, Hwang JJ, Lin JL, et al. Joint effects of N-terminal pro-B-type-natriuretic peptide and C-reactive protein vs angiographic severity in predicting major adverse cardiovascular events and clinical restenosis after coronary angioplasty in patients with stable coronary artery disease. *Circ J.* 2008;72(8):1316–1323.

74. Richards AM, Doughty R, Nicholls MG, et al. Neurohumoral prediction of benefit from carvedilol in ischemic left ventricular dysfunction. Australia-New Zealand Heart Failure Group. *Circulation.* 1999;99(6):786–792.

75. Richards AM, Doughty R, Nicholls MG, et al. Plasma N-terminal pro-brain natriuretic peptide and adrenomedullin: prognostic utility and prediction of benefit from carvedilol in chronic ischemic left ventricular dysfunction. Australia-New Zealand Heart Failure Group. *J Am Coll Cardiol.* 2001;37(7):1781–1787.

76. Mueller C. The use of B-type natriuretic peptides in coronary artery disease: utile or futile? *J Am Coll Cardiol.* 2007;50(3):215–216.

77. Emberson JR, Ng LL, Armitage J, Bowman L, Parish S, Collins R. N-terminal Pro-B-type natriuretic peptide, vascular disease risk, and cholesterol reduction among 20,536 patients in the MRC/BHF heart protection study. *J Am Coll Cardiol.* 2007;49(3):311–319.

78. Omland T, de Lemos JA. Amino-terminal pro-B-type natriuretic peptides in stable and unstable ischemic heart disease. *Am J Cardiol.* 2008;101(3A):61–66.

23 ■ Natriuretic Peptides and Prognostication: Predicting Outcomes Across the Spectrum of Medical Conditions

Sonal Sakariya, MD
Anand V. Iyer, MD
Christopher P. Moriates, MD
Alan S. Maisel, MD, FACC

Introduction

One of the arts in the practice of medicine is the ability to prognosticate, or predict outcomes in the future. Physicians utilize many different methods in order to forecast the course of a disease, the risks and benefits of a given procedure or intervention, or the utility of a hospitalization. As the world of biomarkers continues to explode, the armamentarium of physicians and cardiologists to diagnose, prognosticate, and treat cardiac disease has progressed to a sophisticated level. This knowledge set includes not only evaluating physical signs and symptoms, such as dyspnea and elevated jugular venous pressure (JVP), but also measuring and interpreting an array of endogenous biomarkers. The recent discovery that the natriuretic peptides (NPs) are not only useful for diagnostic purposes but also have profound prognostic implications in heart failure (HF) and a variety of other cardiovascular conditions has promised to revolutionize the practice of cardiology.[1–10]

NP levels—measured in both the Emergency Department (ED) and during hospitalization—predict subsequent cardiac events including rehospitalization, morbidity, and mortality. Furthermore, solid evidence now exists that demonstrates NP levels have a powerful prognostic value across a spectrum of cardiac diseases, including acute and chronic heart failure, stable coronary artery disease (CAD), acute coronary syndrome (ACS), and valvular heart disease. NP levels may indeed be able to provide vital insight into patients with systolic and diastolic dysfunction, along with being able to predict outcomes better than most current modalities, including physical examination, imaging, and routine lab tests.

Stages of Heart Failure

It is useful to consider the value of NP testing for prognosis as a function of the American Heart Association (AHA) Stages of HF, which are defined as: Stage A ("at risk" for HF), Stage B ("established" heart disease without symptoms of HF), Stage C ("symptomatic" HF), and Stage D ("advanced" HF). Given the importance of Stages C and D, we will consider them first, followed by consideration of the use of NPs in Stages A and B.

NP Testing and Prognosis in AHA HF Stages C and D

In recent years, B-type natriuretic peptide (BNP) and N-terminal proBNP (NT-proBNP) have become important prognostic tools in assessing patients with suspected acutely destabilized HF (ADHF).[11–14] Previously, the diagnosis and prognosis of ADHF was based almost solely on nonspecific physical examination findings, such as dyspnea, orthopnea, paroxysmal nocturnal dyspnea (PND), edema, and elevated JVP.[15] Reliance on these factors has proven to be an inaccurate and ultimately costly way to treat ADHF. In fact, currently up to 90% of ADHF patients seen in the ED are admitted to the hospital, lending to the more than one million hospitalizations per year for ADHF in the United States alone.[16,17] In 2007, a total of $33.2 billion was spent on this diagnosis.[18]

NP levels measured in the ED and/or during hospitalization can predict subsequent cardiac events including rehospitalization, morbidity, and mortality.[7–10] A number of studies assessing BNP for prognosis in patients with HF have found that for each 100 pg/mL increase in BNP, there was an associated 35% increase in the relative risk of death.[19] Moreover, NP levels have even proven to be superior to the perception of ED physicians as to the severity of

HF and the prognosis of such patients. In a multicenter, prospective Rapid ED Heart Failure Outpatient Trial (REDHOT), patients sent home from the ED after treatment for ADHF actually had higher BNP levels than those patients that were admitted. However, BNP levels were more strongly related to death and readmission of patients than the perceived severity of outcome. One pointed example is that patients presenting to the ED with acute shortness of breath and BNP less than 200 pg/mL had a much better overall prognosis than those with BNP levels greater than 200 pg/mL (HF-related events and mortality: 9% versus 29%, $P = 0.006$), even when they presented with a perceived NYHA functional class III or IV. This suggests that a "disconnect" exists between the perceived severity of the illness and the actual prognosis as based on BNP values.[20]

NP levels can provide crucial information regarding future cardiac events up to a six-month period following discharge. In a study conducted by Harrison et al., 325 patients were followed for six months after a visit to the ED for dyspnea. Elevated BNP levels, measured in the ED, were strongly correlated to prognosis. Patients with a baseline BNP level greater than 480 pg/mL had a 51% probability of an HF event (e.g., ED visit, cardiac hospital admissions, mortality). Conversely, patients presenting with a BNP of less than 230 pg/mL had only a 2.5% probability of experiencing an event within the specified time period.[8] (Figure 23–1)

In a separate investigation, 72 male patients admitted for HF were studied for a course of 30 days following discharge. During hospitalization, BNP levels were measured within 24 hours of admission, following changes in treatment or patient condition, and within 24 hours of discharge or death. Patients were at a greater risk for mortality or readmission if their BNP concentration increased during hospitalization (239 ± 233 pg/mL).[7] In contrast, patients had better outcomes if their BNP concentration reduced during hospitalization.[10] Of the patients with an increasing BNP during hospitalization, 52% experienced either rehospitalization or cardiac death by the end of the 30-day period.

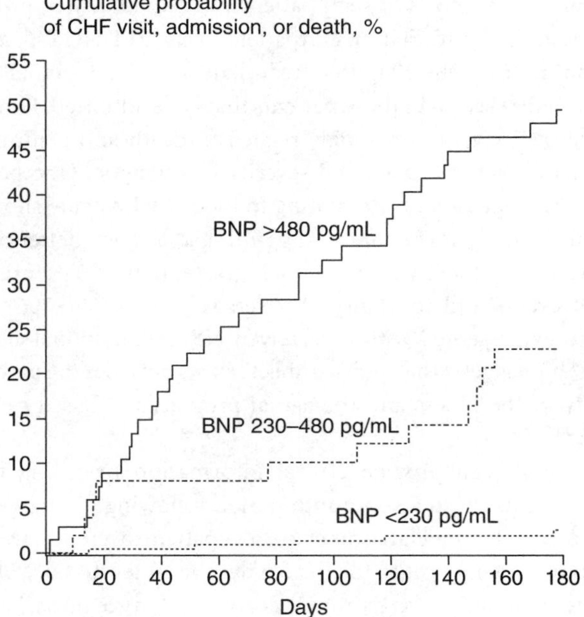

■ **Figure 23–1** Reverse Kaplan-Meier plot showing cumulative risk of any CHF event (ED visit/hospitalization for CHF or death from CHF), stratified by BNP levels. Higher BNP levels are associated with progressively worse prognosis. Patients with BNP levels more than 480 pg/mL had a 6-month cumulative probability of a CHF event of 51%. Patients with BNP levels less than 230 pg/mL had only a 2.5% probability of a CHF event.

However, only 16% of the patients with a decreasing BNP level suffered from such events. While these findings demonstrated that dropping BNP levels were a good prognostic sign, the discharge BNP level was the most significant predictor of 30-day endpoints. A cut point of less than 430 pg/mL was established as having a strong negative predictive value (NPV) for readmission.[7] A larger study examining the efficacy of using serial BNP assays during

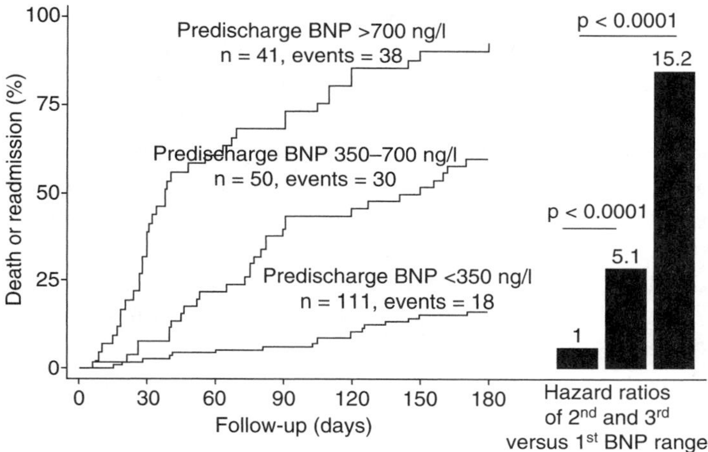

■ **Figure 23–2** Kaplan-Meier curves showing the cumulative incidence of death or re-admission according to predischarge B-type natriuretic peptide (BNP) ranges (<350, 350 to 700, >700 ng/l) in the whole population; $p < 0.001$ for the trend among BNP ranges. On the right, hazard ratios are shown for each BNP range.

hospitalization was conducted by Logeart et al. BNP measurements were performed daily from the time of admission to the time of discharge and events were recorded at a 60-day point in time. Patients with a discharge BNP of less than 350 pg/mL were least at risk for death or readmission and the risk of these events increased incrementally with higher discharge BNP ranges (350–700 ng/l and > 700 pg/mL)[21] (Figure 23–2). Once again, discharge NP levels prevailed as stronger predictors of early outcomes over admission values or changes during hospitalization. Of the patients readmitted, 29% of these events occurred within the first month following discharge. This may be the result of physicians discharging HF patients before congestion was completely relieved. Therefore, a discharge NP level should be part of the solution for improving risk stratification in patients with HF.

The prognostic utility of NT-proBNP has been similarly demonstrated in two convincing studies, the ProBNP Investigation of Dyspnea in the ED (PRIDE) and the International Collaborative of NT-proBNP (ICON) trials. In these two studies, NT-proBNP concentrations at presentation were powerfully prognostic for adverse outcome. In the ICON study,[11] a collaborative study that examined 1256 patients, concentrations of NT-proBNP greater than 5180 pg/mL at presentation were the strongest predictor of death by 76 days in acute HF, superseding other more traditional risk factors, such as age or left ventricular ejection fraction. The PRIDE[22] study resulted in NT-proBNP concentrations that were similarly prognostic, with prognostic importance extending to at least one year associated with values of NT-proBNP in excess of approximately 1000 pg/mL. This prognostic importance was seen in those with and without acute HF, and preliminary data suggest that NT-proBNP remains prognostically meaningful out to four years from enrollment in PRIDE, strongly predicting death and new HF events (JL Januzzi, Personal Communication). Similar to the data by Logeart and colleagues, data exist that show the post-treatment value of NT-proBNP following hospitalization for ADHF to be a more important prognostic variable than presenting concentrations.

While the importance of NPs as a diagnostic and prognostic modality in HF has been recognized, little information is known regarding the timing of obtaining NP levels and its impact on the initiation of treatment. In an analysis of the Acute Decompensated Heart Failure National Registry (ADHERE trial), the medical records of patients admitted with ADHF were retrospectively examined. The authors found a strong association existed between delayed measurement of NP levels and delayed time to treatment. This was likely secondary to the fact that in many of these patients, the diagnosis of HF was not obvious. Delayed treatment was in turn linked to increased in-hospital mortality, independent of other prognostic factors. This adverse impact of delayed treatment was most prominent in patients with greater BNP levels[23] (Figure 23–3).

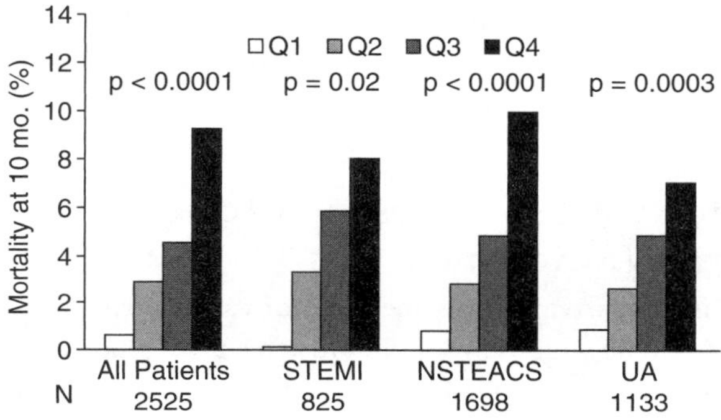

■ **Figure 23–3** Hospital Mortality, Time to Treatment, and iBNP Level. This 3-dimensional plot shows the relationship of hospital mortality (%) to time of initial treatment (quartiles) and initial iBNP levels being drawn (quartiles). iBNP = immunoreactive B-type natriuretic peptide; IV = intravenous.

NP Testing and Prognosis in AHA HF Stage A

Several studies have been executed demonstrating the importance of BNP and NT-proBNP for prognostication in those "at risk" for HF. In the Rancho Bernardo study, measured TnT and NT-proBNP levels in older adults were related to all-cause and cardiovascular disease mortality. Detectable TnT levels were associated with increased risk of all-cause death after adjustments for age, gender, risk factors, and baseline CAD presence. High NT-proBNP levels (>450 pg/mL) were a strong predictor of all-cause and cardiovascular mortality after adjustments. Mortality rates increased in patients with both increased NT-proBNP and detectable TnT.[24] Similar results have been shown for BNP in the Framingham Heart Study.

NP Testing and Prognosis in AHA HF Stage B

Stage B HF is defined as left ventricular dysfunction with asymptomatic HF; it represents a large and growing population of patients in whom symptomatic HF (Stage C and D) is more likely to occur. Accordingly, tools for identifying risk in this population are important.

Coronary Artery Disease and Acute Coronary Syndromes

Biomarkers, particularly in the form of cardiac troponins (cTn) and creatinine kinase-MB (CK-MB), have become the cornerstones of diagnosis and risk stratification in CAD. Recent evidence supports that the NPs can add significant prognostic information for treatments of these diseases, as well as expanding the battery of data points that can be utilized for prognostication.[25–37]

Both BNP and NT-proBNP can serve as prognostic factors for patients with stable CAD.[25] A study of patients diagnosed with stable angina and a greater than 30% coronary artery stenosis demonstrated that a BNP greater than 100 pg/mL gave a 4.4-fold increased risk of cardiovascular death or a nonfatal MI during a mean 2.5-year follow-up.[26] Meta-analyses have shown increased mortality and cardiac events in CAD patients with increased BNP.[28] In a study of 186 patients with stable angina and CAD in Norway, BNP was shown to be a better independent prognostic factor of long-term CAD survival than other risk factors and markers, such as age, gender, left ventricular ejection fraction (LVEF), and diabetes mellitus.[27]

A study of NT-proBNP levels also showed increased mortality in CAD patients with levels greater than 455 pg/mL versus those with values less than 64 pg/mL.[29] Other studies have found increased risk in CHD patients with NT-proBNP greater than 100 pg/mL.[30,31] A study of 345 patients in Taiwan with stable CAD after percutaneous coronary intervention (PCI) showed that patients with NT-proBNP greater than 241 pg/mL had increased risk of major adverse cardiac events; NT-proBNP was a better predictor of mortality than age, LVEF, or C-reactive protein (CRP).[33] A substudy of the Prevention of Events with

Angiotensin-Converting Enzyme Inhibition (PEACE) trial compared BNP and NT-proBNP levels in CAD patients with LVEF greater than 40% prior to receiving trandolapril (an ACE inhibitor) or placebo treatment. After correction for treatment assignment, high BNP was found to be predictive of subsequent HF, while high NT-proBNP was predictive of subsequent cardiovascular mortality, HF, and stroke, superior to BNP for each of these outcome measures.[34]

Emerging data also suggest a link between the ACS prognosis and NP levels.[38-42] It has become standard knowledge that elevated cTn levels suggest a greater severity of disease in patients with ACS, and increasing cTn values are indicative of higher mortality rates and adverse short- and long-term outcomes.[43–51] However, myocardial ischemia, by means of elevated ventricular wall stress, may also trigger the release of NPs.[52–55] A series of clinical trials have demonstrated that NPs are independent predictors of short- and long-term mortality and new-onset heart failure. In a study conducted by Wiviott et al., elevated BNP levels were associated with increased mortality in multiple different presentations of ACS[56] (Figure 23–4).

The effectiveness of NT-proBNP as a prognostic marker was extensively studied in two subanalyses of the Global Utilization of Strategies to open Occluded Arteries (GUSTO)-IV trial. In a substudy of 6809 patients who had baseline NT-proBNP levels measured a median 9.5 hours after ACS symptom onset, NT-proBNP levels were a stronger predictor of 1-year mortality than both troponin T (TnT) and CRP. Heart rate, creatinine clearance, and ST-segment depression also fell short of NT-proBNP's prognostic power.[57] In a subanalysis of GUSTO-IV, 2340 patients with non-ST-elevation MI (NSTEMI) or unstable angina (UA) that were undergoing coronary revascularization within 30 days were examined. Again, elevated NT-proBNP was found to be correlated with 1-year mortality. Furthermore, it was shown that patients with a high baseline NT-proBNP level benefited more from coronary revascularization versus those patients without elevated

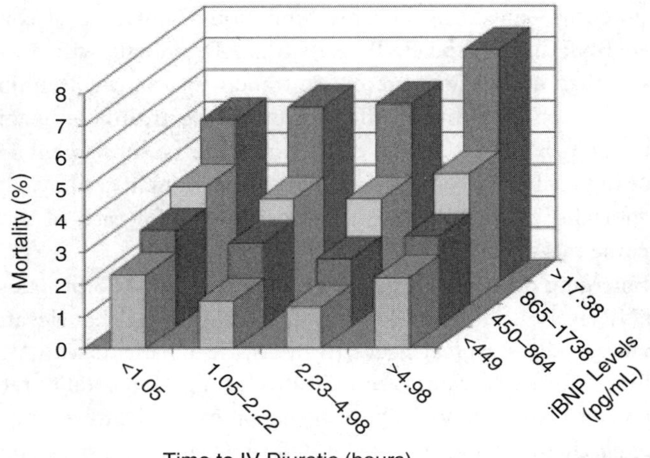

■ **Figure 23–4** Relationship between BNP (quartile) and mortality across the spectrum of patients with ACS. Quartiles of BNP (1: 5.0–43.6 pg/mL, 2: 43.7–81.2 pg/mL, 3: 81.3–137.8 pg/mL, 4: >137.8 pg/mL). STEMI = ST elevation myocardial infarction; NSTEACS = non-ST elevation acute coronary syndrome (unstable angina + non-ST elevation MI); UA = unstable angina.

NT-proBNP.[58] In a similar fashion, in a study of NP levels in the Bad Nauheim ACS Registry (higher risk) and Prognosis in Acute Coronary Syndromes Registry (lower risk), NT-proBNP levels greater than 474 pg/mL were associated with increased six-month mortality.[59] With respect to BNP, a substudy of the Treat Angina with Aggrastat and Determine Cost of Therapy with Invasive or Conservative Strategy-Thrombolysis in Myocardial Infarction (TACTICS-TIMI 18) was conducted to assess whether BNP had a prognostic role in non-ST-elevation ACS. BNP levels were measured in 1676 patients at study enrollment, and levels greater than 80 pg/mL were found to independently predict increased mortality at up to seven days, 30 days, and six months after presentation as well as predict increased incidence and worsening of HF. In addition, the combination of BNP and cTnI values added to risk estimation.[60]

Valvular Disease

Accumulating data suggest that NP levels may provide insight into cardiac conditions beyond those directly involving the myocardium. For example, there is growing evidence that biomarkers can have a substantial complementary role in determining prognoses across the gamut of valvular disorders. Studies have shown prognostic value of NPs in mitral regurgitation (MR), mitral stenosis (MS), aortic regurgitation (AR), and aortic stenosis (AS).

Mitral Regurgitation

NPs can serve as prognostic factors for mitral regurgitation (MR) severity and mortality. Increased BNP and NT-proBNP levels are correlated with increased MR severity and left atrial (LA) dimension, as well as prognosis.[61–64]

Mitral Stenosis

Although the lesion of mitral stenosis is above the left ventricle, one would think that NP levels would be in the normal range, however, studies have demonstrated slightly increased NT-proBNP levels compared to controls.[65] Natriuretic peptide levels also correlate with stenosis severity. NT-proBNP levels inversely correlate with mitral valve surface area.[65] Likewise, BNP levels are significantly higher in those with severe mitral stenosis (valve areas $< 1\ cm^2$) than in those with less severe stenosis.[48] The likely etiology of NP peptide elevations includes the presence of atrial fibrillation leading to diastolic dysfunction, right ventricular dysfunction, and concomitant mitral regurgitation. Following valvulotomy, NP concentrations reduce in parallel with improvements in clinical status and prognosis.[66,67]

Aortic Regurgitation

Increased NP levels have been demonstrated in symptomatic aortic regurgitation (AR) patients versus asymptomatic AR patients.[68] In addition, NP levels correlate with severity of AR, measured by vena contracta width.[69] At a cutoff of 602 pg/mL, NT-proBNP values can predict risk of adverse clinical events in AR patients.[70]

Aortic Stenosis

In aortic stenosis (AS), NP values increase with disease severity: BNP, NT-proBNP, and ANP inversely correlate with aortic valve area, and peptide values are higher in symptomatic patients than in asymptomatic patients.[71,72] Higher BNP values increase the risk of mortality from AS. One-year mortality rates in patients with AS were 6% with BNP less than 296 pg/mL, 34% with BNP between 296 and 819 pg/mL, and 60% with BNP greater than 819 pg/mL.[73] Another study found AS survival rates with BNP greater than 550 pg/mL and less than 550 pg/mL to be 47% and 97%, respectively.[74] In addition, NPs predict the likelihood of symptom development in asymptomatic patients with severe AS; those with NT-proBNP less than 80 pmol/L and BNP less than 130 pg/mL have greater symptom-free survival than those with higher values.[75] Conservatively-treated AS patients also show increased risk for adverse cardiac events if BNP is greater than 640 pg/mL.[76] Thus, in asymptomatic elderly patients with normal left ventricular function, an NP level may tip the scales one way or the other with regards to aortic valve replacement.

The Use of Natriuretic Peptides in Other Diseases

More recently, it has been found that NP levels may play important prognostic roles for extracardiac diseases, such as in cases of pulmonary embolism (PE), adult respiratory distress syndrome (ARDS), and mechanical ventilation. This further identifies the sensitive ability for NPs to elucidate the severity of conditions that may cause strain on the heart.

Pulmonary Embolism

Pulmonary embolism and subsequent right ventricular strain leads to elevation of NP levels and this can in turn serve as a prognostic indicator. Low NP levels (BNP < 50 pg/mL; NT-proBNP < 500 pg/mL) predict a benign hospital course.[77,78] In contrast, meta-analyses have shown that increased BNP and NT-proBNP levels (cutoffs >~100 pg/mL and >~1000 pg/mL, respectively) predict increased mortality, the likelihood of adverse clinical events, and in-hospital complications following PE.[79] NT-proBNP levels greater than 7500 ng/L followed by less than a 50% reduction in the following 24 hours after acute PE strongly predict an increased 30-day mortality compared to patients with PE and low NT-proBNP values.[80] In addition, NP levels may serve as a better prognostic tool for PE mortality than troponin I, though the two markers together may give additive information.[81]

Acute Respiratory Distress Syndrome

Acute respiratory distress syndrome (ARDS) may also prognostically benefit from the measurement of NP levels. High NP values are correlated with unfavorable ARDS outcomes. In ARDS patients, BNP levels predicted mortality with a 1.6 odds ratio for each log increase in BNP.[82] Patients with NT-proBNP levels greater than the 6813 ng/L cutoff point were found to have significantly higher odds of mortality than those below that level.[83]

Mechanical Ventilation

In the future, NPs may have a role in the prediction of safe and successful weaning from mechanical ventilation in ICU settings. Measurements of ANP and BNP one hour after weaning from mechanical ventilation versus measurements at ventilation removal displayed overall ANP increases and increases in BNP in patients with left ventricular dysfunction.[84] Patients on mechanical ventilation with BNP greater than 275 pg/mL experienced longer weaning durations and increased likelihood of weaning failure.[85] In cases of shock or sepsis, however, the data were inconclusive. Some studies have found that BNP and NT-proBNP levels did not correlate with in-hospital mortality or length of stay.[86,87] In contrast, other studies have shown that NPs play a role in prognosis. BNP greater than

Table 23–1: Suggested cutoff values for prognostication using natriuretic peptides.

Marker	Condition	Marker value	Result
BNP	HF or asymptomatic	each 100 pg/mL increase	35% increase in RR of death[22]
BNP	Acute HF	>200 pg/mL	29% mortality (versus 9%)[23]
BNP	Acute dyspnea	>480 pg/mL	51% HF event (versus 2.5%)[24]
BNP	Acute HF	increasing BNP level during hospitalization	52% rehospitalization/ cardiac death (versus 16% decreasing)[7]
BNP	Acute HF	<430 pg/mL	Reduced readmittance (30-day)[7]
BNP	Acute HF	<350 pg/mL	Reduced mortality, rehospitalization (6 months)[26]
NT-proBNP	Acute HF	>5180 pg/mL	Death by 76 days in acute HF[28]
NT-proBNP	Acute HF	>1000 pg/mL	Death by 1 year in acute dyspnea (with or without HF)[27]
NT-proBNP	Older adults	>450 pg/mL	Increased all-cause and cardiovascular mortality (7–9 years)[30]
BNP	CAD; stable angina and stenosis>30%	>100 pg/mL	4.4-fold increased risk of cardiovascular mortality or nonfatal MI in 2.5 year follow-up[32]
BNP	ACS; non-ST elevation	>80 pg/mL	Increased mortality up to 6 months, increased HF incidence[67]

Table 23–1: (Continued)

NT-proBNP	CAD	>455 pg/mL	Increased mortality (median follow-up 9 years)[35]
NT-proBNP	CAD; stable and after PCI	>241 pg/mL	Increased cardiac event risk and artery restenosis risk (18–36 months)[38]
NT-proBNP	ACS; without TnT elevation	>474 pg/mL	Increased 6-month mortality[66]

1290 pg/mL suggested increased risk of mortality in shock patients.[88] In addition, NT-proBNP levels greater than 17,568 pg/mL were shown to be the strongest factor in the prediction of mortality in shock patients.[89] A cutoff of 13,600 pg/mL has also been suggested in septic shock patients.[90] One study showed pro-ANP levels greater than 530 pmol/L indicated increased mortality for sepsis and septic shock patients.[91]

Conclusion

The NPs, besides being excellent tools for diagnosing or excluding HF in patients presenting with dyspnea, have shown incredibly strong prognostic value in many cardiovascular diseases. Further research is bound to more clearly delineate the roles for NPs levels in cardiovascular disease, as well as make them targets for drug and device therapy.

References

1. McCullough PA, Nowak RM, McCord J, et al. B-type natriuretic peptide and clinical judgment in emergency diagnosis of heart failure: analysis from Breathing Not Properly (BNP) Multinational Study. *Circulation*. 2002;106(4):416–422.

2. Davis M, Espiner E, Richards G, et al. Plasma brain natriuretic peptide in assessment of acute dyspnoea. *Lancet*. 1994;343(8895):440–444.

3. Maisel AS, Krishnaswamy P, Nowak RM, et al. Rapid measurement of B-type natriuretic peptide in the emergency diagnosis of heart failure. *N Engl J Med.* 2002;347(3):161–167.

4. McCullough PA, Hollander JE, Nowak RM, et al. Uncovering heart failure in patients with a history of pulmonary disease: rationale for the early use of B-type natriuretic peptide in the emergency department. *Acad Emerg Med.* 2003;10(3):198–204.

5. Morrison LK, Harrison A, Krishnaswamy P, Kazanegra R, Clopton P, Maisel A. Utility of a rapid B-natriuretic peptide assay in differentiating congestive heart failure from lung disease in patients presenting with dyspnea. *J Am Coll Cardiol.* 2002;39(2):202–209.

6. Dao Q, Krishnaswamy P, Kazanegra R, et al. Utility of B-type natriuretic peptide in the diagnosis of congestive heart failure in an urgent-care setting. *J Am Coll Cardiol.* 2001;37(2):379–385.

7. Cheng V, Kazanegra R, Garcia A, et al. A rapid bedside test for B-type peptide predicts treatment outcomes in patients admitted for decompensated heart failure: a pilot study. *J Am Coll Cardiol.* 2001;37(2): 386–391.

8. Harrison A, Morrison LK, Krishnaswamy P, et al. B-type natriuretic peptide predicts future cardiac events in patients presenting to the emergency department with dyspnea. *Ann Emerg Med.* 2002;39(2): 131–139.

9. Maeda K, Tsutamoto T, al AWE. High level of plasma BNP at discharge is an independent risk factor for mortality and morbidity in patients with congestive heart failure. *J Am Coll Cardiol.* 1999; 33:192A.

10. Bettencourt P, Ferreira S, Azevedo A, Ferreira A. Preliminary data on the potential usefulness of B-type natriuretic peptide levels in predicting outcome after hospital discharge in patients with heart failure. *Am J Med.* 2002;113(3):215–219.

11. Januzzi JL, van Kimmenade R, Lainchbury J, et al. NT-proBNP testing for diagnosis and short-term prognosis in acute destabilized heart failure: an international pooled analysis of 1256 patients: the International Collaborative of NT-proBNP Study. *Eur Heart J.* 2006;27: 330–337.

12. Hartmann F, Packer M, Coats AJ, et al. Prognostic impact of plasma N-terminal pro-brain natriuretic peptide in severe chronic congestive heart failure: a substudy of the Carvedilol Prospective Randomized

Cumulative Survival (COPERNICUS) trial, *Circulation*. 2004;110: 1780–1786.

13. Berger R, Huelsman M, Strecker K, et al. B-type natriuretic peptide predicts sudden death in patients with chronic heart failure. *Circulation*. 2002;105:2392–2397.
14. Anand IS, Fisher LD, Chiang YT, et al. Changes in brain natriuretic peptide and norepinephrine over time and mortality and morbidity in the Valsartan Heart Failure Trial (Val-HeFT), *Circulation*. 2003;107:1278–1283.
15. Tresch DD. Clinical manifestations, diagnostic assessment, and etiology of heart failure in elderly patients. *Clin Geriatr Med*. 2000; 16:445–456.
16. Yancy CW. Climbing the mountain of acute decompensated heart failure: the EVEREST Trials. *JAMA*. 2007;297(12):1374–1376.
17. Graff L, Orledge J, Radford MJ, et al. Correlation of the Agency for Health Care Policy and Research congestive heart failure admission guideline with mortality: peer review organization voluntary hospital association initiative to decrease events (PROVIDE) for congestive heart failure. *Ann Emerg Med*. 1999;34(4 Pt 1):429–437.
18. Rosamond W, Flegal K, Friday G, et al. Heart disease and stroke statistics—2007 update: a report from the American Heart Association Statistics Committee and Stroke Statistics Subcommittee. *Circulation*. 2007;115(5):e69–e171.
19. Doust JA, Pietrzak E, Dobson A, Glasziou P. How well does B-type natriuretic peptide predict death and cardiac events in patients with heart failure: systematic review. *BMJ*. 2005;330(7492):625.
20. Maisel A, Hollander JE, Guss D, et al. Primary results of the Rapid Emergency Department Heart Failure Outpatient Trial (REDHOT). A multicenter study of B-type natriuretic peptide levels, emergency department decision making, and outcomes in patients presenting with shortness of breath. *J Am Coll Cardiol*. 2004;44(6):1328–1333.
21. Logeart D, Thabut G, Jourdain P, et al. Predischarge B-type natriuretic peptide assay for identifying patients at high risk of re-admission after decompensated heart failure. *J Am Coll Cardiol*. 2004;43(4):635–641.
22. Januzzi JL, Camargo CA, Anwaruddin S, et al. The N-terminal Pro-BNP investigation of dyspnea in the emergency department (PRIDE) study. *Am J Cardiol*. 2005;95(8):948–954.

23. Maisel AS, Peacock WF, McMullin N, et al. Timing of immunoreactive B-type natriuretic peptide levels and treatment delay in acute decompensated heart failure: an ADHERE (Acute Decompensated Heart Failure National Registry) analysis. *J Am Coll Cardiol.* 2008;52:534–540.

24. Daniels LB, Laughlin GA, Clopton P, Maisel AS, Barrett-Connor E. Minimally elevated cardiac troponin T and elevated N-terminal pro-B-type natriuretic peptide predict mortality in older adults: results from the Rancho Bernardo Study. *J Am Coll Cardiol.* 2008;52(6): 450–459.

25. Richards M, Nicholls MG, Espiner EA, et al. Comparison of B-type natriuretic peptides for assessment of cardiac function and prognosis in stable ischemic heart disease. *J Am Coll Cardiol.* 2006;47(1): 52–60.

26. Schnabel R, Lubos E, Rupprecht HJ, et al. B-type natriuretic peptide and the risk of cardiovascular events and death in patients with stable angina: results from the AtheroGene study. *J Am Coll Cardiol.* 2006;47(3):552–558.

27. Omland T, Richards AM, Wergeland R, Vik-Mo H. B-type natriuretic peptide and long-term survival in patients with stable coronary artery disease. *Am J Cardiol.* 2005;95(1):24–28.

28. Oremus M, Raina PS, Santaguida P, et al. A systematic review of BNP as a predictor of prognosis in persons with coronary artery disease. *Clin Biochem.* 2008;41(4–5):260–265.

29. Kragelund C, Grønning B, Køber L, Hildebrandt P, Steffensen R. N-terminal pro-B-type natriuretic peptide and long-term mortality in stable coronary heart disease. *N Engl J Med.* 2005;352(7): 666–675.

30. Bibbins-Domingo K, Gupta R, Na B, Wu AHB, Schiller NB, Whooley MA. N-terminal fragment of the prohormone brain-type natriuretic peptide (NT-proBNP), cardiovascular events, and mortality in patients with stable coronary heart disease. *JAMA.* 2007;297(2): 169–176.

31. März W, Tiran B, Seelhorst U, et al.; LURIC Study Team. N-terminal pro-B-type natriuretic peptide predicts total and cardiovascular mortality in individuals with or without stable coronary artery disease: the Ludwigshafen Risk and Cardiovascular Health Study. *Clin Chem.* 2007;53(6):1075–1083.

32. Dai D, Hwang J, Lin J, et al. Joint effects of N-terminal pro-B-type-natriuretic peptide and C-reactive protein vs angiographic severity in predicting major adverse cardiovascular events and clinical restenosis after coronary angioplasty in patients with stable coronary artery disease. *Circ J.* 2008;72(8):1316–1323.

33. Ndrepepa G, Braun S, Mehilli J, Schömig A, Kastrati A. Accuracy of N-terminal probrain natriuretic peptide to predict mortality or detect acute ischemia in patients with coronary artery disease. *Cardiology.* 2008;109(4):249–257.

34. Omland T, Sabatine MS, Jablonski KA, et al. Prognostic value of B-Type natriuretic peptides in patients with stable coronary artery disease: the PEACE Trial. *J Am Coll Cardiol.* 2007;50(3):205–214.

35. Kragelund C, Grønning B, Køber L, et al. N-terminal pro-B-type natriuretic peptide and long-term mortality in stable coronary heart disease. *N Engl J Med.* 2005;352:666–675.

36. Sahinarslan A, Cengel A, Okyay K, et al. B-type natriuretic peptide and extent of lesion on coronary angiography in stable coronary artery disease. *Coron Artery Dis.* 2005;16:225–229.

37. Richards M, Nicholls MG, Espiner EA, et al.; Christchurch Cardioendocrine Research Group. Australia-New Zealand Heart Failure Group. Comparison of B-type natriuretic peptides for assessment of cardiac function and prognosis in stable ischemic heart disease. *J Am Coll Cardiol.* 2006;47:52–60.

38. Galvani M, Ferrini MD, Ottani F. Natriuretic peptides for risk stratification of patients with acute coronary syndromes, *Eur Heart J.* 2004;6:327–333.

39. de Lemos JA, Morrow DA. Brain natriuretic peptide measurement in acute coronary syndromes: ready for clinical application? *Circulation.* 2002;106:2868–2870.

40. Omland T, Persson A, Ng L, et al. N-terminal pro-B-type natriuretic peptide and long-term mortality in acute coronary syndromes. *Circulation.* 2002;106:2913–2918.

41. Omland T, de Lemos JA, Morrow DA, Antman EM, et al. Prognostic value of N-terminal pro-atrial and pro-brain natriuretic peptide in patients with acute coronary syndromes. *Am J Cardiol.* 2002;89:463–465.

42. Galvani M, Ottani F, Murena E, et al. N-terminal pro-brain natriuretic peptide on admission has prognostic value across the whole

spectrum of acute coronary syndromes. *J Am Coll Cardiol.* 2003; 41:402.

43. James S, Armstrong P, Califf R, et al. Troponin T levels and risk of 30-day outcomes in patients with the acute coronary syndrome: prospective verification in the GUSTO-IV trial. *Am J Med.* 2003;115: 178–184.

44. Panteghini, M. The new definition of myocardial infarction and the impact of troponin determination on clinical practice. *Int J Cardiol.* 2006;106:298–306.

45. Tsai S, Chu S, Hsu C, et al. Use and interpretation of cardiac troponins in the ED. *Am J Emerg Med.* 2007;26:331–334.

46. Ottani F, Galvani M, Nicolini FA, et al. Elevated cardiac troponin levels predict the risk of adverse outcome in patients with acute coronary syndromes. *Am Heart J.* 2000;140:917–927.

47. Lindahl B, Toss H, Siegbahn A, Venge P, Wallentin L. Markers of myocardial damage and inflammation in relation to long-term mortality in unstable coronary artery disease. *N Engl J Med.* 2000;343: 1139–1147.

48. Jaffe AS, Babuin L, Apple FS. Biomarkers in acute cardiac disease: the present and the future. *J Am Coll Cardiol.* 2006;48:1–11.

49. Bertrand ME, Simoons ML, Fox KA, et al. Management of acute coronary syndromes: acute coronary syndromes without persistent ST segment elevation; recommendations of the Task Force of the European Society of Cardiology. *Eur Heart J.* 2000;21:1406–1432.

50. Braunwald E, Antman EM, Beasley JW, et al. ACC/AHA 2002 guideline update for the management of patients with unstable angina and non–ST-segment elevation myocardial infarction—summary article: a report of the American College of Cardiology/American Heart Association task force on practice guidelines (Committee on the Management of Patients With Unstable Angina). *J Am Coll Cardiol.* 2002;40:1366–1374.

51. Gupta S, de Lemos J. Use and misuse of cardiac troponins in clinical practice. *Prog Cardiovasc Dis.* 2007;50:151–165.

52. Marumoto K, Hamada M, Hiwada K. Increased secretion of atrial and brain natriuretic peptides during acute myocardial ischaemia induced by dynamic exercise in patients with angina pectoris. *Clin Sci (Lond).* 1995;88:551–556.

53. Hama N, Itoh H, Shirakami G, et al. Rapid ventricular induction of brain natriuretic peptide gene expression in experimental acute myocardial infarction. *Circulation.* 1995;92:1558–1564.

54. Morita E, Yasue H, Yoshimura M, et al. Increased plasma levels of brain natriuretic peptide in patients with acute myocardial infarction. *Circulation.*1993;88:82–91.

55. Talwar S, Squire IB, Downie PF, et al. Plasma N terminal pro-brain natriuretic peptide and cardiotrophin 1 are raised in unstable angina. *Heart.* 2000;84:421–424.

56. Wiviott S, de Lemos J, Morrow D. Pathophysiology, prognostic significance and clinical utility of B-type natriuretic peptide in acute coronary syndromes. *Clin Chim Acta.* 2004;346:119–128.

57. James SK, Lindahl B, Siegbahn A, et al. N-terminal pro-brain natriuretic peptide and other risk markers for the separate prediction of mortality and subsequent myocardial infarction in patients with unstable coronary artery disease: a Global Utilization of Strategies To Open occluded arteries (GUSTO)-IV substudy. *Circulation.* 2003;108:275–281.

58. James SK, Lindbäck J, Tilly J, et al. Troponin-T and N-terminal pro-B-type natriuretic peptide predict mortality benefit from coronary revascularization in acute coronary syndromes: a GUSTO-IV substudy. *J Am Coll Cardiol.* 2006;48:1146–1154.

59. Weber M, Bazzino O, Estrada JLN, et al. N-terminal B-type natriuretic peptide assessment provides incremental prognostic information in patients with acute coronary syndromes and normal troponin T values upon admission. *J Am Coll Cardiol.* 2008;51(12):1188–1195.

60. Morrow DA, De Lemos J, Sabatine MS, et al. Evaluation of B-type natriuretic peptide for risk assessment in unstable angina/non-ST-elevation myocardial infarction: B-type natriuretic peptide and prognosis in TACTICS-TIMI 18. *J Am Coll Cardiol.* 2003;41(8):1264–1272.

61. Detaint D, Messika-Zeitoun D, Avierinos J, et al. B-type natriuretic peptide in organic mitral regurgitation: determinants and impact on outcome. *Circulation.* 2005;111(18):2391–2397.

62. Sutton TM, Stewart RAH, Gerber IL, et al. Plasma natriuretic peptide levels increase with symptoms and severity of mitral regurgitation. *J Am Coll Cardiol.* 2003;41(12):2280–2287.

63. Shimamoto K, Kusumoto M, Sakai R, et al. Usefulness of the brain natriuretic peptide to atrial natriuretic peptide ratio in determining the severity of mitral regurgitation. *Can J Cardiol.* 2007;23(4): 295–300.

64. Yusoff R, Clayton N, Keevil B, Morris J, Ray S. Utility of plasma N-terminal brain natriuretic peptide as a marker of functional capacity in patients with chronic severe mitral regurgitation. *Am J Cardiol.* 2006;97(10):1498–1501.

65. Arat-Ozkan A, Kaya A, Yigit Z, et al. Serum N-terminal pro-BNP levels correlate with symptoms and echocardiographic findings in patients with mitral stenosis. *Echocardiography.* 2005;22(6):473–478.

66. Tharaux PL, Dussaule JC, Hubert-Brierre J, Vahanian A, Acar J, Ardaillou R. Plasma atrial and brain natriuretic peptides in mitral stenosis treated by valvulotomy. *Clin Sci (Lond).* 1994;87(6): 671–677.

67. Nakamura M, Kawata Y, Yoshida H, et al. Relationship between plasma atrial and brain natriuretic peptide concentration and hemodynamic parameters during percutaneous transvenous mitral valvulotomy in patients with mitral stenosis. *Am Heart J.* 1992;124(5): 1283–1288.

68. Gerber IL, Stewart RAH, French JK, et al. Associations between plasma natriuretic peptide levels, symptoms, and left ventricular function in patients with chronic aortic regurgitation. *Am J Cardiol.* 2003;92(6):755–758.

69. Ozkan M, Baysan O, Erinc K, et al. Brain natriuretic peptide and the severity of aortic regurgitation: is there any correlation? *J Int Med Res.* 2005;33(4):454–459.

70. Weber M, Hausen M, Arnold R, et al. Diagnostic and prognostic value of N-terminal pro B-type natriuretic peptide (NT-proBNP) in patients with chronic aortic regurgitation. *Int J Cardiol.* 2008;127(3): 321–327.

71. Gerber IL, Stewart RAH, Legget ME, et al. Increased plasma natriuretic peptide levels reflect symptom onset in aortic stenosis. *Circulation.* 2003;107(14):1884–1890.

72. Lim P, Monin JL, Monchi M, et al. Predictors of outcome in patients with severe aortic stenosis and normal left ventricular function: role of B-type natriuretic peptide. *Eur Heart J.* 2004;25(22):2048–2053.

73. Nessmith MG, Fukuta H, Brucks S, Little WC. Usefulness of an elevated B-type natriuretic peptide in predicting survival in patients with aortic stenosis treated without surgery. *Am J Cardiol.* 2005;96(10):1445–1448.

74. Bergler-Klein J, Mundigler G, Pibarot P, et al. B-type natriuretic peptide in low-flow, low-gradient aortic stenosis: relationship to hemodynamics and clinical outcome: results from the Multicenter Truly or Pseudo-Severe Aortic Stenosis (TOPAS) study. *Circulation.* 2007;115(22):2848–2855.

75. Bergler-Klein J, Klaar U, Heger M, et al. Natriuretic peptides predict symptom-free survival and postoperative outcome in severe aortic stenosis. *Circulation.* 2004;109(19):2302–2308.

76. Weber M, Hausen M, Arnold R, et al. Prognostic value of N-terminal pro-B-type natriuretic peptide for conservatively and surgically treated patients with aortic valve stenosis. *Heart.* 2006;92(11):1639–1644.

77. Kucher N, Printzen G, Doernhoefer T, Windecker S, Meier B, Hess OM. Low pro-brain natriuretic peptide levels predict benign clinical outcome in acute pulmonary embolism. *Circulation.* 2003;107(12):1576–1578.

78. Kucher N, Printzen G, Goldhaber SZ. Prognostic role of brain natriuretic peptide in acute pulmonary embolism. *Circulation.* 2003;107(20):2545–2547.

79. Klok FA, Mos ICM, Huisman MV. Brain-type natriuretic peptide levels in the prediction of adverse outcome in patients with pulmonary embolism: a systematic review and meta-analysis. *Am J Respir Crit Care Med.* 2008;178(4):425–430.

80. Kostrubiec M, Pruszczyk P, Kaczynska A, Kucher N. Persistent NT-proBNP elevation in acute pulmonary embolism predicts early death. *Clin Chim Acta.* 2007;382(1–2):124–128.

81. Kline JA, Zeitouni R, Marchick MR, Hernandez-Nino J, Rose GA. Comparison of 8 biomarkers for prediction of right ventricular hypokinesis 6 months after submassive pulmonary embolism. *Am Heart J.* 2008;156(2):308–314.

82. Karmpaliotis D, Kirtane AJ, Ruisi CP, et al. Diagnostic and prognostic utility of brain natriuretic peptide in subjects admitted to the ICU with hypoxic respiratory failure due to noncardiogenic and cardiogenic pulmonary edema. *Chest.* 2007;131(4):964–971.

83. Bajwa EK, Januzzi JL, Gong MN, Thompson BT, Christiani DC. Prognostic value of plasma N-terminal probrain natriuretic peptide levels in the acute respiratory distress syndrome. *Crit Care Med.* 2008;36(8): 2322–2327.
84. Ait-Oufella H, Tharaux P, Baudel J, et al. Variation in natriuretic peptides and mitral flow indexes during successful ventilatory weaning: a preliminary study. *Intensive Care Med.* 2007 Jul;33(7): 1183–1186.
85. Mekontso-Dessap A, Prost ND, Girou E, et al. B-type natriuretic peptide and weaning from mechanical ventilation. *Intensive Care Med.* 2006;32(10):1529–1536.
86. Rudiger A, Gasser S, Fischler M, Hornemann T, Eckardstein AV, Maggiorini M. Comparable increase of B-type natriuretic peptide and amino-terminal pro-B-type natriuretic peptide levels in patients with severe sepsis, septic shock, and acute heart failure. *Crit Care Med.* 2006;34(8):2140–2144.
87. McLean AS, Huang SJ, Hyams S, et al. Prognostic values of B-type natriuretic peptide in severe sepsis and septic shock. *Crit Care Med.* 2007;35(4):1019–1026.
88. Tung RH, Garcia C, Morss AM, et al. Utility of B-type natriuretic peptide for the evaluation of intensive care unit shock. *Crit Care Med.* 2004;32(8):1643–1647.
89. Januzzi JL, Morss A, Tung R, et al. Natriuretic peptide testing for the evaluation of critically ill patients with shock in the intensive care unit: a prospective cohort study. *Crit Care.* 2006;10(1):R37.
90. Roch A, Allardet-Servent J, Michelet P, et al. NH2 terminal pro-brain natriuretic peptide plasma level as an early marker of prognosis and cardiac dysfunction in septic shock patients. *Crit Care Med.* 2005;33(5):1001–1007.
91. Morgenthaler NG, Struck J, Christ-Crain M, Bergmann A, Müller B. Pro-atrial natriuretic peptide is a prognostic marker in sepsis, similar to the APACHE II score: an observational study. *Crit Care.* 2005;9(1): R37–R45.

24 ■ Natriuretic Peptides for Guidance of Acute and Chronic Heart Failure Therapy

A. Mark Richards, MD PhD
Richard W. Troughton, MB ChB PhD
M. Gary Nicholls, MD

Introduction

Both atrial natriuretic peptide (ANP) and the B-type peptides (BNP and/or NT-proBNP) are released from cardiomyocytes in response to stretch.[1–3] Increased intracardiac distending pressures are a consequence of increased cardiac load and adverse ventricular remodelling, which may be secondary to both acute (e.g., acute myocardial infarction) and chronic (e.g., uncontrolled hypertension) cardiac injuries. In addition, natriuretic peptide expression is augmented by a range of neurohormones and cytokines including angiotensin II and endothelin I, all of which are activated in heart failure.[3–6] Plasma levels reflect degrees of both systolic and diastolic dysfunction in both the left and right ventricles, the degree of left and right atrial distension, as well as potential contributions from additional stimuli, such as ischemic burden and any coexistent valve dysfunction.[7] In addition, independent relationships exist among circulating plasma natriuretic peptide levels, and both renal function and age. Hence, plasma concentrations of the B-type peptides provide an integrated signal of many factors, which are consistently and independently related to prognosis in heart failure. They are, thus, excellent candidates as prognostic markers in this syndrome.

B-Type Peptides for In-Hospital Monitoring and Treatment of Acute Heart Failure

Admissions for acute decompensated heart failure (ADHF) are common, constituting 5% of medical hospital admissions in the over-65-year-old age group in Western nations. It is the single most frequent diagnosis for patients admitted to the hospital in this age group, and has serious consequences. Inpatient mortality rates vary between 5–10% and short-term readmission rates are also high—in the vicinity of 25% within three months. The purpose of ADHF management is to attain a compensated status as rapidly as possible, and then institute therapy, which gives the best chance of sustained improvement. However, management of ADHF is far from standardized and guidelines for both treatment and monitoring are still evolving.[8]

Monitoring must incorporate consideration of symptoms, signs, and laboratory tests (Table 24–1). In the majority of cases,

Table 24–1: Laboratory tests in heart failure.

Investigation	*Rationale*
Full blood count	- Anemia, heart failure due to decreased O_2^- carrying capacity
Creatinine and estimated glomerular filtration rate	- Renal failure impairs body fluid volume homeostasis and has important effects upon the efficacy and potential toxicity of cardiac drugs
Electrolytes (Na, K)	- Important derangements may result from heart failure and/or its treatment
Glucose	- Diabetes and its control potentially have far-reaching effects on cardiac perfusion and function
Thyroid function tests (with atrial fibrillation, bradycardia, age > 65y and/or signs of thyroid disease)	- Hypo/hyperthyroidism
BNP/NT-proBNP	- Marker of diagnosis, function, and prognosis in heart failure

it is possible to achieve resolution of dyspnea at rest or on minimal exertion, together with removal of peripheral edema. In association with this, reductions of jugular venous pressure, disappearance of the gallop rhythm, and resolution of pulmonary rales can be expected to occur in 90% or more of patients. At this point, however, the completeness of drug therapy is likely to be incomplete and the attending physician faces the challenge of deciding whether the degree of compensation achieved and the quality of therapy established are sufficient to allow discharge of the patient with a high probability that improvement will be sustained in the outpatient setting. Very high rates of readmission and/or death within the short- and intermediate-term indicate that this is a difficult judgment to make.

Plasma B-type peptides offer the possibility of improving our assessment of the degree and sustainability of compensation achieved. Plasma peptide levels at admission and at discharge and the change between these two values all reflect the degree of compensation achieved during the inpatient stay and the risk of pivotal adverse outcomes in the early and intermediate postdischarge period. Knebel et al. demonstrated that in those patients with ADHF monitored invasively, a substantial fall in left ventricular filling pressures (pulmonary capillary wedge pressure) was associated with a sustained fall in NT-proBNP levels. This became evident within 16 hours from presentation.[9] Failure to demonstrate a favorable hemodynamic response was associated with no fall in B-type peptides. Similarly, Cioffi et al. found that a lack of NT-proBNP response to acute therapy was associated with an absence of improvement in ventricular filling pressures and with adverse prognosis.[10]

In an early report, Cheng et al. studied a group of 72 patients admitted with ADHF and found that those patients destined to suffer death or readmission with heart failure within the next 30 days showed on average no fall in plasma BNP levels, whereas in those that escaped these adverse outcomes, initial BNP levels were lower and plasma concentrations exhibited a clear-cut fall during

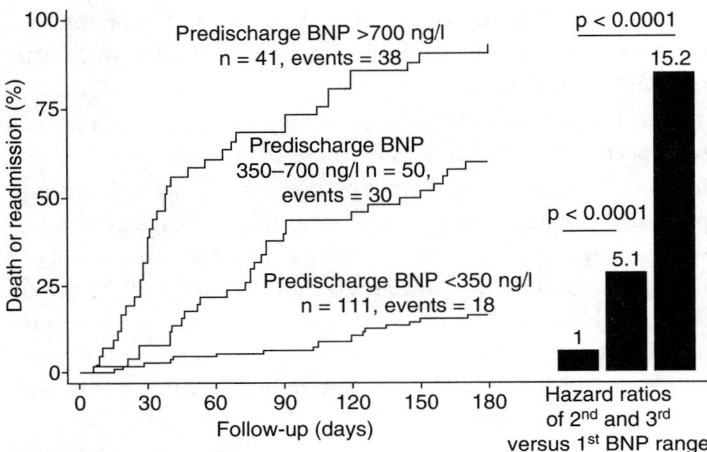

■ **Figure 24–1** Cumulative death or re-admission according to predischarge BNP ranges (<350, 350–700 and >700 ng/l) over 6 months post-discharge in 202 patients admitted and treated for decompensated heart failure. Hazard ratios (bar graphs) are shown for each BNP range.

Reproduced with permission from Elsevier (Logeart et al., *J Am Coll Cardiol* 2004;43(4):635–641).

the hospital stay.[11] Logeart and colleagues extended these findings to a six-month follow-up period. They found on average that post-treatment levels of BNP fell to less than half admission levels. A particularly strong relationship was reported between predischarge BNP levels and the risk of death or readmission over the following six months (Figure 24–1).[12] They reported a steep gradation of risk over a fifteenfold range as predischarge levels of BNP varied from less than 350 to greater than 700 pg/mL. Predischarge BNP levels had good discriminative power by receiver operating characteristic curve (ROC) analysis (area under the curve = 0.80) for the six-month outcomes. BNP remained a significant independent predictor in multivariable analysis and notably performed better than left ventricular ejection fraction assessment and a range of other clinical variables that were poorly predictive of outcomes.

Bayés-Genís et al. and Di Somma et al. both have reported an association between changes in levels of plasma NT-proBNP during acute therapy and achievement of a newly-compensated state. Both reports indicated that over a seven-day period, a fall in plasma NT-proBNP levels of 50% or more was associated with successful treatment for acutely destabilized heart failure. In contrast, those who failed to recompensate and suffered complications or failed to survive the episode of ADHF exhibited no change or typically a less than 15% decrement in plasma B-type peptides.[13–15] Bettencourt et al.[16] pursued this observation in a landmark report relating changes in plasma NT-proBNP in the inpatient period to outcomes over the following six months. Again, levels of NT-proBNP at admission, discharge, and the percent change between these time points were all related to outcomes (Figure 24–2). However, post-treatment values were a stronger predictor of hazard than admission levels. A predischarge level of NT-proBNP greater than 4137 pg/mL was a much stronger predictor of hazard than admission levels of close to 7000 pg/mL. An 8% increase in hazard was associated with each 1000 pg/mL increment of discharge NT-proBNP level with respect to the likelihood of death or readmission.

The remarkable consistency of these data and the independent powerful association of both BNP and NT-proBNP levels with both inpatient and postdischarge outcomes is striking. Although no prospective randomized studies have been undertaken to assess the efficacy or otherwise of altering management and thresholds for discharge according to target levels or target decrements in B-type peptides, existing reports do encourage some simple recommendations:

(A) A fall-from-admission level of plasma BNP and/or NT-proBNP of at least 30%, and preferably 50%, is a reasonable goal.

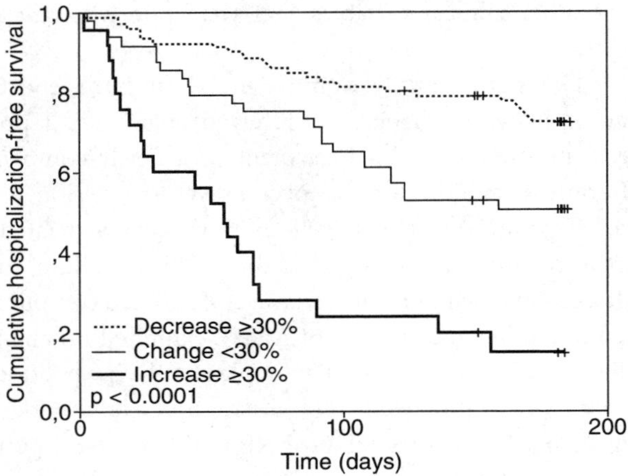

■ **Figure 24–2** Cumulative re-admission free survival over 6 months, according to inpatient NTproBNP response (decreased by ≥30% of baseline, changed <30%, increased ≥30%) in 182 patients admitted with decompensated heart failure. All pairwise comparisons between curves indicate significant differences ($p < 0.007$ for all).

Reproduced with permission from Lippincott Williams & Wilkins (Bettencourt et al., *Circulation* 2004;110(15):2168–2174).

(B) If an initial value is not obtained, predischarge goals of NT-proBNP below 4000 pg/mL and/or BNP below 400 pg/mL are rational.

Achievement of these targets is very likely to be associated with reduced rates of short- and intermediate-term mortality and re-admission with recurrent ADHF.

Clearly, decisions regarding adequacy of compensation and established therapy and the threshold for discharge cannot be based upon B-type peptide measurements in isolation. Biochemical measures (particularly renal function and hemoglobin), symptoms, and signs must also be employed to indicate compensation. At this point, however, careful consideration of the predischarge (i.e., early post-treatment) levels of B-type peptides should be undertaken, and may well influence the timing of discharge, the aggression with which drug therapy (and/or devices) are applied for HF, and the timing and frequency of follow-up.

Outpatient Monitoring and Treatment of Chronic Heart Failure Guided by B-Type Peptide Measurements

What is the optimal monitoring strategy for chronic heart failure? This challenge applies to the management of patients recently discharged from the hospital having survived an episode of ADHF and to those patients whose history has been more gradual with more incipient heart failure, which has nevertheless required the introduction of antiheart failure therapy and surveillance as an outpatient. Provision of optimal treatment for individual patients remains a challenge in part due to the lack of a valid objective marker to guide monitoring and titration of therapy.[17] Effective heart failure monitoring strategies are required, but current tools are crude and tend to be applied in haphazard fashion. Indicators, such as weight and signs on physical examination (including jugular venous pressure and gallop rhythm), have prognostic value, but do not accurately reflect central hemodynamic status or the severity of cardiac dysfunction.[18] Self-reported symptoms, six-minute walk tests, and echocardiographic indices of left ventricular filling pressures may have value for therapy monitoring, but in fact have never been prospectively tested in monitoring strategies and, in any case, they are limited by resource constraints.[19,20] Likewise, implantable hemodynamic monitoring systems are yet to be tested in randomized controlled trials and their expense, together with the need for deployment by highly-skilled staff in tertiary centers, render them relevant for only a very small proportion of patients with chronic heart failure.[21] In this relative vacuum of options, B-type peptides may well come to play an important role in monitoring and optimizing HF therapy.[16,22] The potential utility of serial measurements of B-type peptides as a guide to treatment in chronic heart failure is currently under close scrutiny.

Such an application of serial plasma B-type peptide measurements requires underpinning with an understanding of the relationship between central hemodynamic measurements (particularly left ventricular filling pressures) and concurrent plasma concentrations of B-type peptides. In addition, the inherent variability of plasma B-type peptide measurements is pivotal. In contrast to ADHF where the signal-to-noise ratio of plasma BNP or NT-proBNP is very high, the chronic compensated state is associated with far lower mean peptide concentrations. Therefore, any background variability needs to be understood in order to establish the least significant shift in B-type peptides that can be reliably interpreted as reflecting either improvement or deterioration in cardiac status.

Little data exist on the relationship of plasma B-type peptide concentrations to ventricular filling pressures in the outpatient setting. Studies of ambulatory heart failure subjects with implantable monitoring devices do provide some insight.[21,23] Serial concurrent measurements of hemodynamics and NT-proBNP levels in a group of subjects over several months showed that intersubject differences were profound and sustained, and plots of grouped data did not indicate a significant association between plasma peptide concentrations and either estimated pulmonary artery diastolic or right ventricular systolic pressures. However, serial measurements within single patients demonstrated significant positive correlations between plasma NT-proBNP and estimated pulmonary artery diastolic pressures. This suggests that within individual patients, variation in NT-proBNP reflects concurrent changes in hemodynamic status. It is likely absolute levels of the B-type peptides cannot be used as a surrogate for absolute left ventricular filling pressures, but changes in levels within individuals will reflect changes in hemodynamic status. This implies that within each individual it will be necessary to ascertain the plasma concentration of B-type peptides at the time of the best achievable ("optimized") state. However, within individual patients, the onset of acute decompensation will be reflected in a significant sharp elevation of B-type peptide levels above their customary value.

Variability in Plasma B-Type Peptide Concentrations

Variation in serial test results of plasma peptide concentrations reflects the net effects of analytical accuracy and shifts in secretion and/or clearance.[24] As already suggested, multiple factors contribute to biological variation (cardiac, neurohormonal, renal, etc.). Alternative processing of NT-proBNP or BNP and subsequent variations in immunoreactivity—which may well vary from one immunoassay to another—may also contribute to apparent variation in plasma peptide measurements.[25] A strategy which employs serial measurements of plasma B-type peptides must adhere to a single, well validated, and stable immunoassay within a given individual patient.

These sources of variation must be sufficiently low such that plasma changes triggering a therapeutic response genuinely reflect either improvement or deterioration in heart failure status. An excess of unexplained biological variation could confound the use of serial peptide measurements to adjust treatment.[26] Early studies from small cohorts of normal subjects[27] suggested an intraindividual change of greater than 92% in serial measurements to provide confidence of a meaningful shift relative to background biological variation. However, in healthy subjects peptide levels are low (often at the limits of assay detection) resulting in small, absolute, intermeasurement changes, but high, proportional (percent) magnitude changes of no biological importance. The background variation of relevance in the application of serial measurements of BNP/NT-proBNP in the management of heart failure is that which pertains to chronic stable heart failure. Bruins et al. assessed serial measurements taken within a single day, on consecutive days, and weekly over six weeks in patients with heart failure.[28] The minimum percent change values for within-day, day-to-day, and week-to-week samples were 25, 55, and 98% respectively. Data from larger cohorts in which clinical stability has been more rigorously defined indicate less true variability.[29–31] Schou et al. investigated 20 patients fulfilling 22 inclusion and exclusion criteria defining stability.[30] In this study, a minimum percent change value of only 23% was required. Cortes et al. reported similar findings in 74 stable patients with measurements of NT-proBNP at 12 and 24 months from baseline.[29] A change in NT-proBNP of 22% or more represented a shift in excess of background biological variation. Notably, NT-proBNP secretion is nonlinear and when log transformed peptide levels are assessed in stable patients, variability is less than 10%, although this may be difficult to apply in a simple management algorithm.[30,31]

With current validated immunoassays, analytical factors account for a very small proportion of total variation in serial peptide measurements.[24] Biological variation should not be regarded as random, but rather as the consequence of altered peptide secretion due to active physiological processes, which may include components independent of altered hemodynamic load. Activation by multiple neurohormonal and immunological factors including angiotensin II, endothelin, catecholamines, and ischemia may be relevant.[3–6] These factors are dynamic and contribute to cardiac remodelling, ventricular dysfunction, and eventually to outcomes in heart failure. It has been suggested that variation greater than three times the analytical imprecision of the assay should be regarded as clinically significant.[32]

Serial Plasma B-Type Peptide Testing and Prognosis in Heart Failure

Over the spectrum of heart failure, NT-proBNP and BNP levels measured at a single time point are a powerful independent predictor of mortality in new heart failure events. Serial measurements provide incremental prognostic information over a single baseline measurement. As discussed above, this has been well demonstrated in the setting of ADHF.[11,12,16] However, the same principle clearly applies in the longer term. Within the neurohormonal substudy of the Valsartan Heart Failure Trial (Val-HeFT), changes in plasma BNP and NT-proBNP levels during follow-up independently predicted survival in patients randomized to Valsartan or placebo, in addition to standard therapy which included Angiotensin Converting Enzyme (ACE) inhibitors.[33] Those with B-type peptide levels above the median at baseline, but below the median at four months, had two-year mortality rates similar to those with low peptide levels at both time points (12.8 and 7.9%, respectively). In contrast, those with below-median baseline levels rising above the median at four months incurred mortality similar to those with persistently elevated levels (22.7 and 25.4%, respectively) (Figure 24–3).

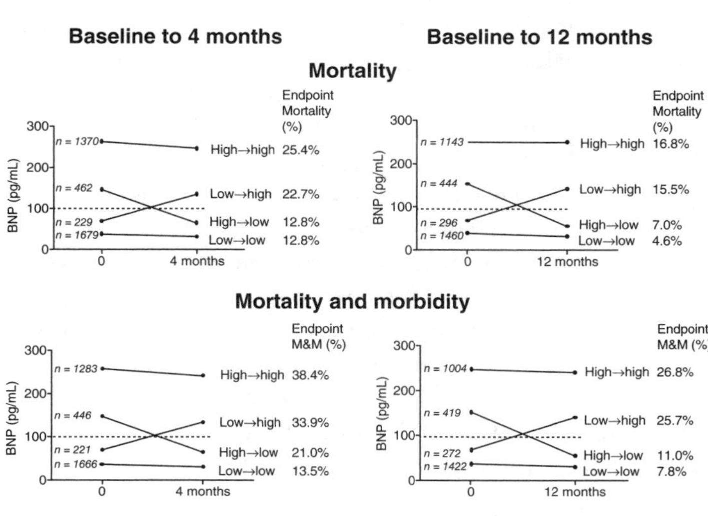

■ **Figure 24–3** Twenty-three month mortality and morbidity in Val-HeFT patients according to change in plasma BNP from baseline to 4 or 12 months categorized by shifts relative to the baseline median values of 97 pg/mL. (M&M = mortality and morbidity).

Reproduced with permission from Elsevier (Latini et al., *Am J Med* 2006;119(1):70.e23–70.e30).

B-Type Peptides as Indicators of Response to Therapy

Improvements in deterioration in heart failure are paralleled by changes in plasma B-type peptide concentrations. They shift following treatment with proven heart failure medications.[34,35] BNP and NT-proBNP levels fall after starting diuretics and vasodilators. Conversely, cessation of diuretics is associated with a rise in peptide levels. Vasodilators, including angiotensin converting enzyme inhibitors and angiotensin II receptor blockers, also produce a fall in peptide levels, as does aldosterone antagonism.[35] Beta blockers induce a more complex response depending on whether the agent used has a vasodilating component to its action and effects will also vary according to the severity and acuity of heart failure at the time of introduction of the beta blocker. Introduction of metoprolol in stable mild heart failure induces a rise in NT-proBNP and BNP levels, reflecting changes in secretion and clearance not due to clinical decompensation.[36,37] In the longer term, beyond two to twelve weeks, B-type peptide levels will fall in parallel with beneficial left ventricular remodelling.[38] Responses to carvedilol (and other vasodilator beta blockers) may differ from metoprolol with an initial fall in natriuretic peptide levels.[39,40] Other beneficial interventions in heart failure are associated with falls in plasma natriuretic peptide levels. Exercise therapy and cardiac resynchronization therapy are both associated with falls in plasma B-type peptide levels in those who benefit from these treatments.[41–45]

Guiding Treatment of Heart Failure with Serial Measurements of B-Type Plasma Natriuretic Peptides

Application of serial measurements of B-type peptides in monitoring and titration of antiheart failure therapy is the subject of intense interest. Murdoch et al. investigated the feasibility of titrating vasodilator therapy in chronic heart failure according to plasma BNP concentrations. They performed a comparison of the hemodynamic and neuroendocrine effects of tailored versus empirical therapy and found they could induce a predictable fall in plasma BNP levels through adjustment in doses of vasodilators, particularly ACE inhibitors.[34] Troughton et al.[46] conducted a landmark pilot study with treatment aimed to achieve NT-proBNP levels of less than 200 pmol/L. This strategy resulted in fewer combined outpatient heart failure decompensations, heart failure admissions, and deaths (Figure 24–4). Compared to clinically-guided treatment, patients randomized to the hormone-guided arm of the trial received higher doses of diuretic and ACE inhibitor therapy. Plasma NT-proBNP levels fell in the hormone-guided group, but not in the clinically-guided group.

Corroboration of these findings was provided by a larger trial undertaken by heart failure specialists working in 17 centers in France.[47] Two hundred and twenty patients with NYHA class II-III heart failure were randomized to treatment according to current guidelines or to treatment influenced by the goal of decreasing BNP plasma levels to less than 100 pg/mL. Trial findings included more frequent changes in anti-heart failure therapy in the first three months within the hormone-guided group. Mean achieved doses of ACE inhibitors and beta blockers were higher in the BNP group. Most importantly, over a median follow-up of 15 months, fewer patients reached the combined endpoint of heart failure-related death or hospital stay for heart failure in the hormone-guided arm of the study (24 versus 52%, $P < 0.001$) (Figure 24–5).

The "STARBRITE" study has been presented in abstract form, but not yet published in full. This study assessed the impact of treatment aimed at achieving an individualized target BNP level during a shorter-term follow-up (90 days).[48] A trend towards reduced mortality and hospital stay did not reach significance, but a more optimal use of proven therapies was observed. Patients under BNP guidance more frequently received trial-based doses of ACE inhibitors and beta blockers and were less likely to have increases in diuretic doses.

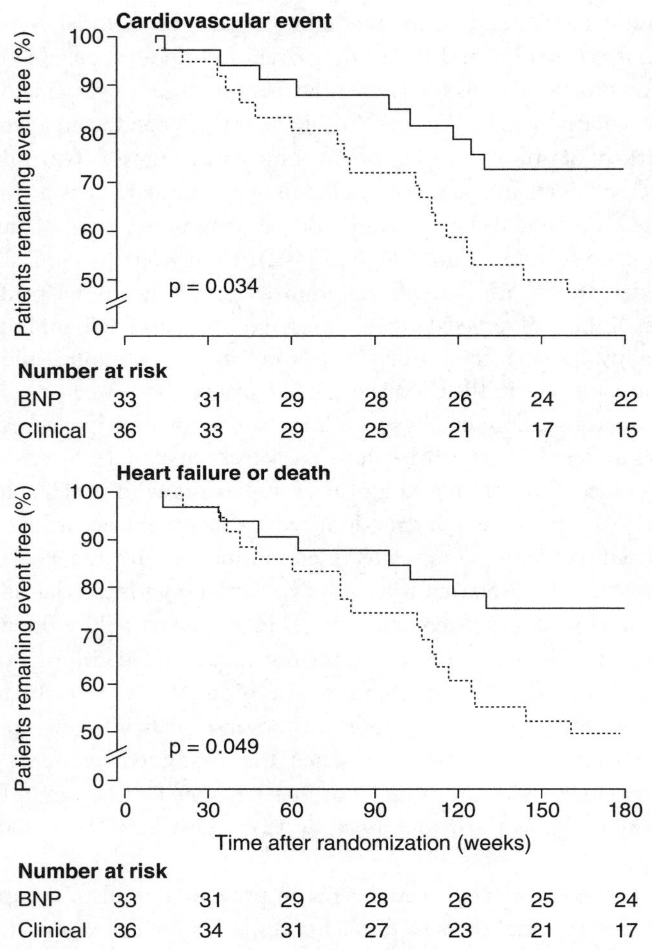

■ **Figure 24–4** Kaplan-Meier event curves for time to first cardiovascular event and to heart failure event or death in patients with treatment guided by serial measurements of NTproBNP (solid line) compared with clinical management (dashed line).

Reproduced with permission from Elsevier (Troughton et al., *Lancet* 2000;355(9210): 1126–1130).

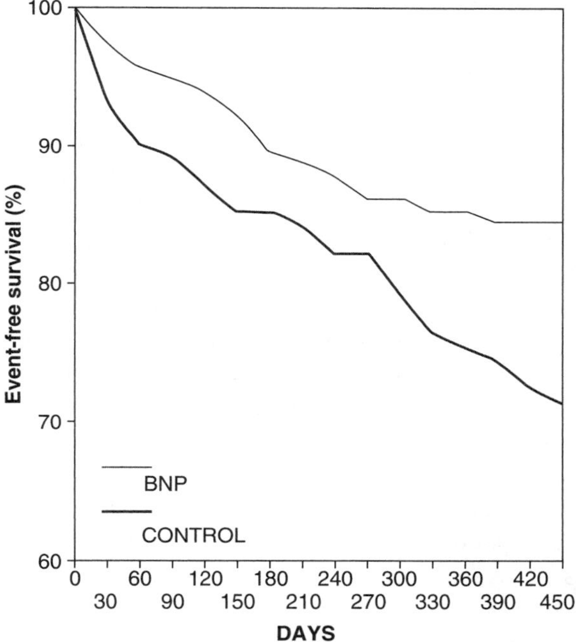

■ **Figure 24–5** Event-free (hospital stay for heart failure or death related to heart failure) survival in patients with treatment guided by serial measurement of BNP (upper line) or by clinical management (lower line) ($p < 0.01$).

Reproduced with permission from Elsevier (Jourdain et al., *J Am Coll Cardiol* 2007;49(16):1733–1739).

Notably, patients recruited to both the Christchurch pilot study[46] and the "BNP-STARS" Trial[47] were relatively young (65–69 years) with trial inclusion criteria requiring systolic dysfunction (i.e., reduced left ventricular ejection fraction). Further trials will address larger numbers of patients more representative of real-life heart failure populations. Methods papers have been published for the "BATTLESCARRED" and "TIME-CHF" Trials,[49,50] and other studies in the United States and in Europe are ongoing. Both

BATTLESCARRED and TIME-CHF have had preliminary results presented. These two trials followed very similar designs, which incorporated stratification according to age (above and below 75 years). Importantly, both have reported benefit in the form of reduced mortality or the composite endpoint of all-cause mortality and hospital admission with heart failure in those less than 75 years of age receiving hormone-guided therapy.

Again, whether an absolute target of BNP or NT-proBNP should be applied across the board or (possibly more rationally) to individualized targets remains uncertain. Knowledge of a patient's B-type peptide status when clinically stable will be valuable for monitoring. Use of a uniform target based on levels associated with increased risk may promote treatment intensification in a greater proportion of patients. However, it may also result in more adverse effects including azotemia or symptomatic hypotension, which may significantly counterbalance benefits in terms of reduced episodes of acute decompensation or heart failure mortality. In any case, serial B-type peptide measurements should always be performed in concert with established standards of assessment of clinical status and biochemical indicators of renal function.[20]

Conclusion

In summary, the B-type peptides are strong and independent prognostic markers across the spectrum of acute and chronic heart failure. Serial peptide measurements provide incremental risk stratification. In stable heart failure, variation in peptide levels between serial measurements is sufficiently small to allow serial monitoring. Peptide levels fall in response to therapies with proven benefits in treating heart failure. Targeting therapy to lower plasma B-type levels may facilitate more optimal use of proven heart failure therapy and may improve outcomes, including overall mortality and reducing inpatient admissions due to heart failure. The optimal application of serial B-type peptide measurements with regard to frequency of testing and whether to use a standard absolute or individualized target peptide level remains to be determined.

References

1. Espiner EA. Physiology of natriuretic peptides. *J Intern Med.* 1994;235:527–541.
2. Magga J, Vuolteenaho O, Tokola H, Marttila M, Ruskoaho H. Involvement of transcriptional and posttranscriptional mechanisms in cardiac overload–induced increase of B-type natriuretic peptide gene expression. *Circ Res.* 1997;81(5):694–702.
3. Wiese S, Breyer T, Dragu A, et al. Gene expression of brain natriuretic peptide in isolated atrial and ventricular human myocardium: influence of angiotensin II and diastolic fiber length. *Circulation.* 2000;102(25):3074–3079.
4. Ruskoaho H, Leskinen H, Magga J, et al. Mechanisms of mechanical load-induced atrial natriuretic peptide secretion: role of endothelin, nitric oxide, and angiotensin II. *J Mol Med.* 1997;75(11):876–885.
5. Liang F, Gardner DG. Autocrine/paracrine determinants of strain-activated brain natriuretic peptide gene expression in cultured cardiac myocytes. *J Biol Chem.* 1998;273(23):14612–14619.
6. He Q, LaPointe MC. Interleukin-1ß regulation of the human brain natriuretic peptide promoter involves Ras-, Rac-, and p38 kinase-dependent pathways in cardiac myocytes. *Hypertension.* 1999;33(1):283–289.
7. Troughton RW, Prior DL, Pereira JJ, Martin M, Fogarty A, Morehead A, et al. Plasma B-type natriuretic peptide levels in systolic heart failure: importance of left ventricular diastolic function and right ventricular systolic function. *J Am Coll Cardiol.* 2004;43(3):416–422.
8. Nieminen MS, Bohm M, Cowie MR, et al. Executive summary of the guidelines on the diagnosis and treatment of acute heart failure: The Task Force on Acute Heart Failure of the European Society of Cardiology. *Eur Heart J.* 2005;26(4):384–416.
9. Knebel F, Schimke I, Pliet K, et al. NT-proBNP in acute heart failure: correlation with invasively measured hemodynamic parameters during recompensation. *J Card Fail.* 2005;11(5, Supplement 1):S38–S41.
10. Cioffi G, Tarantini L, Stefenelli C, et al. Changes in plasma N-terminal proBNP levels and ventricular filling pressures during intensive

unloading therapy in elderly with decompensated congestive heart failure and preserved left ventricular systolic function. *J Card Fail.* 2006;12(8):608–615.

11. Cheng V, Kazanagra R, Garcia A, et al. A rapid bedside test for B-type peptide predicts treatment outcomes in patients admitted for decompensated heart failure: a pilot study. *J Am Coll Cardiol.* 2001;37(2): 386–391.
12. Logeart D, Thabut G, Jourdain P, et al. Predischarge B-type natriuretic peptide assay for identifying patients at high risk of readmission after decompensated heart failure. *J Am Coll Cardiol.* 2004;43(4):635–641.
13. Bayés-Genís A, Santaló-Bel M, Zapico-Muñiz E, et al. N-terminal probrain natriuretic peptide (NT-proBNP) in the emergency diagnosis and in-hospital monitoring of patients with dyspnoea and ventricular dysfunction. *Eur J Heart Fail.* 2004;6(3):301–308.
14. Di Somma S, Magrini L, Mazzone M, et al. Decrease in NTproBNP plasma levels indicates clinical improvement of acute decompensated heart failure. *Am J Emerg Med.* 2007;25(3):335–339.
15. Bayés-Genís A, Pascual-Figal D, Fabregat J, et al. Serial NT-proBNP monitoring and outcomes in outpatients with decompensation of heart failure. *Int J Cardiol.* 2007;120(3):338–343.
16. Bettencourt P, Azevedo A, Pimenta J, Frioes F, Ferreira S, Ferreira A. N-terminal-pro-brain natriuretic peptide predicts outcome after hospital discharge in heart failure patients. *Circulation.* 2004;110(15): 2168–2174.
17. Nicholls GM, Richards AM; Christchurch Cardioendocrine Research Group. Disease monitoring of patients with chronic heart failure. *Heart.* 2007;93(4):519–523.
18. Drazner MH, Rame JE, Stevenson LW, Dries DL. Prognostic importance of elevated jugular venous pressure and a third heart sound in patients with heart failure. *N Engl J Med.* 2001;345(8):574.
19. Tang WHW, Francis GS. The Year in Heart Failure. *J Am Coll Cardiol.* 2005;46(11):2125–2133.
20. Hunt SA. ACC/AHA 2005 Guideline Update for the Diagnosis and Management of Chronic Heart Failure in the Adult: A Report of the American College of Cardiology/American Heart Association Task Force on Practice Guidelines (Writing Committee to Update the 2001

Guidelines for the Evaluation and Management of Heart Failure). *J Am Coll Cardiol.* 2005;46(6):e1–e82.

21. Braunschweig F, Fahrleitner-Pammer A, Mangiavacchi M, et al. Correlation between serial measurements of N-terminal pro brain natriuretic peptide and ambulatory cardiac filling pressures in outpatients with chronic heart failure. *Eur J Heart Fail.* 2006;8(8):797–803.
22. Anand IS, Fisher LD, Chiang Y-T, et al. Changes in brain natriuretic peptide and norepinephrine over time and mortality and morbidity in the Valsartan Heart Failure Trial (Val-HeFT). *Circulation.* 2003;107(9):1278–1283.
23. McClean D, Aragon J, Jamali A, et al. Noninvasive calibration of cardiac pressure transducers in patients with heart failure: an aid to implantable hemodynamic monitoring and therapeutic guidance. *J Card Fail.* 2006;12(7):568–576.
24. Wu AHB. Serial testing of B-type natriuretic peptide and NTpro-BNP for monitoring therapy of heart failure: The role of biologic variation in the interpretation of results. *Am Heart J.* 2006;152(5):828–834.
25. Lam CSP, Burnett Jr JC, Costello-Boerrigter L, Rodeheffer RJ, Redfield MM. Alternate circulating pro-B-type natriuretic peptide and B-type natriuretic peptide forms in the general population. *J Am Coll Cardiol.* 2007;49(11):1193–1202.
26. Richards AM. Variability of NT-proBNP levels in heart failure: implications for clinical application. *Heart.* 2007;93(8):899–900.
27. Wu AHB, Smith A, Wieczorek S, et al. Biological variation for N-terminal pro- and B-type natriuretic peptides and implications for therapeutic monitoring of patients with congestive heart failure. *Am J Cardiol.* 2003;92(5):628–631.
28. Bruins S, Fokkema MR, Romer JWP, et al. High intraindividual variation of B-type natriuretic peptide (BNP) and amino-terminal proBNP in patients with stable chronic heart failure. *Clin Chem.* 2004; 50(11):2052–2058.
29. Cortes R, Rivera M, Salvador A, et al. Variability of NT-proBNP plasma and urine levels in patients with stable heart failure: a 2-year follow-up study. *Heart.* 2007;93(8):957–962.
30. Schou M, Gustafsson F, Kjaer A, Hildebrandt PR. Long-term clinical variation of NT-proBNP in stable chronic heart failure patients. *Eur Heart J.* 2007;28(2):177–182.

31. Schou M, Gustafsson F, Nielsen PH, Madsen LH, Kjaer A, Hildebrandt PR. Unexplained week-to-week variation in BNP and NT-proBNP is low in chronic heart failure patients during steady state. *Eur J Heart Fail.* 2007;9(1):68–74.

32. Masson S, Latini R, Anand IS, et al. Direct comparison of B-type natriuretic peptide (BNP) and amino-terminal proBNP in a large population of patients with chronic and symptomatic heart failure: the Valsartan Heart Failure (Val-HeFT) data. *Clin Chem.* 2006;52(8): 1528–1538.

33. Latini R, Masson S, Wong M, et al. Incremental prognostic value of changes in B-type natriuretic peptide in heart failure. *Am J Med.* 2006;119(1):70.e23–70.e30.

34. Murdoch DR, McDonagh TA, Byrne J, et al. Titration of vasodilator therapy in chronic heart failure according to plasma brain natriuretic peptide concentration: randomized comparison of the hemodynamic and neuroendocrine effects of tailored versus empirical therapy. *Am Heart J.* 1999;138(6):1126–1132.

35. Troughton RW, Richards AM, Yandle TG, Frampton CM, Nicholls MG. The effects of medications on circulating levels of cardiac natriuretic peptides. *Ann Med.* 2007;39(4):242–260.

36. Davis ME, Richards AM, Nicholls MG, Yandle TG, Frampton CM, Troughton RW. Introduction of metoprolol increases plasma B-type cardiac natriuretic peptides in mild, stable heart failure. *Circulation.* 2006;113(7):977–985.

37. The RESOLVD Investigators. Effects of metoprolol CR in patients with ischemic and dilated cardiomyopathy: the randomized evaluation of strategies for left ventricular dysfunction pilot study. *Circulation.* 2000;101(4):378–384.

38. Stanek B, Frey B, Hülsmann M, et al. Prognostic evaluation of neurohumoral plasma levels before and during beta-blocker therapy in advanced left ventricular dysfunction. *J Am Coll Cardiol.* 2001;38(2): 436–442.

39. Hartmann F, Packer M, Coats AJS, et al. Prognostic impact of plasma N-terminal pro-brain natriuretic peptide in severe chronic congestive heart failure: A substudy of the Carvedilol Prospective Randomized Cumulative Survival (COPERNICUS) Trial. *Circulation.* 2004;110(13): 1780–1786.

40. Sanderson JE, Chan WW, Hung YT, et al. Effect of low dose beta blockers on atrial and ventricular (B type) natriuretic factor in heart failure: a double blind, randomised comparison of metoprolol and a third generation vasodilating beta blocker. *Br Heart J.* 1995;74(5): 502–507.
41. Conraads VM, Beckers P, Vaes J, et al. Combined endurance/resistance training reduces NT-proBNP levels in patients with chronic heart failure. *Eur Heart J.* 2004;25(20):1797–1805.
42. Krüger S, Graf J, Merx MW, et al. Brain natriuretic peptide kinetics during dynamic exercise in patients with chronic heart failure. *Int J Cardiol.* 2004;95(1):49–54.
43. Passino C, Severino S, Poletti R, et al. Aerobic training decreases B-type natriuretic peptide expression and adrenergic activation in patients with heart failure. *J Am Coll Cardiol.* 2006;47(9): 1835–1839.
44. Yeh GY, Wood MJ, Lorell BH, et al. Effects of tai chi mind-body movement therapy on functional status and exercise capacity in patients with chronic heart failure: a randomized controlled trial. *Am J Med.* 2004;117(8):541–548.
45. Fruhwald FM, Fahrleitner-Pammer A, Berger R, et al. Early and sustained effects of cardiac resynchronization therapy on N-terminal pro-B-type natriuretic peptide in patients with moderate to severe heart failure and cardiac dyssynchrony. *Eur Heart J.* 2007;28(13): 1592–1597.
46. Troughton RW, Frampton CM, Yandle TG, Espiner EA, Nicholls MG, Richards AM. Treatment of heart failure guided by plasma aminoterminal brain natriuretic peptide (N-BNP) concentrations. *Lancet.* 2000;355(9210):1126–1130.
47. Jourdain P, Jondeau G, Funck F, et al. Plasma brain natriuretic peptide-guided therapy to improve outcome in heart failure: The STARS-BNP Multicenter Study. *J Am Coll Cardiol.* 2007;49(16):1733–1739.
48. Shah MR, Claise KA, Bowers MT, et al. Testing new targets of therapy in advanced heart failure: the design and rationale of the Strategies for Tailoring Advanced Heart Failure Regimens in the Outpatient Setting: BRain NatrIuretic Peptide Versus the Clinical CongesTion ScorE (STARBRITE) trial. *Am Heart J.* 2005;150(5):893–898.
49. Lainchbury JG, Troughton RW, Frampton CM, et al. NTproBNP-guided drug treatment for chronic heart failure: design and methods

in the "BATTLESCARRED" trial. *Eur J Heart Fail.* 2006;8(5): 532–538.

50. Brunner-La Rocca HP, Buser PT, Schindler R, Bernheim A, Rickenbacher P, Pfisterer M. Management of elderly patients with congestive heart failure—Design of the Trial of Intensified versus standard Medical therapy in Elderly patients with Congestive Heart Failure (TIME-CHF). *Am Heart J.* 2006;151(5):949–955.

25 ■ Natriuretic Peptide Testing in Patients with Renal Disease

ROLAND R.J. VAN KIMMENADE MD, PHD
CHRISTOPHER R. DEFILIPPI, MD, FACC
YIGAL M. PINTO, MD, PHD

Introduction

The fact that there is a strong interaction between heart failure and renal impairment has been acknowledged for several decades, even as early as in 1928, when Stewart and McIntosh cited this fact in the *Journal of Clinical Investigation*.[1] Today, 80 years later, this relationship between cardiac and renal dysfunction has become even more relevant because renal impairment not only drastically worsens the prognosis of patients suffering from heart failure, but it also limits the modern physician in his or her therapeutic arsenal. Therefore, some prefer to give heart failure with renal complications its own special identity—the so-called "cardiorenal syndrome."[2,3]

When considering the association between B-type natriuretic peptide (BNP) or amino-terminal proBNP (NT-proBNP) and renal impairment, and realizing that both peptides strongly predict outcomes in heart failure,[4,5] it is only to be expected that high serum concentrations of natriuretic peptides (NPs) are accompanied by a decrease in the glomerular filtration rate (GFR). In fact, the most publications report correlations between BNP or NT-proBNP and GFR with r-values around -0.30 (translating into a r^2-value of only 0.09). These correlations are depicted in Table 25–1.

Although caution is always warranted when interpreting a statistical association as causal, the debate about the correct interpretation of BNP and NT-proBNP's role in renal impairment has at times been blindly biased and fueled by marketing strategies,

Table 25–1: Correlation of natriuretic peptides with estimated glomerular filtration rate.

Author	Population	NT-proBNP	BNP
Mark (n = 296)[66]	Amb CKD		−0.40
DeFilippi (n = 207)[43]	Amb CKD	−0.31	
Khan (n = 54)[67]	Amb CKD	−0.45	−0.38
Vickery (n = 213)[11,34]	Amb CKD	−0.53	−0.36
Austin (n = 171)[35]	Amb CKD	−0.46	−0.36
Richards (n = 1049)[68]	Amb CAD-CM	−0.51	−0.51
Luchner (n = 469)[69]	Amb CAD	−0.29	−0.28
van Kimmenade (n = 165)[24]	Amb HTN	−0.32	−0.32
Anwaruddin (n = 599)[53]	Acute dyspnea	−0.55	
Anwaruddin (n = 209)[53]	Acute HF	−0.34	−0.18
DeFilippi (n = 831)[47]	Acute dyspnea	−0.42	−0.34
McCullough (n = 715)[6]	Acute HF		−0.19
McCullough (n = 737)[6]	Acute dyspnea, non-HF		−0.20
van Kimmenade (n = 720)[25]	Acute HF	−0.34	
Leuchte (n = 118)[70]	Pulm HT	−0.33	No correlation
Spanaus (n = 227)[71]	Amb CKD	−0.61	−0.17
Hogenhuis et al. (n = 541)[72]	Stable HF	−0.27	−0.11
Bruch (n = 341)[73]	Stable HF	−0.32	
Astor (n = 1006)[74]	Hypertensives	−0.21	
Bruch (n = 142)[75,76]	Stable HF	−0.29	

Notes: Amb = ambulatory; CAD = coronary artery disease; CKD = chronic kidney disease; CM = cardiomyopathy; HF = heart failure; HTN = hypertension rather than driven by scientific arguments. In order to provide some clarity in this debate, in this chapter we aim to review data from the diverse observational and interventional studies published so far and we will question what is really known about the association between renal impairment and concentrations of BNP and NT-proBNP. The issues that need to be addressed are:

- What is known about a possible accumulation effect of these peptides in renal impairment?
- What is the *difference* between BNP and NT-proBNP and what are their individual associations with renal function?
- What are the clinical consequences when confronted with an elevated BNP or NT-proBNP concentration in a patient with a decreased renal function?

While these questions may not have complete answers yet, in the last few years several studies have shed light on the mystery of understanding elevated BNP and NT-proBNP concentrations in patients suffering from all different stages of renal impairment, presenting with or without clinical evidence of heart failure.

The Clearance of BNP and NT-proBNP

When the first observational studies demonstrated an association between natriuretic peptides and renal impairment,[6,7] it was hypothesized that this was probably due to accumulation of the peptides, given that both peptides depend on renal clearance for their elimination from the circulation.[8] Furthermore, because BNP (3.5 kDa) has a lower molecular weight than NT-proBNP (8.5 kDa) and—in contrast to NT-proBNP—also cleared by alternative pathways, such as the clearance receptor natriuretic peptide receptor type-C (NPR-C), as well as degraded by neutral endopeptidases, the assumption grew that serum concentrations of NT-proBNP were more influenced by accumulation in renal impairment than BNP.[8] This assumption seemed confirmed by the detection of high concentrations of NT-proBNP in the urine of heart failure patients[9] and the fact that the ratio of NT-proBNP to BNP concentration increases when renal function decreases.[10,11] Taking all these facts together, it was concluded by some authors that perhaps all natriuretic peptide testing, but especially NT-proBNP testing, was unsuitable for application in patients with renal impairment.[8,11,12]

However, rather than assumptions, what was needed in an evidence-based medicine era was a careful evaluation of possible explanations for the association between natriuretic peptide concentrations and renal impairment addressing accumulation, as well as the alternative explanation of a parallel event (not impossible because cardiac and renal dysfunction often coincide), combined with a thorough understanding of renal physiology.

BNP and NT-proBNP in the Kidney

As a first step, it is necessary to look at the clearance of both NP molecules on the glomerular level. Based on their molecular weight, BNP (3.5 kDa) and NT-proBNP (8.5 kDa) are, by definition, Small Molecular Weight Proteins (SMWPs), which include all proteins with a molecular weight ranging from 1 to 50 kDa.[13–15] SMWPs are filtered relatively freely by the glomeruli and catabolized by tubular epithelial cells without any other processing, such as tubular secretion as in creatinine (0.1 kDa) or active reabsorption and return in the circulation as for albumin (69 kDa).

The extraction of a molecule on the level of the glomeruli is called the fractional extraction (FE), and is computed as: [(arterial concentration–venous concentration)/arterial concentration], as measured in the renal arteries and veins, respectively. The FE of a SMWP is mostly determined by its molecular weight, while steric and electrostatic factors may also play a role.[14] When extraction is not hampered at all, the FE equals the filtration fraction, which is in the range of 0.20–0.25 in healthy subjects.[16–18]

Several studies have indeed looked at the FE_{BNP} and $FE_{NT\text{-}proBNP}$ by sampling BNP and NT-proBNP concentrations in the renal arteries and veins (Table 25–2). In these studies, the FE_{BNP} ranged from 13% to 22 %, while the $FE_{NT\text{-}proBNP}$ ranged from 14% to 22%,

Table 25–2: An overview of published fractional extractions of BNP and NT-proBNP.

	Population	FE NT-proBNP	FE BNP
Schou et al.[21]	10 healthy subjects	19%	19%
Goetze et al.[16]	18 hypertensives,	18%	21%
	51 cirrhotic patients,	14%	17%
	18 healthy subjects	16%	14%
Rutten et al.[19]	4 hypertensives	22%	11%
Lainchbury et al.[23]	24 cardiac patients		16%
Richards et al.[22]	16 cardiac patients		21%
Hunt et al.[76]	14 hypertensives	22%	13%
van Kimmenade et al.[24]	165 hypertensives	17%	22%

Note: FE = fractional extraction

depending also on the population being studied.[16,19–24] These FEs may not be equal, but do approximate the above mentioned filtration fraction.

Furthermore, in the largest head-to-head comparison published so far, including 165 hypertensive patients, the measured FEs of both molecules correlated only moderately, but equally, with GFR.[24] However, it should be acknowledged that this was not studied in patients with a GFR less than 30 mL/min/1.73 m^2. These mechanistic studies demonstrate that the *filtration* of BNP and NT-proBNP is only moderately influenced by renal impairment in this population, while on a glomerular level, no differences in renal handling are present.

The absolute, total, renal clearance of a molecule, however, depends not only on the filtration in the glomeruli, but also on the total amount of blood delivered to the kidney in order to be cleared. The latter is reflected by the renal plasma flow (RPF). Therefore, when the RPF decreases, this may also result in a decrease in glomerular filtration rate and lead to a diminished renal clearance. However, this decrease in renal clearance is a nonspecific process and affects BNP, NT-proBNP, and all other peptides or biomarkers, which are renally cleared. Although the impact of a decreased RPF on the clearance of BNP and NT-proBNP has been less studied, when correcting for parameters of renal function (or renal blood flow) in multivariate analyses, it is shown that concentrations of BNP and NT-proBNP remain independently associated with parameters of cardiac structures, function, or outcome, suggesting that elevated concentrations of both peptides in renal impairment resemble cardiac production rather than renal accumulation.[24,25] Furthermore, it was concluded from a similar analysis for lipase (56 kDa) that renal clearance should not affect plasma levels, until the GFR is below 30–40 mL/min.[26–29]

Although the renal clearance of both molecules may be similar, it has been shown that NT-proBNP concentrations rise relatively more in renal impairment when compared to BNP. Several authors have shown that the NT-proBNP/BNP ratio (i.e., the NT-proBNP serum concentration divided by BNP serum concentration) increases when the GFR decreases.[10,11,24] Because this is not caused by differences in renal clearance as discussed above, it is worthwhile to speculate about alternative explanations. Indeed, neutral endopeptidases appear to accumulate in the context of renal failure,[30] while up-regulation of NPR-C has been observed in more advanced disease states as well.[31,32] Both scenarios would further reduce concentrations of BNP relative to NT-proBNP in this context, as has been suggested by several authors.[33,34] However, the relevance of a possible up-regulation of these mechanisms is still undetermined.

Interestingly, rather than looking at the NT-proBNP/BNP ratio, Austin and colleagues looked at the *correlation* between NT-proBNP and BNP in all National Kidney Foundation categories in a study of patients suffering from chronic kidney disease. This correlation remained strong over all categories, with all r-values greater than 0.90 and may be more adequate than a simple ratio.[35]

Urinary Natriuretic Peptide Testing

Another aspect that needs to be addressed is the fact that NT-proBNP was measured in the urine of heart failure patients. Although Togashi and colleagues reported in 1993 that BNP was detectable in urine,[36] the emphasis in the literature has been on the measurement of NT-proBNP in urine and its utility. Ng et al. first demonstrated in a study comparing 34 heart failure patients with 82 healthy controls that NT-proBNP was detectable in urine, while heart failure patients had significantly higher concentrations in their urine compared to controls.[9] This finding was confirmed by several others who also looked at the possible diagnostic role of urinary NT-proBNP testing.[37–39] In all these studies, serum concentrations of NT-proBNP were superior as a diagnostic test to urinary NT-proBNP testing. However, it is worthwhile to briefly discuss urinary NT-proBNP testing and its interpretation.

As discussed previously, SMWPs are filtered freely in the glomeruli followed by catabolization in the brush border of the tubuli, in contrast to creatinine which is only secreted by the tubuli.[13–15] This process of catabolization is nearly complete, and only a minor amount of NT-proBNP is to be expected to "leak" into the urine. This is nicely illustrated as follows: the mean RPF in stable HF patients in a study by Smilde et al. (with a mean GFR 86 mL/min) was 314 mL/min.[40] This means that 1130 L plasma are offered to the kidneys during 24 hours in these patients. Using the median NT-proBNP concentration in serum of the patients from Ng et al. of 5829 *pico*mol/L, this means that 6.5 *micro*mol NT-proBNP arrive in the kidney during these 24 hours. Even with the minimum FE reported of 14% (Table 25–2) this means that at least 0.9 *micro*mol should be found in a 24-hour urine collection. Because the urinary NT-proBNP concentration reported by Ng et al. is only

117 *pico*mol/L, even if the 24-hour diuresis were 5 L, less than 0.1% would be traced back in the urine of these heart failure patients.

Therefore, although NT-proBNP is indeed measurable in urine (with higher concentrations in heart failure patients), caution should be taken in interpreting these (absolute) results as indicative of cardiac disease because there is a strong tubular function interference. BNP is also measurable in urine,[36,41,42] however even more caution should be taken in interpreting results because BNP may be more susceptible to degradation when measured in urine.

Diagnostic Role of Natriuretic Peptides in Acutely Dyspneic CKD Patients

Patients suffering from chronic kidney disease (CKD) who do not (yet) require renal replacement therapy often have elevated NP concentrations that correlate with the different stages of CKD.[11,43] However, elevated concentrations of both BNP and NT-proBNP are also associated with a decreased left ventricular ejection fraction (LVEF), left ventricular hypertrophy (LVH), and other cardiovascular diseases, independent of the GFR or traditional cardiovascular risk factors.[11,43]

The measurement of NT-proBNP and BNP are established methodologies for diagnosing heart failure in patients with acute dyspnea.[5,44] The question is, however, whether the optimal cut-points for BNP and NT-proBNP for diagnosing acute heart failure in patients presenting with acute dyspnea in the emergency department* are also valid in these patients.

As discussed elsewhere, a slightly different cut-point strategy was chosen in each study. These decisions were made arbitrarily and not based on a difference in characteristics of the peptides and both strategies have their own advantages and disadvantages. Initially, a single cut-point for diagnosing heart failure of 100 pg/mL was advocated for BNP.[44] When it was found that BNP

*As established in the Breathing Not Properly (BNP) study and in the International Collaboration on NT-proBNP (ICON) study.

concentrations were elevated in patients with renal impairment, a specific cut-point of 200 pg/mL for patients with a GFR less than 60 mL/min/1.73 m^2 was suggested.[45] Due to clinical experience with BNP testing, it was ultimately advocated to use a general cut-point of 100 pg/mL to rule out heart failure in combination with a general cut-point of 500 pg/mL in order to diagnose heart failure.[46]

For HF, a general NT-proBNP rule-out cut-point (300 pg/mL) with three age-dependent cut-points (<50 years: 450 pg/mL; 50–75 years: 900 pg/mL; >75 years: 1800 pg/mL) was found to be the optimal diagnostic strategy.[5] It was found that the addition of a correction or extra cut-point for decreased renal function did not offer any beneficial value.[5] In addition, a substudy in the ProBNP Investigation of Dyspnea in the Emergency Department (PRIDE) study showed that when applying a single, separate cut-point for patients with a GFR less than 60 mL/min/1.73 m^2, 1200 pg/mL would be that optimal cut-point. In a study of clinician-selected dyspnea patients for NP testing, including 393 with a GFR less than 60 mL/min/1.73 m^2, simultaneous measurements of NT-proBNP and BNP had similar accuracy, while the optimal cutoffs were as reported in the PRIDE and BNP studies.[47]

Importantly, both renal-specific cut-points are within the rule-in and rule-out cut-points—the so-called "gray zone." Therefore, for acute heart failure diagnosis, no extra cut-point is needed for either peptide in CKD patients with renal impairment. However, when confronted with a patient with a "gray zone" NP level combined with renal impairment, the renal cut-point might offer some additional guidance, although the complete clinical picture should dominate the final decision making process.

Predictive Role of Natriuretic Peptides in CKD

Prognosis in Acutely Dyspnoeic Patients

In a subanalysis from the ICON study of 720 patients presenting with acute heart failure, NT-proBNP levels were independently predictive of 60-day outcomes in the setting of impaired renal function.[25] In combination, a GFR less than 60 mL/min/1.73 m^2 and an

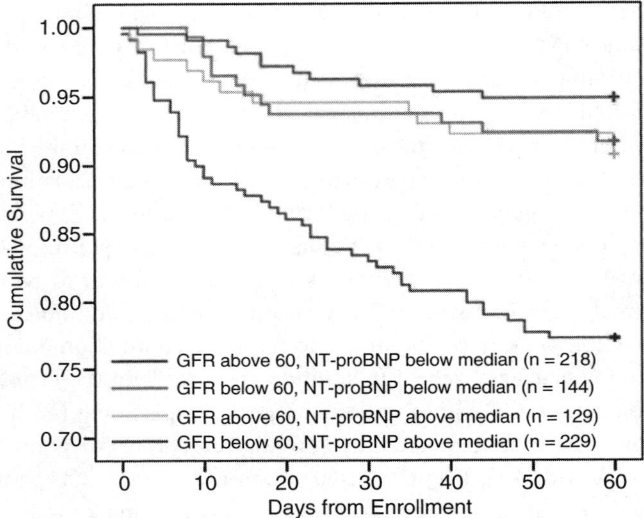

■ **Figure 25–1** Survival curves of HF subjects in ICON as a function of GFR and NT-proBNP concentration on admission (log-rank $p < 0.001$).

Source: van Kimmenade RRJ, Januzzi JL Jr, Baggish AL, et al. Amino-terminal pro-brain natriuretic peptide, renal function and outcomes in acute heart failure; re-defining the cardio-renal interaction? *J Am Coll Cardiol.* 2006;48:1621–1627. Used with permission from Elsevier.

NT-proBNP level above the median (4647 pg/mL) predicted a poor outcome. Intriguingly, it was in fact the combination of both that carried the greatest risk and the absence of either feature resulted in a 60-day outcome similar to patients with an eGFR greater than or equal to 60 mL/min/1.73 m^2 and a NT-proBNP level below the median. This is depicted in Figure 25–1. Furthermore, it is worthwhile mentioning that in fact 273 patients (38%) suffered from only one of these two characteristics (i.e., a GFR less than 60 mL/min/1.73 m^2 and an NT-proBNP level above the median), which is extra support for the argument that an elevated NT-proBNP concentration in renal impairment is not a universal finding.

Unfortunately, to our knowledge, the independent prognostic roles of renal function and BNP have not been studied specifically.

However, DeFilippi et al. did compare BNP and NT-proBNP levels for all-cause mortality in emergency department patients presenting with dyspnea and an eGFR less than 60 mL/min/1.73 m^2.[47] In this study, both peptides were excellent predictors of one-year mortality after adjustment for comorbidities, renal function, and the diagnosis of acute heart failure, and in this analysis the prognostic value of NT-proBNP was superior to that of BNP.

Prognostic Role of Natriuretic Peptides in Non-Dyspneic CKD Patients

In an analysis nearly identical to that of acute heart failure patients in the ICON study, Gardner et al. showed that NT-proBNP was also predictive of outcome in 182 stable heart failure patients, independent of the GFR.[48] Furthermore, in a large head-to-head comparison performed in 3916 stable heart failure patients from the Val-HeFT study population, Masson et al. showed that both BNP and NT-proBNP were—independent of renal function—the strongest predictors of outcome.[49] Again, NT-proBNP seemed to be superior to BNP for the prediction of mortality and morbidity or hospitalization for heart failure in this subanalysis.

Besides outcomes, both BNP and NT-proBNP are also predictive of structural cardiac abnormalities, such echocardiographic abnormalities including a depressed LVEF, LVH, and other parameters of cardiac dysfunction in CKD patients.[43,50–53]

Natriuretic Peptide Testing in Dialysis Patients

Elevated levels of NT-proBNP and BNP are ubiquitous in patients on chronic dialysis therapy.[54–58] Levels of both natriuretic peptides remain elevated in these patients in part because of the presence and severity of structural heart disease, but, importantly, they are also influenced by the type of dialysis membrane used.[54,56,58]

Indeed, in contrast to renal physiology, differences between the clearances of both molecules in patients on dialysis are described. Racek and colleagues found in 94 patients undergoing hemodialysis (HD) on low flux dialysis membranes that BNP levels significantly decreased, whereas NT-proBNP levels significantly increased.

On high flux membranes, HD caused a decrease of both BNP and NT-proBNP.[59] The authors concluded that a decline in NP levels during dialysis seems to be caused by peptide removal rather than be reflective of a decrease in volume overload, and up until now, it is unclear whether NPs could offer any clinical utility in establishing the ideal volume status in HD patients.

Several studies of patients undergoing dialysis have found that NT-proBNP was associated with LV mass, LVEF, K_t/V (extent of dialysis), and cardiovascular events or mortality, but not with the amount of estimated volume overload.[56,60,61] Interestingly, changes over 6 and 12 months in NT-proBNP concentrations also did correlate with changes in left ventricular mass index.[62]

BNP has also been evaluated to determine its utility to guide an HD prescription. Some authors also report that BNP levels correlate poorly with measures of volume status, such as weight and estimated plasma volume,[57,63] however, a smaller study in 32 patients did find a correlation between BNP levels and volume overload.[64]

Data for peritoneal dialysis (PD) are even more sparse than HD. Since fluid shifts in PD are less abrupt than those in HD, NP levels may hypothetically be more reflective of volume status in the PD population. However, although levels of NT-proBNP and BNP were associated with LV mass index and other characteristics of echocardiographic abnormalities,[54] they were also not associated with volume overload.[60,65]

Further studies in this population, as well as in HD patients, are clearly needed in order to find out what the clinical consequences are of these findings. NPs may not be suitable for determination of the optimal fluid status in dialysis patients, but they may eventually be utilized as prognosticators for dialysis patients, along with the analysis of additional biomarkers for myocardial injury or inflammation, such as Troponin T or CRP.[55]

Conclusion

In conclusion, the renal clearance of both BNP and NT-proBNP is equal and serum concentrations seem to be minimally affected by a decrease renal clearance at least until the GFR is not below 30–40 mL/min/1.73 m^2. When applying the standard cut-points, no additional cut-point is needed in order to diagnose acute heart failure in acutely dyspneic patients. When looking for a separate single cut-point for acutely dyspneic patients with a GFR less than 60 mL/min/1.73 m^2, one should use 1200 pg/mL for NT-proBNP and 200 pg/mL for BNP.

For patients on dialysis, NPs seem not to be of additional value in volume estimation; however, they are strongly associated with echocardiographic abnormalities and prognosis in these patients. Importantly, NPs strongly predict outcomes in the complete spectrum of the NKF classes. What is needed now are studies looking at NP-guided therapy in patients with the different degrees of renal function in order to optimally use the highly prognostic information provided by these two biomarkers.

References

1. Stewart H, McIntosh JF. The function of the kidneys in patients suffering from chronic cardiac disease without signs of heart failure. *J Clin Invest.* 1928;6:325–345.
2. Stevenson LW, Nohria A, Mielniczuk L. Torrent or torment from the tubules? Challenge of the cardiorenal connections. *J Am Coll Cardiol.* 2005;45:2004–2007.
3. Shlipak MG, Massie BM. The clinical challenge of cardiorenal syndrome. *Circulation.* 2004;110:1514–1517.
4. Cheng V, Kazanagra R, Garcia A, et al. A rapid bedside test for B-type peptide predicts treatment outcomes in patients admitted for decompensated heart failure: a pilot study. *J Am Coll Cardiol.* 2001;37: 386–391.
5. Januzzi JL Jr, van Kimmenade RRJ, Lainchbury JG, et al. NT-proBNP testing for diagnosis and short-term prognosis in acute congestive heart failure: an international pooled analysis of 1256 patients. The International Collaborative of NT-proBNP (ICON) Study. *Eur Heart J.* 2006;27:330–337.
6. McCullough PA, Duc P, Omland T, et al. B-type natriuretic peptide and renal function in the diagnosis of heart failure: an analysis from

the Breathing Not Properly Multinational Study. *Am J Kidney Dis.* 2003;41:571–579.

7. Luchner A, Hengstenberg C, Lowel H, et al. N-terminal pro-brain natriuretic peptide after myocardial infarction: a marker of cardio-renal function. *Hypertension.* 2002;39:99–104.
8. McCullough PA, Sandberg KR. Sorting out the evidence on natriuretic peptides. *Rev Cardiovasc Med.* 2003;4 (Suppl 4):S13–S19.
9. Ng LL, Geeranavar S, Jennings SC, Loke I, O'Brien RJ. Diagnosis of heart failure using urinary natriuretic peptides. *Clin Sci (Lond).* 2004;106:129–133.
10. Kemperman H, van den Berg M, Kirkels H, de Jonge N. B-type natriuretic peptide (BNP) and N-terminal proBNP in patients with end-stage heart failure supported by a left ventricular assist device. *Clin Chem.* 2004;50:1670–1672.
11. Vickery S, Price CP, John RI, et al. B-type natriuretic peptide (BNP) and amino-terminal proBNP in patients with CKD: relationship to renal function and left ventricular hypertrophy. *Am J Kidney Dis.* 2005;46:610–620.
12. Packer M. Should B-type natriuretic peptide be measured routinely to guide the diagnosis and management of chronic heart failure? *Circulation.* 2003;108:2950–2953.
13. Carone FA, Peterson DR, Oparil S, Pullman TN. Renal tubular transport and catabolism of proteins and peptides. *Kidney Int.* 1979;16: 271–278.
14. Maack T, Johnson V, Kau ST, Figueiredo J, Sigulem D. Renal filtration, transport, and metabolism of low-molecular-weight proteins: a review. *Kidney Int.* 1979;16:251–270.
15. Clark WR, Gao D. Low-molecular weight proteins in end-stage renal disease: potential toxicity and dialytic removal mechanisms. *J Am Soc Nephrol.* 2002;13 (Suppl 1):S41–S47.
16. Goetze JP, Jensen G, Moller S, Bendtsen F, Rehfeld JF, Henriksen JH. BNP and N-terminal proBNP are both extracted in the normal kidney. *Eur J Clin Invest.* 2006;36:8–15.
17. Hollenberg NK, Adams DF, Solomon HS, Rashid A, Abrams HL, Merrill JP. Senescence and the renal vasculature in normal man. *Circ Res.* 1974;34:309–316.

18. Fliser D, Zeier M, Nowack R, Ritz E. Renal functional reserve in healthy elderly subjects. *J Am Soc Nephrol.* 1993;3:1371–1377.

19. Rutten JH, Boomsma F, van den Meiracker AH. Higher renal extraction of ANP compared with NT-proANP, BNP and NT-proBNP. *Eur J Clin Invest.* 2006;36:514–515.

20. Hunt PJ RA, Nicholls MG, Yandle TG, Doughty RN, Espiner EA. Immunoreactive amino-terminal pro-brain natriuretic peptide (NT-PROBNP): a new marker of cardiac impairment. *Clin Endocrinol (Oxf).* 1997;47:287–296.

21. Schou M, Dalsgaard MK, Clemmesen O, et al. Kidneys extract BNP and NT-proBNP in healthy young men. *J Appl Physiol.* 2005;99: 1676–1680.

22. Richards AM, Crozier IG, Yandle TG, Espiner EA, Ikram H, Nicholls MG. Brain natriuretic factor: regional plasma concentrations and correlations with haemodynamic state in cardiac disease. *Br Heart J.* 1993;69:414–417.

23. Lainchbury JG, Nicholls MG, Espiner EA, Ikram H, Yandle TG, Richards AM. Regional plasma levels of cardiac peptides and their response to acute neutral endopeptidase inhibition in man. *Clin Sci (Lond).* 1998;95:547–555.

24. van Kimmenade RRJ, Januzzi JL, Bakker JA, et al. Renal clearance of BNP and NT-proBNP: a mechanistic study in hypertensive subjects. *J Am Coll Cardio*l. 2009;53:884–890.

25. van Kimmenade RRJ, Januzzi JL Jr, Baggish AL, et al. Amino-terminal pro-brain natriuretic peptide, renal function and outcomes in acute heart failure; re-defining the cardio-renal interaction? *J Am Coll Cardiol.* 2006;48:1621–1627.

26. Royse VL, Jensen DM, Corwin HL. Pancreatic enzymes in chronic renal failure. *Arch Intern Med.* 1987;147:537–539.

27. Seno T, Harada H, Ochi K, et al. Serum levels of six pancreatic enzymes as related to the degree of renal dysfunction. *Am J Gastroenterol.* 1995;90:2002–2005.

28. Pitchumoni CS, Arguello P, Agarwal N, Yoo J. Acute pancreatitis in chronic renal failure. *Am J Gastroenterol.* 1996;91:2477–2482.

29. Thierry FX, Dueymes JM, Vernier I, et al. Serum lipase and amylase levels in chronic renal failure: interpretation of results—effects of extrarenal purification. *Nephrologie.* 1988;9:263–267.

30. Deschodt-Lanckman M, Michaux F, De Prez E, Abramowicz D, Vanherweghem JL, Goldman M. Increased serum levels of endopeptidase 24.11 ('enkephalinase') in patients with end-stage renal failure. *Life Sci.* 1989;45:133–141.

31. Kuhn M, Voß M, Mitko D, et al. Left ventricular assist device support reverses altered cardiac expression and function of natriuretic peptides and receptors in end-stage heart failure. *Cardiovascular Res.* 2004;64:308–314.

32. Andreassi MG, Del Ry S, Palmieri C, Clerico A, Biagini A, Giannessi D. Up-regulation of 'clearance' receptors in patients with chronic heart failure: a possible explanation for the resistance to biological effects of cardiac natriuretic hormones. *Eur J Heart Fail.* 2001;3: 407–414.

33. Jaffe AS, Apple FS, Babuin L. Why we don't know the answer may be more important than the specific question. *Clin Chem.* 2004;50: 1495–1497.

34. Vickery S, Webb MC, Price CP, John RI, Abbas NA, Lamb EJ. Prognostic value of cardiac biomarkers for death in a non-dialysis chronic kidney disease population. *Nephrol Dial Transplant.* 2008; 23:3546–3553.

35. Austin WJ, Bhalla V, Hernandez-Arce I, et al. Correlation and prognostic utility of B-type natriuretic peptide and its amino-terminal fragment in patients with chronic kidney disease. *Am J Clin Pathol.* 2006;126:506–512.

36. Togashi K, Fujita S, Kawakami M. Presence of brain natriuretic peptide in urine. *Clin Chem.* 1992;38:322–323.

37. Michielsen EC, Bakker JA, Kimmenade RRJ, Pinto YM, Dieijen-Visser MP. The diagnostic value of serum and urinary NT-proBNP for heart failure. *Ann Clin Biochem.* 2008;45:389–394.

38. Cortes R, Portoles M, Salvador A, et al. Diagnostic and prognostic value of urine NT-proBNP levels in heart failure patients. *Eur J Heart Fail.* 2006;8:621–627.

39. Cortes R, Rivera M, Salvador A, et al. Variability of NT-proBNP plasma and urine levels in patients with stable heart failure: a 2-year follow-up study. *Heart.* 2007;93:957–962.

40. Smilde TD, van Veldhuisen DJ, Navis G, Voors AA, Hillege HL. Drawbacks and prognostic value of formulas estimating renal

function in patients with chronic heart failure and systolic dysfunction. *Circulation.* 2006;114:1572–1580.

41. Totsune K, Takahashi K, Satoh F, et al. Urinary immunoreactive brain natriuretic peptide in patients with renal disease. *Regul Pept.* 1996;63: 141–147.
42. Cortes R, Rivera M, Salvador A, et al. Urinary B-type natriuretic peptide levels in the diagnosis and prognosis of heart failure. *J Card Fail.* 2007;13:549–555.
43. DeFilippi CR, Fink JC, Nass CM, Chen H, Christenson R. N-terminal pro-B-type natriuretic peptide for predicting coronary disease and left ventricular hypertrophy in asymptomatic CKD not requiring dialysis. *Am J Kidney Dis.* 2005;46:35–44.
44. Maisel AS, Krishnaswamy P, Nowak RM, et al. Rapid measurement of B-type natriuretic peptide in the emergency diagnosis of heart failure. *N Engl J Med.* 2002;347:161–167.
45. McCullough PA, Sandberg KR. B-type natriuretic peptide and renal disease. *Heart Fail Rev.* 2003;8:355–358.
46. Knudsen CW, Clopton P, Westheim A, et al. Predictors of elevated B-type natriuretic peptide concentrations in dyspneic patients without heart failure: an analysis from the Breathing Not Properly multinational study. *Ann Emerg Med.* 2005;45:573–580.
47. DeFilippi CR, Seliger SL, Maynard S, Christenson RH. Impact of renal disease on natriuretic peptide testing for diagnosing decompensated heart failure and predicting mortality. *Clin Chem.* 2007;53:1511–1519.
48. Gardner RS, Chong KS, O'Meara E, Jardine A, Ford I, McDonagh TA. Renal dysfunction, as measured by the modification of diet in renal disease equations, and outcome in patients with advanced heart failure. *Eur Heart J.* 2007;28:3027–3033.
49. Masson S, Latini R, Anand IS, et al. Direct comparison of B-type natriuretic peptide (BNP) and amino-terminal proBNP in a large population of patients with chronic and symptomatic heart failure: the Valsartan Heart Failure (Val-HeFT) data. *Clin Chem.* 2006;52: 1528–1538.
50. McKie PM, Rodeheffer RJ, Cataliotti A, et al. Amino-terminal pro-B-type natriuretic peptide and B-type natriuretic peptide: biomarkers for mortality in a large community-based cohort free of heart failure. *Hypertension.* 2006;47:874–880.

51. Eguchi K, Matsui Y, Shibasaki S, et al. Changes in self-monitored pulse pressure correlate with improvements in B-type natriuretic peptide and urinary albumin in treated hypertensive patients. *Am J Hypertens.* 2007;20:1268–1275.

52. Wang TJ, Larson MG, Levy D, et al. Plasma natriuretic peptide levels and the risk of cardiovascular events and death. *N Engl J Med.* 2004;350:655–663.

53. Anwaruddin S, Lloyd-Jones DM, Baggish AL, et al. Renal function, congestive heart failure and NT-proBNP measurement: results from the ProBNP Investigation of Dyspnea in the Emergency Department (PRIDE) Study. *J Am Coll Cardiol.* 2006;47:91–97.

54. Wang AY, Lam CW, Yu CM, et al. N-terminal pro-brain natriuretic peptide: an independent risk predictor of cardiovascular congestion, mortality, and adverse cardiovascular outcomes in chronic peritoneal dialysis patients. *J Am Soc Nephrol.* 2007;18:321–330.

55. Apple FS, Murakami MM, Pearce LA, Herzog CA. Multi-biomarker risk stratification of N-terminal pro-B-type natriuretic peptide, high-sensitivity C-reactive protein, and cardiac troponin T and I in end-stage renal disease for all-cause death. *Clin Chem.* 2004;50: 2279–2285.

56. Madsen LH, Ladefoged S, Corell P, Schou M, Hildebrandt PR, Atar D. N-terminal pro brain natriuretic peptide predicts mortality in patients with end-stage renal disease in hemodialysis. *Kidney Int.* 2007;71:548–554.

57. Sheen V, Bhalla V, Tulua-Tata A, et al. The use of B-type natriuretic peptide to assess volume status in patients with end-stage renal disease. *Am Heart J.* 2007;153:244.e1–e5.

58. Zoccali C, Mallamaci F, Benedetto FA, et al. Cardiac natriuretic peptides are related to left ventricular mass and function and predict mortality in dialysis patients. *J Am Soc Nephrol.* 2001;12:1508–1515.

59. Racek J, Kralova H, Trefil L, Rajdl D, Eiselt J. Brain natriuretic peptide and N-terminal proBNP in chronic haemodialysis patients. *Nephron Clin Pract.* 2006;103:c162–c172.

60. Lee JA, Kim DH, Yoo SJ, Oh DJ, Yu SH, Kang ET. Association between serum n-terminal pro-brain natriuretic peptide concentration and left ventricular dysfunction and extracellular water in continuous ambulatory peritoneal dialysis patients. *Perit Dial Int.* 2006;26:360–365.

61. Winkler K, Wanner C, Drechsler C, Lilienthal J, Marz W, Krane V. Change in N-terminal-pro-B-type-natriuretic-peptide and the risk of sudden death, stroke, myocardial infarction, and all-cause mortality in diabetic dialysis patients. *Eur Heart J.* 2008;29:2092–2099.

62. Choi SY, Lee JE, Jang EH, et al. Association between changes in N-terminal pro-brain natriuretic peptide levels and changes in left ventricular mass index in stable hemodialysis patients. *Nephron Clin Pract.* 2008;110:c93–c100.

63. Bargnoux AS, Klouche K, Fareh J, et al. Prohormone brain natriuretic peptide (proBNP), BNP and N-terminal-proBNP circulating levels in chronic hemodialysis patients. Correlation with ventricular function, fluid removal and effect of hemodiafiltration. *Clin Chem Lab Med.* 2008;46:1019–1024.

64. Fagugli RM, Palumbo B, Ricciardi D, et al. Association between brain natriuretic peptide and extracellular water in hemodialysis patients. *Nephron Clin Pract.* 2003;95:c60–c66.

65. Granja CA, Tailor PT, Gorban-Brennan N, Francis J, Bekui A, Finkelstein FO. Brain natriuretic peptide and impedance cardiography to assess volume status in peritoneal dialysis patients. *Adv Perit Dial.* 2007;23:155–160.

66. Mark PB, Stewart GA, Gansevoort RT, et al. Diagnostic potential of circulating natriuretic peptides in chronic kidney disease. *Nephrol Dial Transplant.* 2006;21:402–410.

67. Khan IA, Fink J, Nass C, Chen H, Christenson R, DeFilippi CR. N-terminal pro-B-type natriuretic peptide and B-type natriuretic peptide for identifying coronary artery disease and left ventricular hypertrophy in ambulatory chronic kidney disease patients. *Am J Cardiol.* 2006;97:1530–1534.

68. Richards AM, Nicholls MG, Espiner EA, et al. Comparison of B-type natriuretic peptides for assessment of cardiac function and prognosis in stable ischemic heart disease. *J Am Coll Cardiol.* 2006;47:52–60.

69. Luchner A, Hengstenberg C, Lowel H, et al. NT-ProBNP in outpatients after myocardial infarction: interaction between symptoms and left ventricular function and optimized cut-points. *J Card Fail.* 2005;11:21–27.

70. Leuchte HH, El Nounou M, Tuerpe JC, et al. N-terminal pro-brain natriuretic peptide and renal insufficiency as predictors of mortality in pulmonary hypertension. *Chest.* 2007;131:402–409.

71. Spanaus KS, Kronenberg F, Ritz E, et al. B-type natriuretic peptide concentrations predict the progression of nondiabetic chronic kidney disease: the Mild-to-Moderate Kidney Disease Study. *Clin Chem.* 2007;53:1264–1272.

72. Hogenhuis J, Voors AA, Jaarsma T, et al. Anaemia and renal dysfunction are independently associated with BNP and NT-proBNP levels in patients with heart failure. *Eur J Heart Fail.* 2007;9:787–794.

73. Bruch C, Fischer C, Sindermann J, Stypmann J, Breithardt G, Gradaus R. Comparison of the prognostic usefulness of N-terminal pro-brain natriuretic peptide in patients with heart failure with versus without chronic kidney disease. *Am J Cardiol.* 2008;102:469–474.

74. Astor BC, Yi S, Hiremath L, et al. N-terminal prohormone brain natriuretic peptide as a predictor of cardiovascular disease and mortality in blacks with hypertensive kidney disease: the African American Study of Kidney Disease and Hypertension (AASK). *Circulation.* 2008;117:1685–1692.

75. Bruch C, Reinecke H, Stypmann J, et al. N-terminal pro-brain natriuretic peptide, kidney disease and outcome in patients with chronic heart failure. *J Heart Lung Transplant.* 2006;25:1135–1141.

76. Hunt PJ, Espiner EA, Nicholls MG, Richards AM, Yandle TG. The role of the circulation in processing pro-brain natriuretic peptide (proBNP) to amino-terminal BNP and BNP-32. *Peptides.* 1997;18: 1475–1481.

26 ■ Emerging Biomarkers of Cardiac Failure

PAUL O. COLLINSON MD, FRCP
T. MCDONAGH, MD FRCP

Introduction

The ability to measure natriuretic peptides, predominantly B-type natriuretic peptides (BNP and amino-terminal pro-B type natriuretic peptide [NT-proBNP]), in the routine laboratory has produced a paradigm shift in the awareness of the value of biomarkers for diagnosis and management of heart failure (HF). Basic science research, the human genome project, and proteomic and genomic studies have generated a plethora of potential molecular biomarkers for the diagnosis. The challenge is now to pick out, amongst the candidates, those which may be clinically useful.

Classification of Biomarkers of HF

Emerging markers in HF can be grouped into six broad categories: inflammatory markers, necrosis markers, markers of extracellular matrix turnover and remodeling, neurohormones, markers of stretch and fibrosis, as well as markers of metabolism/nutrition. Inflammatory and necrosis markers in HF is discussed in Chapter 15.

Markers of Extracellular Matrix Turnover and Remodeling

Vascular endothelial growth factor (VEGF, more properly VEGF-A) is one of a subfamily of platelet-derived growth factors, including placental growth factor (PlGF), VEGF-B, VEGF-C, and VEGF-D. It is involved in angiogenesis and is chemotactic for macrophages and granulocytes and vasodilatation via nitrous oxide release. VEGF is elevated in patients with HF, but does not predict outcome.[1–3] Similarly, elevations of PlGF have been reported and are correlated to severity of cardiac dysfunction.[4]

Hepatocyte growth factor/scatter factor (HGF/SF) is a paracrine cellular growth factor produced by mesenchymal cells. It is secreted as a single inactive polypeptide, is cleaved by serine proteases into a 69-kDa alpha-chain and 34-kDa beta-chain, with a disulfide bond between the alpha and beta chains that produces the active, heterodimeric molecule. It acts primarily upon epithelial and endothelial cells and stimulates mitogenesis, cell motility, and matrix invasion to give it a central role in angiogenesis. HGF/SF is increased in patients with HF, and falls following treatment.[5] Values correlate with disease severity and are independently prognostic of BNP.[2] It is proposed as a biomarker of HF,[6] but further evidence is limited.

Epidermal growth factor (EGF) is a 6045-Da protein. It acts by binding with high affinity to epidermal growth factor receptor (EGFR). EGF has found to be elevated in HF patients,[3] however of major interest is its interaction with angiotensin II and aldosterone,[7–12] suggesting a potential target for therapy. Connective tissue growth factor has also been reported to be elevated in patients with cardiac failure, correlating with indices of diastolic (but not systolic) function, MMP 2, and TIMP 2.[13]

Matrix Metalloproteinases and Their Inhibitors

Matrix metalloproteinases (MMPs) are zinc-dependent endopepetidases collectively capable of degrading extracellular matrix proteins and processing bioactive molecules. They are known to be involved in the cleavage of cell surface receptors, the release of apoptotic ligands (such as the FAS ligand), and chemokine activation and inactivation. They are, therefore, involved in both remodeling and inflammation. There are 28 MMPs, which are inhibited by specific endogenous tissue inhibitors of metalloproteinases (TIMPs); these latter markers comprise a family of four protease inhibitors: TIMP-1, TIMP-2, TIMP-3, and TIMP-4.

After myocardial infarction, MMP 2 levels show an inverse correlation and MMP 9 levels show a positive correlation with ventricular dysfunction.[14] Postinfarct survival and development of HF is predicted by MMP 3,[15] MMP 9,[16,17] and TIMP 1.[17]

In HF, MMP 1,[18] MMP 2,[19,20] MMP 9,[19,20] and TIMP 1,[18,19,21–23] but not MMP 3,[19] are reported as elevated. One large study has reported MMP 9 is not elevated in patients with HF after adjustment for other variables.[23] MMP 1 levels are reduced,[21] but TIMP 2 is not elevated in HF.[20] Norepinephrine correlates with MMP 2 levels in HF and appears to increase its synthesis.[20]

In one analysis, MMP 1—but not TIMP 1—predicted outcome,[21] while in another, TIMP 1 was an outcome predictor.[23] MMP 2—but not MMP 3, MMP 9, or TIMP 1—and BNP correlated with NYHA grade (although not with each other), and were independent outcome predictors.[19] Others have found MMP 3, not MMP 2, and BNP to be independent outcome predictors.[24] MMP 9, despite the ability to predict adverse effects after AMI, appears consistently to be a poor outcome predictor,[19,23–25] in HF patients, especially when compared to BNP[25] or TIMP 1.[23] TIMP 1 remains elevated after mechanical circulatory support, although BNP falls.[22]

Currently MMPs and TIMPs remain ill-understood. Until normal values are defined (including biological determinants of variation), the pathophysiology is more clearly defined,[26] and large studies directly comparing the individual candidates using agreed and validated methods occur, it is unlikely these analytes will achieve clinical application.

Markers of Collagen Turnover

Collagen scar formation relates to infarct size and left ventricular (LV) function. Levels of procollagen III aminopropeptide (PIIINP) correlate with indices of cardiac function.[27] After AMI, PIIINP predicts risk of subsequent death and HF.[28] Measurements of markers of collagen turnover have therefore been studied as potential noninvasive markers of extracellular matrix remodeling in the heart.

Serum concentrations of procollagen type I aminoterminal peptide (PINP),[29] PIIINP,[29–31] type I collagen telopeptide (ICTP),[18,30] and basement membrane laminin (BML)[30] are elevated in patients with cardiac failure. Elevation of procollagen type I carboxyterminal peptide (PICP)[18,22,29,31] and PINP[29,31] does not appear to be a consistent finding. Elevation of PIINP may be dependent on disease severity, as PIIINP levels were not correlated with indices of left ventricular structure or function in ambulatory asymptomatic individuals,[32] unlike BNP.

Elevations of serum PICP,[29] PINP,[29] ICTP,[30,33] and BML[30] are all associated with a worse prognosis in patients with cardiac failure. Elevated PIIINP predicted worse prognosis in multiple studies of HF patients[29,30,34,35] and was additive in prognostication with conventional measures of cardiac function and neurohormones, including aldosterone.[34] Aldosterone blockade with spironolactone is associated with a reduction in PICP, PINP, and PIIINP levels with no response seen in patients with low values of these markers.[29]

Other markers of interest in this category are the tenascins, which are extracellular matrix glycoproteins. There are four members of the tenascin family: tenascin-C (TN-C), tenascin-R (nervous system), tenascin-X (connective tissue), and tenascin-W (kidney). TN-C is a matricellular protein controlling extracellular matrix deposition[36] that has been implicated in transforming growth factor beta-1 (TGFβ1) signaling in various models of fibrosis. It binds to cell-surface receptors, including integrins, as well as to other extracellular matrix proteins, proteases, growth factors, and cytokines, modulating their bioavailability. Unlike other extracellular matrix components, it has no apparent structural role. TN-C is highly expressed during embryonic development, but poorly expressed or absent in the adult heart,[37] except after myocardial infarction[38] when it is involved in active remodeling of the extracellular matrix, resulting in "replacement fibrosis." Elevation of TN-C is associated with ventricular remodeling and a worse outcome after AMI.[39] Enhanced TN-C expression was associated with early cardiac fibrosis and cardiac death in experimental animals.[40] Elevation of TN-C has been observed in patients with cardiac failure.[22,41,42] Levels correlate with the degree of left ventricular dysfunction and indices of cardiac remodeling.[41] Levels fall when there is successful negative cardiac remodeling.[42] There is interest in direct detection of myocardial remodeling by imaging using labeled antibodies to TN-C.[43] It may be a specific indicator for the monitoring of remodeling.

Another marker, osteopontin (secreted phosphoprotein 1 [SPP1], bone sialoprotein I, early T-lymphocyte activation 1) may have a role in HF evaluation. Osteopontin (OPN) is a glycoprotein first identified in osteoblasts and implicated as one important mediator of the profibrotic effects of angiotensin II in the heart by binding to αvβ1, αvβ3, and αvβ5 integrins.[44] In vascular smooth muscle cells, OPN is acutely up-regulated by cytokines and growth factors and contributes to vascular smooth muscle cell migration, adhesion, and spreading. Experimentally, OPN is expressed in cardiac myocytes in HF and expression-inhibited by angiotensin converting enzyme inhibitors (ACE-I).[45] OPN expression is increased in cardiomyocytes in HF patients.[46] Serum[22,47,48] and circulating T cell OPN levels[48] are increased in patients with HF, and values variably correlate[47,48] with the severity of HF. Of note, synthesis of OPN is stimulated by 1,25-dihydroxyvitamin D3. Vitamin D levels are increasingly being recognized as having a role in heart disease[49,50] and it is interesting to speculate that there may be a link between the two.

Galectin-3

Galectin-3 is a 26-kDa α3-galactoside binding lectin. The protein is composed of a small N-terminal domain, a domain consisting of proline- and glycine-rich repeats, and a C-terminal carbohydrate recognition domain. Galectin-3 is expressed in a variety of tissues and cell types and is localized mainly in the cytoplasm. Depending on cell type and proliferation state, a significant amount of the lectin can also be detected in the nucleus, on the cell surface, or in the extracellular environment.[51–53] Galectin-3 overexpression causes changes in the expression levels of cell cycle regulators, including cyclin D1.

Galectin-3 is up-regulated in an experimental model of HF. It is derived from macrophages and induces cardiac fibroblast proliferation, collagen deposition, and ventricular dysfunction.[54] It appears to be an early marker of potential myocyte dysfunction as it is overexpressed before the transition to overt HF. It may, therefore, be a marker of early remodeling and potential dysfunction. Galectin-3 has been studied in patients presenting with acute HF. Levels are elevated, although as an initial diagnostic test, it is inferior to NT-proBNP measurement.[55] As a prognostic marker, however, it is superior to NT-proBNP in the short term, but a combination of the two markers proved to be the best discriminator for an adverse 60-day outcome.[55] Galectin-3 is also elevated in patients with end-stage chronic HF.[22]

Neurohormones

Markers of neurohormonal activation have been shown to be important for prognostication in HF, and span a broad range of physiologies.

Copeptin

In light of the important role of arginine vasopressin (AVP) for regulating water balance in acute and chronic HF, knowledge of endogenous plasma AVP levels might be helpful in diagnosing and monitoring treatment in patients with cardiovascular diseases. Copeptin (also known as the AVP-associated glycopeptide) consists of 39 amino acids and is derived from a 164-amino acid precursor termed preprovasopressin, which consists of a signal peptide, AVP, neurophysin II, and copeptin. Thus, copeptin is the C-terminal part of proAVP (CT-proAVP).[56] Copeptin levels are elevated after acute myocardial infarction (AMI)[57] and are associated with LV dysfunction and remodeling and clinical HF post-AMI.[58] In patients with acute[59] and chronic HF, elevation of copeptin predicts disease severity and poor outcome.[60,61] Copeptin has been said to be superior to[60] and an additive to BNP.[61] Prediction may be dependent on disease severity. Copeptin was found to be the best single predictor of mortality in patients with NYHA functional class II and class III. In NYHA functional class IV, a patient's outcome was best predicted by serum sodium, but again, copeptin added additional independent information.[61]

Adrenomedullin

Adrenomedullin (AM) is a member of the calcitonin gene-related peptide (CGRP) family. It is synthesized as an immature 53-amino acid precursor and modified by amidation into a mature 52-amino acid peptide with an intramolecular disulfide bond. In the heart, AM is present in ventricular tissue. Although mainly produced by vascular endothelial cells, vascular smooth muscle cells, and macrophages, AM can also be produced by fibroblasts, adipocytes, and cardiac myocytes. It does not appear to be stored, so it is probably regulated by transcription triggered by proinflammatory cytokines (TNF-α, IL-1β, IFN, and nitric oxide). The actions of AM are mediated by the seven transmembrane G-protein-coupled calcitonin receptor-like receptor. The potential functions of AM include: vasodilator, natriuretic, diuretic, antiapoptotic, and prosurvival roles, as well as taking part in angiogenesis and modulation of inflammation.[62] The predominant inotropic effect is on the atria.[63]

Adrenomedullin predicts the risk of future cardiovascular events, including HF in an asymptomatic population (where it was found to be superior to CRP measurement)[64] and following AMI.[65] AM levels are raised in the circulation[66,67] and ventricular tissue[67] of patients with congestive HF. Values are proportional to the degree of HF, although elevation does not seem to be marked in NYHA grade I HF.[66] AM has been studied as a prognostic marker in HF and has been compared with BNP. It has been demonstrated to be an independent risk predictor and synergistic with BNP in acute[59] and chronic HF.[68,69]

Apelin

The apelin gene (located on the long arm of the human X chromosome) is transcribed as a 77-amino acid preproprotein.[70,71] This cleaved to shorter active peptides. The full-length mature peptide is comprised of 36 amino acids (apelin-36). A stable 13-amino acid peptide (apelin-13) has been identified with a pyroglutamate substitution at the N-terminus. The pyroglutamated form of apelin-13 is the most potent and may be the most active ligand. The apelin receptor (APJ) has marked similarities to the AT1 receptor. The APJ receptor is a 377-amino acid G-coupled receptor. There is no evidence to date that the apelin-APJ pathway involves more than one receptor. The proposed cardiovascular effects of the apelin-APJ system are the opposite of the effects of the renin-angiotensin system. Human and animal studies suggest that apelin-APJ expression is up-regulated in response to hypoxia/ischemia, maintained or even augmented in conditions of chronic pressure overload and the early stages of HF, but substantially down-regulated in severe HF. Possible factors contributing to the decline of apelinergic expression in severe HF include increased renin-angiotensin-aldosterone activation and myocardial stretch. These changes may be reversible, as cardiac apelin and APJ are up-regulated after mechanical offloading of the left ventricle.[72] In comparison to BNP/NT-proBNP, current data do not suggest a diagnostic or prognostic role for apelin measurement in acute[55] or chronic cardiac failure.[70,71,73–75]

Endothelin

The endothelins (endothelins 1, 2, and 3 [ET-1, ET-2, ET-3]) comprise a family of three peptides. They show sequence homology with four further peptides (sarafotoxins) extracted from the venom of Atractaspis engaddensis.[76–78] ET-1 is the principal cardiovascular isoform and is a 21-amino acid peptide with a hydrophobic C-terminus and 2 cysteine bridges at the N-terminus. ET-1 is produced predominantly by the vascular endothelial and smooth muscle cells, but also by airway epithelial cells, macrophages, fibroblasts, and cardiac myocytes. It is generated from precursor peptides via a two-step proteolytic pathway: preproET-1 is stripped of its signal sequence and secreted into the cytoplasm as proET-1. ProET-1 is further cleaved by a furin-like endopeptidase to the 38-amino acid precursor molecule, "big" ET-1, which circulates in plasma at low concentration, but is not thought to possess significant biological activity.

Endothelial cells produce ET-1 through both constitutive and regulated (rapid release) pathways. The major role of ET-1 is maintenance of vascular tone. In the myocardium, it may be required to maintain myocyte viability.[79] The cardiac tissue endothelin system is activated in experimental, as well as in clinical HF. The expression of cardiac, pulmonary preproET-1, and ET-1 peptides has been found to be increased in various experimental animal HF models and in patients with end-stage ischemic cardiomyopathy. Endothelin stimulates the secretion of neurohormones known to be important in ventricular function and remodeling, such as norepinephrine, angiotensin II, vasopressin, and aldosterone. These neurohormones also stimulate ET production. ET-1 enhances conversion of angiotensin I to angiotensin II.

ET-1 levels are elevated in cardiac failure and are thought to derive from pulmonary congestion and reduced pulmonary clearance. ET-1 and big ET-1 levels are raised in HF patients. Levels are inversely correlated to functional state and survival.[65,78,80–82] ET-1 concentrations correlate with measures of ventricular remodeling in patients with ischemic HF and dilated cardiomyopathy. Cardiac overexpression of ET-1 could be related to increased expression of inflammatory cytokines and an inflammatory cardiomyopathy leading to HF and death. In the largest and best documented cohort to date, ET-1 has been shown to be inferior to BNP,[81] however, there has been considerable interest in ET-1 antagonists for therapy. Unfortunately, the results in clinical studies in HF patients have been uniformly disappointing.[76–78,83]

Relaxin

The relaxin family of peptides is a subgroup of the relaxin-insulin peptide family. They have a two-chain structure, with two interchain and one intrachain-disulfide bond. In the human, there are seven relaxin family peptides. It has been reported that the failing human heart is a relevant source of circulating relaxin peptides, and that myocytes, as well as interstitial cells, produce relaxin. Relaxin is increased in HF. Plasma levels of relaxin correlate with the severity of HF and relaxin levels respond to HF therapy. Elevation of ventricular filling pressure up-regulates relaxin expression and the hormone acts as a potent inhibitor of ET-1 and modulates effects of angiotensin II.[84,85]

Urotensin II

Urotensin II (U-II) is derived from a larger precursor prepropeptide, prepro-U-II, encoded by a single gene. It is a somatostatin-like peptide expressed in the central nervous system and many other tissues, including that of the kidney, spleen, small intestine, thymus, prostate, and pituitary and adrenal glands. It is also present in plasma. U-II is the most potent vasoconstrictor identified to date, with approximately 10-, 100-, and 300-fold greater potency than ET-1, serotonin, and norepinephrine, respectively. In addition to its vascular effects, U-II has trophic and mitogenic actions, and it has been suggested that it may affect myocardial hypertrophy and fibrosis and vascular smooth muscle cell proliferation.[86–89]

Plasma levels of U-II are elevated in HF.[90–93] They correlate positively with plasma ET-1, adrenomedullin, BNP, and NT-proBNP, and negatively with left ventricular ejection fraction. U-II has been suggested to be diagnostically superior to BNP,[91] however this remains in doubt.

Markers of Biomechanical Stretch

Recent studies suggest that there is a gene expression profile that is activated in cardiomyocytes subjected to biomechanical stress in comparison to neurohormonally-induced cardiomyocyte hypertrophy.[94] It has been suggested that this is mediated, at least in part, by angiotensin II–dependent signaling. There are number of potential biomarkers of mechanical stretch of interest. While many are discussed elsewhere in this book, several are worthy to consider here.

Growth-Differentiation Factor 15

Growth-differentiation factor 15 (GDF15), also known as MIC-1, is a secreted member of the transforming growth factor (TGF)-ß superfamily. GDF15 is only detectable in the liver and placenta,[95] but can be induced in the heart by myocardial infarction and pressure overload.[96,97] It has been proposed that GDF15 is a cytokine released in an auto- or paracrine way that displays antihypertrophic and cardioprotective features.[97] The preanalytical and population characteristics of GDF15 have been characterized. It correlates with CRP and cystatin C in the healthy elderly, but not with NT-proBNP.[98] GDF15 is elevated in patients with chronic HF, and correlates with NYHA class. Values are similarly prognostic as NT-proBNP, but both are independent predictors of prognosis.[99] GDF15 may have a role to play in diagnosis and risk stratification in patients with cardiac failure, but more studies are required.

ST2

ST2 (also known as IL1RL1, DER4, T1, and FIT-1) is a member of the Toll-like/IL-1-receptor superfamily. Four isoforms of ST2 exist: soluble (s)ST2, ST2 ligand (ST2L), ST2v, and ST2Lv. The overall structure of ST2L is similar to the structure of the type I IL-1 receptors.

The ligand for ST2 is an 18-kDa protein IL-33 (also known as IL-1F11)—a member of the IL-1 interleukin family. The mode by which IL-33 exerts its effect has not been fully established, but the IL-33/ST2 system might also participate in the fibrotic response to tissue injury. Expression of ST2 is markedly up-regulated upon the application of mechanical strain to cardiac myocytes.[100] IL-33/

ST2 signaling is a mechanically-activated, cardioprotective fibroblast-cardiomyocyte paracrine system.[101]

sST2 is elevated following myocardial infarction[102] and elevated levels predict an adverse outcome independently of NT-proBNP values.[103] In patients with acute HF, elevation of sST2 predicts an adverse outcome and is an independent prognostic marker.[104–107] Interestingly, sST2 predicts an adverse outcome in patients presenting with acute dyspnea regardless of whether they have HF or not[104] and in patients with pulmonary disease.[108]

Metabolic and Nutritional Markers

The risk factors for cardiovascular disease include obesity and metabolic syndrome. Diabetes is considered to be a myocardial infarction risk equivalent. Obesity, metabolic syndrome, and diabetes are therefore linked to the development and progression of cardiovascular disease. Recently, it has been recognized that adipose tissue is also a source of cytokines and other bioactive molecules, usually referred to as adipokines. There is, therefore, a link between the conventional markers of inflammation, cardiovascular risk, and adipose tissue. Finally and paradoxically, end-stage cardiac failure is associated with cachexia. Development of such cardiac cachexia is associated with a poor outcome.

Ghrelin

Human ghrelin is a 28-amino acid peptide[109–111] with a biological role of generating fat tissue by decreasing fat oxidation. Stimulation of motility and gastric emptying induced by ghrelin may involve a local effect, as well as central mechanisms. Ghrelin may also have an immunomodulating role.[112] It inactivates NK-κB, one of the major regulatory pathways of the inflammatory response.[113] The relationship between ghrelin levels and HF is not entirely clear. Initial studies suggested that elevated ghrelin levels are only seen in patients with cardiac cachexia.[114] This affliction is also associated with elevated levels of neuropeptide Y (NPY), one of the putative satiety hormones.[115] There is interest in ghrelin as a marker of abnormal metabolism in cardiac failure and considerable interest in its potential role as a therapeutic agent.[111,116,117]

Leptin

Leptin is a 16 KDa peptide initially identified as produced by the white adipocytes, but subsequently was found to be produced by a wide range of tissues.[110,118,119] Leptin acts centrally to curb appetite and increase energy expenditure. A major target of leptin's central action is NPY, which stimulates food intake, inhibits thermogenesis, and results in increased serum insulin and steroid levels. Leptin receptors are expressed in the heart and leptin itself may act as a cardiac hypertrophic factor.[120]

Increased levels of leptin and leptin receptors occur in patients with HF. Noncachectic patients with HF show increased plasma leptin and soluble leptin receptor levels; in these patients, hyperleptinemia correlates to serum levels of proinflammatory cytokines, such as TNF-α, and also show a positive relationship between plasma leptin and insulin concentrations.[121] In moderate HF, elevated leptin levels and norepinephrine (but not TNF-α) directly and independently predict insulin resistance.[122]

Patients with HF show increased energy expenditure. There is a positive relationship between plasma leptin and insulin concentrations that may be related to the increased energy expenditure observed in patients with congestive HF.[123] This is supported by an association between plasma leptin concentrations and energy expenditure, as well as body energy stores in HF patients, but not in controls.[124] The major limitation of leptin is the strong dependence on body mass index (BMI) and fat mass. Elevated leptin levels, corrected for fat mass, have been observed in patients with HF both with and without cachexia.[125] It has been suggested that lower total fat mass may account for the lower leptin levels found in cardiac failure patients.[126]

The major problem with interpreting studies of leptin measurement in patients with HF is to disentangle interconnectivity between this marker and parallel physiologic issues. Do hormone levels represent change in fat mass (a direct and inappropriate stimulus due to central regulation) or are they part of the generalized response to increased inflammatory signals? Further studies to define the pathobiology need to be undertaken before routine measurement should be implemented.

Adiponectin

Adiponectin is a 244-amino acid fat-derived peptide thought to play an important role in the regulation of energy metabolism.[110] In humans, plasma adiponectin concentrations are inversely correlated with BMI and body fat. Adiponectin may exert anti-inflammatory, antifibrotic, and antiatherogenic effects, particularly in endothelial cells and macrophages.[110,127] A local cardiac adiponectin system has been demonstrated in the heart that is regulated independently of adiponectin and TNF-α levels in the serum. It has been shown that this network is deranged in dilated cardiomyopathy.[128] Local production of adiponectin by the myocardium has been demonstrated in patients with cardiac failure.[129] Plasma adiponectin concentrations are increased in patients with HF. Elevated adiponectin has been consistently related to disease severity[130–132] and is reported to be an outcome predictor.[3,64,130,133–135] All studies where BNP/NT-proBNP were measured suggest strong correlation between these markers and adiponectin; moreover, adiponectin may be additive to BNP/NT-proBNP measurement for prognosis. How effective adiponectin is as an independent predictor of outcome is variable across the different studies and depends on the model used.

Resistin

Human resistin, a 12.5-kDa protein of 92 amino acids, is produced as a 108-amino acid propeptide.[110] Elevated levels of resistin are found in obese individuals compared to lean individuals. One study has examined resistin in patients with HF,[136] and found elevated levels that corresponded to severity of HF and predicted outcome. There was no correlation with BMI or blood glucose level. In this study, resistin was superior to measurement of BNP as an outcome predictor.

Conclusion

In conclusion, there is a plethora of novel markers in HF; the ultimate choice of whether any of these will be used clinically will depend on analytical suitability, plausibility for application, and whether the test will allow for a treatment opportunity. Ultimately, it is most likely that novel markers in HF will complement, rather than recapitulate, those that are already available to the clinician.

References

1. Chin BS, Blann AD, Gibbs CR, Chung NA, Conway DG, Lip GY. Prognostic value of interleukin-6, plasma viscosity, fibrinogen, von Willebrand factor, tissue factor and vascular endothelial growth factor levels in congestive heart failure. *Eur J Clin Invest.* 2003;33(11):941–948.
2. Lamblin N, Susen S, Dagorn J, et al. Prognostic significance of circulating levels of angiogenic cytokines in patients with congestive heart failure. *Am Heart J.* 2005;150(1):137–143.
3. Haugen E, Furukawa Y, Isic A, Fu M. Increased adiponectin level in parallel with increased NT-pro BNP in patients with severe heart failure in the elderly: A hospital cohort study. *Int J Cardiol.* 2008;125(2):216–219.
4. Nakamura T, Funayama H, Kubo N, et al. Elevation of plasma placental growth factor in the patients with ischemic cardiomyopathy. *Int J Cardiol.* 2009;131:186–191.
5. Ueno S, Ikeda U, Hojo Y, et al. Serum hepatocyte growth factor levels are increased in patients with congestive heart failure. *J Card Fail.* 2001;7(4):329–334.
6. Katz JN, Drazner MH. Assessing prognosis in heart failure: is hepatocyte growth factor the next B-type natriuretic peptide? *Am Heart J.* 2005;150(1):1–3.
7. Berk BC. Angiotensin II signal transduction in vascular smooth muscle: pathways activated by specific tyrosine kinases. *J Am Soc Nephrol.* 1999;10 (Suppl 11):S62–S68.

8. Shah BH, Catt KJ. A central role of EGF receptor transactivation in angiotensin II -induced cardiac hypertrophy. *Trends Pharmacol Sci.* 2003;24(5):239–244.
9. Takashima S. Pharmacological role of HB-EGF shedding by angiotensin II in cardiomyocytes. *Nippon Yakurigaku Zasshi.* 2004;124(2): 69–75.
10. Chan HW, Smith NJ, Hannan RD, Thomas WG. Tackling the EGFR in pathological tissue remodelling. *Pulm Pharmacol Ther.* 2006;19(1): 74–78.
11. Fiebeler A, Muller DN, Shagdarsuren E, Luft FC. Aldosterone, mineralocorticoid receptors, and vascular inflammation. *Curr Opin Nephrol Hypertens.* 2007;16(2):134–142.
12. Marney AM, Brown NJ. Aldosterone and end-organ damage. *Clin Sci (Lond).* 2007;113(6):267–278.
13. Koitabashi N, Arai M, Niwano K, et al. Plasma connective tissue growth factor is a novel potential biomarker of cardiac dysfunction in patients with chronic heart failure. *Eur J Heart Fail.* 2008; 10(4):373–379.
14. Squire IB, Evans J, Ng LL, Loftus IM, Thompson MM. Plasma MMP-9 and MMP-2 following acute myocardial infarction in man: correlation with echocardiographic and neurohumoral parameters of left ventricular dysfunction. *J Card Fail.* 2004;10(4):328–333.
15. Kelly D, Khan S, Cockerill G, et al. Circulating stromelysin-1 (MMP-3): a novel predictor of LV dysfunction, remodelling and all-cause mortality after acute myocardial infarction. *Eur J Heart Fail.* 2008; 10(2):133–139.
16. Wagner DR, Delagardelle C, Ernens I, Rouy D, Vaillant M, Beissel J. Matrix metalloproteinase-9 is a marker of heart failure after acute myocardial infarction. *J Card Fail.* 2006;12(1):66–72.
17. Kelly D, Khan SQ, Thompson M, et al. Plasma tissue inhibitor of metalloproteinase-1 and matrix metalloproteinase-9: novel indicators of left ventricular remodelling and prognosis after acute myocardial infarction. *Eur Heart J.* 2008;29:2116–2124.
18. Schwartzkopff B, Fassbach M, Pelzer B, Brehm M, Strauer BE. Elevated serum markers of collagen degradation in patients with mild to moderate dilated cardiomyopathy. *Eur J Heart Fail.* 2002;4(4): 439–444.

19. George J, Patal S, Wexler D, Roth A, Sheps D, Keren G. Circulating matrix metalloproteinase-2 but not matrix metalloproteinase-3, matrix metalloproteinase-9, or tissue inhibitor of metalloproteinase-1 predicts outcome in patients with congestive heart failure. *Am Heart J.* 2005;150(3):484–487.
20. Banfi C, Cavalca V, Veglia F, et al. Neurohormonal activation is associated with increased levels of plasma matrix metalloproteinase-2 in human heart failure. *Eur Heart J.* 2005;26(5):481–488.
21. Jordan A, Roldan V, Garcia M, et al. Matrix metalloproteinase-1 and its inhibitor, TIMP-1, in systolic heart failure: relation to functional data and prognosis. *J Intern Med.* 2007;262(3):385–392.
22. Milting H, Ellinghaus P, Seewald M, et al. Plasma biomarkers of myocardial fibrosis and remodeling in terminal heart failure patients supported by mechanical circulatory support devices. *J Heart Lung Transplant.* 2008;27(6):589–596.
23. Frantz S, Stork S, Michels K, et al. Tissue inhibitor of metalloproteinases levels in patients with chronic heart failure: an independent predictor of mortality. *Eur J Heart Fail.* 2008;10(4):388–395.
24. Ohtsuka T, Nishimura K, Kurata A, Ogimoto A, Okayama H, Higaki J. Serum matrix metalloproteinase-3 as a novel marker for risk stratification of patients with nonischemic dilated cardiomyopathy. *J Card Fail.* 2007;13(9):752–758.
25. Vorovich EE, Chuai S, Li M, et al. Comparison of matrix metalloproteinase 9 and brain natriuretic peptide as clinical biomarkers in chronic heart failure. *Am Heart J.* 2008;155(6):992–997.
26. Agostoni P, Banfi C. Matrix metalloproteinase and heart failure: is it time to move from research to clinical laboratories? *Eur Heart J.* 2007;28(6):659–660.
27. Uusimaa P, Risteli J, Niemela M, et al. Collagen scar formation after acute myocardial infarction: relationships to infarct size, left ventricular function, and coronary artery patency. *Circulation.* 1997; 96(8):2565–2572.
28. Poulsen SH, Host NB, Jensen SE, Egstrup K. Relationship between serum amino-terminal propeptide of type III procollagen and changes of left ventricular function after acute myocardial infarction. *Circulation.* 2000;101(13):1527–1532.
29. Zannad F, Alla F, Dousset B, Perez A, Pitt B; RALES Investigators. Limitation of excessive extracellular matrix turnover may contribute

to survival benefit of spironolactone therapy in patients with congestive heart failure: insights from the randomized aldactone evaluation study (RALES). *Circulation.* 2000;102(22):2700–2706.

30. Klappacher G, Franzen P, Haab D, et al. Measuring extracellular matrix turnover in the serum of patients with idiopathic or ischemic dilated cardiomyopathy and impact on diagnosis and prognosis. *Am J Cardiol.* 1995;75(14):913–918.
31. Alla F, Kearney-Schwartz A, Radauceanu A, Das DS, Dousset B, Zannad F. Early changes in serum markers of cardiac extra-cellular matrix turnover in patients with uncomplicated hypertension and type II diabetes. *Eur J Heart Fail.* 2006;8(2):147–153.
32. Wang TJ, Larson MG, Benjamin EJ, et al. Clinical and echocardiographic correlates of plasma procollagen type III amino-terminal peptide levels in the community. *Am Heart J.* 2007;154(2):291–297.
33. Kitahara T, Takeishi Y, Arimoto T, et al. Serum carboxy-terminal telopeptide of type I collagen (ICTP) predicts cardiac events in chronic heart failure patients with preserved left ventricular systolic function. *Circ J.* 2007;71(6):929–935.
34. Cicoira M, Rossi A, Bonapace S, et al. Independent and additional prognostic value of aminoterminal propeptide of type III procollagen circulating levels in patients with chronic heart failure. *J Card Fail.* 2004;10(5):403–411.
35. Radauceanu A, Ducki C, Virion JM, et al. Extracellular matrix turnover and inflammatory markers independently predict functional status and outcome in chronic heart failure. *J Card Fail.* 2008;14(6):467–474.
36. Tremble P, Chiquet-Ehrismann R, Werb Z. The extracellular matrix ligands fibronectin and tenascin collaborate in regulating collagenase gene expression in fibroblasts. *Mol Biol Cell.* 1994;5(4):439–453.
37. Chuva de Sousa Lopes SM, Feijen A, Korving J, et al. Connective tissue growth factor expression and Smad signaling during mouse heart development and myocardial infarction. *Dev Dyn.* 2004;231(3):542–550.
38. Willems IE, Arends JW, Daemen MJ. Tenascin and fibronectin expression in healing human myocardial scars. *J Pathol.* 1996;179(3):321–325.

39. Sato A, Aonuma K, Imanaka-Yoshida K, et al. Serum tenascin-C might be a novel predictor of left ventricular remodeling and prognosis after acute myocardial infarction. *J Am Coll Cardiol.* 2006; 47(11):2319–2325.

40. Chaulet H, Lin F, Guo J, et al. Sustained augmentation of cardiac alpha1A-adrenergic drive results in pathological remodeling with contractile dysfunction, progressive fibrosis and reactivation of matricellular protein genes. *J Mol Cell Cardiol.* 2006;40(4): 540–552.

41. Terasaki F, Okamoto H, Onishi K, et al. Higher serum tenascin-C levels reflect the severity of heart failure, left ventricular dysfunction and remodeling in patients with dilated cardiomyopathy. *Circ J.* 2007;71(3):327–330.

42. Hessel MH, Bleeker GB, Bax JJ, et al. Reverse ventricular remodelling after cardiac resynchronization therapy is associated with a reduction in serum tenascin-C and plasma matrix metalloproteinase-9 levels. *Eur J Heart Fail.* 2007;9(10):1058–1063.

43. Odaka K, Uehara T, Arano Y, et al. Noninvasive detection of cardiac repair after acute myocardial infarction in rats by 111. In: Fab fragment of monoclonal antibody specific for tenascin-C. *Int Heart J.* 2008;49(4):481–492.

44. Schnee JM, Hsueh WA. Angiotensin II, adhesion, and cardiac fibrosis. *Cardiovasc Res.* 2000;46(2):264–268.

45. Singh K, Sirokman G, Communal C, et al. Myocardial osteopontin expression coincides with the development of heart failure. *Hypertension.* 1999;33(2):663–670.

46. Stawowy P, Blaschke F, Pfautsch P, et al. Increased myocardial expression of osteopontin in patients with advanced heart failure. *Eur J Heart Fail.* 2002;4(2):139–146.

47. Kotlyar E, Vita JA, Winter MR, et al. The relationship between aldosterone, oxidative stress, and inflammation in chronic, stable human heart failure. *J Card Fail.* 2006;12(2):122–127.

48. Soejima H, Irie A, Fukunaga T, et al. Osteopontin expression of circulating T cells and plasma osteopontin levels are increased in relation to severity of heart failure. *Circ J.* 2007;71(12):1879–1884.

49. Zittermann A, Koerfer R. Vitamin D in the prevention and treatment of coronary heart disease. *Curr Opin Clin Nutr Metab Care.* 2008;11(6):752–757.

50. Wang TJ, Pencina MJ, Booth SL, et al. Vitamin D deficiency and risk of cardiovascular disease. *Circulation.* 2008;117(4):503–511.
51. Yang RY, Hsu DK, Liu FT. Expression of galectin-3 modulates T-cell growth and apoptosis. *Proc Natl Acad Sci U S A.* 1996;93(13): 6737–6742.
52. Morris S, Ahmad N, Andre S, et al. Quaternary solution structures of galectins-1, -3, and -7. *Glycobiology.* 2004;14(3):293–300.
53. Leffler H, Carlsson S, Hedlund M, Qian Y, Poirier F. Introduction to galectins. *Glycoconj J.* 2004;19(7–9):433–440.
54. Sharma UC, Pokharel S, van Brakel TJ, et al. Galectin-3 marks activated macrophages in failure-prone hypertrophied hearts and contributes to cardiac dysfunction. *Circulation.* 2004;110(19): 3121–3128.
55. van Kimmenade RRJ, Januzzi JL Jr, Ellinor PT, et al. Utility of amino-terminal pro-brain natriuretic peptide, galectin-3, and apelin for the evaluation of patients with acute heart failure. *J Am Coll Cardiol.* 2006;48(6):1217–1224.
56. Morgenthaler NG, Struck J, Jochberger S, Dunser MW. Copeptin: clinical use of a new biomarker. *Trends Endocrinol Metab.* 2008; 19(2):43–49.
57. Khan SQ, Dhillon OS, O'Brien RJ, et al. C-terminal provasopressin (copeptin) as a novel and prognostic marker in acute myocardial infarction: Leicester Acute Myocardial Infarction Peptide (LAMP) study. *Circulation.* 2007;115(16):2103–2110.
58. Kelly D, Squire IB, Khan SQ, et al. C-terminal provasopressin (copeptin) is associated with left ventricular dysfunction, remodeling, and clinical heart failure in survivors of myocardial infarction. *J Card Fail.* 2008;14(9):739–745.
59. Gegenhuber A, Struck J, Dieplinger B, et al. Comparative evaluation of B-type natriuretic peptide, mid-regional pro-A-type natriuretic peptide, mid-regional pro-adrenomedullin, and Copeptin to predict 1-year mortality in patients with acute destabilized heart failure. *J Card Fail.* 2007;13(1):42–49.
60. Stoiser B, Mortl D, Hulsmann M, et al. Copeptin, a fragment of the vasopressin precursor, as a novel predictor of outcome in heart failure. *Eur J Clin Invest.* 2006;36(11):771–778.
61. Neuhold S, Huelsmann M, Strunk G, et al. Comparison of copeptin, B-type natriuretic peptide, and amino-terminal pro-B-type natriuretic

peptide in patients with chronic heart failure: prediction of death at different stages of the disease. *J Am Coll Cardiol.* 2008;52(4): 266–272.

62. Yanagawa B, Nagaya N. Adrenomedullin: molecular mechanisms and its role in cardiac disease. *Amino Acids.* 2007;32(1):157–164.
63. Bisping E, Tenderich G, Barckhausen P, et al. Atrial myocardium is the predominant inotropic target of adrenomedullin in the human heart. *Am J Physiol Heart Circ Physiol.* 2007;293(5):H3001–H3007.
64. Nishida H, Horio T, Suzuki Y, et al. Plasma adrenomedullin as an independent predictor of future cardiovascular events in high-risk patients: comparison with C-reactive protein and adiponectin. *Peptides.* 2008;29(4):599–605.
65. Khan SQ, Dhillon O, Struck J, et al. C-terminal pro-endothelin-1 offers additional prognostic information in patients after acute myocardial infarction: Leicester Acute Myocardial Infarction Peptide (LAMP) Study. *Am Heart J.* 2007;154(4):736–742.
66. Nishikimi T, Saito Y, Kitamura K, et al. Increased plasma levels of adrenomedullin in patients with heart failure. *J Am Coll Cardiol.* 1995;26(6):1424–1431.
67. Jougasaki M, Wei CM, McKinley LJ, Burnett JC Jr. Elevation of circulating and ventricular adrenomedullin in human congestive heart failure. *Circulation.* 1995;92(3):286–289.
68. Pousset F, Masson F, Chavirovskaia O, et al. Plasma adrenomedullin, a new independent predictor of prognosis in patients with chronic heart failure. *Eur Heart J.* 2000;21(12):1009–1014.
69. Richards AM, Doughty R, Nicholls MG, et al. Plasma N-terminal pro-brain natriuretic peptide and adrenomedullin: prognostic utility and prediction of benefit from carvedilol in chronic ischemic left ventricular dysfunction. Australia-New Zealand Heart Failure Group. *J Am Coll Cardiol.* 2001;37(7):1781–1787.
70. Chandrasekaran B, Dar O, McDonagh T. The role of apelin in cardiovascular function and heart failure. *Eur J Heart Fail.* 2008;10(8): 725–732.
71. Japp AG, Newby DE. The apelin-APJ system in heart failure: pathophysiologic relevance and therapeutic potential. *Biochem Pharmacol.* 2008;75(10):1882–1892.
72. Chen MM, Ashley EA, Deng DX, et al. Novel role for the potent endogenous inotrope apelin in human cardiac dysfunction. *Circulation.* 2003;108(12):1432–1439.

73. Foldes G, Horkay F, Szokodi I, et al. Circulating and cardiac levels of apelin, the novel ligand of the orphan receptor APJ, in patients with heart failure. *Biochem Biophys Res Commun.* 2003;308(3): 480–485.

74. Chong KS, Gardner RS, Morton JJ, Ashley EA, McDonagh TA. Plasma concentrations of the novel peptide apelin are decreased in patients with chronic heart failure. *Eur J Heart Fail.* 2006;8(4): 355–360.

75. Miettinen KH, Magga J, Vuolteenaho O, et al. Utility of plasma apelin and other indices of cardiac dysfunction in the clinical assessment of patients with dilated cardiomyopathy. *Regul Pept.* 2007;140(3):178–184.

76. Barton M, Yanagisawa M. Endothelin: 20 years from discovery to therapy. *Can J Physiol Pharmacol.* 2008;86(8):485–498.

77. Kirkby NS, Hadoke PW, Bagnall AJ, Webb DJ. The endothelin system as a therapeutic target in cardiovascular disease: great expectations or bleak house? *Br J Pharmacol.* 2008;153(6):1105–1119.

78. Motte S, McEntee K, Naeije R. Endothelin receptor antagonists. *Pharmacol Ther.* 2006;110(3):386–414.

79. Zhao XS, Pan W, Bekeredjian R, Shohet RV. Endogenous endothelin-1 is required for cardiomyocyte survival in vivo. *Circulation.* 2006;114(8):830–837.

80. Papassotiriou J, Morgenthaler NG, Struck J, Alonso C, Bergmann A. Immunoluminometric assay for measurement of the C-terminal endothelin-1 precursor fragment in human plasma. *Clin Chem.* 2006;52(6):1144–1151.

81. Masson S, Latini R, Anand IS, et al. The prognostic value of big endothelin-1 in more than 2,300 patients with heart failure enrolled in the Valsartan Heart Failure Trial (Val-HeFT). *J Card Fail.* 2006;12(5):375–380.

82. Frantz RP, Lowes BD, Grayburn PA, et al. Baseline and serial neurohormones in patients with congestive heart failure treated with and without bucindolol: results of the neurohumoral substudy of the Beta-Blocker Evaluation of Survival Study (BEST). *J Card Fail.* 2007;13(6):437–444.

83. De Luca L, Mebazaa A, Filippatos G, et al. Overview of emerging pharmacologic agents for acute heart failure syndromes. *Eur J Heart Fail.* 2008;10(2):201–213.

84. Dschietzig T, Richter C, Bartsch C, et al. The pregnancy hormone relaxin is a player in human heart failure. *FASEB J.* 2001;15(12): 2187–2195.

85. Dschietzig T, Bartsch C, Richter C, Laule M, Baumann G, Stangl K. Relaxin, a pregnancy hormone, is a functional endothelin-1 antagonist: attenuation of endothelin-1-mediated vasoconstriction by stimulation of endothelin type-B receptor expression via ERK-1/2 and nuclear factor-kappaB. *Circ Res.* 2003;92(1):32–40.

86. Russell FD. Emerging roles of urotensin-II in cardiovascular disease. *Pharmacol Ther.* 2004;103(3):223–243.

87. Zhu YC, Zhu YZ, Moore PK. The role of urotensin II in cardiovascular and renal physiology and diseases. *Br J Pharmacol.* 2006; 148(7):884–901.

88. McDonald J, Batuwangala M, Lambert DG. Role of urotensin II and its receptor in health and disease. *J Anesth.* 2007;21(3):378–389.

89. Pakala R. Role of urotensin II in atherosclerotic cardiovascular diseases. *Cardiovasc Revasc Med.* 2008;9(3):166–178.

90. Richards AM, Nicholls MG, Lainchbury JG, Fisher S, Yandle TG. Plasma urotensin II in heart failure. *Lancet.* 2002;360(9332): 545–546.

91. Ng LL, Loke I, O'Brien RJ, Squire IB, Davies JE. Plasma urotensin in human systolic heart failure. *Circulation.* 2002;106(23): 2877–2880.

92. Gruson D, Rousseau MF, Ahn SA, van Linden F, Ketelslegers JM. Circulating urotensin II levels in moderate to severe congestive heart failure: its relations with myocardial function and well established neurohormonal markers. *Peptides.* 2006;27(6):1527–1531.

93. Russell FD, Meyers D, Galbraith AJ, et al. Elevated plasma levels of human urotensin-II immunoreactivity in congestive heart failure. *Am J Physiol Heart Circ Physiol.* 2003;285(4):H1576–H1581.

94. Frank D, Kuhn C, Brors B, et al. Gene expression pattern in biomechanically stretched cardiomyocytes: evidence for a stretch-specific gene program. *Hypertension.* 2008;51(2):309–318.

95. Paralkar VM, Vail AL, Grasser WA, et al. Cloning and characterization of a novel member of the transforming growth factor-beta/bone morphogenetic protein family. *J Biol Chem.* 1998;273(22): 13760–13767.

96. Xu J, Kimball TR, Lorenz JN, et al. GDF15/MIC-1 functions as a protective and antihypertrophic factor released from the myocardium in association with SMAD protein activation. *Circ Res.* 2006;98(3):342–350.

97. Kempf T, Eden M, Strelau J, et al. The transforming growth factor-beta superfamily member growth-differentiation factor-15 protects the heart from ischemia/reperfusion injury. *Circ Res.* 2006;98(3): 351–360.

98. Kempf T, Horn-Wichmann R, Brabant G, et al. Circulating concentrations of growth-differentiation factor 15 in apparently healthy elderly individuals and patients with chronic heart failure as assessed by a new immunoradiometric sandwich assay. *Clin Chem.* 2007;53(2): 284–291.

99. Kempf T, von Haehling S, Peter T, et al. Prognostic utility of growth differentiation factor-15 in patients with chronic heart failure. *J Am Coll Cardiol.* 2007;50(11):1054–1060.

100. Weinberg EO, Shimpo M, De Keulenaer GW, et al. Expression and regulation of ST2, an interleukin-1 receptor family member, in cardiomyocytes and myocardial infarction. *Circulation.* 2002;106(23): 2961–2966.

101. Sanada S, Hakuno D, Higgins LJ, Schreiter ER, McKenzie AN, Lee RT. IL-33 and ST2 comprise a critical biomechanically induced and cardioprotective signaling system. *J Clin Invest.* 2007;117(6): 1538–1549.

102. Shimpo M, Morrow DA, Weinberg EO, et al. Serum levels of the interleukin-1 receptor family member ST2 predict mortality and clinical outcome in acute myocardial infarction. *Circulation.* 2004;109(18):2186–2190.

103. Sabatine MS, Morrow DA, Higgins LJ, et al. Complementary roles for biomarkers of biomechanical strain ST2 and N-terminal prohormone B-type natriuretic peptide in patients with ST-elevation myocardial infarction. *Circulation.* 2008;117(15):1936–1944.

104. Januzzi JL Jr, Peacock WF, Maisel AS, et al. Measurement of the interleukin family member ST2 in patients with acute dyspnea: results from the PRIDE (Pro-Brain Natriuretic Peptide Investigation of Dyspnea in the Emergency Department) study. *J Am Coll Cardiol.* 2007;50(7):607–613.

105. Rehman SU, Martinez-Rumayor A, Mueller T, Januzzi JL Jr. Independent and incremental prognostic value of multimarker testing in acute dyspnea: results from the ProBNP Investigation of Dyspnea in the Emergency Department (PRIDE) study. *Clin Chim Acta.* 2008;392(1–2):41–45.

106. Mueller T, Dieplinger B, Gegenhuber A, Poelz W, Pacher R, Haltmayer M. Increased plasma concentrations of soluble ST2 are predictive for 1-year mortality in patients with acute destabilized heart failure. *Clin Chem.* 2008;54(4):752–756.

107. Boisot S, Beede J, Isakson S, et al. Serial sampling of ST2 predicts 90-day mortality following destabilized heart failure. *J Card Fail.* 2008;14(9):732–738.

108. Martinez-Rumayor A, Camargo CA, Green SM, Baggish AL, O'Donoghue M, Januzzi JL. Soluble ST2 plasma concentrations predict 1-year mortality in acutely dyspneic emergency department patients with pulmonary disease. *Am J Clin Pathol.* 2008;130(4): 578–584.

109. Nagaya N, Kangawa K. Ghrelin, a novel growth hormone-releasing peptide, in the treatment of chronic heart failure. *Regul Pept.* 2003;114(2–3):71–77.

110. Meier U, Gressner AM. Endocrine regulation of energy metabolism: review of pathobiochemical and clinical chemical aspects of leptin, ghrelin, adiponectin, and resistin. *Clin Chem.* 2004;50(9): 1511–1525.

111. Nagaya N, Kojima M, Kangawa K. Ghrelin, a novel growth hormone-releasing peptide, in the treatment of cardiopulmonary-associated cachexia. *Intern Med.* 2006;45(3):127–134.

112. Smith RG, Jiang H, Sun Y. Developments in ghrelin biology and potential clinical relevance. *Trends Endocrinol Metab.* 2005;16(9): 436–442.

113. Li WG, Gavrila D, Liu X, et al. Ghrelin inhibits proinflammatory responses and nuclear factor-kappaB activation in human endothelial cells. *Circulation.* 2004;109(18):2221–2226.

114. Nagaya N, Uematsu M, Kojima M, et al. Elevated circulating level of ghrelin in cachexia associated with chronic heart failure: relationships between ghrelin and anabolic/catabolic factors. *Circulation.* 2001;104(17):2034–2038.

115. le Roux CW, Ghatei MA, Gibbs JS, Bloom SR. The putative satiety hormone PYY is raised in cardiac cachexia associated with primary pulmonary hypertension. *Heart.* 2005;91(2):241–242.

116. Marleau S, Mulumba M, Lamontagne D, Ong H. Cardiac and peripheral actions of growth hormone and its releasing peptides: relevance for the treatment of cardiomyopathies. *Cardiovasc Res.* 2006;69(1):26–35.

117. Strassburg S, Anker SD. Metabolic and immunologic derangements in cardiac cachexia: where to from here? *Heart Fail Rev.* 2006;11(1): 57–64.

118. Ren J. Leptin and hyperleptinemia—from friend to foe for cardiovascular function. *J Endocrinol.* 2004;181(1):1–10.

119. Schulze PC, Kratzsch J. Leptin as a new diagnostic tool in chronic heart failure. *Clin Chim Acta.* 2005;362(1–2):1–11.

120. Karmazyn M, Purdham DM, Rajapurohitam V, Zeidan A. Leptin as a cardiac hypertrophic factor: a potential target for therapeutics. *Trends Cardiovasc Med.* 2007;17(6):206–211.

121. Schulze PC, Kratzsch J, Linke A, et al. Elevated serum levels of leptin and soluble leptin receptor in patients with advanced chronic heart failure. *Eur J Heart Fail.* 2003;5(1):33–40.

122. Doehner W, Rauchhaus M, Godsland IF, et al. Insulin resistance in moderate chronic heart failure is related to hyperleptinaemia, but not to norepinephrine or TNF-alpha. *Int J Cardiol.* 2002;83(1): 73–81.

123. Leyva F, Anker SD, Egerer K, Stevenson JC, Kox WJ, Coats AJ. Hyperleptinaemia in chronic heart failure. Relationships with insulin. *Eur Heart J.* 1998;19(10):1547–1551.

124. Toth MJ, Gottlieb SS, Fisher ML, Ryan AS, Nicklas BJ, Poehlman ET. Plasma leptin concentrations and energy expenditure in heart failure patients. *Metabolism.* 1997;46(4):450–453.

125. Doehner W, Pflaum CD, Rauchhaus M, et al. Leptin, insulin sensitivity and growth hormone binding protein in chronic heart failure with and without cardiac cachexia. *Eur J Endocrinol.* 2001; 145(6):727–735.

126. Murdoch DR, Rooney E, Dargie HJ, Shapiro D, Morton JJ, McMurray JJ. Inappropriately low plasma leptin concentration in the cachexia associated with chronic heart failure. *Heart.* 1999;82(3): 352–356.

127. Hopkins TA, Ouchi N, Shibata R, Walsh K. Adiponectin actions in the cardiovascular system. *Cardiovasc Res.* 2007;74(1):11–18.

128. Skurk C, Wittchen F, Suckau L, et al. Description of a local cardiac adiponectin system and its deregulation in dilated cardiomyopathy. *Eur Heart J.* 2008;29(9):1168–1180.

129. Takano H, Obata JE, Kodama Y, et al. Adiponectin is released from the heart in patients with heart failure. *Int J Cardiol.* 2009;132: 221–226.

130. George J, Patal S, Wexler D, et al. Circulating adiponectin concentrations in patients with congestive heart failure. *Heart.* 2006;92(10): 1420–1424.

131. Nakamura T, Funayama H, Kubo N, et al. Association of hyperadiponectinemia with severity of ventricular dysfunction in congestive heart failure. *Circ J.* 2006;70(12):1557–1562.

132. Tanaka T, Tsutamoto T, Nishiyama K, et al. Impact of oxidative stress on plasma adiponectin in patients with chronic heart failure. *Circ J.* 2008;72(4):563–568.

133. Kistorp C, Faber J, Galatius S, et al. Plasma adiponectin, body mass index, and mortality in patients with chronic heart failure. *Circulation.* 2005;112(12):1756–1762.

134. Tamura T, Furukawa Y, Taniguchi R, et al. Serum adiponectin level as an independent predictor of mortality in patients with congestive heart failure. *Circ J.* 2007;71(5):623–630.

135. Wannamethee SG, Whincup PH, Lennon L, Sattar N. Circulating adiponectin levels and mortality in elderly men with and without cardiovascular disease and heart failure. *Arch Intern Med.* 2007;167(14):1510–1517.

136. Takeishi Y, Niizeki T, Arimoto T, et al. Serum resistin is associated with high risk in patients with congestive heart failure—a novel link between metabolic signals and heart failure. *Circ J.* 2007;71(4): 460–464.

Section IV

Markers of Thrombosis and Hemostasis

27 ▪ Rationale for Measurement of Thrombosis Markers in Cardiology

Mahesh J. Patel, MD
Richard C. Becker, MD

Introduction

Biomarkers hold considerable promise for improving the management of patients with cardiovascular (CV) thrombotic disorders. In this chapter, the current state of thrombosis biomarkers associated with atrial fibrillation (AF), coronary artery disease, and heart failure will be reviewed. In addition, existing and future challenges of employing thrombosis biomarkers in the management of patients with CV disease will also be discussed.

From a clinical perspective, the fundamental role of a biomarker is to aid in medical decision making in order to improve patient outcomes. Specifically among CV diseases, thrombosis biomarkers may help determine an individual's diagnosis or the prognosis of a thrombotic event, in addition to guiding the therapeutic decisions surrounding these events. An ideal thrombosis biomarker is fundamentally characterized by a high degree of accuracy, reproducibility, sensitivity, and specificity, as well as evidence suggesting its measurement would meaningfully contribute to patient management.[1–2]

Biomarkers of Thrombosis

Thrombosis markers can all be conveniently categorized within each of the major branches of the human hemostatic system. The hemostatic system serves to maintain the integrity of the circulation by promoting blood fluidity under normal circumstances, promoting blood clotting at times of vessel wall injury, and reestablishing blood flow after vessel wall healing. Figure 27–1 displays several key cellular and enzymatic components of this system. The

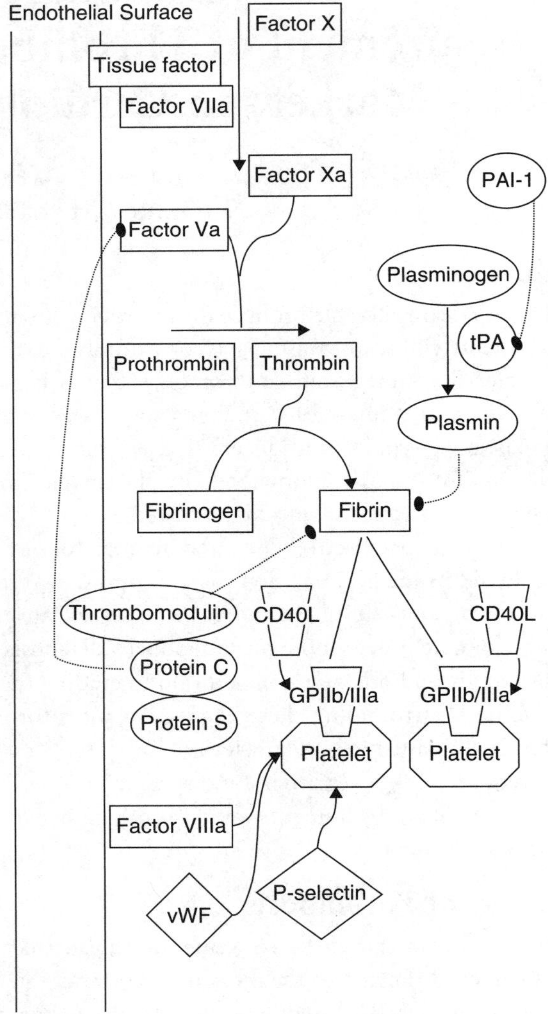

■ **Figure 27–1** Hemostatic System: This figure displays the key cellular and enzymatic components of the human hemostatic system, which are also key thrombosis biomarkers. The rectangular-shaped structures represent coagulation biomarkers, the oval-shaped structures represent anticoagulation biomarkers, the trapezoid-shaped structures represent platelet surface biomarkers, and the diamond-shaped structures represent endothelial cell biomarkers. The solid lines with arrowheads represent pathways of activation and the dotted lines with circular heads represent pathways of de-activation.

major components of this system include the coagulation factors, anticoagulation factors, platelets, and endothelial cells. In addition, gene polymorphisms may also have a role in the future to better understand function of the coagulation system.

Biomarkers of Coagulation

Coagulation factors are activated by mechanical injury to the vessel wall or by systemically-generated mediators that promote thrombus composed of platelets and fibrin. Three proteins with pivotal roles in arterial, venous, and cardiac chamber-associated thrombosis are: thrombin, fibrinogen, and tissue factor (TF). Thrombin is a regulatory protease with numerous cellular and biochemical functions that include the conversion of soluble fibrinogen to insoluble fibrin strands. Thrombin itself is formed by a series of steps initiated by tissue factor found within the subendothelial and subendocardial matrix and microparticles. Tissue factor binds to factor VIIa from the circulation, and this complex activates factor X, which, after further binding with factor Va, converts prothrombin to thrombin.

Biomarkers of Anticoagulation

Naturally-occurring anticoagulant, fibrinolytic, and antifibrinolytic proteins are critical for maintaining blood fluidity, facilitating vascular repair, and regulating thrombus growth and development. Thrombomodulin, an integral membrane protein on endothelial cells, attenuates fibrin formation by binding to thrombin and removing it from the circulation, and it also mediates the anticoagulant activity of protein C. Plasminogen activation inhibitor-1 (PAI-1) regulates the fibrinolytic activity of tissue plasminogen activator (tPA).

Platelet Surface Biomarkers

Platelets have a central role in primary hemostasis and also participate in the pathogenesis of flow-limiting arterial thrombosis. Glycoprotein IIb/IIIa (GpIIb/IIIa) receptors and CD40 ligand

(CD40L) are two important biomarkers found on the surface of platelets. GpIIb/IIIa receptors bind to fibrinogen, which serves as a protein bridge between platelets facilitating platelet aggregation. GPIIb/IIIa receptors are activated by CD40L, which itself is released by activated platelets (as well as inflammatory cells).

Endothelial Cell Biomarkers

Endothelial cells (EC) line the inner surface of the circulatory system. Circulating EC levels, as well as the EC-derived proteins, the von Willebrand factor (vWF), and P-selectin, are potential biomarkers of thrombosis. Circulating endothelial progenitor cells, originating primarily from the bone marrow, replenish damaged ECs in the vasculature. vWF is expressed and released in response to cell injury, binds to numerous proteins (including factor VIII), mediates platelet adhesion and aggregation, and participates in localized thrombus formation. P-selectin, released following platelet activation, contributes to inflammatory responses, specifically platelet-leukocyte aggregate generation.

Gene Polymorphisms

In addition to markers involved functionally in the hemostatic system, polymorphisms of genes encoding these proteins may also serve as biomarkers for thrombosis. These polymorphisms may cause phenotypic variations in thrombosis biomarkers, which may in turn affect individual susceptibility to thrombus formation.

Clinical Applications of Thrombosis Biomarkers

The hallmark of a clinically important biomarker is that it provides novel information, which can guide medical decision making and lead to improved clinical outcomes. There are three potential ways thrombosis biomarkers can be used in the management of cardiovascular diseases to achieve this goal. First, thrombosis biomarkers may help to more rapidly diagnose thrombotic events associated with cardiovascular diseases compared to conventional standards of diagnosis—more rapid diagnosis would allow for earlier initiation of therapy in the course of the thrombotic event. Second, thrombosis biomarkers may help to more accurately prognosticate the risk of developing thrombotic events in patients with cardiovascular diseases—more refined prognostic data would allow for more individualized preventive strategies for thrombotic events. And third, thrombosis biomarkers may help gauge an individual's response to therapies for thrombotic events—subclinical measures of treatment response with thrombosis biomarkers would also allow for a more personalized treatment plan. Thrombosis biomarkers have been extensively evaluated on these three performance measures of biomarkers in several areas of cardiovascular disease.

Atrial Fibrillation

Atrial fibrillation is a common disease associated with significant morbidity and mortality related to thromboembolic events, particularly ischemic stroke. Stagnant blood flow in a fibrillating atrium, as well as a local and systemic prothrombotic state, help explain the risks of thromboembolism associated with atrial fibrillation. Novel biomarkers that more accurately convey the risk of thromboembolism and guide decisions in regards to anticoagulation therapies would significantly enhance the management of atrial fibrillation.

Thrombosis biomarkers may have a role in the diagnosis of thrombosis in patients with atrial fibrillation (Table 27–1). Amongst biomarkers of coagulation, thrombin, fibrinogen, and tissue factor have all been associated with atrial fibrillation.[3–11] However, of these coagulation biomarkers, only markers of thrombin generation or activity (prothrombin fragment 1 + 2 and fibrinopeptide A) have been associated with spontaneous echo contrast in the left atrial appendage—echocardiographic findings that suggest thrombotic potential.[12] The major limitation with this study, aside from its small size, is that it does not demonstrate an association between thrombosis biomarkers and actual evidence of atrial thrombus, only an association with spontaneous echo

Table 27–1: Thrombosis biomarkers in atrial fibrillation.
Part A: Diagnosis of atrial thrombosis

Study	Study design	Study population	Sample size	Outcome	Thrombosis biomarkers	Independent associations
Tsai et al.	Case-control	Chronic nonrheumatic atrial fibrillation	73 cases	Spontaneous echo contrast or atrial thrombus	Prothrombin F1 + 2 Fibrinopeptide A	? ?
Conway et al.	Cross-sectional	Chronic atrial fibrillation	37 cases	Spontaneous echo contrast or atrial thrombosis	Soluble P-selectin vWF* Tissue factor Fibrinogen	No No No No
Heppel et al.	Case-control	Nonrheumatic atrial fibrillation	109 cases	Spontaneous echo contrast or atrial thrombosis	beta-thromboglobulin	Yes

					vWF*	Yes
					Thrombin generation and activity	No
					D-dimer	No
					Platelet factor 4	No
					Fibrinogen	No
					Factor VII	No
					Factor VIII	No

Part B: Prognosis

Study	Study design	Study population	Sample size	Outcome	Thrombosis biomarkers	Independent associations
SPAF III	Subanalysis of randomized trial	Nonvalvular atrial fibrillation	994 cases	Vascular events	vWF*	Yes
					Soluble P-selectin	No
SPAF III	Subanalysis of randomized trial	Nonvalvular atrial fibrillation	1531 cases	Stroke	prothrombin F1 + 2	No
					beta-thromboglobulin	No
					Fibrinogen	No

*vWF = von Willebrand Factor

contrast. As such, inadequate evidence exists for measurement of markers of thrombin generation or activity in routine clinical practice for diagnosis of left atrial thrombosis.

Endothelial cell biomarkers have also been evaluated as markers of thrombosis in patients with atrial fibrillation. The endothelial cell biomarkers P-selectin and vWF have both been associated with atrial fibrillation.[5,7,10–11,13–15] A small study (n = 37) has shown that soluble P-selectin is associated with spontaneous echo contrast; however, the association was not observed after multivariable adjustment.[14] This study was also limited by its small size and association between thrombosis biomarker and spontaneous echo contrast, rather than thrombus. As a result, soluble P-selectin should not be measured in routine clinical practice for diagnosis of left atrial thrombosis.

A study by Heppell et al. does demonstrate an association between thrombosis biomarkers and atrial thrombosis. In this case-control study of 109 patients with nonrheumatic atrial fibrillation, patients with transesophageal echocardiographic evidence of left atrial thrombus had several increased biomarkers of thrombosis, which included markers of coagulation and endothelial cells, compared with subjects without thrombosis. Amongst these biomarkers, only beta-thromboglobulin and vWF were independently associated with left atrial thrombus.[16] Median values (and interquartile ranges) for beta-thromboglobulin and vWF in the group of subjects with left atrial thrombus were 56.8 IU/mL (44.1–77.6) and 1.81 IU/mL (1.4–2.8), respectively. In a model predicting the presence of atrial thrombus in this study, beta-thromboglobulin and vWF had larger partial coefficients than did age or spontaneous echo contrast, but smaller than peak left atrial appendage velocity.[16] Based upon these findings, there may be a role for beta-thromboglobulin and vWF in helping to diagnose atrial thrombus in patients with atrial fibrillation; however, these findings first need to be replicated in different and larger cohorts. Furthermore, cut point levels would need to be defined for vWF and beta-thromboglobulin to maximize the c-statistic for each of these biomarkers in diagnosing atrial thrombus. As a result, vWF and beta-thromboglobulin should not be presently measured in routine clinical practice for diagnosis of atrial thrombosis, however, they may serve a role in screening atrial fibrillation subjects for the need for transesophageal echocardiograms.

Thrombosis markers have also been studied to see if there are specific thrombosis biomarker profiles that correlate with different types of atrial fibrillation, such as acute, paroxysmal, persistent, and permanent.[11,13] Two small studies have suggested that vWF, P-selectin, and fibrinogen levels are higher in permanent atrial fibrillation compared with other subtypes.[19,20] Other studies examining vWF levels[11,13] and platelet biomarkers[17,18] have not reported a difference based on clinical subtypes of atrial fibrillation. Based upon this evidence, there is no clear evidence to suggest that there are distinct thrombosis biomarker profiles associated with different subtypes of atrial fibrillation. Furthermore, given similar rates of stroke in all subtypes of atrial fibrillation, there does not appear to be any clinically useful information that would be ascertained from distinguishing thrombosis biomarkers profiles in these patients, as the anticoagulation strategies would unlikely change based on the findings.

Thrombosis biomarkers have also been investigated in their role in risk assessment in atrial fibrillation for future CV events (Table 27–1). Currently, clinical risk factors are used to assess risk for future thromboembolic events in patients with atrial fibrillation. In the Stroke Prevention in Atrial Fibrillation (SPAF) III study, which was a randomized trial of 1892 subjects with nonvalvular atrial fibrillation comparing adjusted-dose warfarin (to maintain an international normalized ratio [INR] between 2.0 and 3.0) versus fixed low-dose warfarin plus aspirin 325 mg versus aspirin alone, cardiovascular risk factors for stroke (such as advancing age, prior cerebral ischemia, recent heart failure, and diabetes) in atrial fibrillation were associated with vWF and soluble P-selectin.[21] Thrombosis markers have also been shown to be independently associated with future cardiovascular events in patients with atrial fibrillation.[22] In SPAF III, vWF was a significant predictor of both ischemic stroke and vascular events (ischemic stroke, myocardial infarction [MI], or vascular death) in 994 patients with atrial fibrillation receiving aspirin (alone or in combination with fixed low-dose warfarin), and the risk of these events was greatest among those with the highest levels of vWF. After adjustment for traditional risk factors, vWF remained a predictor for vascular events, with an adjusted risk ratio of 2.5 (95% CI 1.2–5.0) for the upper tertile versus the lower tertile; the cut points for vWF tertiles were 131 and 158 IU/dL. No independent associations with stroke or other vascular events were observed with soluble P-selectin.[22] In a separate analysis from SPAF III, levels of prothrombin F1 + 2, beta thromboglobulin, and fibrinogen did not independently predict the risk of future stroke or vascular events.

While vWF may represent an attractive prognostic thrombosis biomarker in low to moderate risk patients, there are several potential limitations. vWF is an acute phase reactant, with levels that rise in the setting of numerous inflammatory conditions and levels that are also influenced by blood type and estrogen levels. Large scale prospective studies are needed to further characterize the association between vWF and future CV events in patients with atrial fibrillation and to establish relevant thresholds for management decisions.

Genetic polymorphisms have also been evaluated for their role in risk assessment in atrial fibrillation. Factor V Leiden and G20210A mutation have both been shown to have an association with atrial fibrillation,[19,23] however neither predicted embolic events.[24]

Thrombosis biomarkers have also been evaluated in their capacity to guide treatment decisions in atrial fibrillation. Cardioversion is commonly used in the management of atrial fibrillation, and several thrombosis markers have been shown to either increase or remain unchanged after electrical or pharmacologic cardioversion into sinus rhythm.[19,22,25,26] This observation is consistent with the recognized risk for stroke after cardioversion in patients with atrial fibrillation. It is conceivable that thrombosis markers could be followed serially to determine the optimal duration of anticoagulant therapy following cardioversion; however, prospective studies must first be performed before these thrombosis biomarkers can be considered for use in clinical practice for guiding anticoagulant therapy after cardioversion to sinus rhythm. Along these lines, biomarkers of thrombosis have been preliminarily evaluated in their ability to guide anticoagulant therapy. Several studies have shown that treatment with either warfarin or heparin in patients with atrial fibrillation improves the prothrombotic profile of biomarkers.[4,6,9,10,27,28] Only one of these studies, however, sought to correlate the thrombosis biomarker profile among those treated with warfarin to clinical outcomes, and in this study an association with CV events was observed for those with persistent elevations in thrombosis biomarkers.[27] A total of 113 subjects with chronic atrial fibrillation were treated with warfarin to a target INR between 2.0 and 3.0. Thrombin activity (prothrombin fragment 1 + 2 and thrombin-antithrombin complexes) and D-dimer decreased with initiation of warfarin therapy; during an average follow-up of 44 months, approximately 20% suffered a CV event (stroke, MI, peripheral vascular occlusion, or vascular death). Higher levels of the anticoagulation biomarkers D-dimer and tPA on warfarin were associated with a higher event rate for the combined endpoint of CV events.[27] After multivariable adjustment, subjects with top versus lower two quartiles of D-dimer levels had a hazard ratio (HR) of 4.78 (95% CI 1.39–16.41) for combined CV events, while tPA antigen as a continuous variable had an HR of 1.01 (95% CI 1.01–1.17). These findings suggest that subjects with atrial fibrillation with INRs between 2.0 and 3.0, but with elevated levels of D-dimer and tPA, are more likely to suffer from recurrent CV events.

Of note, other studies have demonstrated an association between anticoagulation biomarkers, such as thrombomodulin, PAI-1, and tPA, and atrial fibrillation.[7,9,11,29] Treatment algorithms which gauge the intensity of anticoagulant therapy based upon

D-dimer and tPA levels should be investigated prospectively, particularly in patients receiving treatment to an INR range considered therapeutic. Presently, however, there is no clinical role for thrombosis biomarkers in guiding warfarin therapy.

Aspirin and/or clopidogrel have been compared with warfarin to determine their relative effects on thrombosis markers. However, only warfarin has demonstrated a reduction in thrombosis markers.[28,30]

Coronary Artery Disease

The major presentations of coronary artery disease (CAD) are acute coronary syndromes (ACS), which, in a majority of instances, are the end-result of coronary arterial thrombosis and thromboembolism. Several thrombosis biomarkers are associated with ACS and have demonstrated some signs of clinical relevance.

Table 27–2 reviews some of the prospective data evaluating the prognostic information obtained from thrombosis biomarkers in CAD. The coagulation, thrombin, fibrinogen, and tissue factor biomarkers have all been associated with ACS.[31–36] Of these coagulation biomarkers, fibrinogen is one of the most studied, and several analyses demonstrate that it is an independent predictor of CV events in patients with and without known CVD.[33,34,37,38] In a nested case-control study from the Physicians' Health Study, a large prospective study of approximately 15,000 men without a prior history of CVD, baseline fibrinogen was independently associated with future MI. High fibrinogen levels (≥343 mg/dL, the 90th percentile distribution of the control subjects) had a twofold increase in MI risk (age- and smoking-adjusted relative risk = 2.09, 95% CI 1.15–3.78).[33]

Another coagulation biomarker, fibrinopeptide A, which is a marker of thrombin activity, has also been found to be an independent predictor of CV events; however, given its short half-life and long turnaround time for its measurement, it does not have an important role in clinical risk assessment.[32,39,40] Another coagulation biomarker, tissue factor, has not been evaluated prospectively to assess for its role in risk assessment.

Table 27–2: Thrombosis biomarkers in coronary artery disease.

Thrombosis biomarker	Study	Study design	Study population	Sample size	Outcome	Independent associations
Fibrinogen	Physician's Health Study	Subanalysis of randomized trial	No CVD	199 cases	MI	Yes
	PRIME	Prospective cohort	No CVD	10,500 cases	MI, angina, PVD	Yes
	Thompson et al.	Prospective	Angina	3043 cases	MI or sudden death	Yes
Thrombomodulin	ARIC	Case-cohort	No CVD	258 cases	CHD	Yes
	PRIME	Prospective cohort nested case-control	No CVD	296 cases	MI	No
PAI-1	Thogersen et al.	Prospective nested case-control	No CVD	78 cases	MI	No
	ARIC	Case-cohort	No CVD	326 cases	CHD	No
	Collet et al.	Prospective	STEMI	153 cases	Mortality	Yes

Table 27–2: (Continued)

Thrombosis biomarker	Study	Study design	Study population	Sample size	Outcome	Independent associations
tPA	Thogersen et al.	Prospective nested case-control	No CVD	78 cases	MI	No
	Physician's Health Study	Case-control	No CVD	231 cases	MI	No
	ARIC	Case-cohort	No CVD	326 cases	CHD	No
Soluble CD40L	Heeschen et al.	Subanalysis of randomized trial	ACS	1088 cases	Death or MI	Yes
vWF	PRIME	Prospective cohort nested case-control	No CVD	296 cases	MI	Yes
	Thompson et al.	Prospective	Angina	3043 cases	MI or sudden death	Yes
	Whincup et al.	Prospective nested case-control	Men ages 40–59	625 cases	CHD	Yes

Endothelial cell biomarkers may also have a role in risk assessment. vWF, P-selectin, and circulating endothelial cells have all been associated with ACS.[41–45] Of these, vWF is one of the most studied, and several analyses demonstrate that it is an independent predictor of CV events in patients with and without known CVD.[34,41,42] In an analysis from the Prospective Epidemiological Study of Myocardial Infarction (PRIME), a study of over 10,000 men without CVD, vWF was found to be an independent predictor of future MI. Individuals with plasma vWF levels in the highest quartile showed a 3.04-fold increase in the risk for MI compared with those in the lowest quartile (95% CI, 1.08–4.18); cut points for the quartiles were not presented, but the mean ± SD level of vWF in the cases of CHD was 124.5 ± 47.8.[41] A meta-analysis also demonstrates that vWF is an independent predictor of future CV events.[42]

Based on this data, fibrinogen and vWF may both have important roles in risk assessment in patients with and without CVD. However, more research is needed to evaluate whether or not they provide incremental and clinically meaningful prognostic data by an improvement in the C statistic compared to traditional CVD risk assessment tools, such as the Framingham risk score, and other biomarkers, such as high-sensitivity CRP. The C statistic, however, may not be optimal in assessing models that predict future risk or stratify individuals into risk categories.[46]

Biomarkers of anticoagulation have also been evaluated for their role in risk assessment. Thrombomodulin, PAI-1, and tPA are biomarkers of anticoagulation that have all been associated with ACS.[47–51] Of the anticoagulation biomarkers, thrombomodulin has been extensively evaluated in prospective studies; however, there is inconsistent data in regards to its association with future CV events.[41,47] In an analysis from the Atherosclerosis Risk in Communities (ARIC) study, a prospective study of over 14,000 subjects without a history of CVD, thrombomodulin was an independent predictor for future MI with a negative association (adjusted RR of the highest quintile compared with lowest was 0.29

[95% CI 0.15–0.57]).[37] In contrast, an analysis of the PRIME dataset revealed no association between thrombomodulin and future MI.[41] The explanation for the different findings observed for soluble thrombomodulin in ARIC and PRIME is not clear, though it has been postulated to be related to differences in age and ethnicity between the two populations.[41] Given this inconsistent data, thrombomodulin does not presently have a role in risk assessment in routine clinical practice; more prospective studies will be needed to better define the relationship between thrombomodulin and future CV events.

Studies have also demonstrated an inconsistent relationship between another anticoagulation biomarker—PAI-1—and future CV events.[48,51,52] In a study by Collet et al., the change in PAI-1 levels in the setting of a STEMI (between levels at time of presentation and levels 24 hours later) was an independent predictor of 30-day mortality. The increase in PAI-1 among subjects who died was 46.9 ± 26.3 ng/mL versus −0.6 ± 2.8 ng/mL in those who survived.[48] Other studies have demonstrated an association between PAI-1 and future CV events in univariate analyses that were lost after multivariable adjustment.[51,52] In an analysis of the ARIC study, the highest PAI-1 quintile (>30.4 ng/mL) had an RR of 2.32 for future CHD events compared with the lowest quintile (≤6.17 ng/mL); this association was lost, however, after adjustment for known CV risk factors. Based upon these findings, a single measurement of PAI-1 would not provide any new risk assessment insight for CHD. On the other hand, some evidence suggests serial measurements of PAI-1 in the setting of an MI may provide useful prognostic information.

tPA is another anticoagulation biomarker of which levels have also been extensively studied as a prognostic tool.[39,50,51] While tPA has been found to be associated with future CV events in univariate analyses from the Physician's Health Study and ARIC, these associations were abrogated after multivariable adjustment.[50,51]

The platelet-derived biomarker, soluble CD40 ligand, is a promising thrombosis biomarker for risk assessment. It was evaluated by Heeschen et al. in a subanalysis of an ACS randomized controlled trial (c7E3 Fab Antiplatelet Therapy in Unstable Refractory Angina [CAPTURE] trial) comparing treatment with abciximab versus placebo and was found to be strongly associated with nonfatal MI and death.[47] The rate of CV events was highest among patients in the fourth and fifth quintiles of soluble CD40L levels, and the cut point for the fourth quintile was 5.0 mcg/L. In a separate validation sample of patients presenting with chest pain, subjects with soluble CD40L levels greater than 5.0 mcg/L had an adjusted HR of 6.65 (95% CI 3.18–13.89) for future CV events compared to subjects with levels less than 5.0 mcg/L. Major issues regarding the robustness of the analytical method for measurement of CD40L exist, however.

The prognostic significance of various genetic polymorphisms of thrombosis biomarkers associated with future CV events has also been studied, particularly among those known to result in a phenotypic change in the biomarker. Genetic polymorphisms of thrombomodulin (mutation at Ala455Val and mutation leading to Ala25Thr substation)[53–55] and the promoter region for PAI-1 gene (4G/5G insertion/deletion)[56] are associated with an increase in risk for CV events; however, the increase in risk is very modest and, as a result, likely provides no meaningful incremental clinical risk assessment information. There may be subgroups of the population for whom the polymorphism may provide greater risk assessment information. For example, the risk of MI is enhanced in African Americans and young male smokers with the thrombomodulin polymorphisms[54] and in patients at high CV risk with polymorphisms of PAI-1 promoter.[56] Other genetic variations including prothrombin 202010G/A polymorphism,[57] polymorphism of promoter region of tissue factor gene,[58] 311 base pair Alu insertion/deletion mutation of tPA,[59] and PIA1/A2 polymorphism of GPIIb/IIIa receptor[60,61] have shown no association with future CV events in prospective trials and, as a result, have no clinical utility in risk assessment. The reason very few genetic polymorphisms of thrombosis biomarkers have been associated with future

CV events may be a true lack of association, but also a lack of power to detect an association given the low frequency of these polymorphisms in the population.

In addition to prognosis, thrombosis biomarkers may also have a role in guiding treatments in ACS; changes in biomarker profiles may inform management decisions in these patients. One example deals with soluble CD40L levels in a cohort of ACS subjects treated with abciximab. In this trial, soluble CD40L was associated with increased CV risks. Among those treated with abciximab, subjects with the fourth and fifth highest quintiles of soluble CD40L levels had a reduced risk for future CV events compared to subjects with lower levels and a similar reduction in risk was not observed in the placebo arm, suggesting that the benefits of GpIIb/IIIa inhibitors in ACS may be guided by soluble CD40L levels.[62] These findings are very promising, but will need to be evaluated prospectively before they can be considered for routine use in the management of ACS.

Another example of the potential role of thrombosis biomarkers in ACS is the use of thrombin level measurement in a cohort of ACS managed with intravenous unfractionated heparin. Intravenous unfractionated heparin has been associated with decreasing or stabilizing markers of thrombin activity.[57,63,64] Stopping unfractionated heparin therapy has been associated with an increase in these markers.[65] In patients with heparin-resistant increases in thrombin activity, there is angiographic evidence of intracoronary thrombus and ischemic complications in coronary interventions.[51] These results suggest that following markers of thrombin activity levels may help guide decisions in regard to initiation and duration of anticoagulation therapy. However, a prospective study would be needed to evaluate such an approach before it could be clinically utilized.

Congestive Heart Failure

Heart failure (HF) is associated with thrombotic events, such as strokes, left ventricular thrombus, and deep venous thrombosis.

Thrombosis biomarkers have been associated with HF, and these prothrombotic profiles provide a potential mechanistic understanding for the development of thrombotic events in patients with HF and potentially a role in the clinical management of these patients.

Some evidence suggests that there may be distinct prothrombotic biomarker profiles in patients with stable versus decompensated heart failure.[66,67] Amongst biomarkers of coagulation, thrombin, fibrinogen, and tissue factor, all have been associated with HF.[66,68–74] Of these coagulation biomarkers, only higher levels of TF have been associated with acute HF patients versus chronic patients, based on a study by Chin et al. comparing 77 patients with acute HF with 53 patients with chronic stable disease.[66]

Endothelial cell biomarkers have also been evaluated in their role in distinguishing between acute and chronic HF. The endothelial cell biomarkers, circulating endothelial cells, vWF, P-selectin, and E-selectin have all been associated with HF.[66–68,70–72,75–79] In the study by Chin et al. mentioned above, the patients with acute HF had higher levels of vWF; however, in another small study by Chong et al. comparing 35 patients with acute HF and 40 patients with chronic HF, no differences were observed in vWF or E-selectin levels between the two groups.[66,67] Another study of 30 patients with acute HF and 30 patients with chronic HF also showed no evidence of elevated levels of vWF, E-selectin, or circulating endothelial cells in patients with acute versus chronic HF.[77] The small number of patients in each of these studies makes any definitive interpretation of this data difficult, and, given the conflicting data results, sufficient evidence does not exist to support use of endothelial cell biomarkers for distinguishing acute versus chronic HF.

Anticoagulation biomarkers have also been evaluated in their capacity to distinguish between acute and chronic HF. Thrombomodulin and tPA both have been associated with HF.[67,68,75] In a small study by Chong et al., thrombomodulin levels were higher in those with acute HF.[67]

Thrombosis biomarkers have also been associated with the prognosis of HF patients (Table 27–3). In the studies by Chin et al. and Chong et al., HF patients with higher levels of vWF were associated with higher 6-month mortality rates and a combined CV endpoint, respectively.[66,67] However, in a study by Kistorp et al. comparing 195 patients with HF to 116 controls, vWF was elevated in HF patients, but was not associated with future CV events.[76–79]

Several other thrombosis biomarkers have also been evaluated in regards to their prognostic importance in HF. In the analysis by Kistorp et al., elevated levels of E-selectin were associated with risk of recurrent ischemic CV events among HF patients with diabetes.[76] In a study by Marcucci et al., 214 subjects with NYHA Class II–IV HF were followed prospectively and D-dimer was found to be an independent predictor of death at median follow-up of 8.5 months,[80] while in a separate analysis, lower levels of tissue factor in HF patients were associated with improved CV endpoints, including reduced mortality.[66] While these studies demonstrate interesting findings in regards to an association among E-selectin, D-dimer, and TF and future CV events in patients with HF, they are isolated findings in single studies and need further validation in larger and more diverse patient cohorts before they can be considered for use in routine clinical care.

From a therapeutic perspective, as noted, patients with AF are at high risk for embolism, and those with HF and AF are at highest risk. In a single-center randomized placebo controlled trial (n = 76 patients with HF) to test the effects of warfarin on thrombosis biomarkers, warfarin resulted in a decrease in markers of thrombin activity and D-dimer,[73] while in a study of 59 patients with stable HF, anticoagulation with warfarin was associated with greater vWF size and lower levels of markers of thrombin activity, but no change in fibrinogen, TF, or D-dimer levels.[81] Similarly, in a randomized double-blinded placebo-controlled trial evaluating the effects of low molecular weight heparin on thrombosis biomarkers in 100 HF patients, heparin was associated with a decrease in markers of thrombin activity and D-dimer.[82]

Table 27–3: Thrombosis markers in heart failure.

Thrombosis biomarker	Study	Study design	Study population	Sample size	Outcome	Independent associations
vWF	Chin et al.	Case control	Acute HF	130 cases	Mortality	?
	Chong et al.	Case-control	Acute and chronic HF	75 cases	CV death, MI, stroke, cardiac transplant, HF admission	?
	Kistorp et al.	Case-control	Chronic HF	195 cases	Ischemic CV events	No
E-selectin	Chong et al.	Case-control	Acute and chronic HF	75 cases	CV death, MI, stroke, cardiac transplant, HF admission	No
	Kistorp et al.	Case-control	Chronic HF	195 cases	Ischemic CV events	?
Tissue factor	Chin et al.	Case-control	Acute HF	130 cases	Mortality	No
D-dimer	Marcucci et al.	Cohort	Chronic HF	214 cases	Mortality	Yes
Thrombin-antithrombin III complex	Marcucci et al.	Cohort	Chronic HF	214 cases	Mortality	No
Soluble thrombomodulin	Chong et al.	Case-control	Acute and chronic HF	75 cases	CV death, MI, stroke, cardiac transplant, HF admission	No

Conclusion: The Future of Thrombosis Biomarkers

Despite a large body of promising research on thrombosis biomarkers in cardiovascular disease, sufficient evidence does not yet exist to support the use of any of them in the management of cardiovascular disease. Given the low yield of clinically-applicable thrombosis biomarkers in cardiovascular disease to date, considerable challenges still lie ahead in advancing the field of thrombosis biomarkers. Fortunately, advances in research platforms for biomarker discovery and clinical application will help meet these challenges.

Advances in high throughput platforms such as genomics, transcriptomics, proteomics, and metabolomics will increase the pace of the discovery phase of thrombosis biomarker research in an unbiased fashion, as well as provide greater insight into the mechanisms underlying cardiovascular thrombotic disorders. These "-omic" platforms will allow for the development of human biosignatures associated with various disease states of thrombotic events. Genomics will help define a patient's inherent risk of developing future thrombotic events. Transcriptomics, proteomics, and metabolomics will not only help determine a patient's risk of CV events, but will also help diagnose and stage diseases and guide clinical management decisions. For example, in the field of platelet biomarkers, the "-omics" platforms have demonstrated significant potential in fully characterizing platelet biology in atherothrombotic disorders and identifying prothrombotic signatures.[83] Furthermore, integrating "-omics" platforms into drug trials would also improve drug development in multiple ways, such as identifying predictors of response and toxicity to therapy.[84]

References

1. Biomarkers Definitions Working Group. Biomarkers and surrogate endpoints: preferred definitions and conceptual framework. *Clin Pharmacol Ther*. 2001;69(3):89–95.

2. Vasan RS. Biomarkers of cardiovascular disease: molecular basis and practical considerations. *Circulation.* 2006;113(19):2335–2362. Review.

3. Conway DS, Buggins P, Hughes E, Lip GY. Relationship of interleukin-6 and C-reactive protein to the prothrombotic state in chronic atrial fibrillation. *J Am Coll Cardiol.* 2004;43(11):2075–2082.

4. Roldán V, Marín F, Blann AD, et al. Interleukin-6, endothelial activation and thrombogenesis in chronic atrial fibrillation. *Eur Heart J.* 2003;24(14):1373–1380.

5. Li-Saw-Hee FL, Blann AD, Edmunds E, Gibbs CR, Lip GY. Effect of acute exercise on the raised plasma fibrinogen, soluble P-selectin and von Willebrand factor levels in chronic atrial fibrillation. *Clin Cardiol.* 2001;24(5):409–414.

6. Roldán V, Marín F, Marco P, et al. Anticoagulant therapy modifies fibrinolytic dysfunction in chronic atrial fibrillation. *Haemostasis.* 2000;30(4):219–224.

7. Mondillo S, Sabatini L, Agricola E, et al. Correlation between left atrial size, prothrombotic state and markers of endothelial dysfunction in patients with lone chronic nonrheumatic atrial fibrillation. *Int J Cardiol.* 2000;75(2–3):227–232.

8. Kahn SR, Solymoss S, Flegel KM. Nonvalvular atrial fibrillation: evidence for a prothrombotic state. *CMAJ.* 1997;157(6):673–681.

9. Mitusch R, Siemens HJ, Garbe M, Wagner T, Sheikhzadeh A, Diederich KW. Detection of a hypercoagulable state in nonvalvular atrial fibrillation and the effect of anticoagulant therapy. *Thromb Haemost.* 1996;75(2):219–223.

10. Lip GY, Lowe GD, Rumley A, Dunn FG. Increased markers of thrombogenesis in chronic atrial fibrillation: effects of warfarin treatment. *Br Heart J.* 1995;73(6):527–533.

11. Marín F, Roldán V, Climent VE, et al. Plasma von Willebrand factor, soluble thrombomodulin, and fibrin D-dimer concentrations in acute onset non-rheumatic atrial fibrillation. *Heart.* 2004;90(10):1162–1166.

12. Tsai LM, Chen JH, Tsao CJ. Relation of left atrial spontaneous echo contrast with prethrombotic state in atrial fibrillation associated with systemic hypertension, idiopathic dilated cardiomyopathy, or no identifiable cause (lone). *Am J Cardiol.* 1998;81(10):1249–1252.

13. Freestone B, Chong AY, Nuttall S, Blann AD, Lip GY. Soluble E-selectin, von Willebrand factor, soluble thrombomodulin, and total body nitrate/nitrite product as indices of endothelial damage/dysfunction in paroxysmal, persistent, and permanent atrial fibrillation. *Chest.* 2007;132(4):1253–1258. Epub 2007 Sep 21.

14. Conway DS, Buggins P, Hughes E, Lip GY. Relation of interleukin-6, C-reactive protein, and the prothrombotic state to transesophageal echocardiographic findings in atrial fibrillation. *Am J Cardiol.* 2004;93(11):1368–1373, A6.

15. Varughese GI, Patel JV, Tomson J, Lip GY. Effects of blood pressure on the prothrombotic risk in 1235 patients with non-valvular atrial fibrillation. *Heart.* 2007;93(4):495–499. Epub 2006 Sep 27.

16. Heppell RM, Berkin KE, McLenachan JM, Davies JA. Haemostatic and haemodynamic abnormalities associated with left atrial thrombosis in non-rheumatic atrial fibrillation. *Heart.* 1997;77(5):407–411.

17. Choudhury A, Chung I, Blann AD, Lip GY. Elevated platelet microparticle levels in nonvalvular atrial fibrillation: relationship to p-selectin and antithrombotic therapy. *Chest.* 2007;131(3):809–815.

18. Choudhury A, Chung I, Blann AD, Lip GY. Platelet surface CD62P and CD63, mean platelet volume, and soluble/platelet P-selectin as indexes of platelet function in atrial fibrillation: a comparison of "healthy control subjects" and "disease control subjects" in sinus rhythm. *J Am Coll Cardiol.* 2007;49(19):1957–1964. Epub 2007 Apr 30.

19. Hatzinikolaou-Kotsakou E, Kartasis Z, Tziakas D, et al. Atrial fibrillation and hypercoagulability: dependent on clinical factors or/and on genetic alterations? *J Thromb Thrombolysis.* 2003;16(3):155–161.

20. Li-Saw-Hee FL, Blann AD, Gurney D, Lip GY. Plasma von Willebrand factor, fibrinogen and soluble P-selectin levels in paroxysmal, persistent and permanent atrial fibrillation. Effects of cardioversion and return of left atrial function. *Eur Heart J.* 2001;22(18):1741–1747.

21. Conway DS, Pearce LA, Chin BS, Hart RG, Lip GY. Plasma von Willebrand factor and soluble p-selectin as indices of endothelial damage and platelet activation in 1321 patients with nonvalvular atrial fibrillation: relationship to stroke risk factors. *Circulation.* 2002;106(15):1962–1967.

22. Conway DS, Pearce LA, Chin BS, Hart RG, Lip GY. Prognostic value of plasma von Willebrand factor and soluble P-selectin as indices of endothelial damage and platelet activation in 994 patients with nonvalvular atrial fibrillation. *Circulation.* 2003;107(25):3141–3145.

23. Pengo V, Filippi B, Biasiolo A, Pegoraro C, Noventa F, Iliceto S. Association of the G20210A mutation in the factor II gene with systemic embolism in nonvalvular atrial fibrillation. *Am J Cardiol.* 2002;90(5):545–547.

24. Poli D, Antonucci E, Cecchi E, et al. Thrombophilic mutations in high-risk atrial fibrillation patients: high prevalence of prothrombin gene G20210A polymorphism and lack of correlation with thromboembolism. *Thromb Haemost.* 2003;90(6):1158–1162.

25. Jacob K, Talwar S, Copplestone A, Gilbert TJ, Haywood GA. Activation of coagulation occurs after electrical cardioversion in patients with chronic atrial fibrillation despite optimal anticoagulation with warfarin. *Int J Cardiol.* 2004;95(1):83–88.

26. Oltrona L, Broccolino M, Merlini PA, Spinola A, Pezzano A, Mannucci PM. Activation of the hemostatic mechanism after pharmacological cardioversion of acute nonvalvular atrial fibrillation. *Circulation.* 1997;95:2003–2006.

27. Vene N, Mavri A, Kosmelj K, Stegnar M. High D-dimer levels predict cardiovascular events in patients with chronic atrial fibrillation during oral anticoagulant therapy. *Thromb Haemost.* 2003;90(6):1163–1172.

28. Kamath S, Blann AD, Chin BS, Lip GY. A prospective randomized trial of aspirin-clopidogrel combination therapy and dose-adjusted warfarin on indices of thrombogenesis and platelet activation in atrial fibrillation. *J Am Coll Cardiol.* 2002;40(3):484–490.

29. Roldán V, Marín F, Marco P, Martínez JG, Calatayud R, Sogorb F. Hypofibrinolysis in atrial fibrillation. *Am Heart J.* 1998;136(6): 956–960.

30. Li-Saw-Hee FL, Blann AD, Lip GY. Effects of fixed low-dose warfarin, aspirin-warfarin combination therapy, and dose-adjusted warfarin on thrombogenesis in chronic atrial fibrillation. *Stroke.* 2000;31(4): 828–833.

31. Figueras J, Monasterio Y, Lidon RM, Nieto E, Soler-Soler J. Thrombin formation and fibrinolytic activity in patients with acute myocardial

infarction or unstable angina: in-hospital course and relationship with recurrent angina at rest. *J Am Coll Cardiol.* 2000;36:2036–2043.

32. Ardissino D, Merlini PA, Gamba G, et al. Thrombin activity and early outcome in unstable angina pectoris. *Circulation.* 1996;93:1634–1639.

33. Ma J, Hennekens CH, Ridker PM, Stampfer MJ. A prospective study of fibrinogen and risk of myocardial infarction in the Physicians' Health Study. *J Am Coll Cardiol.* 1999;33:1347–1352.

34. Thompson SG, Kienast J, Pyke SD, Haverkate F, van de Loo JC. Hemostatic factors and the risk of myocardial infarction or sudden death in patients with angina pectoris. European Concerted Action on Thrombosis and Disabilities Angina Pectoris Study Group. *N Engl J Med.* 1995;332:635–641.

35. Suefuji H, Ogawa H, Yasue H, et al. Increased plasma tissue factor levels in acute myocardial infarction. *Am Heart J.* 1997;134:253–259.

36. Soejima H, Ogawa H, Yasue H, et al. Heightened tissue factor associated with tissue factor pathway inhibitor and prognosis in patients with unstable angina. *Circulation.* 1999;99:2908–2913.

37. Scarabin PY, Aillaud MF, Amouyel P, et al. Associations of fibrinogen, factor VII and PAI-1 with baseline findings among 10,500 male participants in a prospective study of myocardial infarction—the PRIME Study. Prospective Epidemiological Study of Myocardial Infarction. *Thromb Haemost.* 1998;80(5):749–756.

38. Ernst E, Resch KL. Fibrinogen as a cardiovascular risk factor: a meta-analysis and review of the literature. *Ann Intern Med.* 1993;118(12):956–963.

39. Li YH, Teng JK, Tsai WC, et al. Prognostic significance of elevated hemostatic markers in patients with acute myocardial infarction. *J Am Coll Cardiol.* 1999;33(6):1543–1548.

40. Galvani M, Ferrini D, Ottani F, Eisenberg PR. Early risk stratification of unstable angina/non-Q myocardial infarction: biochemical markers of coronary thrombosis. *Int J Cardiol.* 1999;68 Suppl 1:S55–S61.

41. Morange PE, Simon C, Alessi MC, et al. Endothelial cell markers and the risk of coronary heart disease: the Prospective Epidemiological Study of Myocardial Infarction (PRIME) study. *Circulation.* 2004;109:1343–1348.

42. Whincup PH, Danesh J, Walker M, et al. von Willebrand factor and coronary heart disease: prospective study and meta-analysis. *Eur Heart J.* 2002;23:1764–1770.

43. Gurbel PA, Serebruany VL, Shustov AR, et al. Increased baseline levels of platelet P-selectin, and platelet-endothelial cell adhesion molecule-I in patients with acute myocardial infarction as predictors of unsuccessful thrombolysis. *Coron Artery Dis.* 1998;9:451–456.

44. Francis S. Endothelial progenitor cells and coronary artery disease. *Heart.* 2004;90:591–592.

45. Mutin M, Canavy I, Blann A, Bory M, Sampol J, Dignat-George F. Direct evidence of endothelial injury in acute myocardial infarction and unstable angina by demonstration of circulating endothelial cells. *Blood.* 1999;93:2951–2958.

46. Cook NR. Use and misuse of the receiver operating characteristic curve in risk prediction. *Circulation.* 2007;115:928–935.

47. Salomaa V, Matei C, Aleksic N, et al. Soluble thrombomodulin as a predictor of incident coronary heart disease and symptomless carotid artery atherosclerosis in the Atherosclerosis Risk in Communities (ARIC) Study: a case-cohort study. *Lancet.* 1999;353:1729–1734.

48. Collet JP, Montalescot G, Vicaut E, et al. Acute release of plasminogen activator inhibitor-l in ST-segment elevation myocardial infarction predicts mortality. *Circulation.* 2003;108:391–394.

49. Hamsten A, Wiman B, de Faire U, Blomback M. Increased plasma levels of a rapid inhibitor of tissue plasminogen activator in young survivors of myocardial infarction. *N Engl J Med.* 1985;313:1557–1563.

50. Ridker PM, Vaughan DE, Stampfer MJ, Manson JE, Hennekens, CH. Endogenous tissue-type plasminogen activator and risk of myocardial infarction. *Lancet.* 1993;341:1165–1168.

51. Folsom AR, Aleksic N, Park E, Salomaa V, Juneja H, Wu KK. Prospective study of fibrinolytic factors and incident coronary heart disease: the Atherosclerosis Risk in Communities (ARIC) Study. *Arterioscl Thromb Vasc Biol.* 2001;21:611–617.

52. Thögersen AM, Jansson JH, Boman K, et al. High plasminogen activator inhibitor and tissue plasminogen activator levels in plasma precede a first acute myocardial infarction in both men and women: evidence

for the fibrinolytic system as an independent primary risk factor. *Circulation.* 1998;98(21):2241–2247.

53. Norlund L, Holm J, Zoller B, Ohlin AK. A common thrombomodulin amino acid dimorphism is associated with myocardial infarction. *Thromb Haemost.* 1997;77:248–251.
54. Doggen CJ, Kunz G, Rosendaal FR, et al. A mutation in the thrombomodulin gene, 127G to A coding for Ala25Thr, and the risk of myocardial infarction in men. *Thromb Haemost.* 1998;80:743–748.
55. Wu KK, Aleksic N, Ahn C, et al. Thrombomodulin Ala455Val polymorphism and risk of coronary heart disease. *Circulation.* 2001;103:1386–1389.
56. Iacoviello L, Burzotta F, Di Castelnuovo A, Zito F, Marchioli R, Donati MB. The 4G/5G polymorphism of PAI-l promoter gene and the risk of myocardial infarction: a meta-analysis. *Thromb Haemost.* 1998;80:1029–1030.
57. Reiner AP, Siscovick DS, Rosendaal FR. Hemostatic risk factors and arterial thrombotic disease. *Thromb Haemost.* 2001;85:584–595.
58. Arnaud E, Barbalat V, Nicaud V, et al. Polymorphisms in the 5′ regulatory region of the tissue factor gene and the risk of myocardial infarction and venous thromboembolism: the ECTIM and PATHROS studies. Etude Cas-Témoins de l'Infarctus du Myocarde. Paris Thrombosis case-control Study. *Arterioscl Thromb Vasc Biol.* 2000;20:892–898.
59. Ridker PM, Baker MT, Hennekens CH, Stampfer MJ, Vaughan DE. Alu-repeat polymorphism in the gene coding for tissue-type plasminogen activator (tPA) and risks of myocardial infarction among middle-aged men. *Arterioscl Thromb Vasc Biol.* 1997;17:1687–1690.
60. Ridker PM, Hennekens CH, Schmitz C, Stampfer MJ, Lindpaintner K. PIA1/A2 polymorphism of platelet glycoprotein IIa and risks of myocardial infarction, stroke, and venous thrombosis. *Lancet.* 1997;349:385–388.
61. Poirier O, Georges JL, Ricard S, et al. New polymorphisms of the angiotensin II type I receptor gene and their associations with myocardial infarction and blood pressure: the ECTIM study. Etude Cas-Témoin de 1'1nfarctus du Myocarde. *J Hypertens.* 1998;16:1443–1447.
62. Heeschen C, Dimmeler S, Hamm CW, et al. Soluble CD40 ligand in acute coronary syndromes. *N Engl J Med.* 2003;348:1104–1111.

63. Mombelli G, Marchetti O, Haeberli A, Straub PW. Effect of intravenous heparin infusion on thrombin-antithrombin complex and fibrinopeptide A in unstable angina. *Am Heart J.* 1998;136(6):1106–1113.

64. Granger CB, Becker R, Tracy RP, et al. Thrombin generation, inhibition and clinical outcomes in patients with acute myocardial infarction treated with thrombolytic therapy and heparin: results from the GUSTO-I Trial. GUSTO-I Hemostasis Substudy Group. Global Utilization of Streptokinase and TPA for Occluded Coronary Arteries. *J Am Coll Cardiol.* 1998;31(3):497–505.

65. Granger CB, Miller JM, Bovill EG, et al. Rebound increase in thrombin generation and activity after cessation of intravenous heparin in patients with acute coronary syndromes. *Circulation.* 1995;91(7): 1929–1935.

66. Chin BS, Conway DS, Chung NA, Blann AD, Gibbs CR, Lip GY. Interleukin-6, tissue factor and von Willebrand factor in acute decompensated heart failure: relationship to treatment and prognosis. *Blood Coagul Fibrinolysis.* 2003;14(6):515–521.

67. Chong AY, Freestone B, Patel J, et al. Endothelial activation, dysfunction, and damage in congestive heart failure and the relation to brain natriuretic peptide and outcomes. *Am J Cardiol.* 2006;97(5):671–675. Epub 2006 Jan 10.

68. Cugno M, Mari D, Meroni PL, et al. Haemostatic and inflammatory biomarkers in advanced chronic heart failure: role of oral anticoagulants and successful heart transplantation. *Br J Haematol.* 2004; 126(1):85–92.

69. Banfi C, Brioschi M, Barcella S, et al. Oxidized proteins in plasma of patients with heart failure: role in endothelial damage. *Eur J Heart Fail.* 2008;10(3):244–251.

70. Vila V, Martínez-Sales V, Almenar L, Lázaro IS, Villa P, Reganon E. Inflammation, endothelial dysfunction and angiogenesis markers in chronic heart failure patients. *Int J Cardiol.* 2008;130:276–277.

71. Gibbs CR, Blann AD, Watson RD, Lip GY. Abnormalities of hemorheological, endothelial, and platelet function in patients with chronic heart failure in sinus rhythm: effects of angiotensin-converting enzyme inhibitor and beta-blocker therapy. *Circulation.* 2001; 103(13):1746–1751.

72. Mastroroberto P, Chello M, Perticone F. Elevated circulating levels of von Willebrand factor and D-dimer in patients with heart failure and mechanical prosthesis. *Scand J Thorac Cardiovasc Surg.* 1996;30(2): 77–81.

73. Jafri SM, Mammen EF, Masura J, Goldstein S. Effects of warfarin on markers of hypercoagulability in patients with heart failure. *Am Heart J.* 1997;134(1):27–36.

74. Jafri SM, Ozawa T, Mammen E, Levine TB, Johnson C, Goldstein S. Platelet function, thrombin and fibrinolytic activity in patients with heart failure. *Eur Heart J.* 1993;14(2):205–212.

75. Chong AY, Blann AD, Patel J, Freestone B, Hughes E, Lip GY. Endothelial dysfunction and damage in congestive heart failure: relation of flow-mediated dilation to circulating endothelial cells, plasma indexes of endothelial damage, and brain natriuretic peptide. *Circulation.* 2004;110(13):1794–1798. Epub 2004 Sep 13.

76. Kistorp C, Chong AY, Gustafsson F, et al. Biomarkers of endothelial dysfunction are elevated and related to prognosis in chronic heart failure patients with diabetes but not in those without diabetes. *Eur J Heart Fail.* 2008;10(4):380–387. Epub 2008 Mar 17.

77. Chong AY, Lip GY, Freestone B, Blann AD. Increased circulating endothelial cells in acute heart failure: comparison with von Willebrand factor and soluble E-selectin. *Eur J Heart Fail.* 2006;8(2):167–172. Epub 2005 Sep 26.

78. Lip GY, Pearce LA, Chin BS, Conway DS, Hart RG. Effects of congestive heart failure on plasma von Willebrand factor and soluble P-selectin concentrations in patients with non-valvular atrial fibrillation. *Heart.* 2005;91(6):759–763.

79. Stumpf C, Lehner C, Eskafi S, et al. Enhanced levels of CD154 (CD40 ligand) on platelets in patients with chronic heart failure. *Eur J Heart Fail.* 2003;5(5):629–637.

80. Marcucci R, Gori AM, Giannotti F, et al. Markers of hypercoagulability and inflammation predict mortality in patients with heart failure. *J Thromb Haemost.* 2006;4(5):1017–1022.

81. Vila V, Sales VM, Almenar L, Lázaro IS, Villa P, Reganon E. Effect of oral anticoagulant therapy on thrombospondin-1 and von Willebrand factor in patients with stable heart failure. *Thromb Res.* 2008;121(5):611–615. Epub 2007 Aug 10.

82. De Lorenzo F, Newberry D, Scully M, et al. Low molecular weight heparin (bemiparin sodium) and the coagulation profile of patients with heart failure. *Am Heart J.* 2002;143(4):689.

83. Becker R. Platelets from genome to proteome and beyond. *J Thromb Thrombolysis.* 2007;23(3):245–248.

84. Becker R. A rationale for conducting parallel mechanistic studies in clinical trials of pharmacotherapy. *J Thromb Thrombolysis.* 2008; 25(3):300–302.

28 ■ Markers of Platelet Function and Assessment of Platelet Activation and Aggregation

VICTOR L. SEREBRUANY, MD, PHD

Introduction

New therapies for the treatment of vascular disease are being discovered every day. Considering that platelets play a key role in the development of such diseases, modern antiplatelet regimens are commonly used and necessitate the obvious need for serial assessment of the platelet function. Some have been used for many years, such as conventional platelet aggregometry, and some are quite new and evolving.[1] As new therapies and indications for antiplatelet therapy arise, the importance of reliable methods for monitoring the *in vitro* and *ex vivo* effects of these therapies is estimable. On the other hand, our ability to predict worsened vascular outcomes or excess bleeding risks by the changes of platelet activity biomarkers is very limited, if it exists at all. Trustable biomarkers to measure antiplatelet effect are necessary, but still presently lacking.

Before biomarkers of platelet function are to be used in a more widespread manner, it will be necessary to better comprehend their shortcomings for justification of monitoring antiplatelet regimens. For example, we have no answer yet as to whether or not baseline heightened platelet activity leads to worsened vascular outcomes, and whether inhibiting platelets further will improve outcomes independently from standard intensity platelet activity. While the answers seem simple and obvious, real facts and credible data are mostly lacking.

Another missing piece of the puzzle is the target of platelet inhibition to balance thrombotic and bleeding risks. We do not know, for example, the optimal degree or range of residual platelet activity after aspirin or/and clopidogrel therapy for chronic prevention of vascular occlusive events, while simultaneously optimally avoiding excessive bleeding risks.[2] These data are urgently needed before transition to individual tailoring of antiplatelet regimens based on the serial assessment of platelet activity becomes a reality and can be intelligently advocated.

Platelets and Primary Hemostasis

Human platelets are small and discoid in shape, with dimensions of approximately 2.0–4.0 by 0.5 μm, and a mean volume of 7–11 fl.[1,3] They are the second most numerous cells in the blood normally circulating at between 150–45010^9/l. Platelets are anucleated discoid cells derived from megakaryocytes, and they typically circulate for ten days.[1,4] They have cytoplasmic granules known as dense granules and alpha granules. These organelles contain compounds that amplify the platelet response if they are released or secreted. Their shape and small size enables them to be pushed to the edge of vessels, placing them in the optimal location required to constantly survey the integrity of the vasculature. Platelets are also surprisingly multifunctional and are involved in various pathophysiological activities including: hemostasis and thrombosis, clot retraction, vessel constriction and repair, inflammation (including promotion of atherosclerosis), immunity, and even oncobiology (Figure 28–1).

When a blood vessel wall is damaged, platelets adhere to the wound edges; aggregate; synthesize prostaglandins; and release serotonin, ADP, and ATP. Prostaglandin synthesis and release products cause further aggregation. The coagulation cascade is initiated, thrombin is generated, fibrin is formed, and the platelet plug anchors to the damaged vessel.

The main function of platelets is the maintenance of blood vessel integrity by prevention of red cell migration through the vessel wall. Platelets also prevent vascular leakage by plugging any sites of damage or injury. When wounds expose the

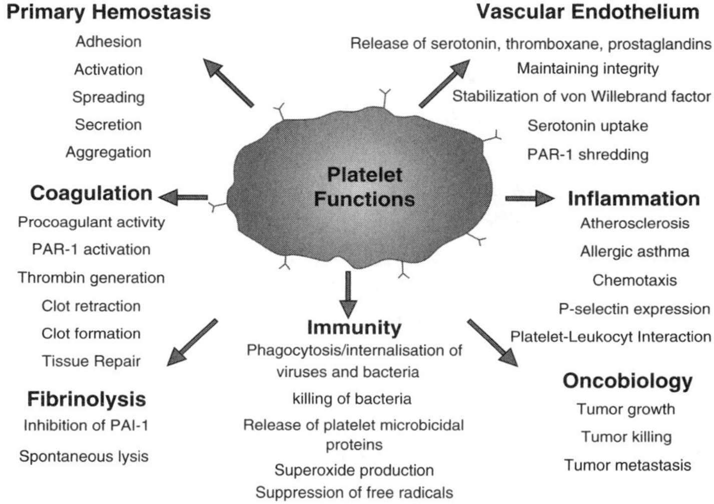

■ **Figure 28–1** The multifunctional platelet.

subendothelium and/or basement membrane, circulating platelets are recruited to the site to form a platelet aggregate. This physiologic reaction is known as the formation of the primary hemostatic plug. Platelets adhere and aggregate at any site of subendothelial exposure. Exposure of the subendothelium results in the unmasking of the structural protein collagen. Platelets adhere to the now-exposed collagen fibrils.[5] The platelets change shape and pseudopods are formed. The shape change and pseudopods result in closer contact with other individual platelets. More platelets are recruited and stimulated to undergo shape change, pseudopod formation, and granule release. This aggregated mass physically prevents leakage at the site. von Willebrand factor (found in the alpha granules of the platelets and circulating in the blood in association with Factor VIII) is classified as an adhesive protein. It interacts with a binding site on the platelet membrane and acts as a cornerstone to strengthen the platelets' adherence to the endothelium.[6]

Platelet Dysfunction

Defects in platelet function due to lack of a cell membrane glycoprotein, cytoplasmic storage granules, platelet enzymes, or a deficiency of plasma factor often result in excessive bleeding after trauma, frequent bruising after shaving and tooth brushing, nosebleeds, or excessive menstrual blood loss.

Upon vessel wall damage, platelets undergo a highly regulated set of functional responses including: adhesion, spreading, release reactions, aggregation, exposure of a procoagulant surface, microparticle formation, and clot retraction (Figure 28–2). All of these responses are mandatory for rapid formation of a hemostatic plug that occludes the site of damage to prevent blood loss.[7,8] When there is a defect in any of these functions and/or platelet quantity, hemostasis is usually impaired and there may be an associated increased risk of bleeding.

In contrast, a marked increase in platelet number or reactivity can lead to excess thrombus formation. Arterial thrombi can also develop within atherosclerotic lesions, resulting in ischemic stroke and myocardial infarction. Antiplatelet therapy can therefore be beneficial in the treatment and prevention of arterial thrombotic conditions, but must be carefully administered to maintain a delicate balance between outcome benefit and risk of bleeding.

The main use of platelet function tests has been traditionally to identify the potential causes of abnormal bleeding,[9] to monitor therapy affecting hemostasis in patients with a high risk of bleeding, and to ensure normal platelet function either prior to or during surgery.[10] However, platelet biomarkers are increasingly being utilized to monitor the efficacy of antiplatelet therapy and to potentially identify platelet hyperfunction to predict thrombosis.[11]

History of Platelet Function Testing

Platelets were first reliably described by the remarkably early observations of Bizzozero in the late 19th century.[12] Not only did he identify platelets as distinct corpuscles within human blood, but

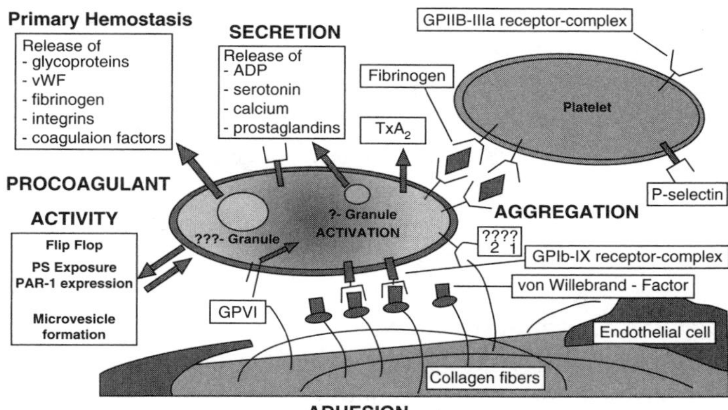

■ **Figure 28–2** The multiple roles, and cornerstone position of platelets in regulation of hemostasis. Vascular wall injury results in exposure of collagen and subendothelial proteins. Initial platelet adhesion is mediated via vWF binding to the Gp Ib/IX/V complex on the platelet surface. Collagen binding to the platelet GPVI results in cellular activation resulting in firm adhesion and spreading through the activated receptors Gp IIb/IIIa and a2b1. Platelet adhesion also results in platelet activation resulting in degranulation. These facilitate further local recruitment of platelets into the vicinity resulting in platelet aggregation mediated by fibrinogen and vWF bridging between activated Gp IIb/IIIa on adjacent cells. The exposure of anionic phospholipid provides a surface upon which platelets can support thrombin generation and fibrin formation resulting in stabilization of the resulting hemostatic plug.

he observed them forming thrombi within damaged areas of vessel wall using real-time optical microscopy. Today, modern imaging methods are capable of capturing in detail the same real-time interactions of platelets with the vessel wall and dynamics of thrombus formation.[13] In contrast to coagulation defects, for which screening tests (e.g., the activated partial thromboplastin time [APTT] and prothrombin time [PT]) are inexpensive, fully automated, and easy to perform, platelet function defects are much more difficult to diagnose because there are no definitive screening tests. Indeed, no current or future platelet function test is likely to be fully sensitive to a specific disease, due to the large number and variety of platelet defects.

The current evaluation of a potential platelet defect usually involves platelet aggregation and/or measurement of granule content/release. Platelet aggregation is labor-intensive, costly, time-consuming, and requires a fair degree of expertise and experience to perform and interpret.

Three major steps were needed for aggregometry to become the "gold standard" for platelet testing. First, in 1962, Born described the aggregation of platelets induced by ADP and modified a conventional colorimeter to continuously monitor this aggregation in platelet-rich plasma (PRP).[14] These modifications also included incubation at 37°C, stirring of the sample, and recording of the change in light transmission over time with a pen recorder. Then, in 1977, Feinman et al. designed an instrument to simultaneously measure platelet aggregation and ATP secretion.[15] This device utilized infrared light and a sensitive photomultiplier at right angles to the aggregation lightpath to measure ATP secretion by firefly luminescence. This was the first model of what is now known as an lumi-aggregometer. Finally, in 1980, Cardinal and Flower described the impedance method for measuring aggregation in whole blood.[16] First, a very small electric current is passed between two electrodes. During initial contact with the blood, the electrodes become coated with a monolayer of platelets. When an aggregating agent is added, platelets aggregate on the monolayer, increasing the impedance. This increase is recorded with a pen, or digitally. The addition of impedance measurement to the lumi-aggregometer rendered it the first whole blood lumi-aggregometer.

Quality Control, Samples, and Anticoagulants

Platelet function testing presents many challenges in ensuring that accurate and meaningful results are obtained. Firstly, unlike with coagulation tests, there are no widely-available internal or external quality control materials available.[17] Most assays are performed on fresh blood and many laboratories establish normal ranges using repeated control volunteer blood and/or assay-known normal samples in parallel to ensure that each test/reagent is viable.

Many platelet function tests, such as those using aggregometry, still remain poorly standardized. Different laboratories often use panels of different agonists, often with different ranges of concentrations. Normal platelet function is also largely calcium-dependent, so anticoagulation of the blood sample through calcium chelation can immediately present a validation problem.[3,17] Most laboratories utilize tests that require citrated blood samples within a narrow time window (<2 hours). Although this is convenient within a coagulation laboratory because citrate tubes are also used for clotting tests, the quality, handling, temperature, and age of the blood sample can also cause significant artifacts in platelet assays. Platelets are inherently prone to artificial activation, but also to desensitization. It is important that these are minimized during phlebotomy, anticoagulation, sample transit, and handling within the laboratory. Present guidelines require the following:

- using a light tourniquet,
- using a needle of at least 21 gauge,
- using a nontraumatic venipuncture with smooth blood flow,
- discarding the first few drops of blood drawn,
- using polypropylene or siliconized glass tubes/syringes,
- ensuring immediate gentle mixing with anticoagulant,
- minimizing delays from sampling to analysis,
- keeping all tubes at room temperature,
- checking that the blood tube is not over- or under-filled, and
- avoiding unnecessary manipulation of the sample (e.g., in the studies of McKenzie et al. and Kottke-Marchant and Corcoran)[18,19]

Therefore, ensuring sample quality is of utmost importance before any platelet aggregation study is performed.

Aggregometry can be performed within commercially-available multichannel aggregometers. Whole blood aggregometers using impedance technology are also available and are sometimes combined with luminometry to simultaneously measure dense granular ADP release. However, in most laboratories, citrated blood is normally centrifuged to obtain PRP, which is stirred within a cuvette incubated at 37°C between a light source and a sensor detector. Upon addition of various concentrations of a panel of agonists (e.g., collagen, ADP, thrombin, ristocetin, adrenaline, etc.), the platelets aggregate and light transmission increases. Classical platelet responses to each agonist can then be monitored including: lag phase, shape change, and primary and secondary aggregation. Parameters measured include the rate (slope) of aggregation and the maximal amplitude (%) or percentage of aggregation after a fixed period of time.

In short, platelet aggregation is at present the most useful *in vitro* test of platelet function presently available. When used correctly, it may be a valid and reliable diagnostic tool, which can provide insight that is difficult or impossible to obtain by other techniques, thus aiding in patient diagnosis and proper selection of treatment or therapy. Experience with this technique has delineated a spectrum of inherited and acquired platelet dysfunctional conditions and has opened up a potential field of biomarker-driven drug therapy options. The platelet-related effects of some medications are outlined in Table 28–1.

Interpretation

The most common cause of platelet dysfunction detected with aggregometry among patients with heart disease in general—and those after acute events in particular—is directly related to medication effects. With aspirin and related compounds, arachidonate aggregation is markedly decreased (below 10%) or almost absent (1–2%), and aggregation induced by other agonists may be variably impaired.[20] A variety of other platelet inhibiting agents, such as P2Y12 inhibitors (e.g., ticlopidine clopidogrel, prasugrel), and

Table 28–1: Diagnostic utility of platelet aggregation for monitoring antiplatelet agents.

ANTIPLATELET AGENT	CHANGES IN AGGREGATION PROFILE
Aspirin	Impaired response to arachidonic acid, epinephrine, collagen
Clopidogrel, ticlopidine, prasugrel	Reduction of ADP-induced aggregation and collagen-induced response slightly after loading dose
Abciximab, eptifibatide, tirofiban	>80% reduction of ADP and collagen-induced aggregation
PAR-1 receptor antagonists	Complete inhibition of TRAP-induced aggregation
Selective serotonin reuptake inhibitors	Diminished serotonin-induced aggregation
Angiotensin receptor blockers	Slight inhibition on ADP and collagen

glycoprotein IIb/IIIa receptor blockers (e.g., abciximab) are well-known to impair platelet aggregation. Indeed, the use of aggregometry may be of special use in monitoring the effects of antiplatelet agents for efficacy (e.g., in the case of "resistance states" when higher doses of antiplatelet drugs are needed to achieve therapeutic effect), or for safety reasons (e.g., monitoring for "wash out" of a P2Y12 inhibitor prior to proceeding with surgical procedures).

A vast number of other medications—including angiotensin receptor blockers, selective serotonin reuptake inhibitors, and statins—have been implicated in impaired platelet aggregation,[21,22] although the clinical significance of these findings is unclear. If a patient is found to have impaired platelet aggregation in this assay, a careful review of prescribed, as well as over-the-counter medications is indicated. Other causes of impaired platelet aggregation include uremia and paraproteinemias. Myeloproliferative disorders can impair platelet aggregation due to epinephrine production, in particular. Hyperaggregation has also been reported with myeloproliferative disorders and various tumors.

Major hereditary platelet dysfunctions are probably far less common than acquired defects. However, the mechanism for development of severe, especially catastrophic hemorrhages is much more complex, and is not entirely dependent on platelet inhibition. Unrecognized latent genetic defects[23] should be considered suspects in cases of massive bleeding events despite average, and even low platelet inhibition after antiplatelet agents.[24,25] A hereditary disorder may be considered in patients with bleeding histories and no obvious acquired etiology to account for an abnormal platelet aggregation study. Ideally, the aggregation study should be repeated on a fresh specimen to determine if the abnormality is reproducible.

Platelet storage pool disorders may variably decrease responses to epinephrine, ADP, and occasionally other agonists. These disorders are characterized by deficiencies in alpha or dense platelet granules. Alpha granules normally store platelet factor 4 (PF4), beta thromboglobulin, and other substances. Alpha granule deficiency is a rare disorder called "gray platelet syndrome" because platelets appear gray with light microscopy due to a lack of such granules. In this syndrome, platelets are large; thrombocytopenia may be present. Dense granules normally contain ADP, serotonin, and other compounds. A research test for dense granule deficiency is the platelet ATP : ADP ratio, which is increased with this abnormality. In rare cases, some patients are deficient in both alpha and dense granules.

Rare genetic disorders may underlie some causes of storage pool deficiency, including Hermansky-Pudlak syndrome (dense granule deficiency with pulmonary fibrosis and albinism syndrome), Chediak-Higashi syndrome, Wiskott-Aldrich syndrome, or thrombocytopenia with absent radius syndrome. Glanzmann thrombasthenia is a rare inherited condition in which platelet glycoprotein IIb/IIIa is deficient; this receptor mediates platelet aggregation via interactions with fibrin. Therefore, in Glanzmann syndrome, aggregation is decreased with all agonists (ADP, collagen, epinephrine, and arachidonate) except risocetin, which agglutinates platelets using von Willebrand factor and platelet GP Ib. Bernard-Soulier disease is a rare inherited disorder characterized by GP Ib deficiency, and therefore decreased ristocetin-induced aggregation, a finding also seen in severe von Willebrand disease.

Conclusion

Platelet aggregation is the "gold standard" for assessing platelet function in the clinical setting. As a result, platelet function testing is increasingly utilized outside of the specialized hematology laboratory, mostly for the purpose of monitoring antiplatelet therapy, and/or predicting such adverse outcomes as rethrombosis or stent thrombosis (Table 28–2). Although this expansion represents an important advancement, validation, reliability, and quality control testing are still of concern. It is highly likely that in the near future important discoveries in the platelet genome[26] and proteome[27] will be made that will lead to many exciting advances in the field, such as platelet-specific microarrays, which may also have a significant impact upon the diagnosis and management of patients with either hemostatic or thrombotic defects.

Despite the established importance of platelet inhibition for treatment or prevention of thrombotic vascular events, recent oral antiplatelet drug development cannot be considered as a uniform success. In fact, the MATCH,[28] CHARISMA,[29] and TRITON[30] trials raise more concerns with regards to the questionable vascular efficacy, and obviously increased bleeding risks due to more potent combination antiplatelet regimens. Therefore, any attempt to identify high-risk cohorts associated with worsened clinical outcomes or potentially-excessive hemorrhagic complications should be undertaken—this being the top priority and direction for further antiplatelet drug development. It is in this setting that platelet aggregometry will have its most important application.

Table 28–2: A list of potential clinical applications for platelet aggregation.

Potential clinical utility	Comments
Screening for platelet dysfunction	Very reliable for screening purposes, rather than definite diagnosis
Monitoring DDAVP therapy	Test needs to detect the influence of released vWF
Monitoring vWF replacement therapy	Some concentrates lack high MW vWF
Monitoring pro-hemostatic therapy	Factor VIIa, platelet concentrates, DDAVP
Monitoring antiplatelet therapy	Increasingly used
Detecting drug resistance	Aspirin and/or thienopyridine resistance
Platelet dysfunction in menorrhagia	
Detection of platelet hyperfunction	Predicting thrombosis and vascular death?
Prediction of surgical bleeding	Can tests predict bleeding reliably?
Control of platelet concentrates	Monitoring the platelet storage quality

References

1. George JN. Platelets. *Lancet.* 2000;355:1531–1539.
2. Serebruany VL. The "clopidogrel resistance" trap. *Am J Cardiol.* 2007;100:1044–1046.
3. Harrison P. Platelet function analysis. *Blood Reviews.* 2005;19: 111–123.
4. Weiss HJ. Platelet physiology and abnormalities of platelet function. *New Eng J Med.* 1975;293:531–541.
5. Michelson AD. *Platelets.* San Diego: Academic Press; 2002.

6. Budde U, Schneppenheim R. Von Willebrand factor and vonWillebrand disease. *Rev Clin Exp Hematol.* 2001;5:335–368.
7. Rodgers GM. Overview of platelet physiology and laboratory evaluation of platelet function. *Clin Obstet Gynecol.* 1999;42:349–359.
8. Ruggeri ZM. Platelets in atherothrombosis. *Nat Med.* 2002;8: 1227–1234.
9. Peerschke EI. The laboratory evaluation of platelet dysfunction. *Clin Lab Med.* 2002;22:405–420.
10. Rand ML, Leung R, Packham MA. Platelet function assays. *Transfus Apheresis Sci.* 2003;28:307–317.
11. Tsiara S, Elisaf M, Jagroop IA, Mikhailidis DP. Platelets as predictors of vascular risk: is there a practical index of platelet activity? *Clin Appl Thromb Hemost.* 2003;9:177–190.
12. de Gaetano G. A new blood corpuscle: an impossible interview with Giulio Bizzozero. *Thromb Haemost.* 2001;86:973–979.
13. Celi A, Merrill-Skoloff G, Gross P, et al. Thrombus formation: direct real-time observation and digital analysis of thrombus assembly in a living mouse by confocal and widefield intravital microscopy. *J Thromb Haemost.* 2003;1:60–68.
14. Born GVR. Quantitative investigations into the aggregation of blood platelets. *J Physiol.* 1962;162:62–67.
15. Feinman RD, Lubowsky J, Charo I, Zabinski MP. The lumi-aggregometer: a new instrument for simultaneous measurement of aggregation and secretion. *J Lab Clin Med.* 1977;90:119–125.
16. Cardinal DC, Flower RJ. The electronic aggregometer: a novel device for assessing platelet behavior in blood. *J Pharmacol Meth.* 1980;3: 135–158.
17. Harrison P. Progress in the assessment of platelet function. *Br J Haematol.* 2000;111:733–744.
18. McKenzie ME, Gurbel PA, Levine DJ, Serebruany VL. Clinical utility of available methods for determining platelet function. *Cardiology.* 1999;92:240–247.
19. Kottke-Marchant K, Corcoran G. The laboratory diagnosis of platelet disorders. *Arch Pathol Lab Med.* 2002;126:133–146.
20. Malinin AI, Atar D, Callahan KP, McKenzie ME, Serebruany VL. Effects of a single dose aspirin on platelets in humans with multiple

risk factors for coronary artery disease. *Europ J Pharm.* 2003;462: 139–143.

21. Malinin A, Ong S, Makarov L, Petuchova E, Serebruany VL. Platelet inhibition beyond conventional antiplatelet agents: expanding role of angiotensin receptor blockers, statins, and selective serotonin reuptake inhibitors. *Int J Clin Pract.* 2006;60:993–1002.
22. Serebruany VL. Use of selective serotonin reuptake inhibitors is associated with increased bleeding risk: are we missing something? *Am J Med.* 2006;119:113–116.
23. Salles II, Feys HB, Iserbyt BF, De Meyer SF, Vanhoorelbeke K, Deckmyn H. Inherited traits affecting platelet function. *Blood Rev.* 2008;22:155–172.
24. Quiroga T, Goycoolea M, Panes O, et al. High prevalence of bleeders of unknown cause among patients with inherited mucocutaneous bleeding. A prospective study of 280 patients and 299 controls. *Haematologica.* 2007;92:357–365.
25. Franchini M, Mannucci PM. Interactions between genotype and phenotype in bleeding and thrombosis. *Haematologica.* 2008;93:649–652.
26. Gnatenko DV, Dunn JJ, McCorkle SR, et al. Transcript profiling of human platelets using microarray and serial analysis of gene expression. *Blood.* 2003;101:2285–2293.
27. Maguire PB, Fitzgerald DJ. Platelet proteomics. *J Thromb Haemost.* 2003;1:1593–1601.
28. Diener HC, Bogousslavsky J, Brass LM, et al. Aspirin and clopidogrel compared with clopidogrel alone after recent ischaemic stroke or transient ischaemic attack in high-risk patients (MATCH): randomised, double-blind, placebo-controlled trial. *Lancet.* 2004;364: 331–337.
29. Bhatt DL, Fox KA, Hacke W, et al. Clopidogrel and aspirin versus aspirin alone for the prevention of atherothrombotic events. *N Engl J Med.* 2006;354:1706–1717.
30. Wiviott SD, Braunwald E, McCabe CH, et al. Prasugrel versus clopidogrel in patients with acute coronary syndromes. *N Engl J Med.* 2007;357:2001–2015.

Section V

Lipid Markers

29 ▪ Contemporary Interpretation of Lipid Guidelines in Modern Medicine

Michael J. Blaha, MD
Roger S. Blumenthal, MD

Introduction

Atherosclerotic cardiovascular disease (CVD), including both coronary heart disease (CHD) and stroke, remains both highly prevalent and highly preventable. There are approximately 1,200,000 heart attacks per year in the United States, which includes 770,000 Americans suffering their first heart attack. Each year, about 780,000 people experience new or recurrent stroke.[1] While the mortality rate from these conditions is decreasing, CVD remains the leading cause of death in the United States—and with the exception of the year 1918, has been the leading cause for over 100 years.[1]

Cholesterol is a prerequisite for the central lesion in CHD, the atherosclerotic plaque. From an early age, dietary and endogenously-produced cholesterol accumulates in the intima and inner media of coronary arteries, leading to inflammation and endothelial dysfunction. Gradually, lipid accumulation leads to plaque growth into the lumen of coronary arteries, disrupting blood flow. An acute coronary syndrome (ACS) occurs when the fibrous cap overlying the lipid core ruptures or becomes disrupted, exposing oxidized lipid and other plaque contents to the bloodstream, leading to thrombosis and acute reduction of coronary perfusion.

Most patients that die of CHD suffer from high blood cholesterol.[2] The Framingham Heart Study, a large population-based cohort study of asymptomatic patients launched in 1948,

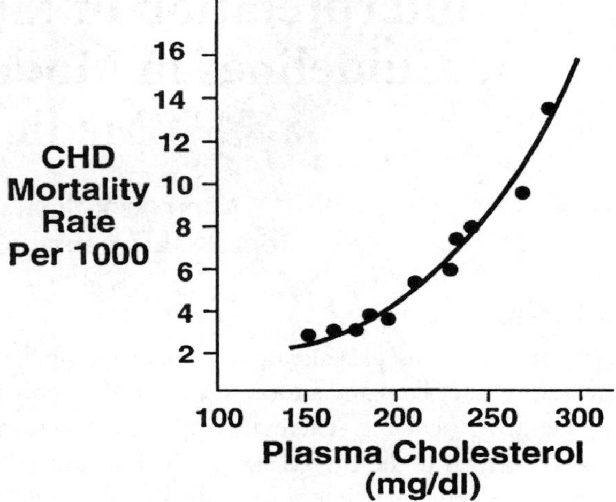

■ **Figure 29–1** The MRFIT study established the curvilinear relationship between total blood cholesterol and CHD mortality.

established the positive association between total cholesterol and CHD amongst both men and women.[3] Subsequently, the Multiple Risk Factor Intervention Trial (MRFIT) demonstrated a robust J-shaped curvilinear relationship between total cholesterol and CVD mortality (Figure 29–1), establishing ≥200 mg/dL as a common threshold for increased risk.[4] The Johns Hopkins Precursor Study[5] and the Bogalosa Heart Study[6] confirmed that early exposure to elevated cholesterol in young adulthood predicts CHD later in life.

From these observations emerged the "lipid hypothesis." Stating that reduction in blood cholesterol should lead to decreased incidence of CHD. First tested in the Lipid Research Clinics Coronary Primary Prevention Trial (LRC-CPPT)[7,8] and the Helsinki Heart Study,[9] and corroborated with data from modern statin trials, the central role of lipid lowering in CHD risk reduction has now been clearly established. Decreasing cholesterol has been shown to reduce initial coronary events, recurrent coronary events, and strokes, as well as to slow progression and induce regression of atherosclerosis.

To guide clinicians in the treatment of hypercholesterolemia, the NHLBI launched the National Cholesterol Education Program (NCEP) and convened the first Expert Panel on the Detection, Evaluation, and Treatment of High Blood Cholesterol in Adults (ATP I) in 1986. Since the publication of the initial guidelines, there has been a flurry of basic science and clinical research, leading to the formation of a distinct investigative and clinical specialty in lipidology. In an attempt to keep pace, the ATP updated their guidelines in 1993 and 2001 (with further modifications in 2004).

Guidelines, however, have lagged behind the latest scientific discoveries. For example, while current guidelines emphasize traditional lipoprotein cholesterol concentrations as measured on the routine lipid profile, much recent investigation has focused on the apolipoproteins and other novel lipid biomarkers that may offer distinct advantages (Table 29–1). In light of this, the modern clinician must be not only conversant in the latest guidelines, but must also anticipate their weaknesses and limitations and be proactive in incorporating the latest discoveries into their practice.

In this chapter, a modern approach to lipid guidelines for the primary and secondary prevention of CVD is discussed. Because the actual guidelines are readily available in online publications and are widely disseminated, focus will be placed on clinical trial data underpinning NCEP ATP guidelines, limitations of current recommendations, and anticipated changes in future iterations. To this end, the present chapter is divided into four parts: 1) The Role of Lipids in Atherosclerosis, 2) History and Evolution of the NCEP ATP Guidelines, 3) Limitations of the NCEP ATP III, and 4) The Future of Lipid Guidelines.

Table 29–1: Components of the routine lipid profile versus emerging lipid biomarkers.

Routine lipid profile	Emerging lipid biomarkers
• Total cholesterol	• Apolipoprotein B
• Triglycerides	• Apolipoprotein A-I
• HDL cholesterol	• VLDL
• LDL cholesterol (calculated value)	• VLDL particle size & density
Non-HDL cholesterol can be calculated by hand, not currently reported	• HDL particle size & density
	• LDL particle size & density
	• LDL particle number (LDL-P)
	• Lp(a)

Note: Many new biomarkers enhance the ability to predict CHD and offer new therapeutic targets, but are not routinely measured in clinical practice. Current guidelines use elements of the routine lipid profile to infer the presence of these emerging lipid risk factors.

The Role of Lipids in Atherosclerosis

Lipid Metabolism

Lipoproteins transport cholesterol and triglycerides to peripheral tissue for maintenance of the cell membrane, generation of cellular energy, and metabolism into new bioactive molecules. Lipoproteins vary in the identity of their constituent apolipoproteins, as well as their relative concentrations of cholesterol and triglycerides (Table 29–2). Even within classes of lipoproteins, densities of cholesterol and triglycerides vary, which impacts the relative size and thus the function of these particles (Figure 29–2).[10,11]

Blood cholesterol is derived from both dietary intake and endogenous production in the liver. Dietary lipids are absorbed in the intestines with the help of apolipoprotein B-48,

Table 29–2: Relative concentrations of triglycerides and cholesterol in the four major classes of lipoproteins.

	CHYLOMICRONS	VLDL	LDL	HDL
% Composition				
➢ Protein	1–2	10	25	50
➢ Triglyceride	90–96	60	5	5
➢ Cholesterol	2–5	12	50	20
➢ Phospholipid	5	18	20	25
Important apolipoproteins in atherogenesis	B-48, E	B-100, E	B-100	A-I, A-II

Note: The apolipoproteins present in the lipoproteins and play important roles in atherogenesis.

a degradation product of apolipoprotein B-100, and incorporated into the interior of chylomicrons. These triglyceride-rich chylomicrons are then absorbed into the bloodstream, where they are rapidly hydrolyzed by lipoprotein lipase at the capillary endothelium. The smaller degradation products are predominantly taken up by the liver; however, they can be taken up by other tissue, including walls of coronary arteries, via mechanisms mediated by apolipoprotein E.

Free fatty acids and cholesterol in the liver are synthesized into an important apolipoprotein B-100-containing lipoprotein termed "very low density lipoprotein" (VLDL). VLDL is the principal carrier of plasma triglycerides. Blood levels of VLDL and triglycerides are highly correlated; for this reason, routine triglycerides measurements can be considered surrogate measures for VLDL concentration. VLDL is broken down into intermediate density lipoprotein (IDL) by lipoprotein lipase; as a result, IDL is also elevated in the setting of high triglycerides. Smaller VLDL particles

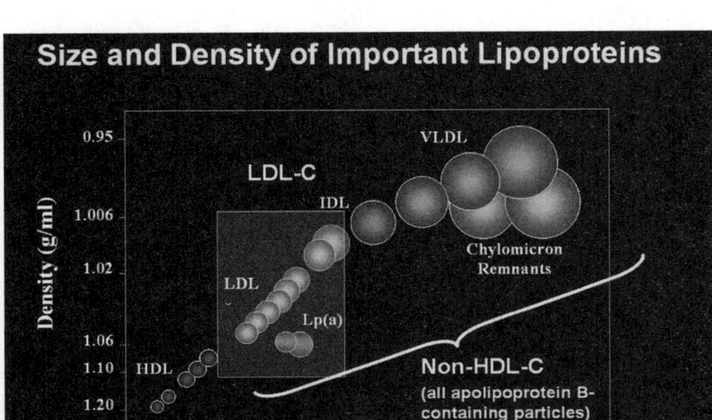

■ **Figure 29–2** Size and density of important lipoproteins. The liver produces VLDL, an apolipoprotein B-containing lipoprotein rich in triglycerides, for transport of lipid material to peripheral tissue. VLDL is broken down into IDL and VLDL remnants, which are all atherogenic lipoproteins. Further breakdown of the triglyceride core produces cholesterol ester enriched LDL, which is the primary determinant of atherosclerosis. HDL, the smallest and least dense lipoprotein, is important for reverse cholesterol transport and is antiatherogenic. Non-HDL-C is a more inclusive laboratory measure of all atherogenic apolipoprotein B-containing lipoproteins as compared to LDL-C.

and IDL may cross into the vessel wall and deliver cholesterol to a growing plaque in processes mediated in part by apolipoprotein B-100 and apolipoprotein E.

Further catabolism of VLDL results in cholesterol-rich low density lipoprotein (LDL), the principal determinant of atherosclerosis. The sole protein component of LDL is apolipoprotein B-100. In a pro-oxidative milieu, LDL is oxidized and made recognizable to type A scavenger receptors present on macrophages in the arterial wall. Oxidized LDL plays other critical roles in atherosclerosis such as increased chemotaxis of inflammatory cells, procoagulation, and reduced responsiveness to nitric oxide-induced vasodilation.[12]

High density lipoprotein (HDL), characterized by apolipoproteins A-I and A-II, is critical for reverse cholesterol transport back to the liver. The ABCA1 protein catalyzes the loading of free cholesterol from peripheral tissue to HDL. The cholesterol in HDL is then esterified, and subsequently taken up by the liver and either excreted or catabolized. In this way, HDL serves a critical role in removing cholesterol present in peripheral tissue from the body. In addition, HDL also has antioxidant and vasodilatory properties.[13]

The Conventional Lipid Profile

Subsequent analyses of the Framingham Heart Study identified high LDL and low HDL as the primary lipoprotein determinants of CHD, even in the context of low LDL[14] The addition of triglycerides, which have been shown in univariate analysis and some multivariate analyses to predict atherosclerotic disease (Figure 29–3),[15] completes the essential elements of the modern lipid panel, which currently drives decision making in clinical lipidology (Table 29–1).

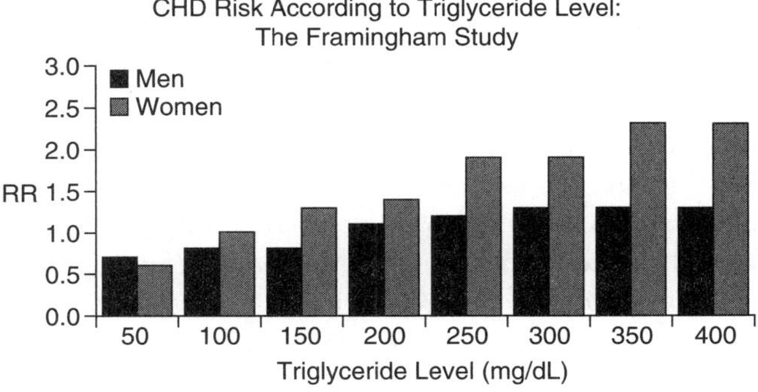

■ **Figure 29–3** The relationship between increasing triglycerides and increasing CHD risk as seen in the Framingham Heart Study.

Routine lipid panels should be drawn in the fasting state, as LDL is routinely a calculated value that relies on the triglyceride concentration according to the Freidewald equation: Total cholesterol–HDL–triglycerides/5 = calculated LDL.[16] Although the Freidewald equation is reasonably accurate in patients with "normal" fasting triglyceride values, it is not accurate in the non-fasting state due to postprandial triglyceride elevation.

Non-HDL Cholesterol and Advanced Lipoprotein Testing

From pioneering epidemiology and basic science work, we now understand the causal relationship between lipoprotein pathophysiology and the atherosclerotic plaque to be an order of magnitude more complicated than can be communicated with the routine lipid profile.[17] Yet little of this new knowledge is routinely reported and, thus, little of it routinely used. Lipoprotein particle sizes, concentrations, or "particle numbers" of lipoprotein classes, and specific apolipoprotein concentrations are emerging as potentially useful clinical parameters, but have heretofore been confined to the research setting or specialized lipid clinics because of expense, unavailability, and incomplete understanding of the clinical importance.[18]

While LDL remains the primary determinant of atherosclerosis, as triglycerides increase, other triglyceride-rich lipoproteins become important determinants of atherosclerosis.[19,20] Non-HDL, obtained by subtracting HDL from total cholesterol on a routine lipid panel, offers the benefit of being an aggregate measure that includes the concentrations of *all* lipoproteins currently thought to contribute to atherosclerosis. Included in this aggregate are all of the above-mentioned apolipoprotein B-containing lipoproteins: VLDL, IDL, chylomicron remnants, Lipoprotein (LP) (a), and LDL (Figure 29–1). Not surprisingly, as triglycerides increase, non-HDL correlates with apolipoprotein B much better than does LDL.[21,22]

Consideration of non-HDL offers several other advantages. Due to its improved correlation with apolipoprotein B, non-HDL outperforms other routine lipid measures in predicting both subclinical atherosclerosis and CHD events. It can be calculated directly from routine lipid panels, incurring no additional expense, and can accurately be derived from a nonfasting specimen; thus, it requires no special preparation by the patient. Finally, the importance of the triglyceride-rich lipoproteins included in the non-HDL measure will likely increase as the population ages and becomes more obese, insulin resistant, and hyperglycemic. Convincing arguments have been made to include non-HDL on the routine lipid profile.[23]

The emerging epidemic of insulin resistance and the metabolic syndrome is also shifting the population towards a small, dense VLDL, LDL, and HDL profile.[24] Increasing activity of cholesterol ester transfer protein (CETP) catalyzes the transfer of triglycerides to these lipoproteins in exchange for cholesterol ester. The triglycerides are then hydrolyzed, resulting in smaller, denser lipoprotein particles. Small, dense LDL more efficiently transports cholesterol into the vessel wall and has a greater susceptibility for oxidation, while the smaller HDL is less efficient at reverse cholesterol transport. Epidemiologic studies confirm increased risk in those with the small, dense "Type B" lipid phenotype.[25] Particle size can be measured with density-gradient ultracentrifugation, gradient gel electrophoresis, or nuclear magnetic resonance (NMR) technology.[18]

For a given LDL value, a small dense LDL phenotype will correlate with a greater total LDL particle (LDL-P) number. Emerging literature suggests that the total LDL-P number is a better cardiovascular risk predictor than LDL concentration,[26] particularly among women. Because one apolipoprotein B particle is present in each LDL particle regardless of cholesterol concentration, LDL-P correlates with apolipoprotein B more closely than does LDL.

In time, direct measurement of apolipoprotein B and apolipoprotein A-I may take on a greater role in clinical management of hyperlipidemia.[27,28] Several studies have shown apolipoprotein B to be superior to traditional lipoprotein measures as predictors of CHD,[29,30] and results from a number of studies suggest that the ratio of apolipoprotein B to apolipoprotein A-I may be the single best metric available for predicting CHD.[31]

Lipoprotein(a) is an apolipoprotein B-100-containing particle largely under genetic control, thus much less affected by available pharmacotherapy. Epidemiologic evidence strongly links lipoprotein(a) to CHD, particularly early CHD in patients with no other discernible risk factors. In addition to contributing to formation of the atherosclerotic plaque, lipoprotein(a) displays homology to plasminogen and may inhibit thrombolysis.[32]

History and Evolution of the NCEP ATP Guidelines

ATP I and ATP II

ATP I, convened in 1986, recommended measuring total blood cholesterol to screen for hypercholesterolemia based on data from Framingham and MRFIT. Values less than 200 mg/dL were deemed desirable; 200–239 mg/dL, borderline high; and greater than 240 mg/dL, high risk. Thereafter, LDL was selected as the primary treatment target, with values greater than 160 mg/dL identifying high risk patients (>130 mg/dL with multiple risk factors, such as smoking), and values less than 130 mg/dL as the target. Emphasis was placed on dietary interventions. While HDL was considered a CHD risk factor, the guidelines did not recommend its measurement when screening patients.

In 1993, ATP II emphasized an assessment of CHD risk status to guide treatment and to determine the appropriate goals of therapy. In particular, patients with a history of CHD were considered the highest risk group. A goal LDL of less than 100 mg/dL wás selected for this population based on smaller trials using less effective agents, although conclusive data had not yet become available to confirm this threshold. In lower risk patients, more emphasis was placed on exercise and weight loss than in the prior report. In addition, ATP II added HDL to its screening guidelines.

Large Event-Driven Clinical Trials

After 1993, the results of several large clinical trials became available which confirmed the safety and efficacy of pharmacologic lipid-lowering, as well as reinforced the importance of LDL. These trials differed from earlier studies by the use of modern pharmacotherapies (statins), the use of clinical events as endpoints rather than angiographic luminal atherosclerosis progression, and their large population size (typically over 5000 patients). The results of these trials played a critical part in influencing ATP III.

Initial trials enrolled higher risk patients for both primary and secondary prevention of CHD. The Scandinavian Simvastatin Survival Study (4S), published in 1994, randomized 4444 patients with a prior history of CHD and total cholesterol between 213 and 309 mg/dL to treatment with 20 mg of simvastatin (subsequently titrated) or placebo with follow-up for median 5.4 years.[33] The sole endpoint was overall mortality. In the simvastatin group, total cholesterol was reduced 26%, LDL was reduced 36%, and there was a 30% decreased overall mortality rate (256 versus 182 deaths). In secondary analysis, CHD mortality was reduced 42%, with similar benefit found across all quartiles of total cholesterol, LDL, and HDL.[34]

The West of Scotland Coronary Prevention Study (WOSCOPS) extended this finding to the high-risk primary prevention population.[35] Published in 1995, WOSCOPS randomized 6595 men with no history of CHD to pravastatin 40 mg or placebo and followed for median 4.9 years. Baseline total cholesterol was 272 mg/dL and baseline LDL was 192 mg/dL. Pravastatin treatment resulted in a 20% reduction in total cholesterol, 26% reduction in LDL, coinciding with a 31% reduction in CHD events (248 versus 174 events).

Subsequent trials focused on individuals who, during that era of lipidology, were considered to have only mild to moderate elevations in cholesterol. The Cholesterol and Recurrent Events Trial (CARE), published in 1996, randomized 4159 patients with a history of heart attack to 40 mg of pravastatin or placebo and followed them for mean of 5 years.[36] Baseline LDL was 139 mg/dL, which was reduced 32% by pravastatin and maintained at about 97 mg/dL throughout the trial. Despite lower baseline LDL levels, the pravastatin group experienced a 24% reduction in major coronary events.

In the Long Term Intervention with Pravastatin in Ischemic Disease (LIPID) trial, published in 1998, 9104 patients with a history of heart attack or unstable angina were randomized to pravastatin 40 mg or placebo and followed for mean of 6 years.[37] Baseline cholesterol varied from 155 mg/dL to 271 mg/dL. Both CHD mortality (24%) and all-cause mortality (22%) declined in the pravastatin group, corresponding to a 25% reduction in LDL relative to placebo.

The landmark Air Force/Texas Coronary Atherosclerosis Primary Prevention Study (AFCAPS/TexCAPS) reinforced the benefit of statins for primary prevention in individuals with "average" cholesterol.[38] Published in 1998, the investigators randomized 6605 participants with mean LDL of 150 mg/dL to lovastatin (initial 20 mg with subsequent titration) or placebo and followed for a mean of 5.2 years. Those in the lovastatin group experienced a 25% reduction in LDL to 115 mg/dL and a 37% reduction in initial major coronary events (183 versus 113 first events). This was the first in a series of trials that have helped redefine optimal LDL.

Global Risk Stratification—The Framingham Risk Score

Throughout the 1990s, there was increasing recognition of the synergistic effect of multiple CHD risk factors on overall CHD risk. This shifted focus away from baseline cholesterol levels as the principal determinant of treatment and toward global assessment of CHD risk.[39] The emerging principle stated that even when blood cholesterol levels are not very high, the presence of several other risk factors, including smoking and diabetes, may justify the use of lipid-lowering therapy. This premise was subsequently tested in the Anglo-Scandinavian Cardiac Outcomes Trial—Lipid Lowering Arm (ASCOT-LLA), published in 2003, which showed a marked prevention of initial coronary events with atorvastatin in patients with hypertension and other risk factors despite an "average" baseline LDL of 133 mg/dL.[40]

Investigators used data from the Framingham Heart Study to assemble a risk-scoring equation designed to calculate a 10-year risk of CHD. The Framingham Risk Score (FRS) uses age, total cholesterol, HDL, smoking, and systolic blood pressure to estimate risk in asymptomatic men and women free of known CHD. The FRS has been validated in external populations, although this model does not include several risk factors that have been shown to predict CHD in other large studies.

ATP III

In 2001, the ATP published their most recent guideline statement, including revised charts of optimal cholesterol values (Table 29–3).[41] ATP III focused on global risk estimates, most notably the FRS, to determine risk level and dictate initiation and goals of treatment. Patients with 10-year risk less than 10% were considered the lowest risk group; 10–20%, intermediate risk; and greater than 20%, high risk. While patients with known CHD are always placed in the highest risk group, the ATP III also identified peripheral artery disease, abdominal aortic aneurysm, and diabetes as CHD risk equivalents. Goal LDL for the highest risk patients was considered to be less than 100 mg/dL (Table 29–4).

The ATP III formally recognizes non-HDL as the preferred method to measure residual risk after LDL-lowering in patients with elevated triglycerides, such as those with metabolic syndrome, diabetes, or known CHD. For patients with triglycerides greater than 200 mg/dL, goal values for non-HDL are set 30 mg/dL higher

Table 29–3: ATP III classification of risk associated with increasing levels of routinely-measured lipids.

Lipid level (mg/dL)	ATP III classification
LDL: ***Primary Target***	
• <100	Optimal
• 100–129	Near or above optimal
• 130–159	Borderline high
• 160–189	High
• ≥190	Very high
Total cholesterol	
• <200	Desirable
• 200–239	Borderline high
• ≥240	High
Triglycerides	
• <150	Normal
• 150–199	Borderline high
• 200–499	High
• ≥500	Very high
HDL	
• <40	Low
• ≥60	High

than the LDL goal for a given risk group. For example, an intermediate risk patient with a few risk factors for coronary disease has an LDL goal of less than 130 mg/dL and a non-HDL goal of less than 160 mg/dL.

The ATP III also recognizes the metabolic syndrome as a distinct clinical entity with a characteristic of "atherogenic dyslipidemia" (high triglycerides, low HDL, yet no direct impact on LDL) (Table 29–5). The metabolic syndrome is an independent

Table 29–4: Recommendations of the NCEP ATP III.

Risk Category	Lifestyle intervention	Consider drug therapy	LDL goal	Non-HDL goal**
1 High risk				
>20% FRS CHD history CHD equivalent†	≥100 mg/dL	≥100 mg/dL *<100: optional, "very high risk"*	<100 mg/dL *<70: optional, "very high risk"*	<130 mg/dL *<100: optional, "very high risk"*
2 Moderately high risk*				
10–20% FRS ≥2 risk factors‡	≥130 mg/dL	≥130 mg/dL *100–129: optional*	<130 mg/dL *<100: optional*	<160 mg/dL *<130: optional*
3 Moderate risk*				
<10% FRS ≥2 risk factors	≥130 mg/dL	≥160 mg/dL	<130 mg/dL	<160 mg/dL
4 Low risk				
0–1 risk factor	≥160 mg/dL	≥190 mg/dL	<160 mg/dL	<190 mg/dL

FDS denotes Framingham Risk Score, CHD denotes coronary heart disease

*Commonly referred to as intermediate-risk patients

**When triglycerides ≥200 mg/dL

†CHD equivalents: peripheral arterial disease, abdominal aortic aneurysm, and carotid artery disease (transient ischemic attacks or stroke of carotid origin or >50% obstruction of a carotid artery), diabetes

‡Risk factors: smoking, hypertension, low HDL cholesterol (<40 mg/dL), family history of premature CHD (CHD in male first-degree relative <55 years of age; CHD in female first-degree relative <65 years of age), and age (men ≥45 years; women ≥55 years)

Table 29–5: ATP III clinical definition of the metabolic syndrome.

Risk factor	Defining level
Abdominal obesity	Waist circumference
Men	>102 cm (>40 inches)
Women	88 cm (>35 inches)
Triglycerides	≥150 mg/dL
HDL cholesterol	
Men	<40 mg/dL
Women	<50 mg/dL
Blood pressure	≥130/85 mmHg
Fasting glucose	≥100 mg/dL

3 of 5 criteria must be present for diagnosis

risk factor for CHD and diabetes that reflects the clustering of individual metabolic risk factors due to abdominal obesity and insulin resistance.[42] This proinflammatory, prothrombotic condition is becoming epidemic as the population ages, exercises less, becomes more obese, and eats more refined carbohydrates.[43] While ATP III raises awareness about this condition, it offers few specific treatment recommendations beyond aggressive lifestyle modification.

New Clinical Trials: Modification to ATP III

In 2002, the landmark Heart Protection Study (HPS) was published.[44] This trial randomized 20,536 subjects to simvastatin and/or antioxidant therapy in a 2 × 2 factorial design and followed them for mean of 5.5 years. Patients were at increased CVD risk (prior CHD, CVD, diabetes, or untreated hypertension) and were not taking lipid-lowering therapy. All patients in this study benefited similarly from simvastatin (~25% event reduction), including women, patients with diabetes, and patients with baseline LDL less than 100 mg/dL. In fact, simvastatin appeared to provide benefit regardless of baseline LDL. The finding in the HPS of near universal benefit for patients with diabetes has since been confirmed in the 2004 Collaborative Atorvastatin Diabetes Study (CARDS), which showed a 37% reduction in major cardiovascular events with atorvastatin despite baseline LDL of 118 mg/dL.[45]

ASCOT-LLA,[40] discussed above, and Pravastatin or Atorvastatin Evaluation and Infection Therapy (PROVE-IT)[46] trial also influenced the modification of ATP III. In PROVE-IT, 4162 patients recently hospitalized for ACS were randomized to atorvastatin 80 mg or pravastatin 40 mg to compare intensive versus "standard" lipid-lowering strategies.[46] Mean LDL at randomization was 106 mg/dL; on treatment, LDL was 95 mg/dL in the pravastatin group, and 62 mg/dL in the atorvastatin group. The benefit of high dose atorvastatin was seen at 30 days and persisted over the two-year follow-up. This study suggested that high-risk patients may benefit from LDL levels far below the 100 mg/dL threshold advocated by ATP III.

In response to observed benefit at lower levels of LDL without added risk, the NCEP added an extensive footnote to the ATP III guidelines.[47] Despite no identifiable lower LDL threshold for benefit from lipid-lowering therapy in these trials, an optional LDL goal of less than 70 mg/dL was selected for patients at "very high risk." On the strength of ASCOT-LLA, an LDL goal of less than 100 mg/dL was listed as a "therapeutic option" for intermediate risk patients with risk factors.

Limitations of the NCEP ATP III Algorithm

Lifetime Risk

A significant limitation of the ATP III algorithm is its reliance on the calculation of 10-year CHD risk via the FRS. With the weight placed on age in the FRS, it is less likely that a younger patient, despite a few risk factors, will qualify for lipid-lowering therapy.[48]

Consider a 50-year-old male with total cholesterol of 220 mg/dL, HDL 39 mg/dL, and systolic blood pressure of 132 mmHg on blood pressure-lowering therapy. The FRS predicts an 8% likelihood of a CHD event in the next ten years, placing the individual in the low risk category with no recommended lipid-lowering therapy. However, the same risk factors in a 60-year-old patient would have doubled the event risk—16%. In two years, at age 52, this patient will have a 10-year risk of 10%.

This case illustrates the concept of lifetime risk.[49] Atherosclerosis is a lifelong disease that takes decades to become clinically significant. It is known the risk factors in young adulthood lead to CHD later in life.[50] The presence of any suboptimally-treated risk factors portends a high likelihood that a patient will die of a cardiovascular disease, even if not in the next ten years.[51,52] Optimally treating risk factors in young adulthood does indeed reduce risk.[53] Therefore, strong arguments have been made advocating early treatment of hyperlipidemia based on advanced "biologic age" or "arterial age,"[54,55] even if the 10-year risk has not yet reached 10%.

Misclassification of Risk: The Low and Intermediate Risk Patient

The FRS results in an imperfect risk estimate.[56] Longitudinal studies indicate that the FRS misclassifies a significant percentage of low and intermediate risk individuals.[57] While misclassifying a low risk patient as an intermediate risk patient may result in unnecessary costly treatment, of more immediate concern is misclassifying the intermediate risk patient as low risk and withholding potentially life-saving therapy. Studies examining the presence of subclinical atherosclerosis in otherwise low risk patients have been informative in this regard.[58] Several modalities, including carotid intima media thickness (cIMT) as measured by B-mode ultrasound, ankle brachial index (ABI), and coronary artery calcification (CAC) as measured by computed tomography, allow for the quantification of plaque burden well before it obstructs the coronary artery lumen. These measures of subclinical atherosclerosis are highly predictive of future coronary events, independent of the FRS.[59–61] Using these techniques, it has been shown that a significant portion of low risk patients have a burden of atherosclerosis more characteristic of higher risk groups.

There have been many ways proposed to adjust for this misclassification. For example, the 2003 American College of Cardiology (ACC) Bethesda conference on atherosclerosis imaging endorsed an expanded intermediate risk category (6–20% 10-year risk) when coronary calcium imaging predicts increased risk not fully captured by the FRS.[62]

Global Risk Calculation: Missing Risk Factors

There are many nonlipid risk factors that independently predict CHD in other populations that have not been included in the FRS model. There are too many to discuss in detail in this chapter, however, two warrant special attention. Others will be discussed more generally under "Future of Lipid Guidelines" below.

A family history of premature CHD has been shown in many studies to predict CVD events. For example, the Framingham Offspring Study demonstrated an overall twofold increased risk, with a particularly marked effect on those at intermediate risk (thus, reclassifying them as high risk).[63] In addition, studies from the Multi-Ethnic Study of Atherosclerosis (MESA) show an independent association between family history and subclinical atherosclerosis.[64] While the NCEP ATP III recognizes family history as a major risk factor, it is not included in the FRS.

Chronic kidney disease (CKD) is very common in the United States, and will become more prevalent as the population ages. CKD is highly associated with accelerated atherosclerosis and increased CVD events. Stage 3B CKD falls just short of increasing risk to the level of a CHD equivalent (>20%).[65] Other early markers of kidney damage, including microalbuminuria, are also highly associated with CVD.

The Metabolic Syndrome

Publication of the NCEP ATP III was critical in raising awareness of the metabolic syndrome, but the guidelines provide little direction on how to use the concept in clinical practice. This is in part due to the limited evidence for therapies that lower triglycerides and raise HDL. Despite this, it remains critical for clinicians to identify the increased *lifetime risk* associated with the metabolic syndrome, as LDL-lowering therapy remains first-line treatment for risk reduction in this population.

The metabolic syndrome is associated with risk not accounted for by the FRS.[43] However, exact estimation of risk is difficult because, by definition, the metabolic syndrome is a *cluster* of individual risk factors, many of which are nonlipid and not routinely measured. For example, impaired glucose tolerance, C-reactive protein (CRP), and plasminogen activator inhibitor-1 (PAI-1) are independent predictors of CHD, but are not measured in routine clinical practice. In addition, because the metabolic syndrome is not a continuous measure (it is either present or is not), it cannot be used as a risk scoring tool and directly compared to the FRS.

Until traditional risk scoring tools are modified, it is most appropriate to use the metabolic syndrome as a tool for identifying the phenotype of abdominal obesity, insulin resistance, and unaccounted-for increased lifetime risk. Some experts recommend an expanded intermediate risk category (6–20%) for lipid-lowering decisions in these patients.[43]

Women

According to National Health and Nutrition Examination Survey (NHANES) III, less than 1% of asymptomatic women are classified as high risk using the ATP III algorithm.[66] Despite this, the lifetime risk of CVD in women is approximately 50% after the age of 40 years. Since just 4% of women have a 10-year risk of 10–20%, a small 5% fraction of the female population is eligible for lipid lowering therapy.[66]

The gap between CVD risk and lipid-lowering therapy in women is being increasingly recognized. Recent studies have documented the increased burden of subclinical atherosclerosis among otherwise low risk women.[67] The American Heart Association currently publishes specific guidelines for risk reduction in women, with a specific focus on improved risk identification.[68]

The Future of Lipid Guidelines

The future for lipid guidelines will no doubt focus on more intensive goals for LDL lowering with a goal of reversal of CHD, as well as combination therapy for residual risk attenuation and the addition of biomarkers such as inflammatory measures to guide lipid therapy.

Further Lowering of LDL

When data from the placebo and treatment groups of recent clinical trials are pooled, a log-linear relationship between LDL and CHD risk becomes evident (Figure 29–4).[69] With each 1 mg/dL drop in LDL, CHD risk is reduced approximately 1%. This is consistent with decades of epidemiologic data. While the modified ATP III guidelines identified less than 70 mg/dL as an optional goal for high risk patients, this value is somewhat arbitrary. There have been no studies that define a lower limit of LDL below which there are no further reductions in CHD risk, while several studies lend support toward removing "optional" from the less than 70 mg/dL recommendation.

In the first of the new clinical endpoint trials, the Treating to New Targets (TNT) trial randomized 10,003 patients with stable coronary disease to atorvastatin 10 mg or atorvastatin 80 mg and followed for a mean of five years.[70] Baseline LDL was 152 mg/dL; on treatment, LDL was 101 mg/dL in the low dose and 77 mg/dL in the high dose group. High dose atorvastatin was associated with a 22% reduction in major coronary events.

Both the "Z" phase of the Aggrastat to Zocor (A to Z) trial[71] and the Incremental Decrease in End Points Through Aggressive

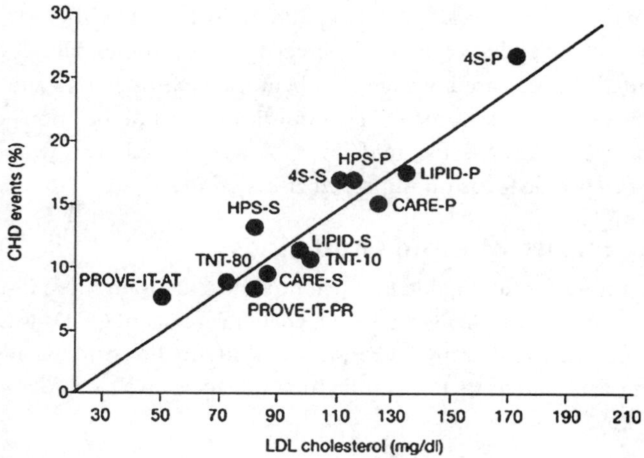

■ **Figure 29–4** Log-linear relationship between LDL-C-lowering and CHD events. A pooled anlaysis of placebo and treatment groups from the large statin trials demonstrates a 1% decrease in CHD risk with each 1% reduction in LDL-C. This observation is consistent with epidemiologic data. This relationship argues for more aggressive LDL-C lowering beyond that currently recommended by the NCEP ATPIII.

Lipid Lowering (IDEAL)[72] trial tested similar low dose versus high dose clinical trial designs in high risk patients. Both showed positive results in prespecified post-hoc analyses. In A to Z, patients followed beginning four months after an ACS had their LDL lowered to 63 mg/dL on high dose statin, which was associated with a 25% reduction in the primary endpoint. In IDEAL, patients with a history of heart attack lowered their LDL to 79 mg/dL on high dose statin, and experienced a 13% reduction in major cardiovascular events plus stroke.

The Reversing Atherosclerosis With Aggressive Lipid Lowering (REVERSAL) trial examined subclinical endpoints in a low dose versus high dose statin study design.[73] A total of 502 patients with symptomatic CHD were randomized to simvastatin 40 mg versus atorvastatin 80 mg and had an intravascular ultrasound (IVUS) assessment of coronary atherosclerosis at baseline and 18 months. High dose atorvastatin resulted in greater lowering of LDL (110 versus 79 mg/dL) and was associated with halted atherosclerosis, while patients receiving simvastatin 40 mg experienced progression in plaque.

Atherosclerosis Regression

Given the difficulty in showing incremental benefit with higher dose versus low dose therapy, as well as the length of time needed to study low risk populations, many recent studies use subclinical assessments of atherosclerosis as study endpoints. Results from these studies have raised the possibility of reversing atherosclerosis by achieving LDL targets much lower than the current ATP III recommendations.[74]

In A Study to Evaluate the Effect of Rosuvastatin on Intravascular Ultrasound-Derived Coronary Atheroma Burden (ASTEROID), 507 patients with angiographic CAD were given rosuvastatin 40 mg in an open-label design.[75] LDL was reduced from baseline 130 mg/dL to 61 mg/dL over two years, with 75% of patients achieving LDL less than 70 mg/dL. At study conclusion, 64% of patients achieved atherosclerosis regression.

The results from the Measuring Effects on Intima-Media Thickness: An Evaluation of Rosuvastatin (METEOR) trial extended the results from ASTEROID into the primary prevention population.[76] In this trial, 984 asymptomatic patients with FRS less than 10% were randomized to rosuvastatin 40 mg or placebo. Patients receiving rosuvastatin had a lower LDL at study completion (152 versus 78 mg/dL), and experienced net atherosclerosis regression versus progression in the placebo group. This trial argues for much more aggressive treatment of lower risk individuals than currently recommended.

Residual Risk—Combination Therapy

Despite risk reduction with aggressive statin therapy, higher risk patients maintain considerable residual risk of CHD.[77] It appears that individuals with metabolic syndrome, diabetes mellitus, high non-HDL, and low HDL have a particularly high residual risk after statins. It is likely that these patients will need a combination of lipid-lowering agents for optimal risk reduction.

The Helsinki Heart Study[9] and the Veterans Affairs High-Density Lipoprotein Cholesterol Intervention Trial (VA-HIT) provided the initial support for the use of fibrates for modest risk reduction in patients with high triglycerides.[78] Secondary analysis of other triglyceride-lowering trials suggests particular benefit in the subgroup with low HDL.[79,80] The ongoing Action to Control Cardiovascular Risk in Diabetes (ACCORD) trial, which will test the efficacy of adding fenofibrate to simvastatin in patients with diabetes, will be critical in determining if fibrates add incremental benefit over statins in patients with presumed high residual risk.[81]

Nicotinic acid raises HDL by 20–35%, providing modest event reduction and slowing atherosclerosis. However, the benefit of adding nicotinic acid to statins has not been adequately tested. The ongoing Atherothrombosis Intervention in Metabolic Syndrome with Low HDL/High Triglycerides and impact on Global Health Outcomes (AIM-HIGH) trial will help answer this question in patients with atherogenic dyslipidemia.[82]

Risk Stratification: The Cardiac Risk Panel

Risk stratification must improve over the present NCEP ATP III algorithm (see "Misclassification of Risk" on page 696). This is particularly true amongst low and intermediate risk patients, for whom the decision to treat with lipid-lowering therapy relies on adequate assessment of risk.

The future of risk stratification will be to measure a "panel" of risk markers, the results of which will provide an adjusted global risk score. The primary criterion for inclusion on this panel will be added calibration to the Framingham model. Several candidates for this "Cardiac Risk Panel" are already well studied. They fall into four broad groups: measures of inflammation, novel lipid-related biomarkers, measures of subclinical atherosclerosis, and genetic markers. Examples from each group are discussed below.

C-Reactive Protein: The JUPITER Trial

C-reactive protein (CRP) is an acute phase reactant produced in the liver that influences numerous proatherogenic and proinflammatory pathways. Measurement of CRP provides prognostic information independent of traditional cardiovascular risk factors and improves FRS calibration. In addition, CRP provides specific improvement in risk classification patients with metabolic syndrome and diabetes—those individuals with the highest residual risk after statin therapy.[83] Statins have been shown to lower CRP by a modest amount, but lifestyle improvements lower it to a much greater degree.

The Justification for the Use of statins in Primary prevention: an Intervention Trial Evaluating Rosuvastatin (JUPITER) trial tested the theory that CRP identifies otherwise low risk patients who will benefit from statin therapy.[84] A total of 17,802 participants with LDL cholesterol less than 130 mg/dL and CRP greater than or equal to 2 mg/L (measured with a high sensitivity CRP method, hsCRP) were randomized to rosuvastatin 20 mg or placebo. Based on traditional assessments of risk, the JUPITER study population was a markedly lower risk group compared to prior primary prevention trials. Despite the low risk, the trial was stopped early on March 31st, 2008 due to unequivocal evidence of benefit and is discussed in Chapter 12 of this text.

Lp-PLA$_2$

Lipoprotein-associated phospholipase A$_2$ (Lp-PLA$_2$) is a critical enzyme in the pathophysiology of the unstable plaque. It is responsible for the hydrolysis of oxidized LDL, generating lysophosphatidylcholine and oxidized free fatty acids, which lead to inflammatory cytokine production, adhesion molecule expression, and chemotaxis of inflammatory cells to the atherosclerotic lesion.

Lp-PLA$_2$ is strongly expressed within macrophages within the necrotic core of vulnerable and ruptured plaques, yet weakly expressed in less advanced lesions.[85]

Serum measurement of Lp-PLA$_2$ appears to uniquely identify patients with rupture-prone plaque. In data from over 25 epidemiologic studies, elevations of this biomarker led to a twofold increase in CVD (independent of traditional Framingham risk factors) and CRP, correlating even more tightly with the incidence of stroke.[86–88] Very low levels correlate highly with stabilized or absent plaque and appear to suggest excellent prognosis. Statins can lower Lp-PLA$_2$ independent of their ability to lower LDL. Based on the growing epidemiologic evidence, a recent expert panel has advocated measurement of this biomarker for further risk stratification on intermediate risk patients.[89]

Coronary Artery Calcification and Carotid Intimal Medial Thickness

There is now a large body of literature suggesting that radiographic measures of subclinical atherosclerosis enhance risk stratification amongst lower risk groups. This concept has face validity—rather than guess the likelihood of atherosclerosis, these techniques measure plaque directly. Coronary artery calcium (CAC) scoring appears to outperform carotid intimal medial thickness (cIMT) in its ability to predict CHD.[90] At high levels, CAC can help reclassify lower risk patients as higher risk patients, while absent CAC predicts an excellent survival and may be used to more appropriately select patients for statin therapy.[91]

The Society for Heart Attack Prevention and Eradication (SHAPE), an organization dedicated to CHD prevention, recently proposed a new algorithm for risk stratification (Figure 29–5).[92] In patients that clinicians identify as "possibly at risk," SHAPE advocates for measurement of subclinical atherosclerosis before any formal calculation of 10-year risk. Based on atherosclerosis burden, SHAPE recommends five risk groups on which to base further global risk stratification and lipid-lowering therapy decisions.

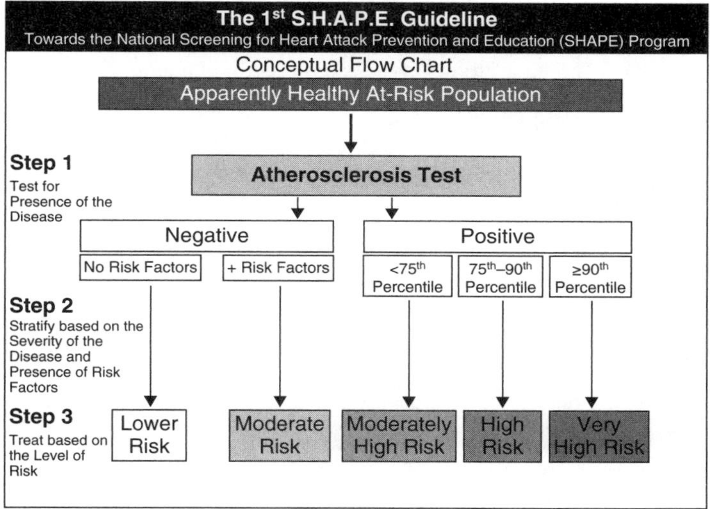

■ **Figure 29–5** The Society for Heart Attack Prevention and Eradication (SHAPE) has recently suggested that atherosclerosis imaging should precede the clinical assessment of risk factors. Global risk assessment can then proceed against a risk background determined by the "atherosclerosis test."

Genetics

Several genetic variants have been linked with increased risk of CHD. Notable among these are polymorphisms in apolipoprotein E and CETP.[93,94] While the relative contribution of each of these mutations to a complicated process, such as atherosclerosis, is small, the frequency of these variants in the population is large. Measured in combination on a cardiovascular genetic profile, they may represent a significant population-attributable risk for CHD.

Variants in the apolipoprotein E allele illustrate the importance of this concept. Apolipoprotein E is a diverse protein that plays a key role in the receptor-mediated uptake of cholesterol and triglycerides in the liver. The most common genotype in the

Table 29–6: Anticipated changes in future lipid guidelines.*

- Remove "optional" from LDL goal <70 mg/dL in high risk, <100 mg/dL in intermediate risk patients
- Further decreases in LDL goals based on new clinical trial evidence
- Optional goal of atherosclerosis regression in higher risk primary prevention population
- Non-HDL reported on all lipid panels
- Measurement of novel lipid biomarkers to characterize residual risk after LDL lowering (see Table 29–1), emphasis on plaque stabilization
- Recommendations for combination lipid-lowering therapy to optimize other lipid parameters, including triglycerides and HDL
- "Cardiac Risk Panel" to more accurately risk stratify patients: inflammatory markers, novel lipid biomarkers, subclinical atherosclerosis measures, genetic variants
- Option to use atherosclerosis imaging to gauge success of therapy

*Some of these will be incorporated into the NCEP ATP IV, due in the Fall of 2009.

population is termed ε3/ε3. Individuals with this genotype have lower cholesterol levels, while individuals with ε4/ε4 have higher cholesterol levels compared to those patients with ε3/ε3. In a recent meta-analysis of 86,067 healthy participants, the ε2/ε2 genotype conferred a 17% reduction in CHD, while ε4/ε4 increased CHD by 22% compared to individuals with ε3/ε3.[93]

Conclusion

Blood cholesterol levels are important in the pathogenesis and epidemiology of CVD. Lipid-lowering guidelines have evolved over the last two decades, with the present ATP III recommendations emphasizing global risk stratification for the appropriate selection of patients and targets for LDL lowering. The current algorithm, however, has many limitations. Future guidelines will advocate for more aggressive LDL-lowering, will emphasize non-traditional lipid measures as potential targets of therapy, and will recommend many new lipid and nonlipid biomarkers for the most accurate risk stratification of patients (Table 29–6). The ATP IV guidelines are due in the fall of 2009.

References

1. Rosamond W, Flegal K, Furie K, et al. American Heart Association Statistics Committee and Stroke Statistics Subcommittee. Heart disease and stroke statistics—2008 update: a report from the American Heart Association Statistics Committee and Stroke Statistics Subcommittee. *Circulation.* 2008;117(4):e25–e146.
2. Greenland P, Knoll MD, Stamler J, et al. Major risk factors as antecedents of fatal and nonfatal coronary heart disease events. *JAMA.* 2003;290:891–897.
3. Kannel WB, Castelli WP, Gordon T, McNamara PM. Serum cholesterol, lipoproteins, and the risk of coronary heart disease. The Framingham Study. *Ann Intern Med.* 1971;74(1):1–12.
4. Neaton JD, Wentworth D. Serum cholesterol, blood pressure, cigarette smoking, and death from coronary heart disease. Overall findings and differences by age for 316,099 white men. Multiple Risk Factor Intervention Trial Research Group. *Arch Intern Med.* 1992; 152:56–64.
5. Pearson TA, LaCroix AZ, Mead LA, et al. The prediction of midlife coronary heart disease and hypertension in young adults: the Johns Hopkins multiple risk equations. *Am J Prev Med.* 1990;6(2 Suppl): 23–28.
6. Berenson GS, Srinivasan SR, Bao W, et al. Association between multiple cardiovascular risk factors and atherosclerosis in children and young adults. *N Engl J Med.* 1998;338:1650–1656.
7. The Lipid Research Clinics Coronary Primary Prevention Trial results. I. Reduction in incidence of coronary heart disease. *JAMA.* 1984; 251(3):351–364.
8. The Lipid Research Clinics Coronary Primary Prevention Trial results. II. Reduction in incidence of coronary heart disease. *JAMA.* 1984; 251(3):365–374.

9. Frick MH, Elo O, Haapa K, et al. Helsinki Heart Study: primary-prevention trial with gemfibrozil in middle-aged men with dyslipidemia. Safety of treatment, changes in risk factors, and incidence of coronary heart disease. *N Engl J Med.* 1987;317(20):1237–1245.
10. Otvos JD, Jeyarajah EJ, Cromwell WC. Measurement issues related to lipoprotein heterogeneity. *Am J Cardiol.* 2002;90(Suppl):22i–29i.
11. Kwiterovich PO. Clinical relevance of the biochemical, metabolic and genetic factors that influence low-density lipoprotein heterogeneity. *Am J Cardiol.* 2002;90(Suppl):30i–45i.
12. Witztum JL, Steinberg D. Role of oxidized low density lipoprotein in atherogenesis. *J Clin Invest.* 1991;88(6):1785–1792.
13. Ashen MD, Blumenthal RS. Clinical practice. Low HDL cholesterol levels. *N Engl J Med.* 2005;353(12):1252–1260.
14. Castelli WP, Garrison RJ, Wilson PWF, et al. Incidence of coronary heart disease and lipoprotein cholesterol levels. The Framingham Heart Study. *JAMA*. 1986;256:2835–2838.
15. Sarwar N, Danesh J, Eiriksdottir G, et al. Triglycerides and the risk of coronary heart disease: 10,158 incident cases among 262,525 participants in 29 Western prospective studies. *Circulation*. 2007;115(4): 450–458.
16. Friedewald WT, Levy RI, Fredrickson DS. Estimation of low-density lipoprotein in plasma without use of preparative ultracentrifuge. *Clin Chem*. 1972;18:499–502.
17. Brunzell JD, Davidson M, Furberg CD, et al. Lipoprotein management in patients with cardiometabolic risk: consensus conference report from the American Diabetes Association and the American College of Cardiology Foundation. *J Am Coll Cardiol.* 2008;51(15): 1512–1524.
18. Mudd JO, Borlaug BA, Johnston PV, et al. Beyond low-density lipoprotein cholesterol: defining the role of low-density lipoprotein heterogeneity in coronary artery disease. *J Am Coll Cardiol.* 2007; 50(18):1735–1741.
19. Austin MA, King M-C, Vranizan KM, Krauss RM. Atherogenic lipoprotein phenotype: a proposed genetic marker for coronary heart disease risk. *Circulation*. 1990;82:495–506.
20. Grundy SM. Non-high-density lipoprotein cholesterol level as potential risk predictor and therapy target. *Arch Intern Med.* 2001;161(11): 1379–1380.

21. Abate N, Vega GL, Grundy SM. Variability in cholesterol content and physical properties of lipoproteins containing apolipoprotein B-100. *Atherosclerosis.* 1993;104:159–171.

22. Ballantyne CM, Andrews TC, Hsia JA, Kramer JH, Shear C; ACCESS Study Group. Atorvastatin Comparative Cholesterol Efficacy and Safety Study. Correlation of non-high-density lipoprotein cholesterol with apolipoprotein B: effect of 5 hydroxymethylglutaryl coenzyme A reductase inhibitors on non-high-density lipoprotein cholesterol levels. *Am J Cardiol.* 2001;88(3):265–269.

23. Blaha MJ, Blumenthal R, Brinton EA, Jacobson TA, on behalf of the National Lipid Association Taskforce on Non-HDL Cholesterol. The importance of non-HDL cholesterol reporting in lipid management. *Jour Clin Lipidol.* 2008;2:267–273.

24. Krauss RM, Siri PW. Metabolic abnormalities: triglyceride and low-density lipoprotein. *Endocrinol Metab Clin North Am.* 2004;33(2): 405–415.

25. Mora S, Szklo M, Otvos J, et al. LDL particle subclasses, LDL particle size, and carotid atherosclerosis in the Multi-Ethnic Study of Atherosclerosis (MESA). *Atherosclerosis.* 2007;192:211–217.

26. Cromwell WC, Otvos JD. Low-density lipoprotein particle number and risk for cardiovascular disease. *Curr Atheroscler Rep.* 2004;6: 381–387.

27. Sniderman AD, Furberg CD, Keech A, et al. Apolipoproteins versus lipids as indices of coronary risk and as targets of statin treatment. *Lancet.* 2003;361:777–780.

28. Sacks FM. The apolipoprotein story. *Atheroscler Suppl.* 2006; 7(Suppl):23–27.

29. Lamarche B, Moorjani S, Lupien PJ, et al. Apolipoprotein A-1 and B levels and the risk of ischemic heart disease during a five-year follow-up of men in the Quebec Cardiovascular Study. *Circulation.* 1996; 94:23–28.

30. Walldius G, Jungner I, Holme I, Aastveit AH, Kolar W, Steiner E. High apolipoprotein B, low apolipoprotein A-I, and improvement in the prediction of fatal myocardial infarction (AMORIS study): a prospective study. *Lancet.* 2001;358:2026–2033.

31. Barter PJ, Ballantyne CM, Carmena R, et al. Apo B versus cholesterol in estimating cardiovascular risk and in guiding therapy: report of

the Thirty-Person/Ten-Country Panel. *J Intern Med.* 2006;259:247–258.

32. Loscalzo J. Lipoprotein(a). A unique risk factor for atherothrombotic disease. *Arteriosclerosis.* 1990;10:672–679.

33. Pedersen TR, Kjekshus J, Berg K, et al. Randomized trial of cholesterol lowering in 4444 patients with coronary heart disease: the Scandinavian Simvastatin Survival Study (4S). *Lancet.* 1994;344:1383–1389. fixed.

34. Baseline serum cholesterol and treatment effect in the Scandinavian Simvastatin Survival Study (4S). *Lancet.* 1995;345:1274–1275.

35. Shepherd J, Cobbe SM, Ford I, et al. Prevention of coronary heart disease with pravastatin in men with hypercholesterolemia. West of Scotland Coronary Prevention Study Group. *N Engl J Med.* 1995; 333:1301–1307.

36. Sacks FM, Pfeffer MA, Moye LA, et al. The effect of pravastatin on coronary events after myocardial infarction in patients with average cholesterol levels. Cholesterol and Recurrent Events Trial investigators. *N Engl J Med.* 1996;335:1001–1009.

37. Prevention of cardiovascular events and death with pravastatin in patients with coronary heart disease and a broad range of initial cholesterol levels. The Long-Term Intervention with Pravastatin in Ischemic Disease (LIPID) Study Group. *N Engl J Med.* 1998;339:1349–1357.

38. Downs JR, Clearfield M, Weis S, et al. Primary prevention of acute coronary events with lovastatin in men and women with average cholesterol levels: results of AFCAPS/TexCAPS. Air Force/Texas Coronary Atherosclerosis Prevention Study. *JAMA.* 1998;279(20): 1615–1622.

39. Grundy SM, Pasternak R, Greenland P, Smith S Jr, Fuster V. AHA/ACC scientific statement: assessment of cardiovascular risk by use of multiple-risk-factor assessment equations: a statement for healthcare professionals from the American Heart Association and American College of Cardiology. *J Am Coll Cardiol.* 1999;34:1348–1359.

40. Sever PS, Dahlof B, Poulter NR, et al. Prevention of coronary and stroke events with atorvastatin in hypertensive patients who have average or lower-than-average cholesterol concentrations, in the Anglo-Scandinavian Cardiac Outcomes Trial-Lipid Lowering Arm

(ASCOT-LLA): a multicentre randomised controlled trial. *Lancet.* 2003;361(9364):1149–1158.

41. Adult Treatment Panel III. Executive summary of the third report of the National Cholesterol Education Program (NCEP) Expert Panel on Detection, Evaluation, and Treatment of High Blood Cholesterol in Adults. *JAMA*. 2001;285:2486–2497.
42. Blaha MJ, Elasy TA. Clinical use of the metabolic syndrome: why the confusion? *Clinical Diabetes*. 2006;24:125–131.
43. Blaha MJ, Bansal S, Rouf R, Golden SH, Blumenthal RS, Defillipis A. An "ABCDE" approach to the metabolic syndrome. *Mayo Clin Proc.* 2008;83:932–941.
44. Heart Protection Study Collaborative Group. MRC/BHF Heart Protection Study of cholesterol lowering with simvastatin in 20,536 high-risk individuals: a randomized placebo-controlled trial. *Lancet.* 2002; 360:7–22.
45. Colhoun HM, Betteridge DJ, Durrington PN, et al.; CARDS investigators. Primary prevention of cardiovascular disease with atorvastatin in type 2 diabetes in the Collaborative Atorvastatin Diabetes Study (CARDS): multicentre randomised placebo-controlled trial. *Lancet.* 2004;364(9435):685–696.
46. Cannon CP, Braunwald E, McCabe CH, et al. Intensive versus moderate lipid lowering with statins after acute coronary syndromes. *N Engl J Med* 2004;350:1495–1504.
47. Grundy SM, Cleeman JI, Merz CN, et al.; National Heart, Lung, and Blood Institute; American College of Cardiology Foundation; American Heart Association. Implications of recent clinical trials for the National Cholesterol Education Program Adult Treatment Panel III guidelines. *Circulation*. 2004;110(2):227–239.
48. Berry JD, Lloyd-Jones DM, Garside DB, Greenland P. Framingham risk score and prediction of coronary heart disease death in young adults. *Am Heart J.* 2007;154(1):80–86.
49. Lloyd-Jones DM, Leip EP, Larson MG, et al. Prediction of lifetime risk for cardiovascular disease by risk factor burden at 50 years of age. *Circulation*. 2006;113(6):791–798.
50. Loria CM, Liu K, Lewis CE, et al. Early adult risk factor levels and subsequent coronary artery calcification: the CARDIA study. *J Am Coll Cardiol.* 2007;49(20):2013–2020.

51. Navas-Nacher EL, Colangelo L, Beam C, Greenland P. Risk factors for coronary heart disease in men 18 to 39 years of age. *Ann Intern Med.* 2001;134(6):433–439.
52. Klag MJ, Ford DE, Mead LA, et al. Serum cholesterol in young men and subsequent cardiovascular disease. *N Engl J Med.* 1993;328(5): 313–318.
53. Bibbins-Domingo K, Coxson P, Pletcher MJ, Lightwood J, Goldman L. Adolescent overweight and future adult coronary heart disease. *N Engl J Med.* 2007;357(23):2371–2379.
54. Shaw LJ, Raggi P, Berman DS, et al. Coronary artery calcium as a measure of biologic age. *Atherosclerosis.* 2006;188:112–119.
55. "Arterial Age Calculator." NIH/NHLBI Multi-Ethnic Study of Atherosclerosis (MESA) website. 2009. Available at: http://www.mesa-nhlbi.org/CACReference.aspx. Accessed 7/29/2009.
56. Hemann BA, Bimson WF, Taylor AJ. The Framingham Risk Score: an appraisal of its benefits and limitations. *Am Heart Hosp J.* 2007; 5(2):91–96.
57. Brindle P, Beswick AD, Fahey T, Ebrahim SB. Accuracy and impact of risk assessment in the primary prevention of cardiovascular disease: a systematic review. *Heart.* 2006;92(12):1752–1759.
58. Greenland P, Smith SC Jr, Grundy SM. Improving coronary heart disease risk assessment in asymptomatic people: role of traditional risk factors and noninvasive cardiovascular tests. *Circulation.* 2001; 104(15):1863–1867.
59. Chambless LE, Folsom AR, Sharrett AR, et al. Coronary heart disease risk prediction in the Atherosclerosis Risk in Communities (ARIC) study. *J Clin Epidemiol.* 2003;56(9):880–890.
60. Greenland P, LaBree L, Azen SP, Doherty TM, Detrano RC. Coronary artery calcium score combined with Framingham score for risk prediction in asymptomatic individuals. *JAMA.* 2004;291(2):210–215.
61. Ankle Brachial Index Collaboration. Ankle brachial index combined with Framingham Risk Score to predict cardiovascular events and mortality: a meta-analysis. *JAMA.* 2008;300:197–208.
62. Taylor AJ, Merz CN, Udelson JE. 34th Bethesda Conference: Executive summary—can atherosclerosis imaging techniques improve the detection of patients at risk for ischemic heart disease? *J Am Coll Cardiol.* 2003;41(11):1860–1862.

63. Lloyd-Jones DM, Nam BH, D'Agostino RB, et al. Parental cardiovascular disease as a risk factor for cardiovascular disease in middle-aged adults: a prospective study of parents and offspring. *JAMA*. 2004; 291:2204–2211.

64. Nasir K, Budoff MJ, Wong ND, et al. Family history of premature coronary heart disease and coronary artery calcification: Multi-Ethnic Study of Atherosclerosis (MESA). *Circulation.* 2007;116(6):619–626.

65. Parikh NI, Hwang SJ, Larson MG, Levy D, Fox CS. Chronic kidney disease as a predictor of cardiovascular disease (from the Framingham Heart Study). *Am J Cardiol.* 2008;102(1):47–53.

66. Ford ES, Giles WH, Mokdad AH. The distribution of 10-year risk for coronary heart disease among US adults: findings from the National Health and Nutrition Examination Survey III. *J Am Coll Cardiol.* 2004;43(10):1791–1796.

67. Lakoski SG, Greenland P, Wong ND, et al. Coronary artery calcium scores and risk for cardiovascular events in women classified as "low risk" based on Framingham risk score: the multi-ethnic study of atherosclerosis (MESA). *Arch Intern Med.* 2007;167(22):2437–2442.

68. Mosca L, Banka CL, Benjamin EJ, et al. Evidence-based guidelines for cardiovascular disease prevention in women: 2007 update. *Circulation*. 2007;115(11):1481–1501.

69. O'Keefe JH Jr, Cordain L, Harris WH, Moe RM, Vogel R. Optimal low-density lipoprotein is 50 to 70 mg/dL: lower is better and physiologically normal. *J Am Coll Cardiol.* 2004;43(11):2142–2146.

70. LaRosa JC, Grundy SM, Waters DD, et al.; Treating to New Targets (TNT) Investigators. Intensive lipid lowering with atorvastatin in patients with stable coronary disease. *N Engl J Med.* 2005;352(14): 1425–1435.

71. de Lemos JA, Blazing MA, Wiviott SD, et al.; Early intensive vs a delayed conservative simvastatin strategy in patients with acute coronary syndromes: phase Z of the A to Z trial. *JAMA* 2004;292: 1307–1316.

72. Pedersen TR, Faergeman O, Kastelein JJ, et al.; IDEAL Study Group. High-dose atorvastatin vs usual-dose simvastatin for secondary prevention after myocardial infarction. *JAMA*. 2005;294(19):2437–2445.

73. Nissen SE, Tuzcu EM, Schoenhagen P, et al.; REVERAL investigators. Effect of intensive compared with moderate lipid-lowering therapy on

progression of coronary atherosclerosis: a randomized controlled trial. *JAMA*. 2004;291(3):1071–1080.

74. Thompson JB, Blaha M, Resar JR, Blumenthal RS, Desai MY. Strategies to reverse atherosclerosis: an imaging perspective. *Curr Treat Options Cardiovasc Med.* 2008;10(4):283–293.

75. Nissen SE, Nicholls SJ, Sipahi I, et al.; ASTERIOD Investigators. Effect of very high-intensity statin therapy on regression of coronary atherosclerosis: the ASTEROID trial. *JAMA*. 2006;295:1556–1565.

76. Crouse JR III, Raichlen JS, Riley WA, et al.; METEOR study group. Effect of rosuvastatin on progression of carotid intima-media thickness in low-risk individuals with subclinical atherosclerosis: the METEOR Trial. *JAMA*. 2007;297:1344–1353.

77. Campbell CY, Rivera JJ, Blumenthal RS. Residual risk in statin-treated patients: future therapeutic options. *Curr Cardiol Rep.* 2007;9(6): 499–505.

78. Rubins HB, Robins SJ, Collins D, et al. Gemfibrozil for the secondary prevention of coronary heart disease in men with low levels of high-density lipoprotein cholesterol. Veterans Affairs High-Density Lipoprotein Cholesterol Intervention Trial Study Group. *N Engl J Med.* 1999;341:410–418.

79. Manninen V, Tenkanen L, Koskinen P, et al. Joint effects of serum triglyceride and LDL cholesterol and HDL cholesterol concentrations on coronary heart disease risk in the Helsinki Heart Study: implications for treatment. *Circulation.* 1992;85(1):37–45.

80. BIP Study Group. Secondary prevention by raising HDL cholesterol and reducing triglycerides in patients with coronary artery disease: the Bezafibrate Infarction Prevention (BIP) study. *Circulation.* 2000; 102(1):21–27.

81. Ginsberg HN, Bonds DE, Lovato LC, et al.; ACCORD Study Group. Evolution of the lipid trial protocol of the Action to Control Cardiovascular Risk in Diabetes (ACCORD) trial. *Am J Cardiol.* 2007; 99(12A):56i–67i.

82. National Institutes of Health. AIM-HIGH: Niacin plus statin to prevent vascular events. ClinicalTrials.gov Web site. Available at: http://clinicaltrials.gov/ct/show/NCT00120289. Accessed June 26, 2008.

83. Abraham J, Campbell CY, Cheema A, Gluckman TJ, Blumenthal RS, Danyi P. C-reactive protein in cardiovascular risk assessment: a review of the evidence. *J Cardiometab Syndr.* 2007;2(2):119–123.

84. Mora S, Ridker PM. Justification for the Use of Statins in Primary Prevention: an Intervention Trial Evaluating Rosuvastatin (JUPITER)—can C-reactive protein be used to target statin therapy in primary prevention? *Am J Cardiol.* 2006;97(2A):33A–41A.

85. Kolodgie FD, Burke AP, Skorija KS, et al. Lipoprotein-associated phospholipase A2 protein expression in the natural progression of human coronary atherosclerosis. *Arterioscler Thromb Vasc Biol.* 2006; 26:2523–2529.

86. Anderson JL. Lp-PLA2: An independent predictor of CHD events in primary and secondary prevention. *Am J Card.* 2008;101:23F–33F.

87. Ballantyne CM, Hoogeveen RC, Bang H, et al. Lipoprotein-associated phospholipase A2, high-sensitivity C-reactive protein, and risk for incident heart disease in middle-aged men and women in the Atherosclerosis Risk in Communities (ARIC) study. *Circulation.* 2004;109: 837–842.

88. Ballantyne CM, Hoogeveen RC, Bang H, et al. Lipoprotein-associated phospholipase A2, high-sensitivity C-reactive protein, and risk for incident ischemic stroke in middle-aged men and women in the Atherosclerosis Risk in Communities (ARIC) study. *Arch Intern Med.* 2005;165:2479–2484.

89. Davidson MH, Alberts MJ, Anderson JL, et al. Consensus panel recommendation for incorporating Lp-PLA2 testing into cardiovascular disease risk assessment guidelines. *Am J Card.* 2008;101:51F–57F.

90. Folsom AR, Kronmal RA, Detrano RC, et al. Coronary artery calcification compared with carotid intima-media thickness in the prediction of cardiovascular disease incidence: the Multi-Ethnic Study of Atherosclerosis (MESA). *Arch Intern Med.* 2008;168(12):1333–1339.

91. Detrano R, Guerci AD, Carr JJ, et al. Coronary calcium as a predictor of coronary events in four racial or ethnic groups. *N Engl J Med.* 2008;358(13):1336–1345.

92. Naghavi M, Falk E, Hecht HS, et al.; SHAPE Task Force. From vulnerable plaque to vulnerable patient, III: executive summary of the Screening for Heart Attack Prevention and Education (SHAPE) Task Force report. *Am J Cardiol.* 2006;98(2A):2H–15H.

93. Bennet AM, Di Angelantonio E, Ye Z; et al. Association of apolipoprotein E genotypes with lipid levels and coronary risk. *JAMA*. 2007;298(11):1300–1311.

94. Thompson A, Di Angelantonio E, Sarwar N, et al. Association of cholesteryl ester transfer protein genotypes with CETP mass and activity, lipid levels, and coronary risk. *JAMA*. 2008;299(23):2777–2788.

30 ■ Biomarkers in the Metabolic Syndrome

Erik Ingelsson, MD, PhD
Ramachandran S. Vasan, MD, PhD

Introduction: Defining the Metabolic Syndrome and Biomarkers

Metabolic risk factors, such as visceral obesity, dyslipidemia, and high blood pressure tend to cluster in individuals, a notion that has been well-known for almost a century (Figure 30–1).[1,2] In 1988, Reaven hypothesized that insulin resistance was the factor linking noninsulin-dependent diabetes mellitus, essential hypertension, and coronary heart disease.[3] He called the clustering of risk factors "syndrome X," but subsequently the terms "insulin resistance syndrome"[4] and the "metabolic syndrome"[5–10] have been increasingly used. Over the past decade, several definitions of the metabolic syndrome (MetS) have been introduced, such as the ones proposed by the World Health Organization (WHO),[5] the European Group for the Study of Insulin Resistance (EGIR),[6] the National Cholesterol Education Program (NCEP) Adult Treatment Panel III,[7] the American Association of Clinical Endocrinologists (AACE),[8] the International Diabetes Federation (IDF),[9] and those modified by the NCEP.[10] At present, the most widely-used definitions for research, as well as clinical practice, seem to be the original and the modified NCEP criteria (Table 30–1).[7,10]

Biomarkers (biological markers) can be defined as measurable and quantifiable biological parameters (e.g., specific enzyme concentration, specific hormone concentration, specific gene phenotype distribution in a population, presence of biological substances) which serve as indices for health- and physiology-related assessments, such as disease risk, psychiatric disorders, environmental exposure and its effects, disease diagnosis, metabolic processes,

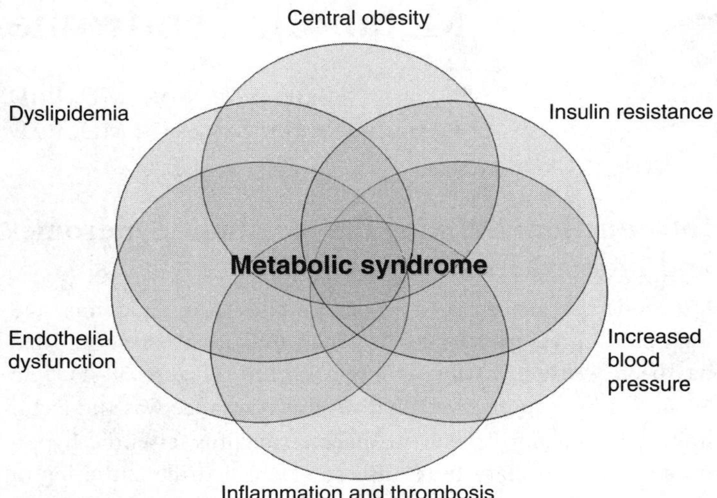

■ **Figure 30–1** Features of the metabolic syndrome.

substance abuse, pregnancy, cell line development, epidemiologic studies, etc.[11] Therefore, biomarkers can be serological (e.g., fasting glucose), structural (e.g., echocardiography), or functional (e.g., blood pressure). Biomarkers can be useful for different purposes in clinical practice: antecedent biomarkers may help identify individuals at risk of developing disease; screening biomarkers assist screening for subclinical disease; diagnostic biomarkers can be used to diagnose existing disease in symptomatic patients; and prognostic biomarkers may help predict recurrences or sequelae of disease, and to monitor treatment.[12] Biomarker studies also serve the purpose to study biological mechanisms leading to diseases or other conditions, and can give rise to new hypotheses that can be tested in other settings, such as experimental studies.

Biomarkers of MetS: An Overview

Insulin resistance is recognized to be a key feature of the MetS,[3,13] but the overlap of the two conditions is only partial.[14] Visceral

Table 30–1: The metabolic syndrome according to the National Cholesterol Education Program (NCEP) Adult Treatment Panel III guidelines.[7]

METABOLIC SYNDROME IS CONSIDERED PRESENT IF 3 OR MORE OF THESE CRITERIA ARE PRESENT	
Abdominal obesity	≥102 cm for men
	≥88 cm for women
Elevated blood pressure	≥130 mm Hg systolic; or
	≥85 mm Hg diastolic; or
	treatment for high blood pressure
Hyperglycemia	Fasting glucose ≥110 mg/dL (6.1 mmol/L);* or treatment with oral hypoglycemic agents or insulin
Hypertriglyceridemia	≥150 mg/dL (1.7 mmol/L); or
	treatment with nicotinic acid or fibrates
Low high-density lipoprotein cholesterol	<40 mg/dL (1.03 mg/dL) in men
	<50 mg/dL (1.3 mg/dL) in women

*In the modified NCEP criteria,[10] the glucose threshold was lowered to 100 mg/dL (5.6 mmol/l).

obesity and hypertriglyceridemia have also been suggested to be of central importance for the development of MetS,[15] along with several other factors, most of which are related to lifestyle factors.[16] Apart from insulin resistance, a range of metabolic, inflammatory, and hormonal abnormalities accompany the MetS. In cross-sectional studies, the MetS has been associated with alterations in circulating concentrations of a wide variety of biomarkers that represent these pathways (Table 30–2). Further, elevation of select biomarkers has been shown to precede the development of other cardiometabolic conditions, such as type 2 diabetes[17–19] and

Table 30–2: Biomarkers known to be associated with the metabolic syndrome.

Categories	Biomarkers
Markers of glucose and insulin metabolism	HOMA-IR
	Proinsulin and split proinsulin
	HbA1c
Markers involved in inflammation and hemostasis	CRP
	Leukocyte count
	IL-6 and other cytokines
	Cell adhesion molecules
	PAI-1
	Fibrinogen and other hemostatic markers
Adipokines and other fat-derived biomarkers	Leptin
	Adiponectin
	Ghrelin
	Retinol-binding protein 4
	Resistin
	Adipose fatty-acid binding protein
	Fetuin-A
Neurohormonal biomarkers	Aldosterone
	Renin
	Natriuretic peptides
Sex hormones	Testosterone
	SHBG
	Estradiol
Renal biomarkers	Cystatin C
	Urinary albumin excretion rate

Notes: HOMA-IR = homeostasis model assessment; HbA1C = hemoglobin A1c; CRP = C-reactive protein; IL-6 = interleukin-6; PAI-1 = plasminogen activator inhibitor-1; SHBG = sex hormone-binding globulin.

hypertension.[20–22] However, there are relatively few studies relating biomarkers to the incidence of the MetS itself.[23–29]

Over the past few years, there has been much debate regarding the usefulness of the MetS concept, both in clinical practice and for research purposes. In part, this controversy was initiated by an opinion paper jointly written by the American Diabetes Association (ADA) and the European Association for the Study of Diabetes (EASD) published in 2005.[30] Several important questions were raised, including:

1) whether such a distinct syndrome exists,
2) what the pathophysiological background of such a putative syndrome is,
3) if defining MetS has any clinical use, and
4) if it leads to unnecessary labeling of, and subsequent medication prescription for, healthy individuals.[30,31]

This ongoing debate notwithstanding, there is general agreement that cardiometabolic risk factors tend to cluster and that such clustering portends an increased risk of cardiovascular disease. Therefore, further characterization of MetS and the underlying pathogenetic mechanisms is important.

In this chapter, we review the current state of knowledge regarding circulating biomarkers related to MetS, with a focus on reported associations and biological mechanisms linking different biomarkers to the syndrome and its individual components. We do not discuss the potential clinical use of different biomarkers in the context of managing the patient with MetS.

Markers of Glucose and Insulin Metabolism in MetS

As disturbances of the glucose and insulin metabolism are the sine qua non of MetS, it is intuitive that biomarkers representing these pathways would be strongly associated with MetS. Fasting glucose is a component of all published definitions of MetS, and measures of insulin resistance, such as the homeostasis model assessment insulin resistance index (HOMA-IR), are part of the WHO,[5] EGIR,[6] and AACE[8] definitions of MetS (or the insulin resistance syndrome), however insulin resistance measures are not a part of the NCEP[7,10] or IDF[9] definitions. Considerable effort over the past few years has been spent on defining and characterizing the MetS as distinct from insulin resistance *per se*, and on the extent of the overlap between these two conditions. There is a broad consensus that different markers of insulin resistance, such as the HOMA-IR, proinsulin, or split proinsulin are all strongly associated with the presence of the MetS—and they are indeed even part of the syndrome according to some definitions of it.

Glycated hemoglobin (HbA1c) is generally used as a proxy for time-averaged blood glucose levels over a period of several weeks, especially in the context of diabetes management. It has been proposed that HbA1c could be used as a simple test to identify individuals at risk for developing MetS, and there are several studies demonstrating cross-sectional associations between higher levels of HbA1c and the presence of the MetS and its components in nondiabetic individuals in the community.[32–34]

Markers of Inflammation and Hemostasis in MetS

Presence of systemic inflammation and disturbances in hemostasis have been proposed to be of major pathophysiological importance for the development of the MetS.[16,25,35] Indeed, biomarkers of inflammation and hemostasis comprise a category that has been the most well-studied in relation to the MetS. Elevated levels of several markers of systemic inflammation, such as C-reactive protein (CRP),[25,35–41] interleukin-6 (IL-6),[40–43] and a peripheral blood leukocyte count[38,44–46] have all been consistently associated with presence of the MetS in different settings. Furthermore, higher CRP levels have also been shown to predict the development of new-onset MetS[25] and diabetes[19,47,48] in normoglycemic individuals, and to predict clinical cardiovascular disease independently of the MetS.[37,41,49] The incremental prognostic information conferred by CRP levels for predicting cardiovascular disease (when added to a multivariable model including all components of MetS) has been questioned.[49] The association between systemic inflammation and presence of the MetS may reflect an ongoing cytokine-mediated acute phase response initiated by the innate immune system in obese and/or insulin resistant individuals. Recently, CRP mRNA was reported to be expressed in human adipose tissue and to be inversely related with adiponectin mRNA levels.[50] Also, IL-6 is partly secreted by the visceral and subcutaneous fat depots, and has an important role in the regulation of glucose and lipid metabolism.[51]

There is less known about associations of MetS and other inflammatory biomarkers, such as novel interleukins, the selectins, or other cell adhesion molecules. Several smaller studies have demonstrated associations between MetS and cell adhesion molecules, such as vascular cell adhesion molecule-1 (VCAM-1),[52,53] intercellular adhesion molecule-1 (ICAM-1),[52,53] and E-selectin.[52,54] More recently, these biomarkers have been shown to be increased in individuals with MetS in two larger community-based samples.[41,55] In one of these studies, the associations of VCAM-1 and E-selectin with presence of the MetS were independent of CRP,[55] emphasizing the importance of cell adhesion molecules in the context of a large panel of inflammatory markers. Inflammation leads to increased expression of cell adhesion molecules and endothelial adhesion. VCAM-1 and ICAM-1 are adhesion receptors involved in the attachment and transendothelial migration of leukocytes,[56] and E-selectin is also involved in leukocyte recruitment and rolling in inflamed tissues. The expression of these cell adhesion molecules can be up-regulated by different stimuli associated with the MetS, including adipokines, other cytokines, advanced glycation end-products, or even increased blood pressure.[56]

Plasminogen activator inhibitor-1 (PAI-1) is the main inhibitor of the two activators of fibrinolysis, tissue plasminogen activator (tPA) and urokinase. Increased circulating levels of PAI-1 have been proposed to be a core feature of the MetS.[57,58] Several cross-sectional studies have demonstrated that PAI-1 is associated with prevalent MetS.[57–59] A recent longitudinal study reported that higher PAI-1 concentrations predicted incident MetS, prospectively.[26] The association of PAI-1 with new-onset MetS and with tracking of several metabolic risk factors is supported by several experimental studies that have highlighted potential mechanisms that could explain the association.[60–64] PAI-1 may have a causal role in the development of obesity and insulin resistance.[60–62] PAI-1-knockout mice demonstrate lower insulin resistance, glucose and triglyceride levels, together with lower body weight compared to wild-type mice when fed a high-energy diet.[61,62] Furthermore, higher PAI-1 levels may reflect endothelial dysfunction,[63] which is considered a key feature of the MetS. Also, higher vascular PAI-1 may accelerate perivascular and medial fibrosis, whereas suppression of PAI-1 protects against the vascular changes in experimental models of hypertension.[64]

Higher fibrinogen has been demonstrated to be associated with the MetS, in both cross-sectional[41,59,65] and longitudinal[27] studies. Alterations in circulating levels of several other hemostatic markers have been reported in patients with the MetS, including changes in factor VII, factor VIII, von Willebrands factor, factor IX, and tPA.[38,66]

Adipokines and Other Fat-Derived Biomarkers in MetS

Leptin

Ever since the discovery of leptin in 1994,[67] considerable research has focused on this adipokine and its role in obesity and insulin resistance. Several community-based studies have demonstrated that higher leptin concentrations are associated not only with obesity,[68–71] but also with elevated blood pressure,[72] type 2 diabetes,[73] and insulin resistance.[71,74] Not surprisingly, leptin levels are elevated in the MetS.[68,75–77] Under normal physiological conditions, leptin acts as a satiety signal, reduces the appetite, and increases the metabolism, but it also has a number of other physiological functions ranging from regulation of puberty, control of placental function, modulation of peripheral insulin sensitivity, and interaction with other hormonal mediators and regulators.[69,78] Nevertheless, in obese individuals leptin fails to suppress appetite or promote weight loss and, as a result, the circulating leptin concentrations increases. This has been termed leptin resistance. Hyperleptinemia[78] has been proposed as a component of the MetS.[76] The exact mechanisms of leptin and its complex interactions with obesity and insulin resistance are not entirely known. Leptin acts as a growth factor for a range of different cell types. It is a mediator of energy expenditure and interacts with other key regulators of energy status and metabolism such as insulin, glucagon, insulin-like growth factors, growth hormone, and glucocorticoids.[69]

Adiponectin

Adiponectin was identified in 1995–96 by four independent groups as an adipocyte-specific factor that is expressed in adipose tissue abundantly.[79–82] Whereas leptin concentrations are positively correlated with body mass index, adiponectin is inversely correlated.[83] This negative correlation is stronger with visceral than with subcutaneous adiposity.[84] Lower adiponectin concentrations have been associated with the development of type 2 diabetes[85] and cardiovascular disease,[86] findings that have been replicated with consistent findings in different study samples.[83] Also, hypoadiponectinemia is associated with high blood pressure[87] and dyslipidemia,[88,89] independent of obesity. In addition to being associated with the individual components of the MetS, there is consistent evidence that hypoadiponectinemia is associated with the syndrome *per se* in a range of different age groups and ethnicities.[90–94] Lower adiponectin concentrations have been shown to precede the onset of type 2 diabetes, paralleled by decreasing insulin sensitivity.[85,95] Adiponectin-knockout mice develop adiponectin deficiency and increased tumor necrosis factor-alpha (TNF-α)

concentrations, resulting in severe diet-induced insulin resistance mediated by reduced fatty-acid transport protein 1 (FATP-1) mRNA and insulin-receptor substrate 1 (IRS-1)-mediated insulin signaling.[96] Furthermore, insulin resistance can be reversed by treatment with adiponectin in physiological doses in mouse models of obesity and lipoatrophy.[97]

Ghrelin

Ghrelin is a stimulator of growth hormone release, and an appetite-stimulating signal that is released from the gut and that acts upon the brain.[98] It counters the appetite-reducing and metabolism-increasing effects of leptin, and is a coordinator of behavioral, metabolic, and gastrointestinal responses to meal patterns. Circulating concentrations of ghrelin have been reported to decrease in individuals with high blood pressure,[68,99] obesity,[68,100,101] insulin resistance,[101] and type 2 diabetes.[99] Ghrelin levels are lower in patients with the MetS,[68,102,103] and the alterations in its levels may contribute to some of the features of the syndrome. Ghrelin is a vasodilator, possibly due to its effects on myocardial and aortic growth hormone secretagogue receptors;[104,105] the injection of ghrelin in healthy individuals can decrease mean arterial pressure and increase cardiac output.[104] Furthermore, ghrelin deficiency may increase insulin resistance by different mechanisms including its somatotrophic effects[106] and its effects on insulin signaling in the peripheral tissues.[107] An alternative explanation to the observed relations of ghrelin and insulin metabolism is that low ghrelin concentrations are secondary to changes in glucose and insulin.[108]

Retinol-Binding Protein 4 and Glucose Transporter 4

Retinol-binding protein 4 (RBP4) is a novel fat-derived adipokine that has been shown to be positively associated with obesity,[109–112] insulin resistance,[109–114] and type 2 diabetes.[109,110,112] RBP4 levels are elevated in the MetS.[110,111] Soluble glucose transporter 4 (GLUT4) is a key regulator of glucose homeostasis, being the major glucose transporter protein that mediates glucose uptake in peripheral tissues.[115] Down-regulation of GLUT4 expression in adipose tissue is a common feature in different insulin-resistant states, such as obesity, type 2 diabetes, and the MetS. In 2005, it was reported that the expression of RBP4 is elevated in adipose tissue of adipose-specific-GLUT4-knockout mice,[112] and that circulating concentrations of RBP4 are elevated in insulin-resistant mice[112] and in humans with obesity and type 2 diabetes.[110,112] Furthermore, fenretinide, a synthetic retinoid that causes increased urinary excretion of RBP4, normalizes circulating RBP4 levels and improves insulin sensitivity in mice with obesity induced by a high-fat diet.[112]

Other Adipose Tissue Associated Biomarkers

There are several other fat-derived biomarkers that are associated with the MetS. Resistin is a member of a family of cysteine-rich proteins secreted by adipocytes in rodents, and it was first established to be linked to insulin resistance in animal models.[116] Data from humans are more inconsistent, but several studies have shown increased concentrations of circulating resistin to be associated with insulin resistance[117,118] and the presence of the MetS.[119,120]

Adipocyte-specific fatty acid-binding protein (A-FABP) belongs to the fatty acid-binding protein superfamily. These tissue-specific proteins are involved in the shuttling of fatty acids to cellular compartments, modulation of intracellular lipid metabolism, and regulation of gene expression.[121] Animal studies have demonstrated that A-FABP-knockout mice develop obesity to the same extent as wild-type controls, but are somewhat protected from insulin resistance, hyperinsulinemia, and the development of diabetes.[122] Also, the acute insulin response and lipolysis after a beta-adrenergic stimulation is suppressed in such A-FABP-deficient mice compared with their wild-type littermates, suggesting that A-FABP may affect systemic insulin sensitivity.[123] In humans, A-FABP has been shown to be higher in individuals with obesity, insulin resistance, and MetS.[124,125] More recently, this biomarker has been demonstrated to predict development of the MetS[28] and type 2 diabetes,[126] independent of adiposity and insulin resistance.

Fetuin-A is a protein found in high concentrations in serum, known to be the natural inhibitor of insulin receptor tyrosine kinase in liver and skeletal muscle.[127] Fetuin-A-knockout mice have enhanced insulin sensitivity and glucose clearance, resistance to weight gain, and lower circulating free fatty acid and triglyceride concentrations.[128] In a sample of patients with coronary heart disease, higher fetuin-A concentrations were strongly associated with the presence of the MetS and an atherogenic lipid profile.[129] Recently, it was demonstrated that fetuin-A can induce low-grade inflammation and decrease adiponectin production in both animals and in humans.[130]

Neurohormonal Biomarkers in MetS

Renin-Angiotensin-Aldosterone System

Activation of the renin-angiotensin-aldosterone (RAAS) system has been proposed to be involved in the development of the MetS.[131] Weight loss can decrease circulating concentrations of several biomarkers representing this system, including levels of aldosterone and renin.[132] Higher aldosterone concentrations have been shown to be associated with a greater prevalence of the MetS, as well as its components, including increased waist circumference, triglycerides, and blood pressure.[133,134] Several cross-sectional studies have reported positive correlations between serum aldosterone and insulin resistance.[134,135] Also, plasma renin activity has been associated inversely with insulin sensitivity assessed by HOMA-IR[133] or with euglycemic clamp techniques[136] in cross-sectional studies. In a recent longitudinal study, higher aldosterone concentrations predicted new-onset MetS prospectively in the community-based Framingham Heart Study sample.[26] In that report, higher aldosterone was positively associated with future increases in systolic blood pressure and was inversely related to changes in high-density lipoprotein cholesterol. Increased aldosterone could cause increased blood pressure through several mechanisms, including increased renal sodium retention, increased angiotensin II action, impaired endothelial function, and decreased vascular compliance.[137] There may also be mechanisms that link aldosterone to the adipose tissue metabolism, which could explain the strong association of this mineralocorticoid with the MetS and with insulin resistance. Indeed, there are in vitro studies that support a role for aldosterone in adipogenesis, by mediating early adipocyte differentiation.[138,139]

Natriuretic Peptides

B-type natriuretic peptide (BNP) and N-terminal proBNP (NT-proBNP) are synthesized in the cardiac ventricles by cleavage of their precursor protein, $proBNP_{108}$. Their circulating concentrations are increased in patients with heart failure and other cardiovascular diseases characterized by pressure or volume overload, and increased cardiac filling pressures.[140] Natriuretic peptides have been demonstrated to predict adverse outcome in individuals with acute coronary syndrome,[141] and incident cardiovascular disease in healthy individuals from the community.[142] Furthermore, increased baseline concentrations of BNP have been associated with blood pressure progression,[20] whereas obese individuals have been shown to have lower concentrations of circulating BNP.[143] This inverse cross-sectional relation with obesity can have several potential explanations, including increased clearance of natriuretic peptides by natriuretic peptide clearance receptors (NPC-Rs) that are abundant in adipose tissue, or reduced bioavailability of natriuretic peptides from impaired myocardial hormone release or synthesis.[143] The inverse association of natriuretic peptides with metabolic risk factors have been confirmed in two other recent studies, where higher N-terminal pro-atrial natriuretic peptide (NT-proANP), BNP, and NT-proBNP concentrations were associated with lower body mass index, waist circumference, fasting insulin, fasting glucose, triglycerides, and total cholesterol.[144,145] Also, the presence of MetS was inversely associated with concentrations of natriuretic peptides in these studies,[144,145] whereas the positive association with blood pressure was confirmed.

Sex Hormones in the MetS

Whereas biomarkers may be differentially associated with the presence of the MetS in men versus women, these gender-related differences are particularly striking when sex hormones are studied in relation to the syndrome.

Androgens

In women, androgen excess has been known to be associated with insulin resistance for several decades, both in rare syndromes of extreme insulin resistance and in the polycystic ovary syndrome, a common condition in premenopausal women characterized by hyperandrogenism and chronic oligo- or anovulation, together with peripheral insulin resistance and hyperinsulinemia.[146] Free androgen index (FAI; total testosterone/sex hormone-binding globulin[SHBG]) is often used as a surrogate for free testosterone, but the accuracy is dependent on appropriate assays for total testosterone and SHBG, and many commercially-available assays lack in accuracy and sensitivity.[147] In postmenopausal women without diabetes, FAI has been shown to correlate positively with fasting glucose and fasting insulin.[148,149] Also, postmenopausal women with the MetS have higher FAI and total testosterone levels together with lower SHBG concentrations.[150,151] The association of hyperandrogenism and MetS in postmenopausal women is strong, with a twelve-fold increase in odds of the MetS in women in the highest tertile of FAI (compared with the lowest), even after adjustment for body mass index in a recent study.[150] Similar findings have also been observed in premenopausal women. Even after exclusion of women with polycystic ovary syndrome, women with the MetS have higher FAI and lower SHBG levels.[152] In fact, the association of hyperandrogenism with insulin resistance may be evident in early adolescence.[153] There are also longitudinal data demonstrating that low SHBG concentrations predict the development of type 2 diabetes in pre- and postmenopausal women, independent of serum insulin, body mass index, and other potential confounders.[154,155] A recent longitudinal study demonstrated that an increase in bioavailable testosterone and a decrease in SHBG levels during the perimenopausal transition increased the odds of developing the MetS after menopause.[29]

In men, the association between androgens and the presence of insulin resistance or the MetS differs from that observed in women. Several studies have demonstrated that low serum testosterone is associated with insulin resistance in men. Insulin sensitivity in hypogonadal men can be improved by testosterone replacement.[156] However, it is unclear whether the primary event is hypoandrogenemia or insulin resistance. In Klinefelter's syndrome, low testosterone concentrations are clinically manifested before hyperinsulinemia develops. Also, lower levels of androgens have been demonstrated to predict central obesity,[157] as well as insulin resistance and type 2 diabetes in men.[158]

Estrogens

There is also substantial evidence that estrogen plays an important role in the regulation of insulin sensitivity and energy homeostasis. However, the directionality of the reported effects has been inconsistent, possibly due to varying effects in different age groups, and the differences in the effects of endogenous versus exogenous estrogen. There are many studies showing reduced prevalence of insulin resistance when postmenopausal women are treated with hormone replacement therapy.[159] Also, estrogen has beneficial effects on adipose tissue and skeletal muscle metabolism in ovariectomized mice.[160] Female mice with estrogen deficiency or absent estrogen action (due to inactivation of the aromatase or ERα estrogen receptor genes) develop the MetS.[161,162] In a large study of women between 50 and 59 years of age, estradiol levels were lower in individuals with MetS, and inversely correlated with total cholesterol and diastolic blood pressure.[163] On the other hand, in a recent study of postmenopausal women, high concentrations of estradiol, along with high levels of testosterone, predicted the incidence of type 2 diabetes on follow-up, independent of HbA1C and other components of the MetS at baseline.[164] Similarly, in another study of postmenopausal women, estradiol concentrations were higher in women with the MetS, obesity, and abnormal glucose regulation.[150] In men, associations between estradiol and obesity, abnormal glucose regulation, and the MetS appear to be be weaker.[158,165,166]

Overall, the relations of sex hormones and the MetS suggest a sexual dimorphism in the relations. These observations are intriguing and should encourage further research to understand the underlying biological mechanisms.

Renal Biomarkers in MetS

Cystatin C

Cystatin C is an endogenous cysteine inhibitor, which is produced by nearly all human cells and is present in all body fluids.[167] It has been suggested to be a superior proxy for glomerular filtration rate (GFR) compared to serum creatinine, although this view is not undisputed and cystatin C has yet to be fully established as the marker of choice for estimating kidney function in clinical practice.[168] Cystatin C has recently been shown to be a strong independent risk factor for death and cardiovascular events in the community.[169–171] Circulating levels of the biomarker have been shown to be increased in individuals with the MetS in small and/or selected study samples.[172–174] In a recent longitudinal study, it was shown that higher baseline insulin sensitivity measured with euglycemic clamp techniques was associated with a lower risk of impaired renal function assessed with cystatin C at follow-up, independent of glucometabolic variables and other confounders at baseline.[175]

Urine Albumin

The urine albumin excretion rate is a marker of microalbuminuria, which can be used as an early sign of subclinical renal damage. It has also been suggested to be a marker of generalized vascular dysfunction,[176] as it mirrors target organ damage caused by hypertension. It has repeatedly been demonstrated to predict incident cardiovascular disease in different study samples,[177–180] even in healthy individuals with levels well below the current microalbuminuria threshold.[177,179] There are several studies demonstrating strong and consistent associations between the MetS and microalbuminuria measured by urinary albumin excretion rate.[181–184]

The MetS and accompanying impairment of insulin sensitivity could be associated with elevation of renal biomarkers via a number of different mechanisms. Hyperinsulinemia can stimulate the expression and activation of insulin-like growth factor 1 and transforming growth factor beta, together with the RAAS system—factors that can activate proliferation of mesangial cells and extracellular matrix expansion in the kidney.[185] Also, insulin resistance may increase oxidative stress,[186] which can promote renal injury by reduced nitric oxide bioavailability,[187] along with increased concentrations of glycoxidation and lipid peroxidation products.[188]

Conclusion

Derangements in circulating levels of biomarkers from a wide variety of pathways are observed in patients with the MetS. One reason that such a diverse set of biomarkers are associated with the MetS is the fact that it is a syndrome by definition—a constellation of signs and symptoms. As such, biomarkers that are associated with one of the components of the MetS are often associated with the syndrome itself. Nonetheless, the MetS constitutes a clustering of metabolic risk factors, which heralds an increased risk of cardiovascular disease. Further elucidation of the mechanisms leading up to the MetS (including perturbations of several key biological pathways) is fundamental to understanding the condition and preventing its sequelae. Studies of biomarkers associated with the MetS may also generate new therapeutic targets, which can be tested in additional studies.

References

1. Kylin E. Studien Über das Hypertonie-Hyperglykämie-Hyperurikämiesyndrom. *Zentralblatt für innere Medizin.* 1923;44:105–127.
2. Maranon G. Ãœber Hypertonie und Zuckerkrankheit. *Zentralblatt fur innere Medizin.* 1922;43:169–176.
3. Reaven GM. Banting lecture 1988. Role of insulin resistance in human disease. *Diabetes.* 1988;37:1595–1607.
4. Haffner SM, Valdez RA, Hazuda HP, Mitchell BD, Morales PA, Stern MP. Prospective analysis of the insulin-resistance syndrome (syndrome X). *Diabetes.* 1992;41:715–722.
5. Alberti KG, Zimmet PZ. Definition, diagnosis and classification of diabetes mellitus and its complications. Part 1: diagnosis and classification of diabetes mellitus provisional report of a WHO consultation. *Diabet Med.* 1998;15:539–553.
6. Balkau B, Charles MA. Comment on the provisional report from the WHO consultation. European Group for the Study of Insulin Resistance (EGIR). *Diabet Med.* 1999;16:442–443.
7. Executive Summary of The Third Report of The National Cholesterol Education Program (NCEP) Expert Panel on Detection, Evaluation, And Treatment of High Blood Cholesterol In Adults (Adult Treatment Panel III). *JAMA.* 2001;285:2486–2497.
8. Einhorn D, Reaven GM, Cobin RH, et al. American College of Endocrinology position statement on the insulin resistance syndrome. *Endocr Pract.* 2003;9:237–252.
9. Alberti KG, Zimmet P, Shaw J. Metabolic syndrome—a new worldwide definition. A Consensus Statement from the International Diabetes Federation. *Diabet Med.* 2006;23:469–480.
10. Grundy SM, Cleeman JI, Daniels SR, et al. Diagnosis and management of the metabolic syndrome: an American Heart Association/National Heart, Lung, and Blood Institute Scientific Statement. *Circulation.* 2005;112:2735–2752.
11. Metabolic Syndrome. National Library of Medicine. http://www.ncbi.nlm.nih.gov/medlineplus/metabolicsyndrome.html. Accessed December 5, 2008.
12. Vasan RS. Biomarkers of cardiovascular disease: molecular basis and practical considerations. *Circulation.* 2006;113:2335–2362.

13. Ferrannini E, Haffner SM, Mitchell BD, Stern MP. Hyperinsulinaemia: the key feature of a cardiovascular and metabolic syndrome. *Diabetologia.* 1991;34:416–422.

14. Reilly MP, Wolfe ML, Rhodes T, Girman C, Mehta N, Rader DJ. Measures of insulin resistance add incremental value to the clinical diagnosis of metabolic syndrome in association with coronary atherosclerosis. *Circulation.* 2004;110:803–809.

15. Lemieux I, Pascot A, Couillard C, et al. Hypertriglyceridemic waist: a marker of the atherogenic metabolic triad (hyperinsulinemia; hyperapolipoprotein B; small, dense LDL) in men? *Circulation.* 2000; 102:179–184.

16. Eckel RH, Grundy SM, Zimmet PZ. The metabolic syndrome. *Lancet.* 2005;365:1415–1428.

17. Festa A, Williams K, Tracy RP, Wagenknecht LE, Haffner SM. Progression of plasminogen activator inhibitor-1 and fibrinogen levels in relation to incident type 2 diabetes. *Circulation.* 2006;113:1753–1759.

18. Meigs JB, Hu FB, Rifai N, Manson JE. Biomarkers of endothelial dysfunction and risk of type 2 diabetes mellitus. *JAMA.* 2004;291: 1978–1986.

19. Pradhan AD, Manson JE, Rifai N, Buring JE, Ridker PM. C-reactive protein, interleukin 6, and risk of developing type 2 diabetes mellitus. *JAMA.* 2001;286:327–334.

20. Freitag MH, Larson MG, Levy D, et al. Plasma brain natriuretic peptide levels and blood pressure tracking in the Framingham Heart Study. *Hypertension.* 2003;41:978–983.

21. Sesso HD, Buring JE, Rifai N, Blake GJ, Gaziano JM, Ridker PM. C-reactive protein and the risk of developing hypertension. *JAMA.* 2003;290:2945–2951.

22. Wang TJ, Evans JC, Meigs JB et al. Low-grade albuminuria and the risks of hypertension and blood pressure progression. *Circulation.* 2005;111:1370–1376.

23. Han TS, Sattar N, Williams K, Gonzalez-Villalpando C, Lean ME, Haffner SM. Prospective study of C-reactive protein in relation to the development of diabetes and metabolic syndrome in the Mexico City Diabetes Study. *Diabetes Care.* 2002;25:2016–2021.

24. Holvoet P, Lee DH, Steffes M, Gross M, Jacobs DR Jr. Association between circulating oxidized low-density lipoprotein and incidence of the metabolic syndrome. *JAMA.* 2008;299:2287–2293.

25. Laaksonen DE, Niskanen L, Nyyssonen K, et al. C-reactive protein and the development of the metabolic syndrome and diabetes in middle-aged men. *Diabetologia.* 2004;47:1403–1410.

26. Ingelsson E, Pencina MJ, Tofler GH, et al. Multimarker approach to evaluate the incidence of the metabolic syndrome and longitudinal changes in metabolic risk factors: the Framingham Offspring Study. *Circulation.* 2007;116:984–992.

27. Onat A, Ozhan H, Erbilen E, et al. Independent prediction of metabolic syndrome by plasma fibrinogen in men, and predictors of elevated levels. *Int J Cardiol.* 2009;135:211–217.

28. Xu A, Tso AW, Cheung BM, et al. Circulating adipocyte-fatty acid binding protein levels predict the development of the metabolic syndrome: a 5-year prospective study. *Circulation.* 2007;115:1537–1543.

29. Janssen I, Powell LH, Crawford S, Lasley B, Sutton-Tyrrell K. Menopause and the metabolic syndrome: the Study of Women's Health Across the Nation. *Arch Intern Med.* 2008;168:1568–1575.

30. Kahn R, Buse J, Ferrannini E, Stern M. The metabolic syndrome: time for a critical appraisal: joint statement from the American Diabetes Association and the European Association for the Study of Diabetes. *Diabetes Care.* 2005;28:2289–2304.

31. Gale EA. The myth of the metabolic syndrome. *Diabetologia.* 2005; 48:1679–1683.

32. Dilley J, Ganesan A, Deepa R, et al. Association of A1C with cardiovascular disease and metabolic syndrome in Asian Indians with normal glucose tolerance. *Diabetes Care.* 2007;30:1527–1532.

33. Osei K, Rhinesmith S, Gaillard T, Schuster D. Is glycosylated hemoglobin A1c a surrogate for metabolic syndrome in nondiabetic, first-degree relatives of African-American patients with type 2 diabetes? *J Clin Endocrinol Metab.* 2003;88:4596–4601.

34. Sung KC, Rhee EJ. Glycated haemoglobin as a predictor for metabolic syndrome in non-diabetic Korean adults. *Diabet Med.* 2007; 24:848–854.

35. Festa A, D'Agostino R Jr, Howard G, Mykkanen L, Tracy RP, Haffner SM. Chronic subclinical inflammation as part of the insulin

resistance syndrome: the Insulin Resistance Atherosclerosis Study (IRAS). *Circulation.* 2000;102:42–47.

36. Fröhlich M, Imhof A, Berg G, et al. Association between C-reactive protein and features of the metabolic syndrome: a population-based study. *Diabetes Care.* 2000;23:1835–1839.
37. Ridker PM, Buring JE, Cook NR, Rifai N. C-reactive protein, the metabolic syndrome, and risk of incident cardiovascular events: an 8-year follow-up of 14,719 initially healthy American women. *Circulation.* 2003;107:391–397.
38. Wannamethee SG, Lowe GD, Shaper AG, Rumley A, Lennon L, Whincup PH. The metabolic syndrome and insulin resistance: relationship to haemostatic and inflammatory markers in older nondiabetic men. *Atherosclerosis.* 2005;181:101–108.
39. Nakanishi N, Shiraishi T, Wada M. C-reactive protein concentration is more strongly related to metabolic syndrome in women than in men: the Minoh Study. *Circ J.* 2005;69:386–391.
40. Van Guilder GP, Hoetzer GL, Greiner JJ, Stauffer BL, Desouza CA. Influence of metabolic syndrome on biomarkers of oxidative stress and inflammation in obese adults. *Obesity (Silver Spring).* 2006;14: 2127–2131.
41. Pischon T, Hu FB, Rexrode KM, Girman CJ, Manson JE, Rimm EB. Inflammation, the metabolic syndrome, and risk of coronary heart disease in women and men. *Atherosclerosis.* 2008;197:392–399.
42. Wannamethee SG, Whincup PH, Rumley A, Lowe GD. Interrelationships of interleukin-6, cardiovascular risk factors and the metabolic syndrome among older men. *J Thromb Haemost.* 2007;5: 1637–1643.
43. Hamid YH, Rose CS, Urhammer SA, et al. Variations of the interleukin-6 promoter are associated with features of the metabolic syndrome in Caucasian Danes. *Diabetologia.* 2005;48:251–260.
44. Lohsoonthorn V, Dhanamun B, Williams MA. Prevalence of metabolic syndrome and its relationship to white blood cell count in a population of Thai men and women receiving routine health examinations. *Am J Hypertens.* 2006;19:339–345.
45. Tsai JC, Sheu SH, Chiu HC, et al. Association of peripheral total and differential leukocyte counts with metabolic syndrome and risk of ischemic cardiovascular diseases in patients with type 2 diabetes mellitus. *Diabetes Metab Res Rev.* 2007;23:111–118.

46. Desai MY, Dalal D, Santos RD, Carvalho JA, Nasir K, Blumenthal RS. Association of body mass index, metabolic syndrome, and leukocyte count. *Am J Cardiol.* 2006;97:835–838.
47. Festa A, D'Agostino R Jr, Tracy RP, Haffner SM. Elevated levels of acute-phase proteins and plasminogen activator inhibitor-1 predict the development of type 2 diabetes: the insulin resistance atherosclerosis study. *Diabetes.* 2002;51:1131–1137.
48. Freeman DJ, Norrie J, Caslake MJ, et al. C-reactive protein is an independent predictor of risk for the development of diabetes in the West of Scotland Coronary Prevention Study. *Diabetes.* 2002;51: 1596–1600.
49. Rutter MK, Meigs JB, Sullivan LM, D'Agostino RB Sr, Wilson PW. C-reactive protein, the metabolic syndrome, and prediction of cardiovascular events in the Framingham Offspring Study. *Circulation.* 2004;110:380–385.
50. Ouchi N, Kihara S, Funahashi T, et al. Reciprocal association of C-reactive protein with adiponectin in blood stream and adipose tissue. *Circulation.* 2003;107:671–674.
51. Lau DC, Dhillon B, Yan H, Szmitko PE, Verma S. Adipokines: molecular links between obesity and atherosclerosis. *Am J Physiol Heart Circ Physiol.* 2005;288:H2031–H2041.
52. Soro-Paavonen A, Westerbacka J, Ehnholm C, Taskinen MR. Metabolic syndrome aggravates the increased endothelial activation and low-grade inflammation in subjects with familial low HDL. *Ann Med.* 2006;38:229–238.
53. Gomez Rosso L, Benitez MB, Fornari MC, et al. Alterations in cell adhesion molecules and other biomarkers of cardiovascular disease in patients with metabolic syndrome. *Atherosclerosis.* 2008;199: 415–423.
54. Miller MA, Cappuccio FP. Cellular adhesion molecules and their relationship with measures of obesity and metabolic syndrome in a multiethnic population. *Int J Obes (Lond).* 2006;30:1176–1182.
55. Ingelsson E, Hulthe J, Lind L. Inflammatory markers in relation to insulin resistance and the metabolic syndrome. *Eur J Clin Invest.* 2008;38:502–509.
56. Schram MT, Stehouwer CD. Endothelial dysfunction, cellular adhesion molecules and the metabolic syndrome. *Horm Metab Res.* 2005;(37 Suppl)1:49–55.

57. Alessi MC, Juhan-Vague I. PAI-1 and the metabolic syndrome: links, causes, and consequences. *Arterioscler Thromb Vasc Biol.* 2006;26: 2200–2207.

58. Mertens I, Verrijken A, Michiels JJ, Van der Planken M, Ruige JB, Van Gaal LF. Among inflammation and coagulation markers, PAI-1 is a true component of the metabolic syndrome. *Int J Obes (Lond).* 2006;30:1308–1314.

59. Kraja AT, Province MA, Arnett D, et al. Do inflammation and procoagulation biomarkers contribute to the metabolic syndrome cluster? *Nutr Metab (Lond).* 2007;4:28.

60. Liang X, Kanjanabuch T, Mao SL, et al. Plasminogen activator inhibitor-1 modulates adipocyte differentiation. *Am J Physiol Endocrinol Metab.* 2006;290:E103–E113.

61. Ma LJ, Mao SL, Taylor KL, et al. Prevention of obesity and insulin resistance in mice lacking plasminogen activator inhibitor 1. *Diabetes.* 2004;53:336–346.

62. Schafer K, Fujisawa K, Konstantinides S, Loskutoff DJ. Disruption of the plasminogen activator inhibitor 1 gene reduces the adiposity and improves the metabolic profile of genetically obese and diabetic ob/ob mice. *FASEB J.* 2001;15:1840–1842.

63. Huvers FC, De Leeuw PW, Houben AJ, et al. Endothelium-dependent vasodilatation, plasma markers of endothelial function, and adrenergic vasoconstrictor responses in type 1 diabetes under near-normoglycemic conditions. *Diabetes.* 1999;48:1300–1307.

64. Kaikita K, Fogo AB, Ma L, Schoenhard JA, Brown NJ, Vaughan DE. Plasminogen activator inhibitor-1 deficiency prevents hypertension and vascular fibrosis in response to long-term nitric oxide synthase inhibition. *Circulation.* 2001;104:839–844.

65. Imperatore G, Riccardi G, Iovine C, Rivellese AA, Vaccaro O. Plasma fibrinogen: a new factor of the metabolic syndrome. A population-based study. *Diabetes Care.* 1998;21:649–654.

66. Mertens I, Van Gaal LF. Obesity, haemostasis and the fibrinolytic system. *Obes Rev.* 2002;3:85–101.

67. Zhang Y, Proenca R, Maffei M, Barone M, Leopold L, Friedman JM. Positional cloning of the mouse obese gene and its human homologue. *Nature.* 1994;372:425–432.

68. Ingelsson E, Larson MG, Yin X, et al. Circulating ghrelin, leptin, and soluble leptin receptor concentrations and cardiometabolic risk

factors in a community-based sample. *J Clin Endocrinol Metab.* 2008;93:3149–3157.

69. Margetic S, Gazzola C, Pegg GG, Hill RA. Leptin: a review of its peripheral actions and interactions. *Int J Obes Relat Metab Disord.* 2002;26:1407–1433.
70. Ruhl CE, Everhart JE. Leptin concentrations in the United States: relations with demographic and anthropometric measures. *Am J Clin Nutr.* 2001;74:295–301.
71. Zimmet P, Hodge A, Nicolson M, et al. Serum leptin concentration, obesity, and insulin resistance in Western Samoans: cross sectional study. *BMJ.* 1996;313:965–969.
72. Beltowski J. Role of leptin in blood pressure regulation and arterial hypertension. *J Hypertens.* 2006;24:789–801.
73. Söderberg S, Zimmet P, Tuomilehto J, et al. Leptin predicts the development of diabetes in Mauritian men, but not women: a population-based study. *Int J Obes (Lond).* 2007;31:1126–1133.
74. Widjaja A, Stratton IM, Horn R, Holman RR, Turner R, Brabant G. UKPDS 20: plasma leptin, obesity, and plasma insulin in type 2 diabetic subjects. *J Clin Endocrinol Metab.* 1997;82:654–657.
75. Franks PW, Brage S, Luan J, et al. Leptin predicts a worsening of the features of the metabolic syndrome independently of obesity. *Obes Res.* 2005;13:1476–1484.
76. Leyva F, Godsland IF, Ghatei M, et al. Hyperleptinemia as a component of a metabolic syndrome of cardiovascular risk. *Arterioscler Thromb Vasc Biol.* 1998;18:928–933.
77. Valle M, Gascon F, Martos R, Bermudo F, Ceballos P, Suanes A. Relationship between high plasma leptin concentrations and metabolic syndrome in obese pre-pubertal children. *Int J Obes Relat Metab Disord.* 2003;27:13–18.
78. Myers MG, Cowley MA, Munzberg H. Mechanisms of leptin action and leptin resistance. *Annu Rev Physiol.* 2008;70:537–556.
79. Hu E, Liang P, Spiegelman BM. AdipoQ is a novel adipose-specific gene dysregulated in obesity. *J Biol Chem.* 1996;271:10697–10703.
80. Maeda K, Okubo K, Shimomura I, Funahashi T, Matsuzawa Y, Matsubara K. cDNA cloning and expression of a novel adipose specific collagen-like factor, apM1 (AdiPose Most abundant Gene transcript 1). *Biochem Biophys Res Commun.* 1996;221:286–289.

81. Nakano Y, Tobe T, Choi-Miura NH, Mazda T, Tomita M. Isolation and characterization of GBP28, a novel gelatin-binding protein purified from human plasma. *J Biochem.* 1996;120:803–812.

82. Scherer PE, Williams S, Fogliano M, Baldini G, Lodish HF. A novel serum protein similar to C1q, produced exclusively in adipocytes. *J Biol Chem.* 1995;270:26746–26749.

83. Okamoto Y, Kihara S, Funahashi T, Matsuzawa Y, Libby P. Adiponectin: a key adipocytokine in metabolic syndrome. *Clin Sci (Lond).* 2006;110:267–278.

84. Cnop M, Havel PJ, Utzschneider KM, et al. Relationship of adiponectin to body fat distribution, insulin sensitivity and plasma lipoproteins: evidence for independent roles of age and sex. *Diabetologia.* 2003;46:459–469.

85. Lindsay RS, Funahashi T, Hanson RL, et al. Adiponectin and development of type 2 diabetes in the Pima Indian population. *Lancet.* 2002;360:57–58.

86. Pischon T, Girman CJ, Hotamisligil GS, Rifai N, Hu FB, Rimm EB. Plasma adiponectin levels and risk of myocardial infarction in men. *JAMA.* 2004;291:1730–1737.

87. Iwashima Y, Katsuya T, Ishikawa K, et al. Hypoadiponectinemia is an independent risk factor for hypertension. *Hypertension.* 2004;43: 1318–1323.

88. Matsubara M, Maruoka S, Katayose S. Decreased plasma adiponectin concentrations in women with dyslipidemia. *J Clin Endocrinol Metab.* 2002;87:2764–2769.

89. Schulze MB, Rimm EB, Shai I, Rifai N, Hu FB. Relationship between adiponectin and glycemic control, blood lipids, and inflammatory markers in men with type 2 diabetes. *Diabetes Care.* 2004;27: 1680–1687.

90. Gilardini L, McTernan PG, Girola A, et al. Adiponectin is a candidate marker of metabolic syndrome in obese children and adolescents. *Atherosclerosis.* 2006;189:401–407.

91. Kim SM, Cho KH, Park HS. Relationship between plasma adiponectin levels and the metabolic syndrome among Korean people. *Endocr J.* 2006;53:247–254.

92. Mohan V, Deepa R, Pradeepa R, et al. Association of low adiponectin levels with the metabolic syndrome—the Chennai Urban Rural Epidemiology Study (CURES-4). *Metabolism.* 2005;54:476–481.

93. Ryo M, Nakamura T, Kihara S, et al. Adiponectin as a biomarker of the metabolic syndrome. *Circ J.* 2004;68:975–981.

94. Wang J, Li H, Franco OH, Yu Z, Liu Y, Lin X. Adiponectin and metabolic syndrome in middle-aged and elderly Chinese. *Obesity (Silver Spring).* 2008;16:172–178.

95. Hotta K, Funahashi T, Bodkin NL, et al. Circulating concentrations of the adipocyte protein adiponectin are decreased in parallel with reduced insulin sensitivity during the progression to type 2 diabetes in rhesus monkeys. *Diabetes.* 2001;50:1126–1133.

96. Maeda N, Shimomura I, Kishida K, et al. Diet-induced insulin resistance in mice lacking adiponectin/ACRP30. *Nat Med.* 2002;8: 731–737.

97. Yamauchi T, Kamon J, Waki H, et al. The fat-derived hormone adiponectin reverses insulin resistance associated with both lipoatrophy and obesity. *Nat Med.* 2001;7:941–946.

98. Pinkney J, Williams G. Ghrelin gets hungry. *Lancet.* 2002;359: 1360–1361.

99. Poykko SM, Kellokoski E, Horkko S, Kauma H, Kesaniemi YA, Ukkola O. Low plasma ghrelin is associated with insulin resistance, hypertension, and the prevalence of type 2 diabetes. *Diabetes.* 2003;52:2546–2553.

100. Choi KM, Lee J, Lee KW, et al. The associations between plasma adiponectin, ghrelin levels and cardiovascular risk factors. *Eur J Endocrinol.* 2004;150:715–718.

101. Katsuki A, Urakawa H, Gabazza EC, et al. Circulating levels of active ghrelin is associated with abdominal adiposity, hyperinsulinemia and insulin resistance in patients with type 2 diabetes mellitus. *Eur J Endocrinol.* 2004;151:573–577.

102. Langenberg C, Bergstrom J, Laughlin GA, Barrett-Connor E. Ghrelin and the metabolic syndrome in older adults. *J Clin Endocrinol Metab.* 2005;90:6448–6453.

103. Ukkola O, Pöykkö SM, Antero Kesäniemi Y. Low plasma ghrelin concentration is an indicator of the metabolic syndrome. *Ann Med.* 2006;38:274–279.

104. Nagaya N, Kojima M, Uematsu M, et al. Hemodynamic and hormonal effects of human ghrelin in healthy volunteers. *Am J Physiol Regul Integr Comp Physiol.* 2001;280:R1483–R1487.

105. Okumura H, Nagaya N, Enomoto M, Nakagawa E, Oya H, Kangawa K. Vasodilatory effect of ghrelin, an endogenous peptide from the stomach. *J Cardiovasc Pharmacol.* 2002;39:779–783.

106. Gil-Campos M, Aguilera CM, Canete R, Gil A. Ghrelin: a hormone regulating food intake and energy homeostasis. *Br J Nutr.* 2006;96:201–226.

107. Murata M, Okimura Y, Iida K, et al. Ghrelin modulates the downstream molecules of insulin signaling in hepatoma cells. *J Biol Chem.* 2002;277:5667–5674.

108. Murdolo G, Lucidi P, Di Loreto C, et al. Insulin is required for prandial ghrelin suppression in humans. *Diabetes.* 2003;52:2923–2927.

109. Cho YM, Youn BS, Lee H, et al. Plasma retinol-binding protein-4 concentrations are elevated in human subjects with impaired glucose tolerance and type 2 diabetes. *Diabetes Care.* 2006;29:2457–2461.

110. Graham TE, Yang Q, Bluher M, et al. Retinol-binding protein 4 and insulin resistance in lean, obese, and diabetic subjects. *N Engl J Med.* 2006;354:2552–2563.

111. Qi Q, Yu Z, Ye X, et al. Elevated retinol-binding protein 4 levels are associated with metabolic syndrome in Chinese people. *J Clin Endocrinol Metab.* 2007;92:4827–4834.

112. Yang Q, Graham TE, Mody N, et al. Serum retinol binding protein 4 contributes to insulin resistance in obesity and type 2 diabetes. *Nature.* 2005;436:356–362.

113. Gavi S, Stuart LM, Kelly P, et al. Retinol-binding protein 4 is associated with insulin resistance and body fat distribution in nonobese subjects without type 2 diabetes. *J Clin Endocrinol Metab.* 2007;92:1886–1890.

114. Jia W, Wu H, Bao Y, et al. Association of serum retinol-binding protein 4 and visceral adiposity in Chinese subjects with and without type 2 diabetes. *J Clin Endocrinol Metab.* 2007;92:3224–3229.

115. Huang S, Czech MP. The GLUT4 glucose transporter. *Cell Metab.* 2007;5:237–252.

116. Steppan CM, Bailey ST, Bhat S, et al. The hormone resistin links obesity to diabetes. *Nature.* 2001;409:307–312.

117. Hivert MF, Sullivan LM, Fox CS, et al. Associations of adiponectin, resistin, and tumor necrosis factor-alpha with insulin resistance. *J Clin Endocrinol Metab.* 2008;93:3165–3172.

118. Osawa H, Tabara Y, Kawamoto R, et al. Plasma resistin, associated with single nucleotide polymorphism -420, is correlated with insulin resistance, lower HDL cholesterol, and high-sensitivity C-reactive protein in the Japanese general population. *Diabetes Care.* 2007;30: 1501–1506.
119. Aquilante CL, Kosmiski LA, Knutsen SD, Zineh I. Relationship between plasma resistin concentrations, inflammatory chemokines, and components of the metabolic syndrome in adults. *Metabolism.* 2008;57:494–501.
120. Norata GD, Ongari M, Garlaschelli K, Raselli S, Grigore L, Catapano AL. Plasma resistin levels correlate with determinants of the metabolic syndrome. *Eur J Endocrinol.* 2007;156:279–284.
121. Boord JB, Fazio S, Linton MF. Cytoplasmic fatty acid-binding proteins: emerging roles in metabolism and atherosclerosis. *Curr Opin Lipidol.* 2002;13:141–147.
122. Hotamisligil GS, Johnson RS, Distel RJ, Ellis R, Papaioannou VE, Spiegelman BM. Uncoupling of obesity from insulin resistance through a targeted mutation in aP2, the adipocyte fatty acid binding protein. *Science.* 1996;274:1377–1379.
123. Scheja L, Makowski L, Uysal KT, et al. Altered insulin secretion associated with reduced lipolytic efficiency in aP2-/- mice. *Diabetes.* 1999;48:1987–1994.
124. Stejskal D, Karpisek M. Adipocyte fatty acid binding protein in a Caucasian population: a new marker of metabolic syndrome? *Eur J Clin Invest.* 2006;36:621–625.
125. Xu A, Wang Y, Xu JY, et al. Adipocyte fatty acid-binding protein is a plasma biomarker closely associated with obesity and metabolic syndrome. *Clin Chem.* 2006;52:405–413.
126. Tso AW, Xu A, Sham PC, et al. Serum adipocyte fatty acid binding protein as a new biomarker predicting the development of type 2 diabetes: a 10-year prospective study in a Chinese cohort. *Diabetes Care.* 2007;30:2667–2672.
127. Auberger P, Falquerho L, Contreres JO, et al. Characterization of a natural inhibitor of the insulin receptor tyrosine kinase: cDNA cloning, purification, and anti-mitogenic activity. *Cell.* 1989;58: 631–640.
128. Mathews ST, Singh GP, Ranalletta M, et al. Improved insulin sensitivity and resistance to weight gain in mice null for the Ahsg gene. *Diabetes.* 2002;51:2450–2458.

129. Ix JH, Shlipak MG, Brandenburg VM, Ali S, Ketteler M, Whooley MA. Association between human fetuin-A and the metabolic syndrome: data from the Heart and Soul Study. *Circulation.* 2006;113: 1760–1767.

130. Hennige AM, Staiger H, Wicke C, et al. Fetuin-A induces cytokine expression and suppresses adiponectin production. *PLoS ONE.* 2008;3:e1765.

131. Prasad A, Quyyumi AA. Renin-angiotensin system and angiotensin receptor blockers in the metabolic syndrome. *Circulation.* 2004;110: 1507–1512.

132. Engeli S, Bohnke J, Gorzelniak K, et al. Weight loss and the renin-angiotensin-aldosterone system. *Hypertension.* 2005;45:356–362.

133. Egan BM, Papademetriou V, Wofford M, et al. Metabolic syndrome and insulin resistance in the TROPHY sub-study: contrasting views in patients with high-normal blood pressure. *Am J Hypertens.* 2005; 18:3–12.

134. Kidambi S, Kotchen JM, Grim CE, et al. Association of adrenal steroids with hypertension and the metabolic syndrome in blacks. *Hypertension.* 2007;49:704–711.

135. Giacchetti G, Ronconi V, Turchi F, et al. Aldosterone as a key mediator of the cardiometabolic syndrome in primary aldosteronism: an observational study. *J Hypertens.* 2007;25:177–186.

136. Lind L, Reneland R, Andersson PE, Haenni A, Lithell H. Insulin resistance in essential hypertension is related to plasma renin activity. *J Hum Hypertens.* 1998;12:379–382.

137. Vasan RS, Evans JC, Larson MG, et al. Serum aldosterone and the incidence of hypertension in nonhypertensive persons. *N Engl J Med.* 2004;351:33–41.

138. Penfornis P, Viengchareun S, Le Menuet D, Cluzeaud F, Zennaro MC, Lombes M. The mineralocorticoid receptor mediates aldosterone-induced differentiation of T37i cells into brown adipocytes. *Am J Physiol Endocrinol Metab.* 2000;279:E386–E394.

139. Rondinone CM, Rodbard D, Baker ME. Aldosterone stimulated differentiation of mouse 3T3-L1 cells into adipocytes. *Endocrinology.* 1993;132:2421–2426.

140. Daniels LB, Maisel AS. Natriuretic peptides. *J Am Coll Cardiol.* 2007;50:2357–2368.

141. de Lemos JA, Morrow DA, Bentley JH, et al. The prognostic value of B-type natriuretic peptide in patients with acute coronary syndromes. *N Engl J Med.* 2001;345:1014–1021.

142. Wang TJ, Larson MG, Levy D, et al. Plasma natriuretic peptide levels and the risk of cardiovascular events and death. *N Engl J Med.* 2004;350:655–663.

143. Wang TJ, Larson MG, Levy D, et al. Impact of obesity on plasma natriuretic peptide levels. *Circulation.* 2004;109:594–600.

144. Olsen MH, Hansen TW, Christensen MK, et al. N-terminal pro brain natriuretic peptide is inversely related to metabolic cardiovascular risk factors and the metabolic syndrome. *Hypertension.* 2005;46: 660–666.

145. Wang TJ, Larson MG, Keyes MJ, Levy D, Benjamin EJ, Vasan RS. Association of plasma natriuretic peptide levels with metabolic risk factors in ambulatory individuals. *Circulation.* 2007;115:1345–1353.

146. Corbould A. Effects of androgens on insulin action in women: is androgen excess a component of female metabolic syndrome? *Diabetes Metab Res Rev.* 2008;24:520–532.

147. Rosner W, Auchus RJ, Azziz R, Sluss PM, Raff H. Position statement: Utility, limitations, and pitfalls in measuring testosterone: an Endocrine Society position statement. *J Clin Endocrinol Metab.* 2007;92: 405–413.

148. Khaw KT, Barrett-Connor E. Fasting plasma glucose levels and endogenous androgens in non-diabetic postmenopausal women. *Clin Sci (Lond).* 1991;80:199–203.

149. Maturana MA, Spritzer PM. Association between hyperinsulinemia and endogenous androgen levels in peri- and postmenopausal women. *Metabolism.* 2002;51:238–243.

150. Weinberg ME, Manson JE, Buring JE, et al. Low sex hormone-binding globulin is associated with the metabolic syndrome in postmenopausal women. *Metabolism.* 2006;55:1473–1480.

151. Golden SH, Ding J, Szklo M, Schmidt MI, Duncan BB, Dobs A. Glucose and insulin components of the metabolic syndrome are associated with hyperandrogenism in postmenopausal women: the atherosclerosis risk in communities study. *Am J Epidemiol.* 2004;160: 540–548.

152. Korhonen S, Hippelainen M, Vanhala M, Heinonen S, Niskanen L. The androgenic sex hormone profile is an essential feature of metabolic syndrome in premenopausal women: a controlled community-based study. *Fertil Steril.* 2003;79:1327–1334.

153. McCartney CR, Prendergast KA, Chhabra S, et al. The association of obesity and hyperandrogenemia during the pubertal transition in girls: obesity as a potential factor in the genesis of postpubertal hyperandrogenism. *J Clin Endocrinol Metab.* 2006;91:1714–1722.

154. Haffner SM, Valdez RA, Morales PA, Hazuda HP, Stern MP. Decreased sex hormone-binding globulin predicts noninsulin-dependent diabetes mellitus in women but not in men. *J Clin Endocrinol Metab.* 1993;77:56–60.

155. Lindstedt G, Lundberg PA, Lapidus L, Lundgren H, Bengtsson C, Bjorntorp P. Low sex-hormone-binding globulin concentration as independent risk factor for development of NIDDM. 12-yr follow-up of population study of women in Gothenburg, Sweden. *Diabetes.* 1991;40:123–128.

156. Kapoor D, Malkin CJ, Channer KS, Jones TH. Androgens, insulin resistance and vascular disease in men. *Clin Endocrinol (Oxf).* 2005;63:239–250.

157. Khaw KT, Barrett-Connor E. Lower endogenous androgens predict central adiposity in men. *Ann Epidemiol.* 1992;2:675–682.

158. Oh JY, Barrett-Connor E, Wedick NM, Wingard DL. Endogenous sex hormones and the development of type 2 diabetes in older men and women: the Rancho Bernardo study. *Diabetes Care.* 2002;25: 55–60.

159. Salpeter SR, Walsh JM, Ormiston TM, Greyber E, Buckley NS, Salpeter EE. Meta-analysis: effect of hormone-replacement therapy on components of the metabolic syndrome in postmenopausal women. *Diabetes Obes Metab.* 2006;8:538–554.

160. D'Eon TM, Souza SC, Aronovitz M, Obin MS, Fried SK, Greenberg AS. Estrogen regulation of adiposity and fuel partitioning. Evidence of genomic and non-genomic regulation of lipogenic and oxidative pathways. *J Biol Chem.* 2005;280:35983–35991.

161. Couse JF, Korach KS. Estrogen receptor null mice: what have we learned and where will they lead us? *Endocr Rev.* 1999;20:358–417.

162. Misso ML, Murata Y, Boon WC, Jones ME, Britt KL, Simpson ER. Cellular and molecular characterization of the adipose phenotype

of the aromatase-deficient mouse. *Endocrinology.* 2003;144:1474–1480.

163. Shakir YA, Samsioe G, Nyberg P, Lidfeldt J, Nerbrand C, Agardh CD. Do sex hormones influence features of the metabolic syndrome in middle-aged women? A population-based study of Swedish women: the Women's Health in the Lund Area (WHILA) Study. *Fertil Steril.* 2007;88:163–171.

164. Ding EL, Song Y, Manson JE, Rifai N, Buring JE, Liu S. Plasma sex steroid hormones and risk of developing type 2 diabetes in women: a prospective study. *Diabetologia.* 2007;50:2076–2084.

165. Goodman-Gruen D, Barrett-Connor E. Sex differences in the association of endogenous sex hormone levels and glucose tolerance status in older men and women. *Diabetes Care.* 2000;23:912–918.

166. Muller M, Grobbee DE, den Tonkelaar I, Lamberts SW, van der Schouw YT. Endogenous sex hormones and metabolic syndrome in aging men. *J Clin Endocrinol Metab.* 2005;90:2618–2623.

167. Mussap M, Plebani M. Biochemistry and clinical role of human cystatin C. *Crit Rev Clin Lab Sci.* 2004;41:467–550.

168. Massey D. Commentary: clinical diagnostic use of cystatin C. *J Clin Lab Anal.* 2004;18:55–60.

169. Sarnak MJ, Katz R, Stehman-Breen CO, et al. Cystatin C concentration as a risk factor for heart failure in older adults. *Ann Intern Med.* 2005;142:497–505.

170. Shlipak MG, Sarnak MJ, Katz R, et al. Cystatin C and the risk of death and cardiovascular events among elderly persons. *N Engl J Med.* 2005;352:2049–2060.

171. Zethelius B, Berglund L, Sundstrom J, et al. Use of multiple biomarkers to improve the prediction of death from cardiovascular causes. *N Engl J Med.* 2008;358:2107–2116.

172. Demircan N, Gurel A, Armutcu F, Unalacak M, Aktunc E, Atmaca H. The evaluation of serum cystatin C, malondialdehyde, and total antioxidant status in patients with metabolic syndrome. *Med Sci Monit.* 2008;14:CR97–CR101.

173. Retnakaran R, Connelly PW, Harris SB, Zinman B, Hanley AJ. Cystatin C is associated with cardiovascular risk factors and metabolic syndrome in Aboriginal youth. *Pediatr Nephrol.* 2007;22:1007–1013.

174. Servais A, Giral P, Bernard M, Bruckert E, Deray G, Isnard Bagnis C. Is serum cystatin-C a reliable marker for metabolic syndrome? *Am J Med.* 2008;121:426–432.

175. Nerpin E, Riserus U, Ingelsson E, et al. Insulin sensitivity measured with euglycemic clamp is independently associated with glomerular filtration rate in a community-based cohort. *Diabetes Care.* 2008;31:1550–1555.

176. Deckert T, Feldt-Rasmussen B, Borch-Johnsen K, Jensen T, Kofoed-Enevoldsen A. Albuminuria reflects widespread vascular damage. The Steno hypothesis. *Diabetologia.* 1989;32:219–226.

177. Arnlov J, Evans JC, Meigs JB, et al. Low-grade albuminuria and incidence of cardiovascular disease events in nonhypertensive and nondiabetic individuals: the Framingham Heart Study. *Circulation.* 2005;112:969–975.

178. Borch-Johnsen K, Feldt-Rasmussen B, Strandgaard S, Schroll M, Jensen JS. Urinary albumin excretion. An independent predictor of ischemic heart disease. *Arterioscler Thromb Vasc Biol.* 1999;19: 1992–1997.

179. Ingelsson E, Sundstrom J, Lind L, et al. Low-grade albuminuria and the incidence of heart failure in a community-based cohort of elderly men. *Eur Heart J.* 2007;28:1739–1745.

180. Miettinen H, Haffner SM, Lehto S, Ronnemaa T, Pyorala K, Laakso M. Proteinuria predicts stroke and other atherosclerotic vascular disease events in nondiabetic and non-insulin-dependent diabetic subjects. *Stroke.* 1996;27:2033–2039.

181. Abuaisha B, Kumar S, Malik R, Boulton AJ. Relationship of elevated urinary albumin excretion to components of the metabolic syndrome in non-insulin-dependent diabetes mellitus. *Diabetes Res Clin Pract.* 1998;39:93–99.

182. Lin CC, Liu CS, Li TC, Chen CC, Li CI, Lin WY. Microalbuminuria and the metabolic syndrome and its components in the Chinese population. *Eur J Clin Invest.* 2007;37:783–790.

183. Klausen KP, Parving HH, Scharling H, Jensen JS. The association between metabolic syndrome, microalbuminuria and impaired renal function in the general population: impact on cardiovascular disease and mortality. *J Intern Med.* 2007;262:470–478.

184. Hao Z, Konta T, Takasaki S, et al. The association between microalbuminuria and metabolic syndrome in the general population in Japan: the Takahata study. *Intern Med.* 2007;46:341–346.

185. Sarafidis PA, Ruilope LM. Insulin resistance, hyperinsulinemia, and renal injury: mechanisms and implications. *Am J Nephrol.* 2006;26: 232–244.

186. Riserus U, Basu S, Jovinge S, Fredrikson GN, Arnlov J, Vessby B. Supplementation with conjugated linoleic acid causes isomer-dependent oxidative stress and elevated C-reactive protein: a potential link to fatty acid-induced insulin resistance. *Circulation.* 2002;106:1925–1929.

187. Prabhakar SS. Role of nitric oxide in diabetic nephropathy. *Semin Nephrol.* 2004;24:333–344.

188. Horie K, Miyata T, Maeda K, et al. Immunohistochemical colocalization of glycoxidation products and lipid peroxidation products in diabetic renal glomerular lesions. Implication for glycoxidative stress in the pathogenesis of diabetic nephropathy. *J Clin Invest.* 1997;100: 2995–3004.

31 ▪ Emerging Lipid-based Biomarkers

NATALIE KHUSEYINOVA, MD
WOLFGANG KOENIG, MD, PHD

Introduction

In the era of "global risk assessment," cardiovascular disease (CVD) risk stratification in primary prevention is usually done on the basis of one of the available risk scores, such as the Framingham Risk Score, the PROCAM Score, or the European Society of Cardiology SCORE. Among other risk factors, the atherogenic lipoprotein phenotype (characterized by increased levels of total cholesterol [TC]), low-density lipoprotein-cholesterol (LDL-C), non-high-density lipoprotein-cholesterol (HDL-C) as well as low concentrations of HDL-C remain to be integral parts of coronary heart disease (CHD) risk assessment. Moreover, it is routinely used for monitoring of standard-of-care treatment. Nonetheless, risk stratification for CVD remains suboptimal even after the introduction of global risk assessment. This has prompted a search for new biomarkers which may further aid in identifying individuals at high risk for CVD. Additional lipid-related molecules, such as lipoprotein-associated phospholipase A_2 (Lp-PLA_2), secretory phospholipase A_2 (sPLA_2), or oxidized LDL are emerging biomarkers that may improve our ability to predict risk of future CVD. This chapter summarizes our current knowledge based on observations from experimental and clinical studies, with emphasis on potential pathophysiological mechanisms of action and on the clinical relevance of various lipid-based biomarkers.

Lipoprotein-Associated Phospholipase A_2

Biology and Potential Atherogenic Mechanisms

Lipoprotein-associated phospholipase A_2 (Lp-PLA_2) has recently emerged as a promising biomarker for atherosclerotic disease.

Lp-PLA_2, a 45.4 kDa calcium-independent member of the phospholipase A_2 family, is secreted largely by cells of hematopoietic origin, such as monocytes/macrophages, T-lymphocytes, and mast and liver cells.[1] Lp-PLA_2 has been detected in both rabbit and human noncoronary atherosclerotic lesions, as well as in human coronary atherosclerotic plaque, especially in complex phenotypes.[1] It has been suggested that Lp-PLA_2 represents both a specific marker and a causal mediator of plaque progression and instability.[2] A major mechanism by which Lp-PLA_2 promotes atherogenesis may be related to its involvement in the cleavage of oxidized LDL.[1] In the bloodstream, two-thirds of Lp-PLA_2 circulates primarily bound to LDL; the remaining third is distributed between HDL and/or very low density lipoprotein (VLDL). LDL represents the circulating reservoir in which Lp-PLA_2 remains inactive until LDL undergoes oxidative modification. After LDL oxidation within the arterial wall, a short acyl group at the sn-2 position of phospholipids becomes susceptible to the hydrolytic action of Lp-PLA_2 that cleaves an oxidized phosphatidylcholine component of the lipoprotein particle, generating two potent proinflammatory and proatherogenic mediators, namely lysophosphatidylcholine (LysoPC) and oxidized fatty acid (oxFA).[1] Proinflammatory actions of LysoPC, as well as those of oxFA, trigger a cascade of events, which directly promote atherogenesis. LysoPC is a potent chemoattractant for T-cells and monocytes, promotes endothelial dysfunction (ED), stimulates macrophage proliferation, and induces apoptosis in smooth muscle cells (SMCs) and macrophages.[2] Thus, Lp-PLA_2 may represent an important "missing link" between the oxidative modification of LDL in the subintimal layer of the arterial wall and local inflammatory processes within the atherosclerotic plaque.

Epidemiology of Lp-PLA_2

Over the past eight years, a large body of evidence has accumulated which shows that increased circulating concentrations of Lp-PLA_2 mass or elevated activity are positively associated with various cardiovascular endpoints.[3] To date, there are more than 25 prospective studies (12 of them conducted in primary prevention settings) demonstrating Lp-PLA_2 as an independent and clinically relevant long-term risk marker for CHD and probably also for stroke (Figure 31–1).[3] A recent meta-analysis including 14 eligible studies with a total of 20,549 participants[4] showed elevated Lp-PLA_2 concentrations resulted in a 60% increased risk of CVD after adjustment for conventional risk factors.

Data from multiple analyses investigating the role of Lp-PLA_2 in the prediction of future CHD in primary prevention revealed consistent results despite various differences in these populations[5]; in this analysis, a 1 SD increase in Lp-PLA_2 concentration was associated with an approximately 20% increased risk of CHD among hypercholesterolemic men, as well as in middle-aged men or in older subjects (aged 55 years and above) with moderately increased TC, respectively.[5] In addition, within the Atherosclerosis Risk in Communities (ARIC) study, Lp-PLA_2 significantly and independently predicted CHD even in subjects with low LDL-C (<130 mg/dL).[5]

Lp-PLA_2 has also been found to be a potent predictor of CVD risk even in settings where conventional lipid measures or other biomarkers often lose their prognostic ability, namely in the elderly.[6–8] However, the magnitude of such association seems to be slightly smaller than that observed in middle-aged subjects. For instance, results from the Rancho Bernardo Study[6] in 1077 apparently healthy community-dwelling older men and women with no history of CHD at baseline showed Lp-PLA_2 as an independent predictor of future CHD events with a 60 to 90% increased risk across extreme quartiles. Furthermore, in the Cardiovascular Health Study (CHS),[7] as well as in the Prospective Study of Pravastatin in the Elderly at Risk (PROSPER) trial,[8] Lp-PLA_2 mass was found to be significantly related to future CHD risk.

On the other hand, clinical data on the predictive value of Lp-PLA_2 in the setting of the acute coronary syndrome (ACS) are scarce and remain to be established.[5] Moreover, controversial

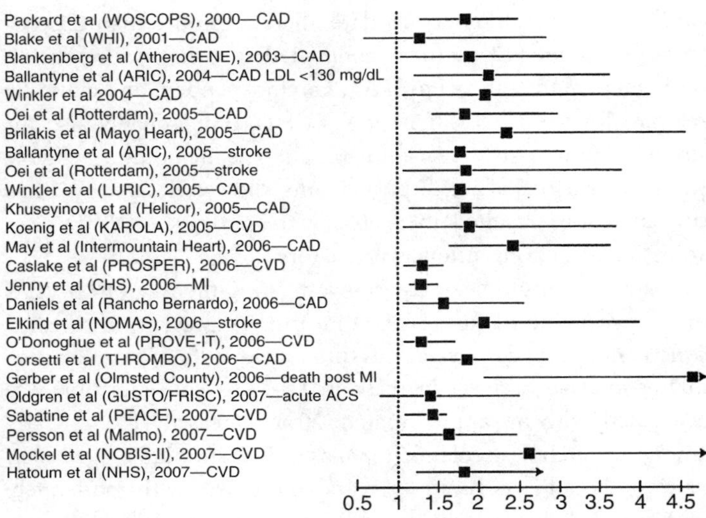

■ **Figure 31–1** Lipoprotein-associated Phospholipase A2 (Lp-PLA2) and Risk of Cardiovascular Disease (CVD). Published prospective epidemiologic studies show the association of elevated Lp-PLA2 (top quantile vs bottom quantile) with cardiovascular risk. A fairly consistent near doubling of risk is associated with elevated Lp-PLA2. Results are fully adjusted for traditional risk factors, lipids, and often for body mass index and high-sensitivity C-reactive protein. Legend: ACS = acute coronary syndrome; ARIC = Atherosclerosis Risk in Communities; CAD = coronary artery disease; CHS = Cardiovascular Health Study; GUSTO/FRISC = Global Use of Strategies to Open Occluded Coronary Arteries/Fragmin During Instability in Coronary Artery Disease; KAROLA = Langzeiterfolge der Kardiologischen Anschlussheil-Behandlung; LDL = low-density lipoprotein cholesterol; LURIC = Ludwigshafen Risk and Cardiovascular Health Study; MI = myocardial infarction; NHS = Nurse's Health Study; NOBIS-II = North Wuerttemberg and Berlin Infarction Study–II; NOMAS = Northern Manhattan Study; PEACE = Prevention of Events with Angiotensin-Converting Enzyme Inhibition; PROSPER = Prospective Study of Pravastatin in the Elderly at Risk; PROVE-IT = Pravastatin or Atorvastatin and Infection Therapy; THROMBO = Thrombogenic Factors and Recurrent Coronary Events; WHI = Women's Health Initiative; WOSCOPS = West of Scotland Coronary Prevention Study.

Source: Corson et al. *Am J Cardiol.* 2008;101(Suppl):41F–50F with permission.

results were found for the association of Lp-PLA_2 with subclinical atherosclerotic disease. However, a recent paper[9] showed Lp-PLA_2 to be independently associated with coronary artery ED. In addition, the same researchers[10] showed local production of Lp-PLA_2 in early atherosclerosis and LysoPC, the active product of Lp-PLA_2, to be associated with ED. Thus, such data argue for a direct involvement of Lp-PLA_2 in the atherosclerotic process.

Lp-PLA_2 as a Potential Therapeutic Target

Another issue, which seems to be pivotal from a clinical point of view, is related to the fact that Lp-PLA_2 could represent an attractive novel therapeutic target. Indeed, azetidinones, a new class of compounds acting as acylating inhibitors of the enzymatic activity of Lp-PLA_2, have shown the ability to interfere with the biological (toxic) sequelae of oxLDL, namely chemoattraction of monocytes and apoptosis in macrophages.[2–11] Decreased accumulation of LysoPC and oxFA contents were also seen with this compound. Moreover, experimental studies in Watanabe heritable hyperlipidemic (WHHL) rabbits have shown that inhibition of Lp-PLA_2 leads to a reduction of atherosclerotic lesion formation.[5] In addition to azetidinones, another class of compounds, namely pyrimidones, being noncovalent Lp-PLA_2 inhibitors, also prevented the production of LysoPC and subsequent monocyte chemotaxis in vitro.[11]

In addition, administration of SB-480848 (darapladib) to diabetic and hypercholesterolemic swine resulted in a considerable decrease in plaque area and a markedly reduced necrotic core area and medial destruction thereby consequently stabilizing atherosclerotic lesions. Moreover, the expression of 24 genes associated with macrophage and T-lymphocyte functioning was also significantly reduced under selective inhibition of Lp-PLA_2 with darapladib.[12]

In vivo studies showed that oral administration of an Lp-PLA_2 inhibitor to healthy volunteers in a phase I clinical trial resulted in dose-dependent reductions in Lp-PLA_2 activity of up to 95%, thereby identifying this compound as a potent Lp-PLA_2 inhibitor with a suitable profile for evaluation in humans.[11] Furthermore, results from an early phase II trial showed that administration of 40 and 80 mg of darapladib to patients for 14 days prior to carotid endarterectomy resulted in the inhibition of Lp-PLA_2 plasma and plaque activity in a dose-dependent manner up to 80%, compared with placebo.[11] More recently, Mohler et al.[13] reported data from a large multicenter, randomized, double-blind, placebo-controlled trial investigating the effect of darapladib on Lp-PLA_2 activity and a panel of biomarkers, reflecting different pathways of the pathophysiology of atherosclerosis. The study population comprised 959 patients with stable CHD or CHD risk equivalents; all were treated with three different doses of darapladib (40, 80, and 160 mg) over 12 weeks against a background of 20 and 80 mg of atorvastatin. Darapladib inhibited Lp-PLA_2 activity in a dose-dependent manner in both statin groups at different LDL-C levels, but did not affect LDL-C levels. At 12 weeks, darapladib in the highest dose significantly decreased interleukin-6 and showed a trend to decreased C-reactive protein (CRP) concentrations, with no effects on myeloperoxidase and matrix metalloproteinase-9. In summary, the study by Mohler et al. showed that darapladib substantially inhibits plasma Lp-PLA_2 activity and suggests a modulation of the systemic inflammatory response in the presence of intensive statin therapy. This study, however, does not provide information about what is going on inside the vessel wall itself after inhibition of Lp-PLA_2 activity. This issue was addressed in the Integrated Biomarker and Imaging Study (IBIS-2) trial[14] using intravascular ultrasound (IVUS) grey scale information, virtual histology, and palpography in 330 patients with angiographically-documented CHD, who were treated with darapladib 160 mg/day or placebo for 12 months. Although no significant differences between groups were found with respect to primary endpoints, such as coronary atheroma deformability determined by IVUS-derived palpography or levels of CRP, key secondary endpoints showed significant effects of darapladib on plaque composition and plasma levels of

Lp-PLA$_2$ activity. After 12 months, patients treated with placebo experienced a significant increase in the necrotic core volume, despite a high level of standard-of-care treatment, while darapladib-treated patients demonstrated no further necrotic core expansion and, consequently, experienced stabilization of atherosclerotic plaque.

Lp-PLA$_2$ as a Marker for Improved Risk Stratification in Clinical Practice

The last point to be mentioned here is a practical consideration of Lp-PLA$_2$ measurements, which might be a critical component for the implementation of Lp-PLA$_2$ biomarker analysis in routine clinical practice. Lp-PLA$_2$, in contrast to other emerging biomarkers related to inflammation, has several distinct features. First, unlike other inflammatory biomarkers, such as CRP, fibrinogen, IL-6, or sPLA$_2$—another well-studied member of the phospholipase superfamily—Lp-PLA$_2$ is not an acute phase reactant, and thus, seems to be unaffected by systemic inflammatory processes (e.g., osteoarthritis or chronic obstructive pulmonary disease).[15] Consequently, Lp-PLA$_2$ is only minimally correlated with systemic inflammatory and hemostatic markers,[16] whereas most of the acute phase reactants are highly correlated among each other. Moreover, Lp-PLA$_2$ may represent a more specific marker of vascular wall inflammation because results from the MONICA/KORA Augsburg cohort showed that increased concentrations of Lp-PLA$_2$ were strongly predictive for incident CHD,[5] but not for incident type 2 diabetes mellitus (T2DM).[17] This is in contrast to several other markers of inflammation, which have been found to be predictive for the mentioned afflictions.

Before more widespread use of Lp-PLA$_2$ testing in clinical practice can be recommended, several important requirements should be fulfilled, including determining what the population-based reference values are for this analyte in order to define normality. Recently, cutoff values for Lp-PLA$_2$ have been proposed, ranging for men and women between 230 and 250 ng/mL, with desirable

Lp-PLA_2 concentrations being less than 235 ng/mL.[18] However, more data in representative populations with the latest Lp-PLA_2 assay generation are needed. Furthermore, data on the biological variability of Lp-PLA_2 are crucial for the correct classification of individuals over time. Recently, it has been demonstrated that the medium-term variability of Lp-PLA_2 was relatively low with a biological variability of 15% and between-subject variation of 22%, thereby comparable to that of commonly-measured lipid parameters.[19] Another important issue is the determination of Lp-PLA_2 in blood. Circulating Lp-PLA_2 might be measured by different assays, e.g., by the PLAC™ test, a simple enzyme-linked immunosorbent assay (ELISA) used for the direct measurement of Lp-PLA_2 mass, and by various activity assays, the most common of them measuring the release of a radioactive isotopic label from a tritiated PAF substrate. However, there is only a moderate correlation between mass-based and activity-based measurements of Lp-PLA_2, so it is difficult to predict whether these two approaches will be equivalent or possibly complementary in predicting CHD risk. In addition, rigorous standardization of assays must be carried out to ensure adequate reproducibility of Lp-PLA_2 measurements, and imprecision of such assays should be low enough to enable reliable and accurate risk assessment with only one or two samples. Therefore, to date, Lp-PLA_2 measurements in unselected populations cannot be recommended to the physician until the above-mentioned requirements have been fulfilled.

Nonetheless, Lp-PLA_2 represents a potent and promising biomarker for the prediction of future CVD. Because specific inhibitors of Lp-PLA_2 are currently under evaluation in randomized clinical trials, modulation of Lp-PLA_2 in plasma and/or the vessel wall might represent a promising novel strategy for the treatment of atherosclerosis. Unfortunately, no study so far has evaluated the effect of systemic lowering of Lp-PLA_2 concentrations on clinical outcomes, which is ultimately needed to prove or disprove a causal involvement of Lp-PLA_2 in atherogenesis. However, a comprehensive meta-analysis based on individual data from prospective Lp-PLA_2 studies is underway (Emerging Risk Factor Collaboration [ERFC] Study)[20] that might be able to generate even more precise risk estimates for subjects in important subgroups.

Type II Secretory Phospholipase A_2

Biology and Potential Atherogenic Mechanisms

Type II secretory phospholipase (sPLA_2) is another well-studied member of the phospholipase 2 family which is highly expressed in hepatocytes, macrophages, endothelial cells, platelets, and vascular SMCs.[21] In contrast to Lp-PLA_2, sPLA_2 is Ca^{2+}-dependent, has a molecular mass of 14 kDa, and belongs to the group of acute phase reactants (Table 31–1). Indeed, circulating levels of sPLA_2 increase largely during systemic inflammatory conditions, such as sepsis, rheumatoid arthritis, or inflammatory bowel disease.[21] Possible atherogenic mechanisms of sPLA_2 might consist of increased release of various lipid mediators at the site of lipoprotein retention in the arterial wall upon hydrolytic action of sPLA_2. This, in turn, may trigger local inflammatory cellular responses. Furthermore, in arterial tissue, sPLA_2 may also directly modify LDL particles to become more atherogenic, thereby making sPLA_2-II-treated lipoproteins more susceptible to further lipid oxidation and enzymatic modification.[21] In addition, sPLA_2 may potentiate the binding and retention of LDL by increasing the affinity of apoB-100 on LDL to glycosaminglycans and proteoglycans.[22,23] SPLA_2 is also implicated in the production of isoprostanes which exhibit strong mitogenic activity and induce platelet aggregation and vasoconstriction.[21] In vivo studies in transgenic mice overexpressing human sPLA_2 showed an enhanced formation of bioactive oxidized phospholipids, as well as increased formation of atherosclerotic lesions.[21]

Epidemiology of sPLA_2

The existing epidemiological database of research for sPLA_2 in atherosclerosis is not as large as for Lp-PLA_2. To date, only a few prospective studies are available that have examined the potential

Table 31–1: Essential characteristics of lipoprotein-associated phospholipase A_2 (Lp-PLA_2) and secretory phospholipase A_2 ($sPLA_2$).

	Lp-PLA_2	$sPLA_2$
Molecular weight	50 kDa	14 kDa
Gene location	6p21.2–p12	1p34–36
Ca^{++} dependency	No	Yes
Production mainly by	Macrophages, T cells, mast cells	Wall SMC and macrophages
Acute phase reactant	No	Yes
Responsiveness to IL-1, IL-6, TNF-α	No	Yes
Substrate	Oxidatively-modified phospholipids only	Unmodified phospholipids
Catalytic activity at	Short acyl group at the sn-2 position of phospholipids	Acyl group at the sn-2 position of glycerophospholipids
Generated products	Lysophosphatidylcholine and oxidized fatty acid	Lysophospholipids and fatty acid
Presence in atherosclerotic lesions	+	+
Epidemiological evidence	+++	+
Selective inhibitor available	Darapladip	Varespladib
Variability study	Yes	No

$^{+}$less strong.
$^{+++}$very strong.
Notes: kDa = kilo Dalton; IL = Interleukin; TNF-α = tumor necrosis factor-α.

role of $sPLA_2$ in CVD in initially healthy subjects, as well as in subjects with clinically manifest disease, and particularly in those with ACS (Table 31–2). The predictive value of $sPLA_2$ in asymptomatic subjects at high risk for the development of future CVD has been evaluated in two nested case-control studies conducted within the European Prospective Investigation of Cancer (EPIC)-Norfolk cohort. The first study,[24] measuring $sPLA_2$ concentrations (mass), comprised 1105 subjects who subsequently developed fatal and nonfatal CHD events during six years of follow-up and 2209 age-, sex-, and enrollment time-matched controls that remained free of disease. The second study[25] included 2797 subjects (991 subjects with incident coronary artery disease (CAD) and 1806 event-free controls), among whom activity of this enzyme was determined at baseline. Both elevated $sPLA_2$ mass and increased activity predicted coronary events: a 34% increased risk for future CHD events in multivariable analyses across extreme quartiles was seen in association with elevated $sPLA_2$ concentrations (mass), whereas a stronger, 65% increased risk was seen with increased $sPLA_2$ activity after adjustment for the same variables, including CRP. Based on these differing results, the authors concluded that $sPLA_2$ activity, which encompasses several types of $sPLA_2$—including types IIA, V, and X—may better reflect the causative role of $sPLA_2$ in the atherogenetic process.[25]

There are also a few studies that evaluated the role of $sPLA_2$ in patients with manifest atherosclerosis. Elevated plasma levels of $sPLA_2$ were significant and independent predictors of future CV events in a small study including 142 consecutive patients with angiographically-proven, stable CHD and 93 controls.[26] At baseline, significantly higher $sPLA_2$ levels were seen in cases compared with controls. Furthermore, CAD patients were followed for a mean duration of 17.2 months, during which 48 coronary events occurred. Kaplan-Meier analysis, as well as Cox models, revealed that subjects with higher levels of $sPLA_2$ (>366 ng/dL) had a significantly higher risk of developing future coronary events, as compared to those with the lowest concentration (≤246 ng/dL). In

Table 31–2: Secretory phospholipase A_2 ($sPLA_2$) and risk of cardiovascular disease (CVD).

Authors	Design	Mass or activity	Cohort	Number of subjects	Follow up	Endpoint	Risk estimates (95% CI)	References
Kugiyama et al.	Nested case-control	Mass	CHD	142/93	17.2 Mos	PCI, CABG, MI, coronary death	OR 3.46 (1.4–8.3) T3 vs T1*	*Am J Cardiol.* 2000;86:718–722.
Liu et al.	Nested case-control	Mass	CHD	247/100	19.3 Mos	Coronary events	OR 2.1 (1.4–7.0) >450 ng/dL vs ≤450 ng/dL*	*Eur Heart J.* 2003;24: 1824–1832.
Mallat et al.	Full cohort	Activity	ACS	446	6.5 Mos	MACE	HR 3.08 (1.37–6.91)* T3 vs T1+T2	*J Am Coll Cardiol.* 2005;46: 1249–1257.

Koenig et al.	Full cohort	Mass and activity	Post-MI	1,032	4.1 Yrs	Fatal and nonfatal MI and stroke	Mass HR 2.11 (1.20–3.72) Activity HR 1.65 (1.12–2.42) T3 vs T1*	*Eur Heart J.* 2008;28:Abstract.
Boekholdt et al.	Nested case-control	Mass	EPIC	707/1396	6 Yrs	Fatal and nonfatal CHD	OR 1.34 (1.02–1.71) Q4 vs Q1**	*ATVB.* 2005;25:839–846.
Mallat et al.	Nested case-control	Activity	EPIC	991/1806	6 Yrs	Incident CHD	OR 1.65 (1.27–2.12) Q4 vs Q1**	*ATVB.* 2007;27: 1177–1183.

*Adjusted for various traditional CV risk factors.

**Adjusted for traditional CV risk factors and CRP.

Notes: Pts = patients; CHD = coronary heart disease; PCI = percutaneous coronary intervention; CABG = coronary artery bypass graft; MI = myocardial infarction; OR = odds ratio; T = tertile; GRACE = Global Registry of Acute Coronary Events; ACS = acute coronary syndrome; MACE = major adverse coronary events; HR = Hazard ratio; KAROLA = Langzeiterfolge der Kardiologischen Anschlussheil-Behandlung; EPIC = European Prospective Investigation of Cancer; m/w = men/women; Q = quartile.

another study from the same group, conducted in 52 patients with unstable angina, 107 stable CHD patients, and 96 controls,[27] $sPLA_2$ levels were measured and follow-up was done in the unstable angina group over a two-year period. In multivariate models, the odds ratio (OR) for a coronary event varied between 3.0 (95% CI 1.2–7.4) and 5.1 (95% CI 1.4–18.6) depending upon the underlying coronary anatomy and whether or not patients had suffered a previous myocardial infarction (MI). The very large confidence intervals reflect the small sample size in the various subgroups studied. Furthermore, in a study with 247 consecutive CHD undergoing percutaneous coronary intervention (PCI) and 100 controls, increased $sPLA_2$ (>450 ng/dL) measured after the intervention independently predicted outcome after two years (OR 2.1; 95% CI 1.4–7.0; $p = 0.025$).[28] Finally, Mallat et al.[29] studied 446 patients with severe ACS from the Global Registry of Acute Coronary Events (GRACE) and followed them for a median of 5.6 months. In multivariable analysis, only $sPLA_2$ activity—not mass—was strongly associated with the composite endpoint of death or MI (hazard ratio [HR] 3.08; 95% CI 1.37–6.91). However, the number of hard endpoints was small ($n = 43$), and thus, the risk associated with increased $sPLA_2$ activity may have been overestimated.

Because most of the above studies (although showing fairly consistent results) were relatively small with heterogeneous cohorts, we decided to investigate whether $sPLA_2$ was associated with prognosis in a large cohort of patients with clinically-overt CHD. Within KAROLA,[30] plasma $sPLA_2$ mass and activity were measured at baseline in a cohort of 1032 patients aged 30–70 years with CHD participating in an inpatient rehabilitation program after acute coronary syndrome (ACS) or coronary artery bypass grafting (CABG). During 4.1-years of follow-up, 95 patients (9.0%) experienced a secondary CVD event. Baseline levels of $sPLA_2$ mass and activity were higher in subjects who experienced an event compared to event-free subjects. In a multivariate model, $sPLA_2$ mass and activity were associated with an increased HR of future CV events. After controlling for age, gender, body mass index (BMI), smoking, history of MI and diabetes mellitus, initial management of CHD, HDL-C, LDL-C, and statin use, the HR was 2.11 (95% CI, 1.20–3.72) and 1.65 (95% CI 1.12–2.42) for mass and activity, respectively, when the top tertiles were compared to the bottom tertiles. Further adjustment for cystatin C, NT-proBNP, CRP, and Lp-PLA$_2$ attenuated the associations still showing a positive trend for mass, but a less clear pattern for sPLA$_2$ activity (HR 1.75 (95% CI 0.96–3.20), p for trend 0.007 and 1.43 (95% CI 0.81–2.52), p for trend 0.22, respectively). However, when sPLA$_2$ mass and activity were analyzed as continuous variables, both still showed a statistically significant increase in risk. Thus, sPLA$_2$ mass and activity appear to be predictive of secondary CVD events in patients with manifest CHD, but larger studies are needed to clearly distinguish effects from other biomarkers reflecting inflammation, renal function, and hemodynamic stress.

Potential Therapeutic Implication of sPLA$_2$ Inhibition

Another issue to be mentioned here is the potential for therapeutic modulation of sPLA$_2$ concentrations by a direct sPLA$_2$ inhibitor, called varespladib (A-002). A phase II trial of this novel sPLA$_2$ inhibitor called Phospholipase Levels And Serological Markers of Atherosclerosis (PLASMA) was recently presented at American College of Cardiology 57th Annual Scientific Session in March 2008.[31] PLASMA is a multicenter, randomized, double-blind, placebo-controlled trial that enrolled approximately 400 patients with stable CHD in the United States and Ukraine. Subjects were randomized to receive one of four different doses of A-002 or placebo for up to eight weeks in addition to standard-of-care therapies. The primary endpoint was a reduction in sPLA$_2$, which was achieved with a high degree of statistical significance. The study also evaluated the effect of varespladib on cholesterol levels (LDL-C, non-HDL, and TC), which, in contrast to the selective Lp-PLA$_2$ inhibitor, darapladib, was clinically meaningful and statistically significant in decreasing traditional lipid parameters.

Furthermore, a significant decrease in the inflammatory response, as measured by circulating levels of CRP, was also observed in this patient population. To date, another trial with A-002 is underway—the so-called Fewer Recurrent Acute coronary events with Near-term Cardiovascular Inflammation Suppression (FRANCIS)—which is designed to evaluate the impact of oral varespladib on known biological markers of cardiovascular risk in ACS patients with elevated LDL and CRP. FRANCIS will also provide first insight into the prevention of secondary major adverse cardiovascular events (MACE) over the duration of the six-month trial.

sPLA$_2$ as a Potential Biomarker in Clinical Practice

Although sPLA$_2$ in several studies was independently associated with increased risk for future CVD events and represents an attractive therapeutic target, no clear recommendation on its clinical usefulness can be given until further data document its incremental value in addition to identifying traditional risk factors. Furthermore, no data on the variability of sPLA$_2$ exist, which is crucial to correctly classify individuals. As in the case of Lp-PLA$_2$, it is also not entirely clear whether measuring sPLA$_2$ mass or activity alone or a combination of both is more informative. Results of the above-discussed studies must be replicated in other cohorts until the clinical usefulness of sPLA$_2$ in the prediction of CHD can be established. Moreover, no study so far has investigated the potential value of sPLA$_2$ in the prediction of cerebrovascular risk. Thus, larger studies in diverse populations are certainly needed using assays with high precision and an established standard to enable direct comparison of the results among studies.

Oxidized LDL

Biology and Potential Atherogenic Mechanisms

Primary events in the pathogenesis of atherosclerosis include the accumulation and subsequent modification of LDL in the subendothelial matrix. To become atherogenic, trapped native LDL particles undergo modification, including lipolysis, proteolysis, glycation, or aggregation. However, the oxidative modification hypothesis proposes that the most significant event in early lesion formation is lipid oxidation, placing oxLDL in a central role for atherogenesis.[32] Minimally-modified LDL (mmLDL), which is still recognized by the LDL receptors, stimulates endothelial cells to produce several cellular adhesion molecules (CAMs), as well as monocyte chemoattractant protein (MCP)–1, and macrophage colony-stimulating factor (M-CSF),[32] resulting in the adhesion of monocytes to the endothelium and subsequent recruitment into the vessel wall. By releasing M-CSF from endothelial cells, mmLDLs also favor monocyte proliferation and differentiation into tissue macrophages, a critical step which could be responsible in turn for converting mmLDL into intensively modified oxLDL. OxLDL has a large number of biological actions and consequences, including injuring endothelial cells, expressing adhesion molecules, recruiting leukocytes and retaining them, as well as forming foam cell and initiating thrombus formation.[33] Proatherogenic properties of oxLDL are summarized in Table 31–3.

Epidemiology of oxLDL

To date, a number of cross-sectional studies have examined the involvement of oxidative modification of LDL in subjects with clinical evidence of CVD. Clinical studies[34,35] have demonstrated that patients with both stable CHD and ACS show elevated plasma levels of oxLDL compared with apparently healthy controls. A positive association between oxLDL and the severity of ACS was found by Ehara et al.,[36] who reported oxLDL concentrations to be significantly higher in patients with MI than in patients with unstable or stable angina pectoris or age-matched control subjects. Findings from other studies suggest that plasma levels of oxLDL represent a more sensitive marker for the presence of CAD than the Global Risk Assessment Score (GRAS),[37] and that oxLDL also correlates with the extent of CAD in heart transplant recipients.[38]

Table 31–3: Proatherogenic properties of oxidized LDL.

Biological effect	Possible mechanism
Foam cell formation	Direct uptake of cholesterol by scavenger receptors, as well as inhibition of their export from macrophages
Chemoattraction of monocytes, T-lymphocytes	Increased expression of MCP-1 and direct chemotactic effect
Macrophage trapping within the intima	Inhibition of the motility of macrophages
Impaired vascular function (vasocon-strictor effect)	Inhibition of nitric oxide release or function
Adhesion of monocytes to endothelium	Increased expression of adhesion molecules
Plaque rupture	Enhanced formation of matrix metalloproteinases
Cell proliferation	Induction of growth factors
Thrombogenesis	Promotion of platelet aggregation and increased tissue factor activity
Increased cellular death	Induction of Fas-mediated apoptosis
Induction of proinflammatory genes	Activation of nuclear factor-κB
Increased antigenicity	Induction of autoantibody (IgG) formation

Note: MCP-1 = monocyte chemoattractant protein-1.

More recently, Tsimikas et al. assessed the association between the oxidized phospholipid : apoB-100 ratio in plasma and the presence of angiographically-confirmed CHD.[39] In 504 CHD patients, an increase in the oxidized phospholipid : apoB-100 ratio was an independent predictor of obstructive CAD, revealing an OR per ratio doubling of 1.21 (95% CI 1.05–1.39; $p = 0.007$).

Salonen et al.[40] were the first to conduct a prospective, population-based, nested case-control study among 30 Finnish men with accelerated progression of carotid atherosclerosis and 30 age-matched controls without progression during a follow up of two years. They found the titer of autoantibodies to oxLDL to be an independent predictor for the progression of carotid atherosclerosis. Another small prospective nested case-control study demonstrated that oxLDL concentrations might be associated with acute MI.[41] During a follow-up of 2.6 years, 26 cases and 26 matched controls and a further 26 controls with LDL >5.0 mmol/L were studied. The oxLDL/plasma cholesterol ratio was higher among cases compared with controls and also higher compared with hypercholesterolemic subjects free of an event, suggesting that the high plasma oxLDL/total cholesterol ratio might serve as a possible indicator of increased risk of MI.

More recently, data of a prospective nested case-control study from two population-based MONICA/KORA Augsburg surveys showed that plasma oxLDL was the strongest predictor of CHD events compared to a conventional lipoprotein profile, and other traditional risk factors for CHD.[42] The association between plasma oxLDL and risk of acute CHD events was investigated in 88 men aged 45–74 with an incident CHD event and 258 age-matched controls during a mean follow-up of 5.6 years. After adjustment for traditional CV risk factors, the HR for a future CHD across extreme tertiles of the oxLDL distribution was 3.79 (95% CI, 2.07–6.95; $p < 0.001$). Plasma oxLDL was the strongest predictor of CHD events compared with a conventional lipoprotein profile and with other traditional risk factors for CHD. More recently, Holvoet et al.,[43] using the Coronary Artery Risk Development in Young Adults (CARDIA) study as a database, investigated the longitudinal association between oxLDL and incident metabolic syndrome (MetS). Within this study, a 3.5-fold increased risk to develop a MetS among 1889 participants after five years' follow-up was seen when the top quintile of oxLDL was compared with the bottom one in the fully adjusted model.[43]

Thus, it seems justified to conclude that oxLDL may indeed play a key role in the generation of inflammatory processes in atherosclerotic lesions. This is supported by a recent prospective study showing that increased antioxidative capacity, as assessed by glutathione peroxidase 1 levels, was associated with improved outcome.[44]

Clinical Relevance of oxLDL Measurements

Despite the above cited evidence, further studies are clearly warranted to establish the clinical relevance of oxLDL measurement in various stages of the atherosclerotic process and to identify in detail the specific pathophysiological mechanisms by which oxLDL exerts it deleterious effects.

Lipoprotein Lipase

Biology and Potential Proatherogenic Mechanisms

Lipoprotein lipase (LPL), a member of the lipase gene family,[45] is a 52-kDa hydrophilic enzyme, which may play a central role in lipid metabolism. The major sources of LPL synthesis are skeletal and heart muscle, as well as adipose tissue, from which the mature enzyme is then secreted and transported to the vascular endothelium—the physiological site of the enzyme's action.[45,46] To achieve its highest catalytic activity, LPL requires a specific cofactor, apoCII, which is found in chylomicrons, whereas apoCIII seems to inhibit the action of the enzyme.[45–47] The efficient lipolysis of triglyceride-rich lipoproteins (with their removal from the circulation) and the generation of material for HDL formation are viewed as antiatherogenic effects of LPL.

LPL is synthesized by macrophages and macrophage-derived foam cells in atherosclerotic lesions (i.e., vessel wall LPL),[45,46] and this fraction of the enzyme has been linked to LPL-related proatherogenic effects. Indeed, local LPL activity on the vascular endothelium leads to a decrease in lipid size and to the production of smaller cholesterol-rich remnants and LDLs, facilitating their penetration of the endothelium. In addition, *in vitro* studies showed that lipolysis could increase the permeability of the endothelial barrier. In the intima, such smaller lipoproteins can be rapidly taken up by macrophages,[47] thereby enhancing deposition of cholesterol esters within macrophages and their subsequent transformation into foam cells.

Apart from its lipolytic activity, LPL has been shown to possess a noncatalytic activity ability on lipoproteins, such as molecular bridging.[46] Bridging function of the enzyme consists of the ability of LPL to anchor lipid particles because the enzyme can interact simultaneously with both lipoproteins and proteoglycans via separate domains. As a result, increased binding and retention of LDL cholesterol by proteoglycans of the subendothelial matrix occurs, thereby proposing LPL activity in the arterial wall to promote atherosclerosis.

Epidemiologic Evidence for LPL as a Predictor of CVD or CHD

Epidemiological evidence of the potential role of LPL in CHD remains scarce and controversial. The association between LPL activity and mass and the presence of CAD were studied in a large cohort of CAD patients participating in the Regression Growth Evaluation Statin Study (REGRESS).[48] Patients with the lowest LPL activity reported more severe angina pectoris according to NYHA classification, compared with patients in the highest quartile of the LPL distribution. The results of a small study from Japan also showed considerably lower levels of preheparin serum LPL mass in male patients with coronary atherosclerosis, compared with those in healthy men.[49] Another case-control study[50] included 194 patients with and without angiographically-proven CAD (n = 158/36, respectively) and demonstrated no differences in LPL activity or concentration between these groups. In addition, no association between LPL quartile distribution and severity and extension of CAD, as assessed by various coronary scores, was found.

Thus, at present, inconsistencies in cross-sectional studies and absence of prospective studies do not support LPL as a useful marker of cardiovascular risk.

Lipoprotein(a)

Biology and Potential Proatherogenic Mechanisms

Lipoprotein(a) (Lp(a)), a cholesteryl ester-rich lipoprotein, is comprised of the glycoprotein apolipoprotein(a) (apo(a)), which is linked by a single disulfide bridge on a 1:1 molar basis to the apoB-100 component of an LDL-like particle.[51] This unique molecular structure seems to be responsible for the dual pathophysiological role of Lp(a), with a role in both atherosclerosis and thrombosis (Figure 31–2): on the one hand, Lp(a), due to its similarity to LDL, is considered a strong proatherogenic agent. Indeed, LDL-like moiety of Lp(a) is virtually indistinguishable from true LDL particles, and therefore is subject to modification by oxidative processes and by the action of lipolytic and proteolytic enzymes.[52] Furthermore, proinflammatory oxidized phospholipids are preferentially bound to Lp(a) and are taken up by macrophages that contribute to foam cell formation, and possibly to plaque rupture.[51,52] More interestingly, Lp(a) is immunodetectable only in atherosclerotic[53]—but not in normal—vessel walls and ED might be an important mechanism responsible for the transport of Lp(a) to the arterial subendothelial space.[51] This is in agreement with numerous findings reporting that in early atherosclerotic lesions, Lp(a) is located within endothelial cells, whereas in advanced lesions, Lp(a) significantly colocalizes with plaque macrophages. In addition, Lp(a) is an acute phase reactant and possesses growth factor-like properties that result in proliferation of vascular smooth muscle cells (VSMC).[51,52] Lp(a) is suggested to induce monocyte chemotactic activity in human vascular endothelial cells.[54] Recently, Fan et al.[55] showed that increased levels of Lp(a) enhanced the development of atherosclerosis in the setting of hypercholesterolemia in WHHL transgenic rabbits expressing human apo(a). On the other hand, apo(a) contains multiple

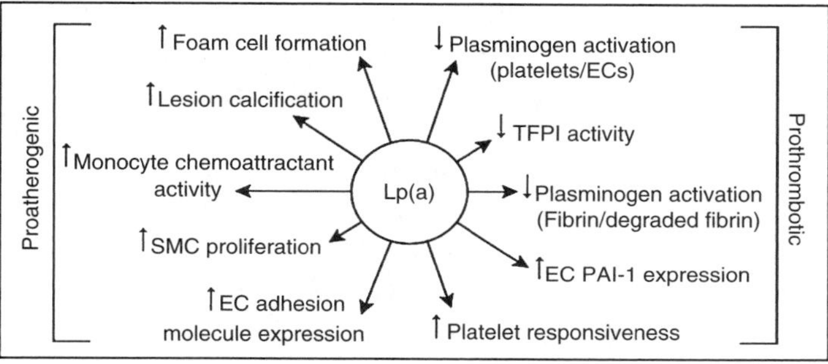

■ **Figure 31–2** Potential Pathogenic Mechanisms of Lipoprotein (a). Lp(a) has been considered to possess both proatherogenic properties, by virtue of its similarity to LDL, as well as prothrombotic properties, by virtue of the similarity of apolipoprotein(a) (apo(a)) to plasminogen. Shown on this diagram are the effects of Lp(a) that have been demonstrated by in-vitro studies or in animal models of apo(a)/Lp(a). Mechanisms that are potentially proatherogenic are shown to the left and those that are potentially prothrombotic are shown to the right. Importantly, none of these mechanisms has been directly demonstrated to be mediated by Lp(a) in human disease. Legend: EC, endothelial cell; SMC, smooth muscle cell; PAI-1, plasminogen activator inhibitor-1; TFPI, tissue factor pathway inhibitor.

Source: Marcovina et al. *Curr Opin Lipidol* 2003:14(4);361–366 with permission.

repeated loop-shaped units called kringle domains, which make them strikingly homologous to the fibrinolytic proenzyme plasminogen—they share up to 89% sequence homology—thereby accounting for the prothrombotic and/or antifibrinolytic role of Lp(a).[51] Indeed, apo(a) is able to inhibit activation of plasminogen due to its interaction with tissue-type plasminogen activator, as well as possibly due to successful competition with plasminogen for binding sites on fibrin.[56] Interestingly, several studies have shown that smaller isoforms of Lp(a) bind aggressively to fibrin thereby providing better inhibition of plasminogen.[56] In addition, stimulation of human endothelial cell PAI-1 synthesis and activity has been suggested as another mechanism by which Lp(a) might inhibit fibrinolysis.[56] In line with the experimental observations, a number of clinical studies confirm—at least in part—the role of Lp(a) in thrombogenesis.

Another hallmark of this lipoprotein is its heterogeneity. Lp(a) is noted to have a molecular weight that can vary between 300 and 800 kDa. It has been suggested that almost 90% of the variation in plasma Lp(a) concentrations is referred to the variation in the number of repeated kringle units in the apo(a) molecule.[57] The high variability of apo(a) is a result of the strong genetic control of apo(a); with a total of over 30 well-characterized alleles, it can strongly influence circulating Lp(a) levels.

Epidemiology of Lp(a)

Concerning the predictive role of Lp(a) for atherosclerotic disorders, there are several meta-analyses to date, indicating a significant association between Lp(a) and CHD. Earlier formal meta-analysis of 27 prospective studies, comprising 5436 CHD cases observed during a mean follow-up of ten years, clearly demonstrated an association between Lp(a) levels and CHD with a combined risk ratio of 1.6 (95% CI 1.4–1.8) for incident CHD if the top third of Lp(a) was compared to the bottom third.[58] The more recently published paper by Bennet et al.[59]—an updated meta-analysis of 31 long-term prospective studies—suggests only modest heterogeneity in the OR for CHD with Lp(a) levels despite diversity of assay methods and variability in Lp(a) levels across populations (Figure 31–3). However, some studies have failed to confirm a relationship between Lp(a) and the risk of CHD. Thus, among 27,791 healthy, mostly Caucasian women in the Women's Health Study who were followed for ten years, the association of Lp(a) with total cardiovascular events remained significant only at extremely high Lp(a) concentrations (≥44 mg/dL).[60] Recent results from the Copenhagen City Heart Study, examining 9330 men and women from the general population, among whom 498 participants developed an MI during ten years of follow-up, confirmed

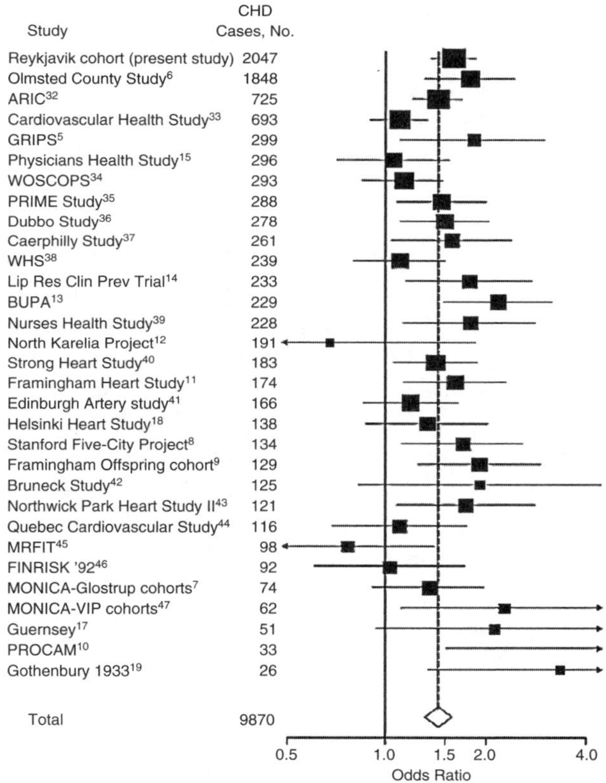

■ **Figure 31–3** Odds Ratios for Coronary Heart Disease (CHD)* in Each of 31 Published Prospective Studies of Lipoprotein(a) in Essentially General Populations. Legend: *(top third vs bottom third) Heterogeneity: $\chi 230 = 52.6$; $P = 0.007$: $I2 = 43\%$ (95% confidence interval [CI], 12%-63%). ARIC indicates Atherosclerosis Risk in Communities; BUPA, British United Provident Association; GRIPS, Göttingen Risk, Incidence and Prevalence Study; Lip Res Clin Prev Trial, Lipid Research Clinics Coronary Primary Prevention Trial; MONICA, Monitoring Trends and Determinants in Cardiovascular Disease; MRFIT, Multiple Risk Factor Intervention Trial; PRIME, Prospective Epidemiological Study of Myocardial Infarction; PROCAM, Prospective Cardiovascular Münster Study; VIP, Västerbotten Intervention Project; WHS, Women's Health Study; and WOSCOPS, West of Scotland Coronary Prevention Study. Error bars represent 95% CIs.

Source: Bennet et al. *Arch Intern Med.* 2008;168(6):598–608 with permission.

that extreme Lp(a) levels ≥95th percentile (≥120 mg/dL) predict a three- to fourfold increase in the risk of MI and an absolute 10-year risk of 20% and 35% in high-risk women and men.[61] Therefore, these data are not supporting generalized screening for Lp(a) because only extremely high levels were associated with cardiovascular risk.

Potential Therapeutic Implications of Elevated Lp(a)

Another important point to mention here is that, unlike other plasma lipoproteins, Lp(a) is very resistant to changes by diet and lipid-lowering medication. Only high doses of nicotinic acid (3–4 g/d) are effective in lowering Lp(a), resulting in a shift from small dense particles to relatively benign, large particles, along with a parallel shift within the class of LDL. Statins are not effective in reducing levels of Lp(a) and fibrates lower it very little. However, Maher et al.[62] demonstrated that modification of the excess CV risk associated with elevated Lp(a) can be achieved via aggressive LDL-C lowering, suggesting that when Lp(a) levels are elevated, the primary objective should be to treat elevated LDL-C more aggressively either with a statin or with niacin.

Role of Lp(a) in Clinical Practice

All of these above-mentioned issues limit the widespread measurement of Lp(a) in clinical practice. Furthermore, there is no clinical evidence that lowering Lp(a) levels lowers cardiovascular risk. However, measurements of Lp(a) might help to identify selected individuals at particularly high risk, who could benefit from aggressive lipid-lowering therapy.

Conclusion

In conclusion, the importance of non-lipoprotein cholesterol as well as oxidize variants of lipoproteins is likely to increase with a better understanding of their pathophysiology and with the derivation of specific therapeutic agents to address their elevation.

References

1. Zalewski A, Macphee C. Role of lipoprotein-associated phospholipase A_2 in atherosclerosis: biology, epidemiology, and possible therapeutic target. *Arterioscler Thromb Vasc Biol.* 2005;25:923–931.
2. Kolodgie FD, Burke AP, Skorija KS, et al. Lipoprotein-associated phospholipase A_2 protein expression in the natural progression of human coronary atherosclerosis. *Arterioscler Thromb Vasc Biol.* 2006; 26:2523–2529.
3. Corson MA, Jones PH, Davidson MH. Review of the evidence for the clinical utility of lipoprotein-associated phospholipase A_2 as a cardiovascular risk marker. *Am J Cardiol.* 2008;101(Suppl):41F–50F.
4. Garza CA, Montori VM, McConnell JP, et al. Association between lipoprotein-associated phospholipase A_2 and cardiovascular disease: a systematic review. *Mayo Clin Proc.* 2007;82:159–165.
5. Khuseyinova N, Koenig W. Predicting the risk of cardiovascular disease: where does lipoprotein-associated phospholipase A2 fit in? *Mol Diagn Ther.* 2007;11:203–217.
6. Daniels LB, Laughlin GA, Sarno MJ, et al. Lipoprotein-associated phospholipase A2 is an independent predictor of incident coronary heart disease in an apparently healthy older population: the Rancho Bernardo Study. *J Am Coll Cardiol.* 2008;51:913–919.
7. Jenny NS, Solomon C, Cushman M, et al. Lipoprotein-associated phospholipase A2 and cardiovascular disease: results from the Cardiovascular Health Study. *Circulation.* 2006;113:E–332 (Abstract).
8. Caslake MJ, Cooney J, Murray E, et al. Lipoprotein-associated phospholipase A_2 as a risk factor for coronary vascular disease in the elderly. *Atherosclerosis Suppl.* 2006;7:484 (Abstract).
9. Yang EH, McConnell JP, Lennon RJ, et al. Lipoprotein-associated phospholipase A2 is an independent marker for coronary endothelial dysfunction in humans. *Arterioscler Thromb Vasc Biol.* 2006;26:106–111.
10. Lavi S, McConnell JP, Rihal CS, et al. Local production of lipoprotein-associated phospholipase A2 and lysophosphatidylcholine in the coronary circulation: association with early coronary atherosclerosis and endothelial dysfunction in humans. *Circulation.* 2007;115:2715–2721.
11. Zalewski A, Macphee C, Nelson JJ. Lipoprotein-associated phospholipase A_2: a potential therapeutic target for atherosclerosis. *Curr Drug Targets Cardiovasc Haematol Disord.* 2005;5:527–532.

12. Wilensky RL, Shi Y, Mohler ER III, et al. Inhibition of lipoprotein-associated phospholipase A2 reduces complex coronary atherosclerotic plaque development. *Nat Med.* 2008;14:1059–1066.

13. Mohler ER III, Ballantyne CM, Davidson MH, et al. The effect of darapladib on plasma lipoprotein-associated phospholipase A2 activity and cardiovascular biomarkers in patients with stable coronary heart disease or coronary heart disease risk equivalent: the results of a multicenter, randomized, double-blind, placebo-controlled study. *J Am Coll Cardiol.* 2008;51:1632–1641.

14. Serruys PW, García-García HM, Buszman P, et al. Effects of the direct lipoprotein-associated phospholipase A2 inhibitor darapladib on human coronary atherosclerotic plaque. *Circulation.* 2008;118:1172–1182.

15. Wolfert RL, Kim NW, Selby RG, et al. Biological variability and specificity of lipoprotein-associated phospholipase A_2, a novel marker of cardiovascular risk. *Circulation.* 2004:110(Suppl III), III–309 (Abstract).

16. Khuseyinova N, Imhof A, Rothenbacher D, et al. Association between Lp-PLA_2 and coronary artery disease: focus on its relationship with lipoproteins and markers of inflammation and hemostasis. *Atherosclerosis.* 2005;182:181–188.

17. Khuseyinova N, Baumert J, Trischler G, et al. Lipoprotein-associated phospholipase A_2 does not predict risk of incident type 2 diabetes mellitus in apparently healthy middle-aged men: a more specific marker for vascular inflammation? AHA Scientific Sessions 2006, Chicago, USA, *Circulation.* 2006;(Abstract Supplement):(Abst 8113).

18. Lanman RB, Wolfert RL, Fleming JK, et al. Lipoprotein-associated phospholipase A_2: review and recommendation of a clinical cut point for adults. *Prev Card.* 2006;9:138–143.

19. Khuseyinova N, Greven S, Rückerl R, et al. Variability of serial lipoprotein-associated phospholipase A_2 measurements in post myocardial infarction patients: results from the AIRGENE Study Center Augsburg. *Clin Chem.* 2008;54:124–130.

20. The Lp-PLA_2 Studies Collaboration. Collaborative meta-analysis of individual participant data from observational studies of Lp-PLA_2 and cardiovascular diseases. *Eur J Cardiovasc Prev Rehabil.* 2007;14:3–11.

21. Jönsson-Rylander AC, Lundin S, Rosengren B, et al. Role of secretory phospholipases in atherogenesis. *Curr Atheroscler Rep.* 2008;10:252–259.

22. Sartipy P, Bondjers G, Hurt-Camejo E. Phospholipase A_2 type II binds to extracellular matrix biglycan: modulation of its activity on LDL by colocalization in glycosaminoglycan matrixes. *Arterioscler Thromb Vasc Biol.* 1998;18:1934–1941.

23. Sartipy P, Camejo G, Svensson L, et al. Phospholipase $A(_2)$ modification of low density lipoproteins forms small high density particles with increased affinity for proteoglycans and glycosaminoglycans. *J Biol Chem.* 1999;274:25913–25920.

24. Boekholdt SM, Keller TT, Wareham NJ, et al. Serum levels of type II secretory phospholipase A_2 and the risk of future coronary artery disease in apparently healthy men and women: the EPIC-Norfolk Prospective Population Study. *Arterioscler Thromb Vasc Biol.* 2005; 25:839–846.

25. Mallat Z, Benessiano J, Simon T, et al. Circulating secretory phospholipase A_2 activity and risk of incident coronary events in healthy men and women. The EPIC-NORFOLK Study. *Arterioscler Thromb Vasc Biol.* 2007;27:1177–1183.

26. Kugiyama K, Ota Y, Takazoe K, et al. Circulating levels of secretory type II phospholipase A_2 predict coronary events in patients with coronary artery disease. *Circulation.* 1999;100:1280–1284.

27. Kugiyama K, Ota Y, Sugiyama S, et al. Prognostic value of plasma levels of secretory type II phospholipase A_2 in patients with unstable angina pectoris. *Am J Cardiol.* 2000;86:718–722.

28. Liu PY, Li YH, Tsai WC, et al. Prognostic value and the changes of plasma levels of secretory type II phospholipase A_2 in patients with coronary artery disease undergoing percutaneous coronary intervention. *Eur Heart J.* 2003;24:1824–1832.

29. Mallat Z, Steg PG, Benessiano J, et al. Circulating secretory phospholipase A_2 activity predicts recurrent events in patients with severe acute coronary syndromes. *J Am Coll Cardiol.* 2005;46:1249–1257.

30. Koenig W, Vossen CY, Mallat Z, et al. Association between type II secretory phospholipase A_2 plasma concentrations and activity and cardiovascular events in patients with coronary heart disease. *Eur Heart J.* 2008;28(Abstract Supplement).

31. Rosenson RS for PLASMA Investigators. Effects of a selective inhibitor of secretory phospholipase A2 on low density lipoproteins and inflammatory pathways. *J Am Coll Cardiol.* 2008;51(Suppl A):A328 (Abstract 1021–1224).

32. Steinberg D. Low density lipoprotein oxidation and its pathobiological significance. *J Biol Chem.* 1997;272:20963–20966.

33. Jessup W, Kritharides L, Stocker R. Lipid oxidation in atherogenesis: an overview. *Biochem Soc Trans.* 2004;32:134–138.

34. Holvoet P, Vanhaecke J, Janssens S, et al. Oxidized LDL and malondialdehyde-modified LDL in patients with acute coronary syndromes and stable coronary artery disease. *Circulation.* 1998;98:1487–1494.

35. Toshima S, Hasegawa A, Kurabayashi M, et al. Circulating oxidized low density lipoprotein levels: a biochemical risk marker for coronary heart disease. *Arterioscler Thromb Vasc Biol.* 2000;20:2243–2247.

36. Ehara S, Ueda M, Naruko T, et al. Elevated levels of oxidized low density lipoprotein show a positive relationship with the severity of acute coronary syndromes. *Circulation.* 2001;103:1955–1960.

37. Holvoet P, Mertens A, Verhamme P, et al. Circulating oxidized LDL is a useful marker for identifying patients with coronary artery disease. *Arterioscler Thromb Vasc Biol.* 2001;21:844–848.

38. Holvoet P, Stassen JM, Van Cleemput J, et al. Oxidized low density lipoproteins in patients with transplant-associated coronary artery disease. *Arterioscler Thromb Vasc Biol.* 1998;18:100–107.

39. Tsimikas S, Brilakis ES, Miller ER, et al. Oxidized phospholipids, Lp(a) lipoprotein, and coronary artery disease. *N Engl J Med.* 2005;353:46–57.

40. Salonen JT, Yla-Herttuala S, Yamamoto R, et al. Autoantibody against oxidised LDL and progression of carotid atherosclerosis. *Lancet.* 1992;339:883–887.

41. Fredrikson NG, Hedblad B, Berglund G, et al. Plasma oxidized LDL: a predictor for acute myocardial infarction? *J Intern Med.* 2003;253:425–429.

42. Meisinger C, Baumert J, Khuseyinova N, et al. Plasma oxidized low-density lipoprotein, a strong predictor for acute coronary heart disease events in apparently healthy, middle-aged men from the general population. *Circulation.* 2005;112:651–657.

43. Holvoet P, Lee DH, Steffes M, et al. Association between circulating oxidized low-density lipoprotein and incidence of the metabolic syndrome. *JAMA.* 2008;299:2287–2293.

44. Blankenberg S, Rupprecht HJ, Bickel C, et al. Glutathione peroxidase 1 activity and cardiovascular events in patients with coronary artery disease. *N Engl J Med.* 2003;349:1605–1613.

45. Mead JR, Irvine SA, Ramji DP. Lipoprotein lipase: structure, function, regulation, and role in disease. *J Mol Med.* 2002;80:753–769.

46. Mead JR, Ramji DP. The pivotal role of lipoprotein lipase in atherosclerosis. *Cardiovasc Res.* 2002;55:261–269

47. Lindqvist P, Ostlund-Lindqvist AM, Witztum JL, et al. The role of lipoprotein lipase in the metabolism of triglyceride-rich lipoproteins by macrophages. *J Biol Chem.* 1983;258:9086–9092.

48. Kastelein JJ, Jukema JW, Zwinderman AH, et al. Lipoprotein lipase activity is associated with severity of angina pectoris. REGRESS Study Group. *Circulation.* 2000;102:1629–1633.

49. Hitsumoto T, Ohsawa H, Uchi T, et al. Preheparin serum lipoprotein lipase mass is negatively related to coronary atherosclerosis. *Atherosclerosis.* 2000;153:391–396.

50. Dugi KA, Schmidt N, Brandauer K, et al. Activity and concentration of lipoprotein lipase in post-heparin plasma and the extent of coronary artery disease. *Atherosclerosis.* 2002;163:127–134.

51. Scanu AM. Lipoprotein(a) and the atherothrombotic process: mechanistic insights and clinical implications. *Curr Atheroscler Rep.* 2003; 5:106–113.

52. Berglund L, Ramakrishnan R. Lipoprotein(a): an elusive cardiovascular risk factor. *Arterioscler Thromb Vasc Biol.* 2004;24:2219–2226.

53. Cambillau M, Simon A, Amar J, et al. Serum Lp(a) as a discriminant marker of early atherosclerotic plaque at three extracoronary sites in hypercholesterolemic men. *Arterioscler Thromb.* 1992;12:1346–1352.

54. Poon M, Zhang X, Dunsky KG et al. Apolipoprotein(a) induces monocyte chemotactic activity in human vascular endothelial cells. *Circulation.* 1997;96:2514–2519.

55. Fan J, Sun H, Unoki H, et al. Enhanced atherosclerosis in Lp(a) WHHL transgenic rabbits. *Ann N Y Acad Sci.* 2001;947:362–365.

56. Marcovina SM, Koschinsky ML. Evaluation of lipoprotein(a) as a prothrombotic factor: progress from bench to bedside. *Curr Opin Lipidol.* 2003;14:361–366.

57. Boerwinkle E, Leffert CC, Lin J, et al. Apolipoprotein (a) gene accounts for greater than 90% of the variation in plasma lipoprotein (a) concentrations. *J Clin Invest.* 1992;90:52–60.

58. Danesh J, Collins R, Peto R. Lipoprotein(a) and coronary heart disease. Meta-analysis of prospective studies. *Circulation.* 2000;102: 1082–1085.

59. Bennet A, Di Angelantonio E, Erqou S, et al. Lipoprotein(a) levels and risk of future coronary heart disease: large-scale prospective data. *Arch Intern Med.* 2008;168:598–608.

60. Suk Danik J, Rifai N, Buring JE, et al. Lipoprotein(a), measured with an assay independent of apolipoprotein(a) isoform size, and risk of future cardiovascular events among initially healthy women. *JAMA.* 2006;296:1363–1370.

61. Kamstrup PR, Benn M, Tybaerg-Hansen A, et al. Extreme lipoprotein(a) levels and risk of myocardial infarction in the general population: the Copenhagen City Heart Study. *Circulation.* 2008; 117:176–184.

62. Maher VM, Brown BG, Marcovina SM, et al. Effects of lowering elevated LDL cholesterol on the cardiovascular risk of lipoprotein(a). *JAMA.* 1995;274:1771–1774.

Section VI

The "-omics": Genomic, Metabolomic, and Proteomic Markers

32 ■ Genetic Biomarkers

Rajat Gupta, MD
Sekar Kathiresan, MD

Introduction

Understanding the inherited basis for cardiovascular diseases began with research focused on rare Mendelian disorders. Investigators uncovered the genetic basis for diseases ranging from monogenic hypercholesterolemia to long QT syndrome. In the process, they elucidated basic mechanisms of disease and demonstrated the power of gene-based approaches in understanding clinical disorders. Advances in genomics over the past decade, including the sequencing of the human genome, are expanding the clinical applications of genetic testing. This chapter will catalog the advances in the genetics of single-gene cardiovascular disorders and describe the more recent progress in genetic mapping for complex diseases, quantitative risk factors, and pharmacogenetic phenotypes.

Mendelian Diseases

Though many single-gene cardiovascular disorders have been characterized, genetic testing for these disorders has not found widespread use in the clinical setting. Therefore, a large portion of this discussion is regarding future possibilities. For example, this chapter will discuss the numerous mutations known to cause hypertrophic cardiomyopathy and at the same time discuss the obstacles to clinical testing. For many Mendelian disorders, genetic discoveries illustrated the mechanism behind the disease, and they are now providing an opportunity to design effective therapy. In recent years, the number of mutations responsible for familial forms of cardiovascular disease has risen dramatically. In this chapter, we will discuss three cardiovascular diseases—monogenic hypercholesterolemia, hypertrophic cardiomyopathy, and long QT syndrome. There are, however, many more familial diseases for which genetic screening is on the horizon, such as: Brugada syndrome, numerous dilated cardiomyopathies, familial sick sinus syndrome, arrhythmogenic right ventricular dysplasia, and atrial fibrillation.

Monogenic Hypercholesterolemia

Familial Hypercholesterolemia

Familial hypercholesterolemia (FH) was first described in 1938 by Swedish physician C. Muller who noted familial clustering of cutaneous xanthomas, elevated cholesterol, and premature coronary artery disease.[1] In the early 1970s and 1980s, Michael Brown and Joseph Goldstein demonstrated that FH was due to ineffective binding of low-density lipoprotein (LDL) with its receptor on accounts of mutations in the LDL receptor gene.[2] Now over 1000 unique allelic variants in the *LDLR* gene have been catalogued. However, the diagnosis of FH remains clinical, as genetic testing for these numerous mutations is only available in research laboratories.[3]

The diagnosis of familial hypercholesterolemia is made on the basis of elevated total serum cholesterol level, along with presence of tendon xanthomas, inferior corneal arcus, and/or coronary artery disease before the age of 50. Because total cholesterol levels increase with age, the cut points for screening of FH in individuals with a family history of the disease is a first-degree relative range from greater than 220 mg/dL for patients younger than age 20, and less than 290 mg/dL for patients older than age 40. Despite these objective criteria, there is wide variability in the phenotype of the disease.[3]

The phenotypic variability is in part explained by the large number of genetic variants identified. The *LDLR* gene maps to the short arm of chromosome 19, spans 45 kb, and has 18 exons. There have been over 1000 *LDLR* variants identified in subjects with FH, although not all have been proven to be functional.[4] Many of these variants have been characterized in human fibroblasts and classified based on how they affect LDL receptor intracellular trafficking or function. Class 1 variants result in inability to synthesize LDLR, largely due to deletions in the promoter region or splice defects. With class 2 variants, the receptor is synthesized, but not transported to the cell surface, due to mutations in the epidermal growth factor (EGF) precursor homology domain. Class 3 variants are mutations in the ligand-binding domain, resulting in inability to bind LDL cholesterol. With class 4 variants, LDL cholesterol is effectively bound at the cell surface, but due to mutations in the receptor's cytoplasmic tail, coated pits cannot be localized and endocytosis does not occur. Finally, class 5 variants are often deletions of the EGF precursor homology domain, which impair the ability of the cell to recycle LDLR.[5]

The clinical impact of genetic characterization of FH variants is seen in treatment options. When homozygous FH is identified it is generally treated with LDL apheresis, as cholesterol lowering medications are ineffective. Heterozygous FH, however, is effectively treated with early initiation of HMG-CoA reductase inhibitors. The development of HMG-coA reductase inhibitors (statins) was in fact a direct result of research in FH. Specifically, the discovery that expression of *LDLR* is regulated by cellular sterol contributed to the development of statins.[6] Future therapeutic options such as gene therapy will similarly be built on characterization of the full range of causative genetic variants.

Familial Defective Apolipoprotein B-100 (apoB-100)

A second relatively common cause of hypercholesterolemia is familial defective apoB (FDB). The prevalence is approximately 1 in 1000 among individuals of Northern European descent. The clinical course is less severe compared with FH due to *LDLR* mutations. Patients with heterozygous FDB present with plasma cholesterol levels in the 275–350 mg/dL range. FDB homozygotes have plasma cholesterol levels comparable to that of FH heterozygotes, and onset of clinical coronary artery disease occurs, on average, in the fifth decade of life.[7]

Familial defective apoB-100 usually results from a missense mutation in the *LDLR* binding domain of apoB.[8] Genetic testing for this Arg3500Gln variant is relatively straightforward and performed after patients have found to have normal *LDLR* expression and function.

PCSK9 Nonsense Mutations

A third form of autosomal dominant familial hypercholesterolemia is a recently characterized mutation in the proprotein convertase subtilisin/kexin type 9 (*PCSK9*) gene. In a cohort of 23 French families with hypercholesterolemia in whom LDLR and apoB sequence variants were excluded, Abifadel and colleagues identified two missense mutations, S127R and F216L, that resulted in gain of function mutation.[9] Subjects with the S127R and F216L mutations displayed LDL cholesterol levels which were two- to fivefold higher than age-matched controls. Functional studies have shown *PCSK9* is integral in posttranslational regulation of *LDLR* processing, reducing the LDLR number.[10]

Hypertrophic Cardiomyopathy

Hypertrophic cardiomyopathy (HCM) can be defined clinically as cardiac hypertrophy in the absence of an increased external load and a hyperdynamic left ventricle with a small chamber. This diagnosis, which is primarily based on echocardiographic findings of cardiac hypertrophy, has significant shortcomings.[11] For example, the presence of systemic hypertension excludes the diagnosis of HCM, as it is an alternate cause of cardiac hypertrophy. However, systemic hypertension is a common disease and could be present concomitantly in patients with HCM and even contribute to the phenotypic expression of HCM. Due to these difficulties with the clinical diagnosis, it is expected that genetic-based testing will become more predominant as molecular genetic techniques are most cost-effective.[12]

The prevalence of HCM is approximately 1 in 500 in the general population.[11] This is based on left ventricular wall thickness of

15 mm or greater on an echocardiogram in 25-to-35-year-old individuals. However, many cases of HCM have a milder degree of cardiac hypertrophy, and many mutations are nonpenetrant in the above age group.

Hypertrophic cardiomyopathy is considered a disease of mutant sarcomeric proteins. Familial aggregation of HCM was described over 50 years ago,[13] but the molecular basis was unknown until the identification of the R403Q mutation in the beta-myosin heavy chain in a family of affected subjects.[14] The most common causal genes are *MYH7*, *MYBPC3*, *TNNT2*, and *TNNI3*, which encode the beta-myosin heavy chain, myosin binding protein-C, cardiac troponin T and I, respectively.[15–19] Of these mutations, those in *MYH7* and *MYBPC3* are the most common, each accounting for 30% of HCM cases.[15–17] Mutations in *TNNT2* and *TNNI3* are less common, although they still account for another 10–15% of the cases of HCM.

Role for Genetic Screening

Patients with HCM exhibit variable clinical manifestations. The variability in phenotype is seen among individuals of different mutations, as well as among individuals with identical causal mutations.[20] Even members of a single family who share the same causal mutation exhibit considerable variability in phenotypic expression of disease. There are many hypotheses for this heterogeneity. It is possible that multiple mutations, in genes that are related to myocardial function and in seemingly unrelated genes, account for the variability.[21,22] However, the odds of each individual having multiple mutations is exceedingly rare. It is likely that environmental factors, such as heavy physical exercise, contribute to the phenotypic expression of HCM.

Early diagnosis through genetic screening would allow identification of individuals at risk, followed by counseling, which together could prevent the clinical manifestations of disease altogether. Additionally, genetic screening would better identify the true prevalence of HCM. Despite the need for screening, routine testing has not been feasible. The diversity of the causal mutations and the low frequency of each specific mutation are the major limiting factors. Furthermore, the screening technique would need to be highly sensitive and specific while remaining cost-effective. The current gold standard is direct sequencing of genomic DNA, which has an excellent sensitivity and specificity. In the case of HCM, it would be necessary to sequence at least all coding exons of a dozen sarcomeric genes. The current sequencing technology is far too expensive and labor intensive to make this approach feasible. Sequencing technology, however, is rapidly evolving and in the next few years direct sequencing may be available for early diagnosis of HCM.

Long QT Syndrome

Congenital long QT syndrome (LQTS) is one of the many heart rhythm disorders in which genetic characterization has led to a better understanding of pathophysiology. Until the first genetic loci responsible for the syndrome were identified in the 1990s, clinical and experimental studies suggested that LQTS might be caused by an imbalance of sympathetic nerve activity. The "sympathetic imbalance" theory was initially favored because of reports that the QT interval could be prolonged by right stellate ganglionectomy or by stimulating the left stellate ganglion.[23,24] This hypothesis was quickly replaced when mutations in eight genes were identified and confirmed to cause congenital LQTS. These include the genes for the cardiac sodium current, I_{Na},[25] multiple genes contributing to the rapid and slow components of the delayed rectifier potassium currents, I_{Kr} and I_{Ks},[26,27] the Ki2.1 channel,[28] and the L-type calcium channel.[29]

Given the fact that each of these mutations responsible for congenital LQTS are involved in ion channel conduction, investigators began studying membrane repolarization abnormalities. Mechanistic insights gained from studying ion channels isolated from Drosophila eventually converged with powerful genetic techniques applied to large families.

Now, there are eight distinct LQTS genes, though testing for these polymorphisms has little role in clinical diagnosis. The classic electrocardiogram (ECG) feature of LQTS patients is prolongation of the rate-corrected QT interval (QTc). The standard QTc value of 440 ms was often used as an index for diagnosis. However, the ECG changes in LQTS are not limited to prolongation of the QTc interval, but may also include factors, such as: T and U wave abnormalities, bradycardia, episodic polymorphic ventricular tachycardia, and unheralded syncope. As a result, diagnostic criteria for LQTS were refined based on a scoring system of clinical criteria including ECG findings and clinical and family histories.[30]

Role for Genetic Screening

Genetic screening plays a limited role in initial diagnosis of LQTS, largely because of the cost- and labor-intensive nature of sequencing each potential culprit gene. There may be, however, a role for more reliable and earlier screening, as death is tragically the first symptom in 10–15% of patients who die of complications from LQTS.

Genetic testing is often used to guide therapy for LQTS, as the clinical course and response to treatment is markedly different for each subtype of the disease. For example, the incidence of a first cardiac event (syncope, cardiac arrest, and sudden death) before the age of 40, and prior to initiation of therapy, also differs among genotypes. It is lower for LQT1 (30%) than for LQT2 (46%) or LQT3 (42%).[31] It was found that triggers of cardiac events differ among the genotypes: LQT1 patients experience the majority of their events during exercise or conditions associated with elevated sympathetic activity, but rarely during rest or sleep. In contrast, this is reversed in LQT2 and LQT3 patients.[31]

As for treatment, there are again differences based on genotype. LQT1 is caused by mutations in the *KCNQ1* gene, resulting in impairment of the slow delayed rectifier potassium channel (I_{Ks}). The first choice in therapy is prescription of beta blockers. Clinical trials have shown suppression of cardiac events by beta blockers is more frequent in patients with LQT1 (81%) than with LQT2 (59%) and LQT3 (50%).[31] A gain of functional defect in the sodium-channel gene, *SCN5A*, is responsible for LQT3. Therefore, treatment with sodium-channel blockade using mexilitine is logically more efficacious. Preliminary clinical and basic experimental data do show that this is case.[32] There are five more long QT syndromes (LQT4–8), however, genotype-specific treatment has not been determined because of the small number of cases. Again, reduction in the cost of genetic screening will allow greater characterization of these diseases, as well as earlier diagnosis of all patients at risk for development of long QT syndrome.

Common/Complex Cardiovascular Disease

Discovery of novel genetic markers for common cardiovascular diseases has dramatically increased since the completion of the Human Genome Project in 2001. The two predominant approaches are candidate gene studies that focus on single genes of known biologic interest or genetic mapping using a set of polymorphisms across the entire genome. Genome-wide association studies (GWASs) test the association of sets of common single nucleotide polymorphisms (SNPs) across the genome for a role in disease or quantitative risk factors for disease.

GWASs are of particular interest because they have proven fruitful in discovering genetic variants contributing to complex traits. For complex traits, the expectation is that many genes contribute—each with a modest effect. In certain circumstances, these markers may have functional consequences, such as altering the expression or function of a gene that directly contributes to development of disease. Alternatively, a marker may have no functional consequences, but may be coinherited with a functional variant by means of linkage disequilibrium. A majority of the reported genetic markers are thought to be of this second type, and studies are underway to determine the genes of functional importance. While this work continues, these coinherited genetic markers can be used for disease prediction. The early attempts to use genetic biomarkers to create genetic risk scores for common diseases, such as atherosclerosis and myocardial infarction, will be reviewed in this section.

Coronary Artery Disease

To date, seven GWASs for coronary artery disease (CAD) in individuals of European ancestry have been published and these have identified 12 loci influencing the risk the disease (Table 32–1).[33–39] The 9p21 locus was the first identified using the GWAS approach and is the most widely-replicated locus, as well as being the locus that confers the highest population attributable risk for CAD in whites, independent of traditional risk factors.[33,34] The locus is not only associated with clinical CAD, but also with subclinical CAD as estimated by coronary calcium, ischemic stroke, and peripheral arterial disease, including abdominal aortic aneurysm.[33,40] Curiously, the lead SNPs at the 9p21 locus have also been found to increase the risk of intracranial arterial (berry) aneurysms.[40] This key discovery supports the hypothesis that the locus is affecting the integrity of the vessel wall and consequently predisposing it to plaque deposition and/or aneurysm formation. The 9p21 locus is near the *CDKN2A* and *CDKN2B* genes and overlaps the recently-discovered antisense noncoding RNA, *ANRIL*.[33,34]

Two interesting observations apply to the remaining eleven CAD susceptibility loci discovered to date. First, four of these loci, 19p13, 1p32, 1p13, and 6q26–q27, appear to be influencing the risk of CAD through known risk factors. The first three loci associate with LDL levels and are near genes that are known or suspected to be important in lipid metabolism (*LDLR*, *PCSK9*, and *CELSR2-PSRC1-SORT1* cluster, respectively).[41] The fourth locus includes the *LPA* gene that determines the level of lipoprotein(a) (Lp(a)), a highly heritable biomarker which is also known to positively correlate with the risk of CAD.[32] Second, similar to 9p21, the *PHACTR1* locus may lead to myocardial infarction by directly promoting the development of atherosclerosis in the coronary

Table 32–1: Coronary artery disease susceptibility loci mapped using the genome-wide association approach.

SNP	Locus	Risk Allele Frequency	Positional Candidate Genes at Locus	OR (95% CI)	P Value
rs4977574	9p21	0.56	*CDKN2A, CDKN2B*	1.29 (1.25–1.34)	2.7×10^{-44}
rs646776	1p13	0.81	*CELSR2, PSRC1, SORT1*	1.19 (1.13–1.26)	7.9×10^{-12}
rs17465637	1q41	0.72	*MIA3*	1.14 (1.10–1.19)	1.4×10^{-9}
rs1746048	10q11	0.84	*CXCL12*	1.17 (1.11–1.24)	7.4×10^{-9}
rs9982601	21q22	0.13	*SLC5A3, MRPS6, KCNE2*	1.20 (1.14–1.27)	6.4×10^{-11}
rs12526453	6q24	0.65	*PHACTR1*	1.12 (1.08–1.17)	1.3×10^{-9}
rs6725887	2q33	0.14	*WDR12*	1.17 (1.11–1.23)	1.3×10^{-8}
rs1122608	19p13	0.75	*LDLR*	1.15 (1.10–1.20)	1.9×10^{-9}
rs11206510	1p32	0.81	*PCSK9*	1.15 (1.10–1.21)	9.6×10^{-9}
rs9818870	3q22	0.15	*MRAS*	1.15 (1.11–1.19)	7.4×10^{-13}
CCTC haplotype	6q26–6q27	0.02	*SLC22A3, LPAL2, LPA*	1.82 (1.57–2.11)	4.2×10^{-15}

arteries. In an independent GWAS for coronary artery calcification in more than 10,000 participants from six prospective cohort studies, *PHACTR1* SNPs were associated with coronary artery calcification at genome-wide significance.[37]

Similar GWASs have been completed for a range of cardiovascular diseases and traits including: myocardial infarction, blood lipid concentrations, type 2 diabetes mellitus, hypertension, body mass index, electrocardiographic QT interval, and atrial fibrillation, among others. Over 200 validated associations have been published recently. A curated database of validated genotype-phenotype associations is available at: http://www.genome.gov/26525384.[42]

Clinical Application of GWAS Findings: Cardiovascular Risk Prediction

Genetic variants may be useful in identifying individuals at higher risk for cardiovascular disease in order to guide treatment decisions. The variants identified so far for clinical diseases or risk factor traits each individually confer a modest risk for disease. Thus, researchers have explored whether a combination of variants, a so-called multi-locus genetic risk profile, can stratify risk. Our group recently showed that the additive effect of five common variants related to LDL cholesterol can stratify individuals across a range from 151 mg/dL to 170 mg/dL and that four common variants related to HDL cholesterol can stratify from 51 mg/dL to 60 mg/dL.[43] We constructed a genotype score derived from these nine variants and evaluated whether this genotype score can be useful in the prediction of cardiovascular disease. In a sample of 5414 individuals free of cardiovascular disease at baseline and followed for an average of 10.6 years, genotype score predicted incident cardiovascular disease. Notably, genotype score remained an independent predictor even after accounting for the baseline level of blood lipids. In a separate study, we showed that the additive effect of nine variants identified for myocardial infarction can identify 20% of the population at a greater than twofold increased risk for myocardial infarction.[44]

For specific clinical applications, a panel of SNPs may prove useful. A key unanswered question in the primary prevention of cardiovascular disease is the appropriate targeting of effective preventive interventions like statins. Specifically, should statins be started at an early age in some individuals and if so, how should these individuals be identified? The cumulative effect of long-term exposure to elevated LDL cholesterol concentration is a key determinant of atherosclerosis and, as such, lifelong reductions in LDL cholesterol levels that include tailored dietary recommendations or early use of statins may be critical to reducing the burden of cardiovascular disease. One hypothesis that merits testing is whether or not young individuals who are dyslipidemic based on a collection of common genetic variants may derive the great benefit from early use of statins. Clinical trials are needed to test such a hypothesis and to demonstrate that management using a set of genotypes can improve outcomes. Such trials are needed prior to use of genotypes in clinical practice.

Pharmacogenomics

Testing for genetic variants has already begun to have clinical significance in the field of pharmacogenomics. Side effects and clinical profiles differ dramatically between patients and these differences may have a genetic basis. There are two main aims of this line of investigation. First, pharmacogenomic testing can be used to decrease the rate of adverse events. This can be done by guiding dosing or determining which patients are at risk for specific side effects. Second, pharmacogenomic testing can determine efficacy of medications in individual patients. The longer term goal is to personalize medication regimens to individual patients based on their pharmacogenomic profile.

There are many efforts underway to better understand individual differences in response to medication that may make personalized medicine possible. The National Institutes of Health has supported a consortium of scientists who are studying how genetic variation contributes to differences in drug response among patients—this consortium is called the Pharmacogenetics Research Network (PGRN).[45] The collected information from this research about specific proteins, genes, and pathways is being integrated into the Pharmacogenetics and Pharmacogenomics Knowledge Base (http://www.pharmgkb.org). As will be discussed below, one of the initial efforts to apply pharamcogenomic information clinically is with warfarin dosing. Towards this end, several investigators have formed the Internal Warfarin Pharmacogenomics Consortium (http://www.pharmgkb.org/views/project.jsp?pId=56). The ultimate goal is for all investigators in this group to share clinical and genetic data to develop a consensus model for drug administration. Finally, researchers who are conducting ancillary pharmacogenomic studies in ongoing or completed clinical research projects supported by the National Heart, Lung, and Blood Institute (NHLBI) have developed a free Web-based tool for health care professionals to estimate the starting warfarin dose (http://www.warfarindosing.org).[46]

In many of the cases where pharmacogenomic data is being used to potentially guide clinical practice, the mechanism by which variants affect drug metabolism or other metabolic pathways is unknown. In several cases, the variants being used to predict clinical response were identified through genome-wide association studies. These large-scale genetic epidemiology studies apply new technological advances that make it possible to identify millions of DNA sequence variations and correlate them with phenotypic characteristics.

Though there are many ongoing trials in the field, three recent papers are of particular interest to cardiovascular medicine. Two of these aim to improve the safety of medications—warfarin and statins. The third tests the efficacy of clopidogrel based on whether genetic polymorphisms change the ability of certain patients to metabolize the drug into its active metabolite. As each of these studies represents a seminal advance in the field of cardiovascular pharmacogenomics, we will discuss them in further detail.

Warfarin Dosing

Recent clinical studies have shown polymorphisms in two genes that contribute to variability in sensitivity to warfarin. Cytochrome P450 2C9 (*CYP2C9*) is the enzyme primarily responsible for the metabolic clearance of the S-enantiomer of warfarin.[47,48] Patients with certain common genetic variants of *CYP2C9* require a lower dose of warfarin and a longer time to reach a stable dose.[49,50] Vitamin K epoxide reductase (*VKORC1*) is a second gene in which polymorphisms are associated with different clinical response. This enzyme recycles vitamin K epoxide to the reduced form of vitamin K, an essential cofactor in the formation of the active clotting factors II, VII, IX, and Z through gamma-glutamyl carboxylation.[51] On the basis of these observations, the FDA approved a labeling change for warfarin that describes the reported effects of *VKORC1* and *CYP2C9* on dose requirements. Little is known, however, on the relative contributions of these genetic variants.

Schwarz and colleagues provide prospective data on variability in the response to initial warfarin therapy on the basis of *CYP2C9* genotypes and *VKORC1* haplotypes.[52] The investigators examined the effects of variants of *CYP2C9* and *VKORC1* on initial warfarin dose requirements in a cohort of 297 patients who were undergoing anticoagulation therapy. They found genetic variation in *VKORC1*, but not in *CYP2C9*, modulates the early response to warfarin. Patients carrying the *VKORC1* haplotype A had significantly higher international normalized ratio values in the first week than did non-A homozygotes. Larger-scale studies are now underway to determine if testing for the *VKORC1* haplotype A can guide warfarin dosing.

Statin Myopathy

Statin therapy has been shown to reduce the incidence of heart disease in several large-scale, randomized trials. The statins are not only efficacious, but also remarkably safe. However, in rare cases, statins can cause muscle pain or weakness, and occasionally lead to rhabdomyolysis. Investigators in the Study of Effectiveness of Additional Reductions in Cholesterol and Homocysteine (SEARCH) Collaborative Group at Oxford University conducted a genome-wide association study in 85 subjects with definite or incipient myopathy and 90 controls, all of whom were taking 80 mg of simvastatin.[53] This genome-wide scan showed a single strong association of myopathy with an SNP (rs436357) located within *SLCO1B1* on chromosome 12. *SLCO1B1* encodes the organic anion-transporting polypeptide OATP1B1, which has been shown to regulate the hepatic uptake of statins. Their results indicate that statin blood concentrations are higher in individuals with the *SLCO1B1* C allele, though not to a statistically significant level. This is consistent with the clinical finding that higher statin doses tend to provoke a higher incidence of statin myopathy. In fact, at simvastatin doses of 20 to 40 mg, the incidence of myopathy is typically only 1 case per 10,000 patients per year. At higher doses, however, this rate significantly increases.[54] Genotyping for *SLCO1B1* polymorphisms may be useful in the future for tailoring the statin dose and monitoring medication safety in people at risk for myopathy.

Clopidogrel Efficacy

While the previous two examples were uses of pharmacogenomic testing to improve the safety of a medication, recent studies have used this approach to better predict the efficacy of the antiplatelet drug, clopidogrel. In the large number of people who are on clopidogrel (for such indications as during acute coronary syndrome, after a percutaneous coronary intervention, or secondary prophylaxis for stroke), interpatient variability has been well described.[55] At least part of this variability is due to polymorphisms in the cytochrome P450 (CYP) genes responsible for converting clopidogrel to its active metabolite. Mega and colleagues tested the association between functional genetic variants in CYP genes, plasma concentrations of active drug metabolite, and platelet inhibition in response to clopidogrel in 162 healthy subjects.[56] Among these healthy subjects, carriers of the *CYP2C19* reduced-function allele had a relative reduction of 32.4% in plasma exposure to the active metabolite of clopidogrel, corresponding with a statistically significant increase in platelet aggregation in response to the drug. The clinical significance of this was shown by testing association between genetic variants (such as the *CYP2C19* polymorphism) and cardiovascular outcomes in a separate cohort of 1477 subjects with acute coronary syndromes who were treated with clopidogrel in the Trial to Assess Improvement in Therapeutic Outcomes by Optimizing Platelet Inhibition with Prasugrel–Thrombolysis in Myocardial Infarction (TRITON–TIMI).[38] Among the clopidogrel-treated subjects in this cohort, carriers had a relative increase of 53% in the composite primary efficacy outcome of the risk of death from cardiovascular causes, myocardial infarction, or stroke (as compared with noncarriers) and an increase by a factor of three in the risk of stent thrombosis. Taken together, these results show that the *CYP2C19* allele lowers the level of active metabolite of clopidogrel, leading to diminished platelet inhibition and a higher rate of major adverse cardiovascular events. Testing for this variant prior to initiation of clopidogrel treatment, or in patients who have shown recurrence of coronary events despite clopidogrel treatment, is of great clinical interest.

Conclusion

Over the past two decades, there has been remarkable progress in our understanding of the inherited basis for phenotypes that segregate in a Mendelian fashion, as well as for common polygenic cardiovascular disorders. Scores of genes have been mapped and a spectrum of mutations has been identified for several disorders. The application of this knowledge to clinical practice is just beginning. With continued investigation, it should be possible to define specific clinical scenarios where a genetic variant or a panel of variants can meaningfully guide clinical treatment decisions.

References

1. Müller C. Xanthoma, hypercholesterolemia, angina pectoris. *Acta Med Scand.* 1938;89:75.
2. Brown MS, Goldstein JL. Receptor-mediated control of cholesterol metabolism. *Science.* 1976;191:150–154.
3. Rader DJ, Cohen J, Hobbs HH. Monogenic hypercholesterolemia: new insights in pathogenesis and treatment. *J Clin Invest.* 2003;111: 1795–1803.
4. Heath KE, Gahan M, Whittall A, Humphries SE. Low-density lipoprotein receptor gene (LDLR) word-wide website in familiar hypercholesterolaemia: update, new features and mutation analysis. *Atherosclerosis.* 2001;154:243–246.
5. Hobbs H, Russell DW, Brown MS, and Goldstein JL. The LDL receptor locus in familial hypercholesterolemia: mutational analysis of a membrane protein. *Ann Rev Genetics.* 1990;24:133–170.
6. Goldstein JL, Brown MS. Regulation of the mevalonate pathway. *Nature.* 1990;343:425–430.
7. Myant NB. Familial defective apolipoprotein B-100: A review, including some comparisons with familial hypercholesterolemia. *Atherosclerosis.* 1993;104:1–18.
8. Borén J, Ekström U, Agen B, Nilsson-Ehle P, Inneraity TL. The molecular mechanism for the genetic disorder familial defective apolipoprotein B100. *J Biol Chem.* 2001;276:9214–9218.
9. Abifadel M, Varret M, Rabes JP, et al. Mutations in PCSK9 cause autosomique dominant hypercholesterolemia. *Nat Genet.* 2003;34: 154–156.
10. Park SW, Moon YA, Horton JD. Post-transcriptional regulation of low density lipoprotein receptor protein by proprotein convertase subtilisin/kexin type 9a in mouse liver. *J Biol Chem.* 2004;279: 50630–50638.
11. Maron BJ. Hypertrophic cardiomyopathy: a systematic review. *JAMA.* 2002;287:1308–1320.
12. Marian AJ. Hypertrophic cardiomyopathy. In: Dzau VJ, Liew CC, eds. *Cardiovascular Genetics and Genomics for the Cardiologist.* Malden, MA: Blackwell Futura. 2007:30–54.
13. Davies LG. A familial heart disease. *Br Heart J.* 1952;14:206–212.

14. Geisterfer-Lowrance AA, Kass S, Tanigawa G, et al. A molecular basis for familial hypertrophic cardiomyopathy: a beta cardiac myosin heavy chain gene missense mutation. *Cell.* 1990;62:999–1006.
15. Richard P, Charon P, Carrier L, et al. Hypertrophic cardiomyopathy: distribution of disease genes, spectrum of mutations, and implications for a molecular diagnosis strategy. *Circulation.* 2003;107:2227–2232.
16. Erdmann J, Raible J, Maki-Abadi J, et al. Spectrum of clinical phenotypes and gene variants in cardiac myosin-binding protein C mutation carriers with hypertrophic cardiomyopathy. *J Am Coll Cardiol.* 2001;38:322–330.
17. Mogensen J, Murphy RT, Kubo T, et al. Frequency and clinical expression of cardiac troponin I mutations in 748 consecutive families with hypertrophic cardiomyopathy. *J Am Coll Cardiol.* 2004;44:2315–2325.
18. Andersen PS, Havndrup O, Bundgaard H, et al. Genetic and phenotypic characterization of mutations in myosin-binding protein C (MYBPC3) in 81 families with familial hypertrophic cardiomyopathy: total or partial haploinsufficiency. *Eur J Hum Genet.* 2004;12:673–677.
19. Torricelli F, Girolami F, Olivotto I, et al. Prevalence and clinical profile of troponin T mutations among patients with hypertrophic cardiomyopathy in Tuscany. *Am J Cardiol.* 2003;92:1358–1362.
20. Marian AJ. On genetic and phenotypic variability of hypertrophic cardiomyopathy: nature versus nurture. *J Am Coll Cardiol.* 2001;38: 331–334.
21. Blair E, Price SJ, Baty CJ, Ostman-Smith I, Watkins H. Mutations in cis can confound genotype-phenotype correlations in hypertrophic cardiomyopathy. *J Med Genet.* 2001;38:385–388.
22. Van Driest SL, Vasile VC, Ommen SR, et al. Myosin binding protein C mutations and compound heterozygosity in hypertrophic cardiomyopathy. *J Am Coll Cardiol.* 2004;44:1903–1910.
23. Chiang CE, Roden DM. The long QT syndromes: genetic basis and clinical implications. *J Am Coll Cardiol.* 2000;36:1–12.
24. Yanowitz F, Preston JB, Abildskov JA. Functional distribution of right and left stellate innervation to the ventricles. Production of neurogenic electrocardiographic changes by unilateral alteration of sympathetic tone. *Circ Res.* 1966;18:416–428.

25. Wang Q, Shen J, Slawski I, et al. SCN5A mutations associated with an inherited cardiac arrhythmia, long QT syndrome. *Cell.* 1995;80: 805–811.

26. Curran ME, Splawski I, Timothy KW, et al. A molecular basis for cardiac arrhythmia: HERG mutations cause long QT syndrome. *Cell.* 1995;80:795–803.

27. Wang Q, Curran ME, Splawski I, et al. Positional cloning of a novel potassium channel gene: KVLQT1 mutations cause cardiac arrhythmias. *Nat Genet.* 1996;12:17–23.

28. Plaster NM, Tawil R, Tristani-Firouzi M, et al. Mutations in Kir2.1 cause developmental and episodic electrical phenotypes in Andersen's syndrome. *Cell.* 2001;105:511–519.

29. Splawski I, Timothy KW, Sharpe LM, et al. Ca (V)1.2 calcium channel dysfunction causes a multisystem disorder including arrhythmia and autism. *Cell.* 2004;119:19–31.

30. Schwartz PJ, Moss AJ, Vincent GM, et al. Diagnostic criteria for the long QT syndrome. *Circulation.* 1993;88:782–784.

31. Schwartz PJ, Priori SG, Spazzolini C, et al. Genotype-phenotype correlation in the long T syndrome: gene-specific triggers for life-threatening arrhythmias. *Circulation.* 2001;103:89–95.

32. Wang DW, Yazawa K, Makita N, et al. Pharmacological targeting of long QT mutant sodium channels. *J Clin Invest.* 1997;99:1714–1720.

33. Helgadottir A, Thorleifsson G, Manolescu A, et al. A common variant on chromosome 9p21 affects the risk of myocardial infarction. *Science.* 2007;317:1322–1324.

34. McPherson R, Pertsemlidis A, Kavaslar N, et al. A common allele on chromosome 9 associated with coronary heart disease. *Science.* 2007; 316:1488–1491.

35. Samani NJ, Erdmann J, Hall AS, et al. Genomewide association analysis of coronary artery disease. *N Engl J Med.* 2007;357:436–439.

36. Erdmann J, Grosshennig A, Braund PS, et al. New susceptibility locus for coronary artery disease on chromosome 3q22.3. *Nat Genet.* 2009; 41:280–282.

37. Soranzo N, Rendon A, Gieger C, et al. A novel variant on chromosome 7q22.3 associated with mean platelet volume, counts, and function. *Blood.* 2009;113:3831–3837.

38. Trégouët DA, König IR, Erdmann J, et al. Genome-wide haplotype association study identifies the SLC22A3-LPAL2-LPA gene cluster as a risk locus for coronary artery disease. *Nat Genet.* 2009;41:283–285.

39. Gudbjartsson DF, Bjornsdottir US, Halapi E, et al. Sequence variants affecting eosinophil numbers associate with asthma and myocardial infarction. *Nat Genet.* 2009;41:342–347.

40. Helgadottir A, Thorleifsson G, Magnusson KP. The same sequence variant on 9p21 associates with myocardial infarction, abdominal aortic aneurysm and intracranial aneurysm. *Nat Genet.* 2008;40: 217–224.

41. Kathiresan S, Melander O, Guiducci C, et al.; Siz new loci associated with blood low-density lipoprotein cholesterol, high density lipoprotein cholesterol or triglycerides in humans. *Nat Genet.* 2008;40: 189–197.

42. Willer CJ, Speliotes EK, Loss RJ, et al.; Six new loci associated with body mass index highlight a neuronal influence on body weight regulation. *Nat Genet.* 2009;41:25–34.

43. Kathiresan S, Melander O, Anevski D, et al. Polymorphisms associated with cholesterol and risk of cardiovascular events. *N Engl J Med.* 2008;359:92–93.

44. Kathiresan S, Voight BF, Purcell S, et al. Genome-wide association of early-onset myocardial infarction with single nucleotide polymorphisms and copy number variants. *Nat Genet.* 2009;41:334–341.

45. Shurin SB, Nabel EG. Pharmacogenomics: ready for prime time? *N Engl J Med.* 2008;358(10):1061–1063.

46. Gage BF, Eby C, Milligan PE, Banet GA, Duncan JR, McLeod HL. Use of pharmacogenetics and clinical factors to predict the maintenance dose of warfarin. *Thromb Haemost.* 2004;91:87–94.

47. Takahashi H, Wilkinson GR, Padrini R, Echizen H. CYP2C9 and oral anticoagulation therapy with acenocoumarol and warfarin: similarities and differences. *Clin Pharmacol Ther.* 2004;75:376–380.

48. Kaminsky LS, Zhang ZY. Human P450 metabolism of warfarin. *Pharmacol Ther.* 1997;73:67–74.

49. Higashi MK, Veenstra DL, Kondo LM, et al. Association between CYP2C9 genetic variants and anticoagulation-related outcomes during warfarin therapy. *JAMA.* 2002;287:1690–1698.

50. Veenstra DL, Blough DK, Higashi MK, et al. CYP2C9 haplotype structure in European American warfarin patients and association with clinical outcomes. *Clin Pharmacol Ther.* 2005;77:353–364.

51. Cain D, Hutson SM, Wallin R. Assembly of the warfarin-sensitive vitamin K 2,3-epoxide reductase enzyme complex in the endoplasmic reticulum membrane. *J Biol Chem.* 1997;272:29068–29075.

52. Schwarz UI, Ritchie MD, Bradford Y, et al. Genetic determinants of response to warfarin during initial anticoagulation. *N Eng J Med.* 2008;358:999–1008.

53. The SEARCH Collaborative Group. SLCO1B1 variants and statin-induced myopathy—a genomewide study. *N Eng J Med.* 2008;359: 789–799.

54. Law M, Rudnicka AR. Statin safety: a systematic review. *Am J Cardiol.* 2006;97:S52C–S60C.

55. Gurbel PA, Bliden KP, Hiatt BL, O'Connor CM. Clopidogrel for coronary stenting: response variability, drug resistance, and the effect of pretreatment platelet reactivity. *Circulation.* 2003;107:2908–2913.

56. Mega JL, Close SL, Wiviott SD, et al. Cytochrome P-450 polymorphisms and response to clopidogrel. *N Engl J Med.* 2009;360:354–362.

33 ■ The Search for New Cardiovascular Biomarkers: Application of Metabolomics to Cardiovascular Biomarker and Pathway Discovery

Gregory D. Lewis, MD
Aarti Asnani, BS
Robert E. Gerszten, MD

Acknowledgments

Funding sources: The authors gratefully acknowledge support from the NIH (R01 HL072872 and U01HL083141), the Donald W. Reynolds Foundation, the Foundation Leducq to REG, the Heart Failure Society of America (GDL), the Harvard/MIT Clinical Investigator Training Program (GDL) and the American Heart Association Fellow-to-Faculty Award (GDL), as well as a pre-doctoral award from the Sarnoff Cardiovascular Research Foundation (AA).

Introduction

Metabolism refers to the body's conversion of food stores into energy currencies that can be utilized to perform work. While decades of research in biochemistry, nutrition, and physiology have revealed specific metabolic pathways, systematic surveys of pathways altered in human disease states, such as diabetes, obesity, and cardiovascular disease, have yet to be performed. An emerging set of tools, based on mass spectrometry (MS), nuclear magnetic resonance (NMR), and other technologies, enable the monitoring of dozens to hundreds of metabolites from biological samples. Though these technologies are still under development, they complement other functional genomic approaches, such as high-throughput genome sequencing, RNA expression analysis, and proteomics, and promise to transform our ability to profile samples with the goal of illuminating biology and discovering valuable clinical biomarkers.

The Birth of Metabolomics

Small biochemicals are the end result of all the regulatory complexity present in the cell, tissue, or organism, including transcriptional regulation, translational regulation, and posttranslational modification (Figure 33–1). Metabolic changes are thus the most proximal reporters of alterations in the body in response to a disease process or drug therapy. In 1971, Arthur Robinson and Linus Pauling conceived the core idea that information-rich data reflecting the functional status of a complex biological system reside in the quantitative and qualitative pattern of metabolites in

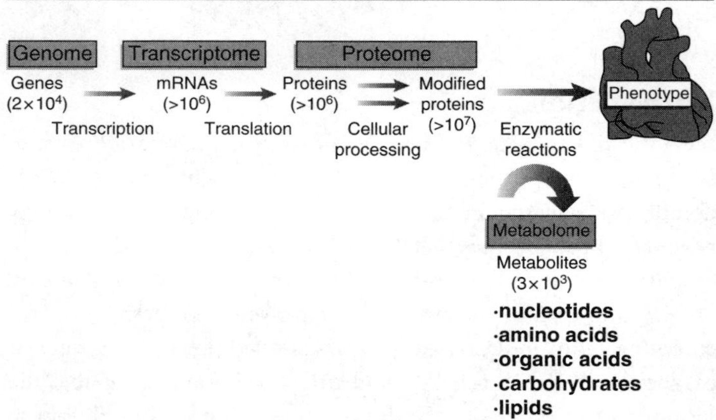

■ **Figure 33–1** Integration of metabolomics with other -omics approaches and relationship to phenotype.

body fluids.[1] In the same year, Horning and Horning[2] first used the term "metabolic profiling" to describe the output of a gas chromatogram from a patient sample. This emerging approach to the quantitative metabolic profiling of large numbers of small molecules in biofluids was ultimately termed "metabonomics" by Nicholson et al.,[3] and "metabolomics" by others. Recently, more focused analyses of specific metabolite families or subsets have even given rise to new terms such as "lipidomics." While the majority of biomarkers have emerged as extensions of "targeted" physiological studies, it has become evident that a metabolite profile derived in an unbiased manner may be informative even if the relationship of these metabolites to the target disease are initially unknown.

To date, the majority of metabolomics studies have been performed in model organisms. Studies have elucidated the genetic control of metabolites in plants, such as arabidopsis, and have determined "metabolic footprints" of genetically-altered yeast (*S. cerevisiae).*[4,5] In the latter report, metabolic profiling of conditioned media was used to "diagnose" otherwise silent mutant phenotypes. Tandem MS has also been used to profile 36 acylcarnitine species in mice over-expressing hepatic malonyl-CoA decarboxylase, yielding novel information regarding muscle beta-hydroxybutyrate levels and insulin sensitivity.[6]

The vision for metabolic profiling to diagnose human disease, however, extends from seminal studies of inborn errors of metabolism in infants. Roe and colleagues pioneered the use of tandem MS-based methods for monitoring fatty acid oxidation, as well as organic and selected amino acids.[7] Their work has culminated in universal neonatal screening for metabolism disorders in the state of North Carolina.[8] It is anticipated that a global metabolomic analysis of more common diseases might identify new biomarkers or spotlight pathways for dietary or drug modulation. The application of metabolomics to complex cardiovascular diseases, however, is likely to be more difficult than its application to inherited inborn errors of metabolism.

Technologies to Define the Human Metabolome

The global collection of metabolites in a cell or organism is often called the metabolome—this refers to all small molecules that exclude nucleic acids and proteins (see Figure 33–1). Present estimates from the Human Metabolome Project and the Kyoto Encyclopedia of Genes and Genomes (KEGG) suggest that the human metabolome consists of approximately 3000 endogenous metabolites (See http://www.hmdb.ca and http://www.genome.jp/kegg/). As with the human genome, the exact size of the human metabolome remains under debate. Estimates of the metabolome size will likely be revised as technologies to detect metabolites become more sensitive and comprehensive. Moreover, some argue that nutritional compounds, xenobiotics modified by human enzymes, as well as microbial metabolites present in the gut, must also be taken into consideration when defining the human metabolome.

The metabolome spans a variety of chemical compound classes, including those that are anionic versus cationic and lipidic versus hydrophilic (Table 33–1). Metabolites in tissue or body fluids are present across a broad range of concentrations. Therefore, no single analytical method is capable of analyzing all metabolites. However, capturing a subset of "sentinel" metabolites in critical pathways may prove to be a more tractable problem than proteomics. Estimates suggest that posttranslational modifications may bring the total number of protein species to greater than 10^6, and perhaps 10^8–10^9 if immunoglobulins are included. Thus, the metabolome may be less complex than the human proteome. Cellular metabolic pathways are highly conserved across species. Therefore, once metabolic changes are identified in humans, complementary functional studies in model organisms may rapidly provide insight into homeostatic and disease pathways.

Metabolites can be measured by several available analytical methods (for reviews of metabolomics technologies, see articles by Dunn WB[9,10] and Lindon JC[11]). Chromatographic procedures,

Table 33–1: Endogenous compounds profiled with current metabolomics technologies.[37]

Metabolite Class
Acetylcarnitines
Acylglycines
Alcohols
Aldehydes
Alkanes/Alkenes
Amides/Amines
Amino Acids
Aromatics
Bile Acids
Branched-Chain Hydrocarbons
Carbohydrates
Carnitines
Catecholamines
Cholesterols
Coenzyme A Derivatives
Esters
Ethers
Fatty Acids/Alcohols
Glycerols/Glycerophospholipids
Glycols/Glycolipids
Heterocyclics
Histidine Metabolites
Hydroxyacids
Imidazoles
Isoprenoids
Ketones
Lactams
Lactones
Lipids
Minerals
Nitrogenous Compounds
Nucleosides/Nucleotides
Organic Acids
Peptides
Phenols
Phosphates
Porphyrins
Prostaglandins
Pterins
Purines
Pyrimidines
Quinones
Sphingolipids
Steroids/Sterols
Sugars
Sulfates
Thiols
Vitamins

such as gas chromatography (GC), high performance liquid chromatography (LC), and capillary electrophoresis have been utilized to identify and quantitate specific metabolite subsets (e.g., amino acids[12,13] or purine metabolites[13,14]), but are best utilized for initial compound separation in combination with other detection techniques. Recently, two high-throughput technologies have garnered the most use for profiling a large number of metabolites simultaneously: NMR spectroscopy and mass spectrometry. The latter distinguishes metabolites on the basis of mass/charge ratio (m/z) and requires a separation of the metabolite components using either GC after chemical derivitization, or LC, with a new method of ultra performance LC (UPLC) being used increasingly. Mass spectrometry also permits absolute quantification of metabolite levels via the standard addition method, which entails using spiked-in, internal standards across a range of concentrations. When available, isotope-labeled standards can be easily differentiated from the endogenous metabolite by the appropriate number of mass units.

Nuclear magnetic resonance spectroscopy utilizes magnetic properties of nuclei to determine the number and type of chemical entities in a molecule. Proton (^{1}H) NMR spectroscopy can detect soluble proton-containing molecules with a molecular weight of approximately 20 kDa or less. The NMR spectra serve as the raw material for pattern recognition analyses, which simplifies the complex multivariate data into two or three dimensions that can be readily understood and evaluated. Both NMR and liquid chromatography-mass spectrometry (LC-MS) systems can be applied to in vivo tissues or to human biological fluids such as serum, plasma, urine, etc.[15] The advantages of NMR are that it requires relatively little sample preparation, is nondestructive, and can provide information about the precise structure of metabolites.[4] However, NMR sensitivity is related to magnet strength, and presently-available instrumentation can unambiguously detect only the most abundant metabolites in plasma. However, more sensitive systems are rapidly evolving.

In contrast, the most important advantage of mass spectrometry coupled with upfront chromatography is far greater sensitivity than NMR MS-based systems have been used to resolve compounds in the nanomole to picomole and even femtomole range, whereas identification of compounds by ^{1}H-NMR requires concentrations of 1 nanomole or higher.[16] In human plasma, limits of detection between 0.1 and 1 μM for a series of compounds analyzed by GC-MS have been described. Normal plasma concentrations for these metabolites are in the micromolar range, well above the limits of detection established for most MS technologies.

Targeted Versus Pattern Recognition Analyses

Perturbations of the metabolome that arise either as a cause or consequence of disease manifest as particular patterns of metabolites in a tissue or body fluid. This patterning concept has been the basis for recent efforts to discover proteomic or metabolomic "signatures" in tissue or serum. Mass spectrometers and NMR techniques can rapidly generate well-defined sets of peaks from a sample across a broad range of mass and charge. A growing controversy is whether such "metabolite signatures" can be used to accurately distinguish disease states from normal. A significant time advantage of direct profile comparisons derives from skipping the far more laborious task of unambiguously identifying the entities that underlie the peaks. Thus, rapid screening of patient samples is possible.

Using a pattern of peaks to diagnose disease without knowing the represented metabolites, however, raises some concerns. One issue is that of reproducibility. Because most mass spectrometers or NMR instruments were not designed as clinical tools, it is hard to generate consistent results from machine to machine or from operator to operator. Some contend that the patterns are mostly "noise" and do not discriminate biologically meaningful information. Without unequivocal identifications, one cannot independently confirm findings with complementary technologies. Others contend that the peaks profiled by the methodologies used to date only represent the most abundant plasma or tissue constituents. The most important consequence of not unequivocally identifying spectral peaks, however, is that little insight is gained into the biology, either to understand disease pathways through basic cellular mechanisms or as a check on the biological consistency and reasonableness of the data. Over-fitting of data is also a common problem when algorithms are generated from hundreds or thousands of peaks. Blinded prospective studies must ultimately be organized to better address the controversy.

Human metabolomics studies are also complicated by potentially confounding clinical variables, such as diet or drug effects, particularly if NMR- or mass spectrometry-based profiling techniques are used in which metabolite peaks are not unambiguously identified. Because of the various limitations inherent to *pattern discovery*, many have championed metabolomics applications in *targeted* approaches. The user targets a predefined set of metabolites to be quantified by monitoring specific chromatographic retention times, as well as parent and daughter mass-to-charge ratios of analytes. The targeted approach is more focused—relying on a predefined set of entities—thus researchers have more confidence in the end results because they know what is giving rise to the signals. Although this approach has many advantages, it is blind to changes in metabolites with retention times and MS characteristics that have not been incorporated into the analysis method. As efforts to define the human metabolome grow, we anticipate increasingly comprehensive targeted platforms for biomarkers and pathway discovery. Improvements in mass spectrometry and databases to enable identification of unknown peaks will also be critical.

Statistical Approaches to Metabolomic Data Reduction and Pathway Analysis

Although a high-throughput metabolomics approach to biomarker discovery brings many advantages, it also brings a danger of generating false positive associations due to multiple testing and over-fitting of data as noted above. Application of traditional statistical approaches (e.g., Bonferroni correction) in this setting tends to levy an insurmountable statistical penalty that can obscure biologically-relevant associations. Even newer statistical techniques, such as advanced resampling methods or control of the false discovery rate,[17] do not address adequately the fundamental problem of how to detect subtle, but important, changes in multiple variables identified in an "-omics" approach.

For metabolites participating in known biological pathways, a bioinformatics approach using pathways analysis can harness the vast information gathered in genomics or metabolomics experiments and turn it into a strength. Specifically, although measurement error in the marker discovery phase often prevents high confidence in any one particular metabolite's correlation, the observation that multiple metabolites in a particular biological pathway are moving in tandem brings confidence that a particular pathway, and hence any biomarkers in that pathway, truly are correlated with the perturbation. By utilizing a more principled selection process for candidate marker triage, this approach increases the likelihood that candidate biomarkers will be validated in subsequent prospective validation studies. This approach also enhances one's ability to use the metabolomic data collected in the biomarker discovery phase to gain insight into disease biology.

Systematic analysis of functional trends has become widespread and important in the analysis of DNA microarray data from model organisms.[18] The value of this approach in human studies was illustrated in a recent analysis of high-throughput differential mRNA expression.[19] Expression of mRNA was assessed on over 22,000 genes comparing patients with type 2 diabetes mellitus and unaffected controls (patients with normal glucose tolerance). A group of genes with depressed expression in diabetes versus controls was identified and tested for association with a collection of other gene characteristics. It was found that this gene set was enriched for genes involved in oxidative phosphorylation. Although *individual* oxidative phosphorylation genes were not dramatically reduced in expression, as a group, the trend was highly significant. Furthermore, the effect was attributable to a subset of oxidative phosphorylation genes regulated by peroxisome proliferator-activated receptor coactivator 1, a regulator of mitochondrial biogenesis. Thus, the analysis of trends among differentially expressed genes led directly to insight into altered metabolism in diabetes patients and hinted at therapeutic hypotheses involving the modulation of oxidative phosphorylation pathways.

There are several statistical issues complicating functional trends analysis of high-throughput data that have been rigorously addressed in software under development, including "FuncAssociate", recently described by Berriz and Roth.[20] Although the analysis software was developed for use with high-throughput mRNA expression data, this general approach may be used in conjunction with essentially any high-throughput experimental approach for identifying or ranking "interesting genes." FuncAssociate has generally been used in conjunction with controlled-vocabulary functional annotation, e.g., Gene Ontology (GO) annotation, but can be used in conjunction with many different sources of gene/protein/metabolite annotation, e.g., expression pattern in other studies, phenotype, protein complex membership, disease association, or phylogenetic profile.

Several data reduction strategies utilizing supervised learning multivariate analysis can be used to construct multivariate metabolite biomarker profiles.[21] In supervised learning, an algorithm is used to transform the multivariate data from metabolite profiles into a lower dimensionality with biological interest (e.g., health versus disease). Metabolite data (inputs) and disease status (outputs or targets) form pairs that are used in the calibration of the model with the goal of the model being to correctly associate the inputs with the targets. Discriminant analysis is a cluster-analysis based algorithm for categorical variables,[22] whereas partial least squares (PLS) is a popular linear regression-based method, and artificial neural networks offer the advantage of a machine-based method that can learn nonlinear mappings.[23]

Principal components analysis (PCA) applies raw data to a normalized matrix, which is then projected onto a specific scoring schema.[4,24] This schema is based upon a series of orthogonal principal components, the first of which describes the maximum variance in the original data set. PCA can be used for dimensionality reduction in a data set by retaining those characteristics of the data set that contribute most to its variance, by keeping lower-order principal components and ignoring higher-order ones. Similarly, Fisher discriminant analysis (FDA) creates normalized data matrices which decrease sample variability within a specific condition (e.g., cells grown aerobically), while maximizing sample variability between different conditions (e.g., aerobic versus anaerobic growth).[25] These relatively unbiased methods of reducing large datasets have the potential to define previously-unknown relationships between metabolites in a given physiologic state.

A limitation of current analytical approaches in metabolomics is that they rely on the relative or absolute concentrations of a metabolite in a given tissue or plasma sample and do not take into account varying enzymatic activities controlling metabolic flux through biological pathways. Studies examining metabolic flux incorporate isotope-labeled metabolites to map the fate of enzymatic substrates. Studies of tricarboxylic acid (TCA) cycle anaplerosis in energy metabolism[26] and the fractional synthetic rate of fatty acids and cholesterol[27] have generally focused on small, well-characterized pathways in specific tissues, such as muscle or liver. The integration of current analytical methods with assessment of enzymatic activities contributing to metabolic flux will help to elucidate biologically relevant metabolic changes.

Emerging "Nontraditional" Roles for Metabolites in Human Physiology

Secreted, small ligands, such as catecholamines, play central roles in cardiovascular physiology. A growing body of literature suggests previously unanticipated roles for metabolites that have been traditionally thought to function exclusively as intracellular signals. He et al. recently discovered that the "orphan" G-protein-coupled receptors, *GPR91* and *GPR99*, which are highly expressed in the kidney, bind to the TCA cycle intermediates succinate and α ketoglutarate, respectively.[28] Injection of succinate into mice caused increased renin secretion and a significant rise in blood pressure. The working hypothesis is that a local mismatch of energy supply and demand, altered metabolism of TCA-cycle intermediates, or injury, leads to mitochondrial dysfunction and the release of succinate and α–ketoglutarate from tissues. Once released into the circulation, the metabolites function in a hormone-like manner. They bind their receptors in the renal cortex, triggering the release of renin and activation of the renin-angiotensin system. In the case of tissue-ischemia from volume loss, this process might be adaptive to match metabolic demands. In other conditions associated with high succinate production, such as congestive heart failure, resultant increases in blood pressure might prove maladaptive. This recent work highlights roles for new types of circulating metabolites functioning as hormones in the body.

Application of Metabolomics to Unique Human Cardiovascular Disease Models

Novel metabolomics techniques still suffer from signal-to-noise issues, however, and applications to humans may be limited by interindividual variability. While recent studies have evaluated the diurnal and even seasonal variation of hemostatic and inflammatory proteins (e.g., fibrinogen, D-dimer, C-reactive protein), systematic studies have yet to be performed for metabolites in humans. Studies to identify novel disease-related pathways are also restricted by the inherent unpredictability of the onset of pathological states. As noted previously, human metabolomics studies are also at high risk for potential clinical confounders, such as diet or drug effects, as well as age, gender, and comorbidities. It has been advocated that the analysis of samples from large patient cohorts, stratified by known risk factors or exposures, may minimize the impact of clinical confounding variables.[29] However, the throughput of most current metabolomics technologies, particularly those that are MS-based, precludes the analysis of large patient cohorts.

To help circumvent these problems, investigators have begun to apply these emerging technologies to unique clinical scenarios where serial sampling can be performed in patients both before and after a controlled perturbation, thereby allowing each patient to serve as his or her own biological control. Clinical cardiology is uniquely suited for such investigation. As proof of principle, a targeted MS-based metabolomics platform was applied to patents undergoing exercise stress testing with myocardial perfusion imaging.[30] A metabolic risk score differentiated ischemic patients from controls with a high degree of accuracy. Similarly, a targeted MS-based metabolomics platform was applied to patients undergoing alcohol septal ablation treatment for hypertrophic obstructive cardiomyopathy, a human model of "planned" myocardial infarction (PMI).[31] Serial blood samples were obtained before and serially after PMI. A PMI-derived metabolic signature consisting of aconitic acid, hypoxanthine, trimethylamine-N-oxide (TMNO), and threonine differentiated cases of spontaneous MI from patients undergoing diagnostic coronary angiography with high accuracy. This study identified changes in circulating metabolites as soon as ten minutes after myocardial injury, a time frame in which no currently-used plasma biomarkers are elevated and which—together with other studies—paves the way for novel metabolic biomarkers to be studied for the diagnosis of myocardial injury and related pathologies.

Strategies emphasizing the in-depth analysis of small, extremely well-phenotyped patient cohorts are ideal in light of current technological limitations. However, such an approach has potential limitations that should be considered. First, although serial sampling in patients serving as their own biological controls helps diminish interindividual variability and signal-to-noise issues, populations studied to date are nevertheless small. Further testing in larger cohorts may be powered to detect more subtle metabolic changes and will provide sufficient precision in the estimates of the utility of each marker to allow for appropriate relative weighting of each component.

Second, while metabolite profiling of serum or plasma offers the advantage of simple sample collection and may reflect the sum of metabolic changes occurring throughout the body, sampling specific tissues that serve as proximal sources of metabolites[32,33] enables localization of metabolic changes and may help to gauge the sensitivity and specificity of signature metabolic profiles in plasma. Alternatively, for metabolites that are rapidly cleared from the circulation, it may be more appropriate to perform metabolic profiling on urine samples.

Integration of Metabolomics with Other "-omics" Technologies in a Systems Biology Approach to Cardiovascular Disease

The identification of new pathways and biomarkers in cardiovascular disease will depend on the complementary power of genetics, transcriptional profiling, proteomics, and metabolomics. For example, Mayr et al. recently utilized metabolomics and proteomics to characterize metabolic profiles of atrial tissue that predispose patients to the development of atrial fibrillation.[33] Genome-wide association studies (GWASs) that provide an unbiased scan of genomic sequence variants will also catalyze integrative "omics" approaches. For example, three groups recently identified several loci, including chromosome 9p21, associated with early onset myocardial infarction.[34–36] The chromosomal regions identified to date do not contain genes recognizably associated with established coronary heart disease risk factors, such as plasma lipoproteins. However, the integration of metabolic and proteomic data from these same patients may provide clues as to how the variants modulate the atherosclerotic process.

Conclusion

In conclusion, an emerging set of analytical and bioinformatics tools have made it possible to profile hundreds of metabolites in complex mixtures, such as plasma. Though these technologies are still under development, when coupled with other functional genomic approaches, metabolomics promises to transform our ability to profile samples with the goal of elucidating biological pathways and discovering valuable clinical biomarkers.

References

1. Pauling L, Robinson AB, Teranishi R, Cary P. Quantitative analysis of urine vapor and breath by gas-liquid partition chromatography. *Proc Natl Acad Sci U S A*. 1971;68:2374–2376.
2. Horning EC, Horning MG. Metabolic profiles: gas-phase methods for analysis of metabolites. *Clin Chem*. 1971;17:802–809.
3. Nicholson JK, Lindon JC, Holmes E. 'Metabonomics': understanding the metabolic responses of living systems to pathophysiological stimuli via multivariate statistical analysis of biological NMR spectroscopic data. *Xenobiotica*. 1999;29:1181–1189.
4. Raamsdonk LM, Teusink B, Broadhurst D, et al. A functional genomics strategy that uses metabolome data to reveal the phenotype of silent mutations. *Nat Biotechnol*. 2001;19:45–50.
5. Allen J, Davey HM, Broadhurst D, et al. High-throughput classification of yeast mutants for functional genomics using metabolic footprinting. *Nat Biotechnol*. 2003;21:692–696.
6. An J, Muoio DM, Shiota M, et al. Hepatic expression of malonyl-CoA decarboxylase reverses muscle, liver and whole-animal insulin resistance. *Nat Med*. 2004;10:268–274.
7. Roe CR, Millington DS, Maltby DA. Identification of 3-methylglutarylcarnitine. A new diagnostic metabolite of 3-hydroxy-3-methylglutaryl-coenzyme A lyase deficiency. *J Clin Invest*. 1986;77:1391–1394.
8. Frazier DM, Millington DS, McCandless SE, et al. The tandem mass spectrometry newborn screening experience in North Carolina: 1997–2005. *J Inherit Metab Dis*. 2006;29:76–85.
9. Dunn WB, Bailey NJ, Johnson HE. Measuring the metabolome: current analytical technologies. *Analyst*. 2005;130:606–625.

10. Dunn WB, Ellis D. Metabolomics: current analytical platforms and methodologies. *Trends Analyt Chem.* 2005;4:285–294.
11. Lindon JC, Holmes E, Nicholson JK. Metabonomics techniques and applications to pharmaceutical research & development. *Pharm Res.* 2006;23:1075–1088.
12. Backstrom T, Goiny M, Lockowandt U, Liska J, Franco-Cereceda A. Cardiac outflow of amino acids and purines during myocardial ischemia and reperfusion. *J Appl Physiol.* 2003;94:1122–1128.
13. Mei DA, Gross GJ, Nithipatikom K. Simultaneous determination of adenosine, inosine, hypoxanthine, xanthine, and uric acid in microdialysis samples using microbore column high-performance liquid chromatography with a diode array detector. *Anal Biochem.* 1996; 238:34–39.
14. Zemgulis V, Ronquist G, Bjerner T, et al. Energy-related metabolites during and after induced myocardial infarction with special emphasis on the reperfusion injury after extracorporeal circulation. *Acta Physiol Scand.* 2001;171:129–143.
15. Cheng LL, Chang IW, Louis DN, Gonzalez RG. Correlation of high-resolution magic angle spinning proton magnetic resonance spectroscopy with histopathology of intact human brain tumor specimens. *Cancer Res.* 1998;58:1825–1832.
16. Zhang X, Wei D, Yap Y, Li L, Guo S, Chen F. Mass spectrometry-based "omics" technologies in cancer diagnostics. *Mass Spectrom Rev.* 2007;26:403–431.
17. Storey JD, Tibshirani R. Statistical significance for genomewide studies. *Proc Natl Acad Sci U S A.* 2003;100:9440–9445.
18. Tavazoie S, Hughes JD, Campbell MJ, Cho RJ, Church GM. Systematic determination of genetic network architecture. *Nat Genet.* 1999; 22:281–285.
19. Mootha VK, Lindgren CM, Eriksson KF, et al. PGC-1alpha-responsive genes involved in oxidative phosphorylation are coordinately downregulated in human diabetes. *Nat Genet.* 2003;34: 267–273.
20. Berriz GF, King OD, Bryant B, Sander C, Roth FP. Characterizing gene sets with FuncAssociate. *Bioinformatics.* 2003;19:2502–2504.
21. van der Greef J, Stroobant P, van der Heijden R. The role of analytical sciences in medical systems biology. *Curr Opin Chem Biol.* 2004;8: 559–565.

22. Manly B. *Multivariable Statistical Methods: A Primer*. London: Chapman & Hall; 1994.

23. Bishop C. *Neural Networks for Pattern Recognition*. Oxford: Clarendon Press; 1995.

24. Baxter IR, Borevitz JO. Mapping a plant's chemical vocabulary. *Nat Genet*. 2006;38:737–738.

25. Villas-Boas SG, Moxley JF, Akesson M, Stephanopoulos G, Nielsen J. High-throughput metabolic state analysis: the missing link in integrated functional genomics of yeasts. *Biochem J*. 2005;388:669–677.

26. Gibala MJ, Young ME, Taegtmeyer H. Anaplerosis of the citric acid cycle: role in energy metabolism of heart and skeletal muscle. *Acta Physiol Scand*. 2000;168:657–665.

27. Bederman IR, Reszko AE, Kasumov T, et al. Zonation of labeling of lipogenic acetyl-CoA across the liver: implications for studies of lipogenesis by mass isotopomer analysis. *J Biol Chem*. 2004;279:43207–43216.

28. He W, Miao FJ, Lin DC, et al. Citric acid cycle intermediates as ligands for orphan G-protein-coupled receptors. *Nature*. 2004;429:188–193.

29. Kirschenlohr HL, Griffin JL, Clarke SC, et al. Proton NMR analysis of plasma is a weak predictor of coronary artery disease. *Nat Med*. 2006;12:705–710.

30. Sabatine MS, Liu E, Morrow DA, et al. Metabolomic identification of novel biomarkers of myocardial ischemia. *Circulation*. 2005;112:3868–3875.

31. Lewis GD, Wei R, Liu E, et al. Metabolite profiling of blood from individuals undergoing planned myocardial infarction reveals early markers of myocardial injury. *J Clin Invest*. 2008;118:3503–3512.

32. Howarth KR, LeBlanc PJ, Heigenhauser GJ, Gibala MJ. Effect of endurance training on muscle TCA cycle metabolism during exercise in humans. *J Appl Physiol*. 2004;97:579–584.

33. Mayr M, Yusuf S, Weir G, et al. Combined metabolomic and proteomic analysis of human atrial fibrillation. *J Am Coll Cardiol*. 2008;51:585–594.

34. Samani NJ, Erdmann J, Hall AS, et al. Genomewide association analysis of coronary artery disease. *N Engl J Med*. 2007;357:443–453.

35. McPherson R, Pertsemlidis A, Kavaslar N, et al. A common allele on chromosome 9 associated with coronary heart disease. *Science.* 2007;316:1488–1491.

36. Helgadottir A, Thorleifsson G, Manolescu A, et al. A common variant on chromosome 9p21 affects the risk of myocardial infarction. *Science.* 2007;316:1491–1493.

Index

C

- differential diagnosis of elevated troponin in non-ACS patients and, 138*t*
- iatrogenic causes of troponin elevation and, 154*t*

D

F

H

J

K

L

M

S

Color Plates

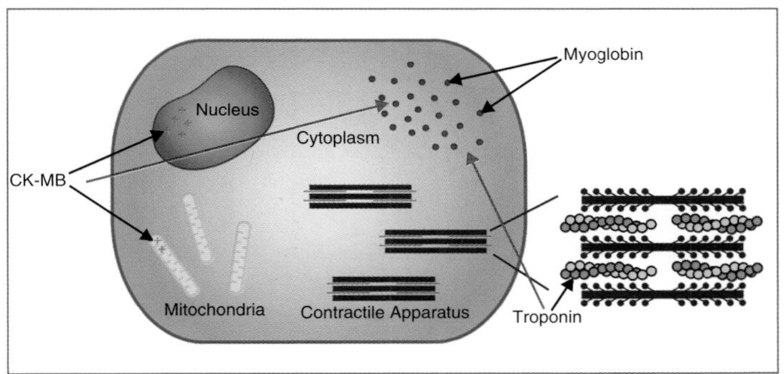

■ **Plate 1 (Figure 1–1) Cellular distribution of cardiac troponin, creatine kinase MB and myoglobin in structural and cytoplasm components.**

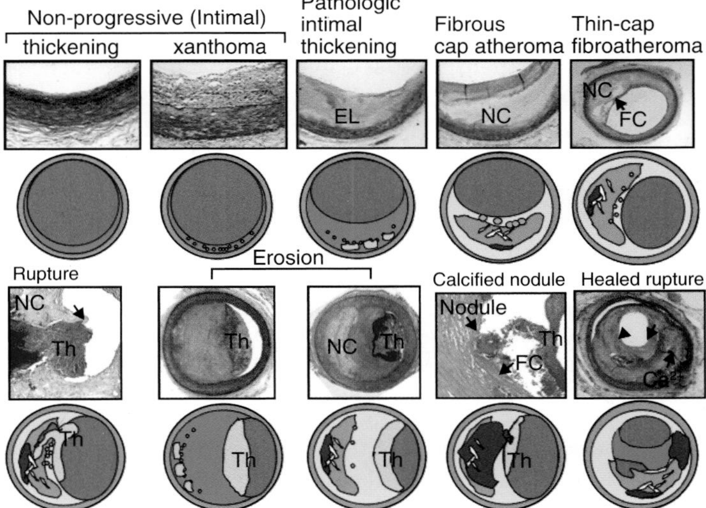

■ **Plate 2 (Figure 12–1) Spectrum of representative coronary lesion morphologies seen in our sudden coronary death population forming the basis for our modified AHA descriptive classification.**

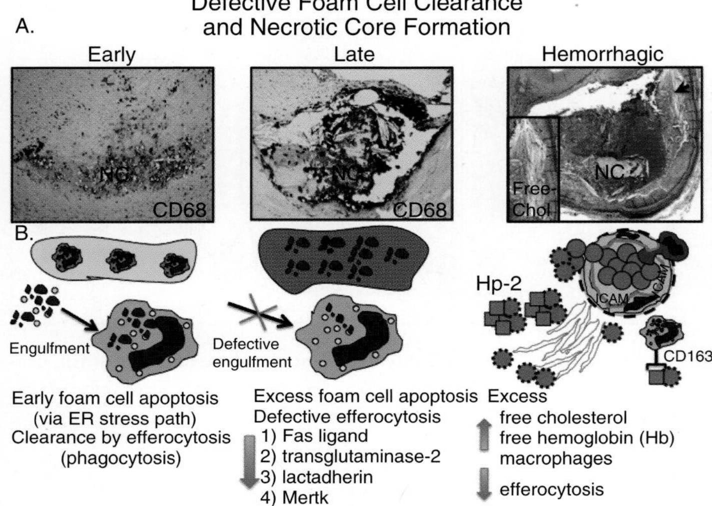

■ **Plate 3 (Figure 12–3) Putative mechanism(s) of necrotic core formation in humans, in part, guided by mouse models of atherosclerosis.**

Panel A shows representative micrographs of human coronary plaques illustrating early, late, and hemorrhagic necrosis. Early necrosis is marked by the infiltration of CD68-positive macrophages within lipid pools whereas late necrosis is represented by increased macrophage death, cell lysis, and loss of extracellular matrix. Hemorrhagic necrosis is accompanied by accumulated free-cholesterol (Free-Chol, arrow), presumably derived from erythrocyte membranes, and is thought to lead to the relatively rapid expansion of the necrotic core. Panel B is a diagrammatic representation of necrotic core formation, highlighted by defective efferocytosis (phagocytosis). The bulk of literature describing pathways of cell death, defective clearance, and mediators of efferocytosis is derived from mouse models of atherosclerosis. Abbreviations: Mertk = Mer receptor tyrosine kinase, FAS = apoptosis stimulating fragment, HP-2 = haptoglobin protein type 2 allele.

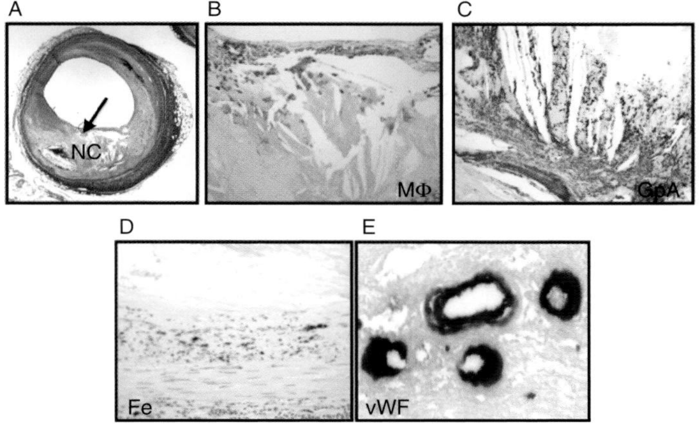

■ **Plate 4 (Figure 12–4) Representative thin-cap fibroatheroma selectively stained for macrophages, glycophorin A, iron and von Willebrand factor.**

Panel A, Thin-cap fibroatheroma identified by the thin fibrous cap (arrow) and relatively large necrotic core (NC); section stained by Movat pentachrome. Panel B, immunostaining against CD68 showing extensive macrophage infiltration (MF) in the peri-core and fibrous cap area. Panel C, extensive accumulation of red blood cell membranes in the necrotic core is shown by specific glycophorin A staining (GpA). Panel D, accumulated iron is also found in macrophages surrounding the necrotic core. Panel E, immunostaining against von Willebrand factor-related antigen shows diffuse staining of intraplaque microvessels near shoulder regions suggesting endothelial leakage.

Modified form Kolodgie FD et al. *N Engl J Med* 2003;349:2316–25.

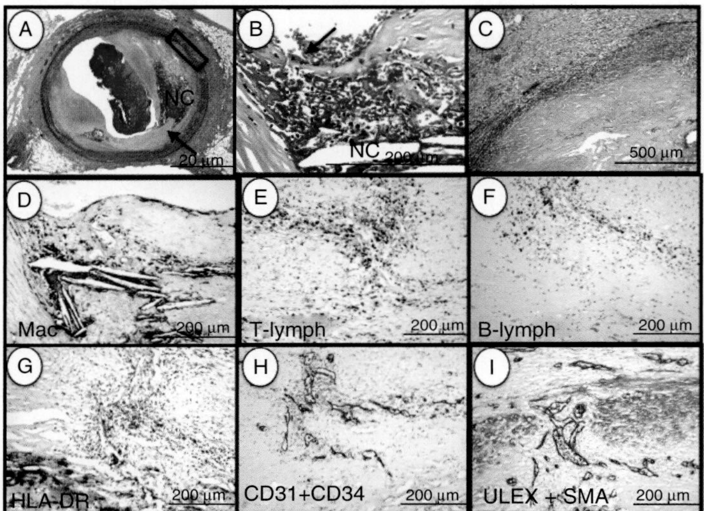

■ **Plate 5 (Figure 12–5)** **Plaque rupture and inflammation.**

Left main coronary artery with plaque rupture and luminal thrombus (A). Note high power view of the ruptured thin fibrous cap (arrow) with an underlying necrotic core (NC) in B. C. Shows the media adventitial border boxed in A with medial destruction and chronic inflammation. D. Shows the cap rupture site stained for macrophages (Mac). E, F, and G serial sections in the pericore region shown in A by an arrow stained for T and B-lymphocytes and G is stained for HLA-DR, respectively. H. Shows an area of medial destruction highlighting angiogenesis by CD 31 + CD34 stain whereas section I is double stained by both ULEX (endothelial marker) and a-smooth muscle actin (SMA) stain, for smooth muscle cells showing focal destruction of the media.

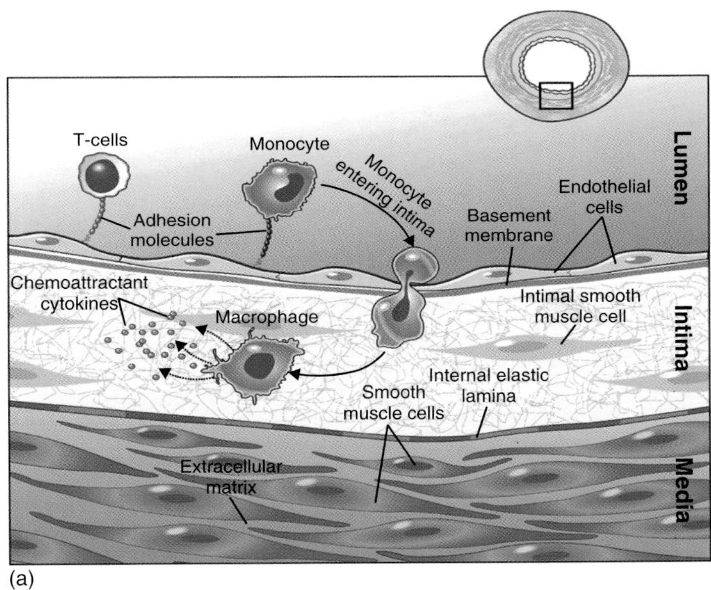

(a)

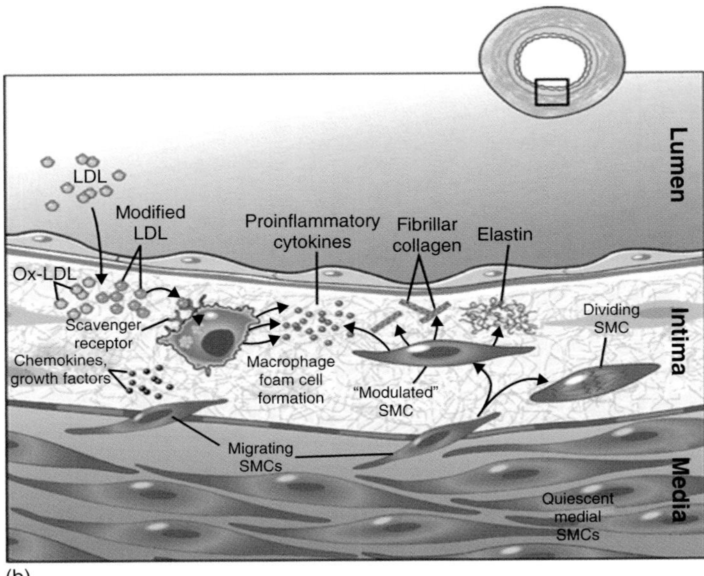

(b)

■ **Plate 6 (Figure 13–1)**

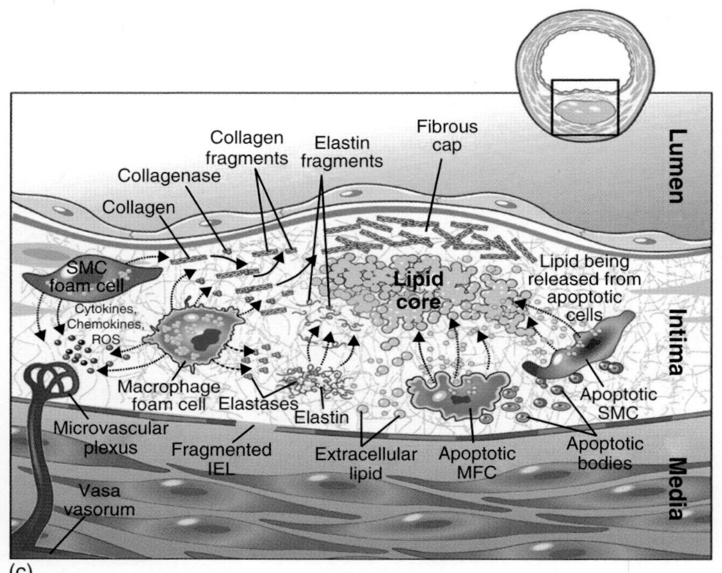

(c)

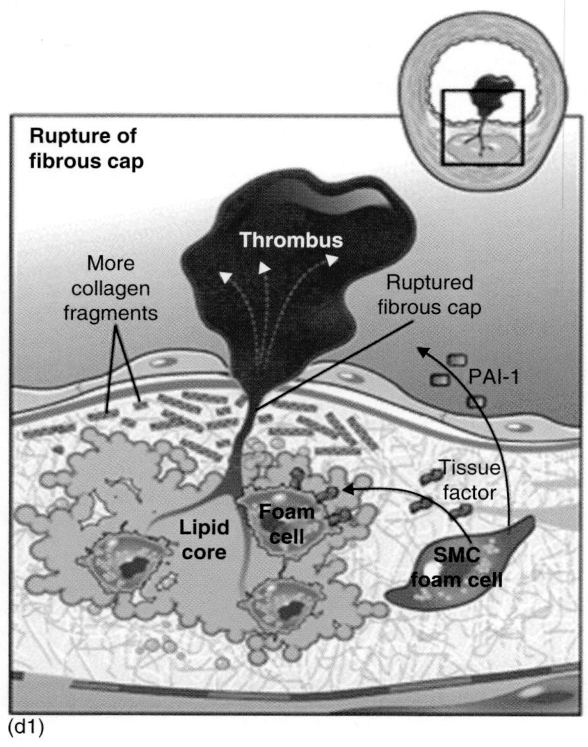

(d1)

■ **Plate 6 (Figure 13–1) (Continued)**

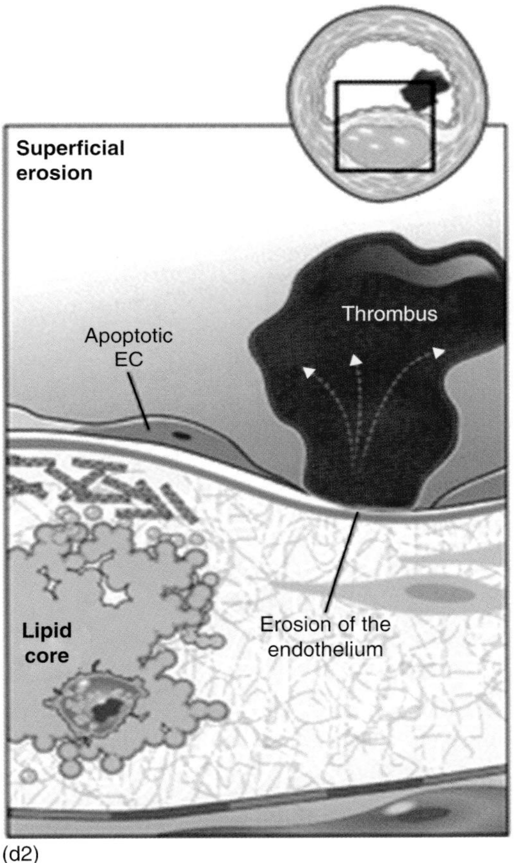

■ **Plate 6 (Figure 13–1)** Mechanisms of plaque formation and rupture (A) Transition from the normal artery wall to an atherosclerotic lesion: Molecules associated with risk factors stimulate inflammatory stress and induce the expression of adhesion molecules for leukocytes and chemoattractants that draw leukocytes into the intimal layer. (B) Formation of the plaque: Mononuclear phagocytes ingest ox-LDL through scavenger receptors to form foam cells. Macrophages in the lesions release chemoattractant cytokines, proinflammatory mediators, and small lipid molecules such as leukotrienes and prostaglandins, as well as reactive oxygen species. (C) Maturation of the atherosclerotic plaque: Proinflammatory mediators released from activated white cells, endothelial cells, and smooth muscle cells (SMCs) potentiate cell death. SMCs disappear and fewer remain to renew the extracellular matrix in the plaque's fibrous cap. (D) The thrombotic complications of atherosclerosis. Finally, the plaque's fibrous cap ruptures, either from mechanical causes or superficial erosion of the endothelial cells caused by desquamation and endothelial apoptosis. This permits blood and its coagulation factors to contact tissue factor, activate the clotting cascade, and form a thrombus.

Source: Libby, P. and P.M. Ridker. Inflammation and atherothrombosis from population biology and bench research to clinical practice. *J Am Coll Cardiol.* 2006; 48(9 Suppl):A33–46.

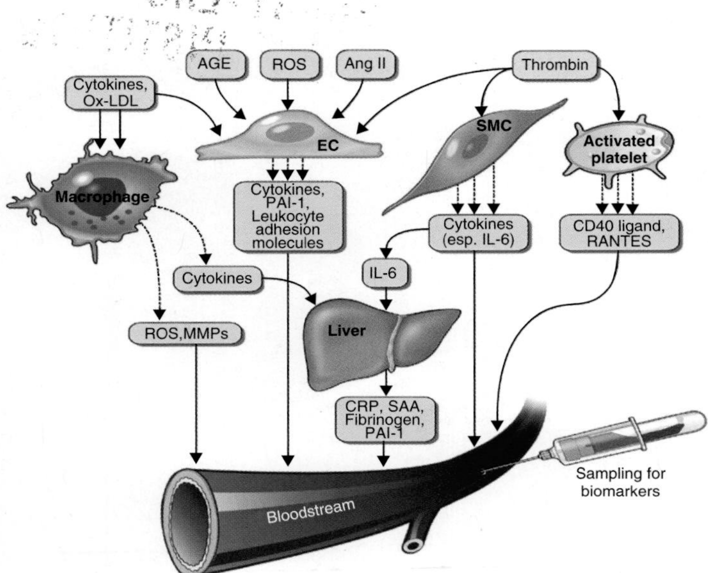

■ **Plate 7 (Figure 13–2)** The inflammatory hypothesis: The primary pro-inflammatory risk factors depicted on the top of this diagram activate the various cell types prominent in the atherosclerotic plaque, including the macrophage, endothelial cells (EC), smooth muscle cells (SMC), and in complicated lesions, the activated platelet. These various cell types in turn secrete inflammatory mediators and reactive oxygen species (ROS). The primary proinflammatory cytokines, including interleukin-1 (IL-1) and TNF-α, can stimulate large amounts of IL-6 production by intrinsic vascular wall cells. IL-6 functions as a messenger and acts on the liver to elicit the acute-phase response. The acute-phase reactants include C-reactive protein (CRP), serum amyloid A (SAA), fibrinogen, and plasminogen activator inhibitor-1.

Source: Libby, P. and P.M. Ridker. Inflammation and atherothrombosis from population biology and bench research to clinical practice. *J Am Coll Cardiol.* 2006; 48(9 Suppl):A33–46.